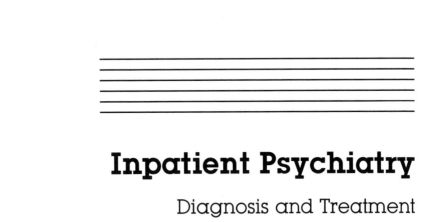

Inpatient Psychiatry

Diagnosis and Treatment

Third Edition

Inpatient Psychiatry

Diagnosis and Treatment

Third Edition

Editor

Lloyd I. Sederer, M.D.

McLean Hospital
Harvard Medical School
Belmont, Massachusetts

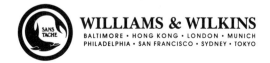

WILLIAMS & WILKINS
BALTIMORE · HONG KONG · LONDON · MUNICH
PHILADELPHIA · SAN FRANCISCO · SYDNEY · TOKYO

Editor: Michael G. Fisher
Associate Editor: Carol Eckhart
Copy Editor: Virginia Gerhart
Designer: Wilma E. Rosenberger
Illustration Planner: Ray Lowman
Production Coordinator: Charles E. Zeller

Although accurate indications, adverse reactions, and dosage schedules for drugs are provided in this book, it is possible that they may change. The reader is urged to review the package information data of the manufacturers of the medications mentioned.

Printed in the United States of America

Library of Congress Cataloging in Publication Data
Inpatient psychiatry : diagnosis and treatment / editor, Lloyd I. Sederer. — 3rd ed.
    p. cm.
   Includes index.
   ISBN 0-683-07629-9
   1. Psychiatric hospital care. 2. Psychiatry. I. Sederer, Lloyd I.
   [DNLM: 1. Mental Disorders—diagnosis. 2. Mental Disorders—therapy. 3. Psychiatry—methods. WM 100 I56]
   RC439.I5 1991
   616.89—dc20
   DNLM/DLC
   for Library of Congress   90-12728
                                         CIP

91 92 93 94
1 2 3 4 5 6 7 8 9 10

To My Son

Preface

I offer this third edition of *Inpatient Psychiatry: Diagnosis and Treatment* with pride and with concern. My pride lies in the quality of the work offered by the contributors to this volume and in the march of progress that has occurred in psychiatry and in inpatient psychiatry, in particular, since the last edition of this text. We have seen refinement in our diagnostic capabilities through descriptive studies, neuroimaging, and epidemiologic inquiry. Treatment precision has advanced on the shoulders of empirical research and accumulated clinical wisdom. Stigma, an enemy of vast proportions, has been subject to the remedial processes of public education and societal enlightenment. Never before, for example, has depression been recognized in its ubiquity; its lack of class, age, and racial distinction; and in its remarkable responsiveness to psychiatric intervention.

Were I able to stop after this incomplete list of successes there would be no need for concern. However, fundamental questions about the future of medicine, of psychiatry, and of hospital treatment in particular are legion and compelling. It is hardly possible to enter into a clinical discussion without ending up in talk about regulation, litigation, managed care, and the prospect of a health care system becoming bankrupt because costs have outstripped the gears of our economy. The landscape of medical practice is changing radically. We can be assured of change, but the nature of that change is, I believe, beyond our best efforts at prognostication.

Inpatient Psychiatry: Diagnosis and Treatment is offered from the perspective of the inpatient unit as the site of acute, intensive care. The inpatient unit has become, in effect, the intensive care unit within a continuum of psychiatric services. Acute treatment occurs in all inpatient psychiatric settings, including the private sector, general hospitals, public mental hospitals, and the Veteran's Administration system. Though each of these sites may show variation in the populations it treats, the illnesses remain the same and the approaches to acute care are fundamentally the same.

The authors of this edition offer a philosophy of treatment based on providing patients with specific interventions in the least restrictive environment. The goals of hospitalization are those of diagnosis and treatment aimed at enabling the patient to successfully leave the hospital for further care. In order to maintain its credibility and its fiscal and clinical responsibility, the inpatient unit must provide no more care, and no less, than is needed.

We offer an approach to the patient that respects disease, person, and circumstance. The patient's biology, character, and situation become the parameters of our understanding and intervention. Though the 1990s have been identified as the Decade of the Brain, a treatment approach that singularly addresses the brain is incomplete. In the tradition of William Osler, this text aspires to psychiatric care that encompasses both science and humanity. As Osler put it, "The human heart has a hidden want which science cannot supply."

The format of the third edition holds to its original design of two principal sections. Section I takes a disorder-specific approach to diagnosis and treatment. Section II identifies specific aspects of inpatient psychiatry and aims toward articulating them in their rich and complex detail.

The third edition has introduced many new authors and important new chapters. Furthermore, each chapter in the first section of the book identifies and discusses major controversies in the hospital care of the disorder identified in that chapter. DSM-IIIR is used throughout the text, but with an appreciation that change will come through DSM-IV which will be introduced sometime after the publication of this text. Careful attention is still given to symptom and syndromal diagnosis, but without requiring the reader to employ only the nosology of DSM-IIIR. All authors have sought to enhance their discussions of in-

patient psychiatric management. Many chapters pay particular attention to the presence of alcohol and substance abuse as a concurrent disorder in the diagnosis and treatment of another psychiatric condition. No generic chapter on personality disorder is offered. There is a chapter on the borderline personality, since this is the primary Axis II disorder found in patients requiring hospital level of care and since borderline patients are a perennial source of clinical problems for hospital-based clinicians.

I want to extend my gratitude to the clinicians, students, and patients who have educated me and my collaborators. I want to extend my appreciation to my editors at Williams and Wilkins, Michael Fisher and Carol Eckhart, for their support and for the confidence they had in commissioning this third edition. My special thanks to Gayle Kissell and Jill Shuman for their assistance in preparing this text. Once again, I want to thank the contributors to this text for their work well done and for the pleasure of allowing me to serve as their editor. Finally, I want to thank my family for enduring the process of book production once again.

LIS
Belmont, Massachusetts

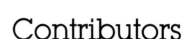

Contributors

Steven A. Adelman, MD
Director, Ambulatory Psychiatry Services
University of Massachusetts Medical Center
Worcester, Massachusetts
Assistant Professor of Psychiatry
University of Massachusetts Medical School
Worcester, Massachusetts

Robert B. Aranow, MD
Psychiatrist in Charge, Clinical Evaluation Unit
McLean Hospital
Belmont, Massachusetts
Associate Director of Postgraduate and Continuing
Medical Education
McLean Hospital
Belmont, Massachusetts
Clinical Instructor in Psychiatry
Harvard Medical School
Boston, Massachusetts

Jay Baer, MD
Assistant Clinical Professor of Psychiatry
Tufts University School of Medicine
Boston, Massachusetts

Harold Bursztajn, MD
Co-Director, Program in Psychiatry and the Law
Massachusetts Mental Health Center
Boston, Massachusetts
Assistant Clinical Professor of Psychiatry
Harvard Medical School
Boston, Massachusetts

John F. Clarkin, PhD
Director of Psychology
The New York Hospital–Cornell Medical Center,
Westchester Division
White Plains, New York
Professor of Clinical Psychology in Psychiatry
Cornell University Medical College
New York, New York

Nancy S. Cotton, PhD
Consultant in Child Psychiatry
The Cambridge Hospital
Cambridge, Massachusetts
Principal Consultant to School-age Patients for the
Division of Child and Adolescent Services
Massachusetts Department of Mental Health
Boston, Massachusetts
Instructor in Psychology
Harvard Medical School
Boston, Massachusetts

Bonnie Cummins
Former Research Associate, Program in Psychiatry
and the Law
Massachusetts Mental Health Center
Boston, Massachusetts

R. L. Ehrenkranz, MD
Assistant Professor, Department of Medicine
Columbia University, College of Physicians and
Surgeons
New York, New York

Barry S. Fogel, MD
Associate Professor of Psychiatry and Human
Behavior
Brown University
Providence, Rhode Island

Marshall Forstein, MD
Director of HIV Mental Health Services, Department
of Psychiatry
The Cambridge Hospital
Cambridge, Massachusetts
Instructor in Psychiatry
Harvard Medical School
Boston, Massachusetts

Ira D. Glick, MD
Associate Medical Director
Payne Whitney Clinic
New York, New York

ix

Senior Science Advisor for Clinical Services
National Institute of Mental Health
Rockville, Maryland
Professor of Psychiatry
Cornell University Medical College
New York, New York

Mark S. Gold, MD
Director of Research
Fair Oaks Hospital
Delray Beach, Florida, and Summit, New Jersey

Tana A. Grady, MD
Medical Staff Fellow, Clinical Neuroendocrinology Branch
National Institute of Mental Health
Bethesda, Maryland

Thomas G. Gutheil, MD
Co-Director, Program in Psychiatry and the Law
Massachusetts Mental Health Center
Associate Professor of Psychiatry
Harvard Medical School
Boston, Massachusetts

Gordon P. Harper, MD
Director of Inpatient Psychiatry
The Children's Hospital
Assistant Professor of Psychiatry
Harvard Medical School
Boston, Massachusetts

Peter Herridge, MD
Associate Director, Neuropsychiatric Evaluation Center
Fair Oaks Hospital
Summit, New Jersey

Janet Abeles Kahane, MEd, OTR/L
Director, Rehabilitation Services
Charles River Hospital
Wellesley, Massachusetts

Steven Mattis, PhD
Associate Professor of Clinical Psychology
New York Hospital–Cornell Medical Center
White Plains, New York

Margaret S. McKenna, MD
Director, Eating Disorder Program
Harvard University Health Services
Boston, Massachusetts
Cambridge, Massachusetts
Associate Psychiatrist
McLean Hospital
Belmont, Massachusetts
Clinical Instructor in Psychiatry
Harvard Medical School
Boston, Massachusetts

John M. Oldham, MD
Acting Director
New York State Psychiatric Institute
New York, New York
Chief Medical Officer
New York State Office of Mental Health
New York, New York
Professor of Clinical Psychiatry
Columbia University, College of Physicians and Surgeons
New York, New York

A. Carter Pottash, MD
Executive Medical Director
Fair Oaks Hospital
Delray Beach, Florida, and Summit, New Jersey

L. Mark Russakoff, MD
Clinical Director and Acting Deputy Director
New York State Psychiatric Institute
New York, New York
Associate Professor of Clinical Psychiatry
Columbia University, College of Physicians and Surgeons
New York, New York

Sharan L. Schwartzberg, EdD, OTR, FAOTA
Associate Staff, Department of Psychiatry, and Adjunct Occupational Therapy Staff
Mount Auburn Hospital
Cambridge, Massachusetts
Professor and Chairperson
Tufts University–Boston School of Occupational Therapy
Medford, Massachusetts

Lloyd I. Sederer, MD
Associate General Director
McLean Hospital
Belmont, Massachusetts
Assistant Professor of Psychiatry
Harvard Medical School
Boston, Massachusetts

Jane Thorbeck, EdD
Assistant Psychologist
Massachusetts General Hospital
Boston, Massachusetts
Instructor in Psychology
Harvard Medical School
Boston, Massachusetts

Roger D. Weiss, MD
Clinical Director, Alcohol and Drug Abuse Program
McLean Hospital
Belmont, Massachusetts
Associate Professor of Psychiatry
Harvard Medical School
Boston, Massachusetts

Contents

Section II. Specific Aspects of Inpatient Psychiatry

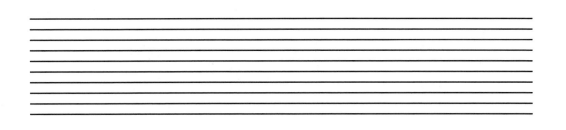

Section I

Inpatient Diagnosis and Treatment

Depression[a]

Tana A. Grady, MD
Lloyd I. Sederer, MD

DEFINITION

Depression is the most common of the major psychiatric disorders. It has been estimated that more than 15% of all adults will experience a depressive episode at some point in the course of their lives (1–3). Depression is also the most common cause for psychiatric hospitalization (4). Furthermore, depression is found widely among medically and surgically hospitalized patients.

When depression is severe, persistent, and disabling of everyday physical and social functioning, it is easily discernible. At other times, the distinction between a normal fluctuation of mood and a depression may not be very clear. Feelings of sadness, blueness, frustration, and discouragement are part of the normal range of human emotions. However, these fluctuations in mood tend to be short-lived, do not become over-whelming in their experience, do not impair reality testing, do not profoundly alter self-esteem, and do not generate suicidal thoughts or behavior. In addition, normal mood fluctuations do not produce persistent disturbances in sleep, appetite, or motoric activity.

The central feature of clinical depression generally is a subjective experience of sadness, despondency, hopelessness, or gloom. This feeling of depressed mood is accompanied by a loss of interest and pleasure in life and its activities and responsibilities. In some cases anxiety may be the predominant mood disturbance, whereas the major complaint in other cases may be one of agitation. Some patients may report no disturbance of mood despite the presence of several other symptoms and clear cause for a mood alteration.

A feeling of lowered self-esteem is common, as are feelings of helplessness. Depressed patients show an inability to perform even the simplest daily tasks. They frequently are preoccupied (perhaps even obsessed) with work, family, money, and their own health. They approach these matters with marked pessimism and hopeless-

[a]The pronouns "he," "him," and "his" as employed at various points in this text are not meant to convey the masculine gender alone. Use of these terms in their generic sense, to denote persons of both sexes, is intended solely to avoid redundancy and awkwardness in expression.

ness. The combination of hopelessness, pessimism, low self-esteem, and guilt may prompt morbid and/or suicidal thoughts.

The majority of depressed patients experience loss of appetite and weight loss associated with their mood disturbance. However, there is a subset of patients who present with increased appetite (hyperphagia), weight gain, increased sleep (hypersomnia), and rejection sensitivity. These patients usually are young women and may have somewhat milder mood disturbances (5, 6).

Sleep disturbance is a very common symptom of depression. Disturbances of sleep include difficulty falling asleep, difficulty remaining asleep, and/or early morning awakening (initial, middle, and terminal insomnia, respectively). Psychomotor disturbances also may be present in the depressed patient. Some may have an increase in psychomotor activity and are described as having agitation. Examples of this include an inability to remain still, hand wringing, nail biting, and incessant smoking or talking. Other patients demonstrate decreased psychomotor activity and are termed psychomotor retarded. These patients typically complain of lethargy and fatigue. Objectively, their body movements are slowed and limited, and their speech has a poverty, monotony and latency. In some severely retarded patients, a clinical syndrome approaching catatonia may occur. In these cases the patient is virtually mute and is without spontaneous movement (7). Catatonic patients show no interest in eating or taking care of their bodily needs.

Additional signs and symptoms associated with depression include decreased libido, diminished interests, inability to experience pleasure (anhedonia), poor concentration, and feelings of guilt. These symptoms frequently result in neglect of work, play, friends, and family. In fact, patients with depression usually are quite isolated.

Cognitive changes also may occur.

Thinking may be slowed and indecision frequent. Previously, depressed patients with significant cognitive alterations were described as having depressive pseudodementia (8). Recent neuropsychological tests have shown actual reversible cognitive deficits related to attention, concentration, memory retrieval, and motivation in patients with major depression. Hence, this syndrome is now referred to more accurately as depression with secondary cognitive impairment (9).

Furthermore, many depressed patients verbalize multiple somatic complaints. Gastrointestinal disturbances, headache, backache, and urinary difficulties are common. Often, patients with a mild preexisting medical condition will present with an exacerbation of that symptomatology. Patients who complain primarily of physical problems typically will present to their internist or primary care physician. With careful examination, the diagnosis of depression aggravating their preexisting disorder can be made.

In a small number of depressed patients, disturbances in reality functioning may occur. These are called delusional or psychotic depressions. These patients show delusions and/or hallucinations that may reflect the person's sense of self-reproach or pessimism. Examples include somatic delusions or auditory hallucinations that are highly critical.

Recent studies have demonstrated another subgroup of depressed patients with a seasonal component to their illness. Seasonal Affective Disorder Syndrome (SADS) has been characterized by a recurrent depressed mood associated with hypersomnia, overeating, and carbohydrate craving (10). A predictable annual onset occurs in the fall and winter with remission in the spring and summer (or vice versa). Changes in climate and latitude may be remedial. The prevalence of this subgroup has not yet been determined (11). An important exclusionary criterion to the diagnosis of SADS is the presence of any environmental change concurrent in time with the onset of symptoms (e.g., change in employment status).

In essence, depression is a syndrome characterized by a persistent, severe, and abnormal mood disturbance, with neurovegetative symptomatology, with or without psychosis, and with or without a seasonal component. The syndrome of depression has varied etiologies that are discussed later in this chapter.

DIAGNOSIS

The revised *Diagnostic and Statistical Manual of Mental Disorders* (DSM-IIIR) of the American Psychiatric Association (12) provides criteria for the diagnosis of depression. Major depression is classified under "Mood Disorders" along with dysthymia, cyclothymia, and the bipolar disorders. In addition to either depressed mood or loss of interest or pleasure, one must have at least four other neurovegetative signs or symptoms of at least two weeks' duration. Exclusionary criteria include (*a*) the presence of an organic factor that may be contributing to presentation; (*b*) normal grief reaction; (*c*) the presence of delusions or hallucinations

in the absence of prominent mood symptoms; and (*d*) the presence of a psychotic disorder (e.g., schizophrenia, schizophreniform disorder, delusional disorder or psychotic disorder not otherwise specified).

In summary, the DSM-IIIR defines depression as a particular constellation of symptoms lasting for at least two or more weeks. DSM-IIIR does allow for distinctions between psychotic and nonpsychotic depressions and those with or without a seasonal component. However, it does not concern itself with specific syndromal or etiological differences between these subtypes of depression.

Nosological research in psychiatry during recent years has attempted to develop valid and reliable systems for the classification of psychiatric disorders. This work remains in progress. In fact, clinicians and investigators are now reviewing the current criteria for the mood disorders and will propose updated criteria for these and other psychiatric disorders to be included in the upcoming DSM-IV and the tenth edition of the International Classification of Disorders (ICD-10).

The accepted nosology of mood disorders to date is outlined in Figure 1.1. This

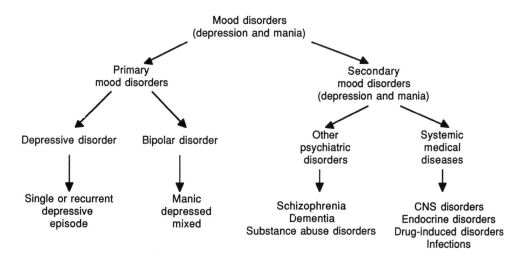

Figure 1.1. Nosology of depression.

classification distinguishes between primary and secondary mood disorders. Primary mood disorders (whether depressive or bipolar in nature) have no previous history of another psychiatric disorder and are not secondary to any systemic medical illness. Secondary mood disorders may be caused by other psychiatric illnesses or an organic illness. The latter currently is classified as an organic mood disorder. Table 1.1 lists conditions that may commonly present as a mood disturbance.

The primary-secondary diagnostic distinction grew out of efforts to enhance research on depressive disorders (13–15). This distinction allows the researcher to examine the depressive syndrome on the basis of etiologic differences. Questions of reactive versus endogenous depression and psychotic versus neurotic depression do not pertain to this diagnostic scheme. The unipolar and bipolar distinctions have become increasingly important, especially with regard to treatment issues. More than a half century ago Gillespie (16) proposed a nosology of depression in which the terms *reactive* and *endogenous* were applied. These terms continue to be used but are less popular and create some semantic confusion. Klerman (17) has suggested that the term

Table 1.1.   Some Organic Causes of Depression

Neurological Disorders
  Parkinson's disease
  Huntington's disease
  Multiple sclerosis
  Primary degenerative dementia
Metabolic Abnormalities and Endocrinopathies

Hyper-or hypothyroidism	Diabetes
Hyponatremia	Uremia
Hypokalemia	Cushing's disease
Pernicious anemia	Addison's disease
Pellagra	Hepatic disease
Hyperparathyroidism	Wernicke-Korsakoff syndrome

Neoplastic Disease
  Pancreatic carcinoma
  Primary cerebral tumor
  Cerebral metastasis
Drugs and Poisons

Alcohol	Sedatives
Amphetamine	Digitalis
Cocaine	Steroids
Barbiturates	Oral contraceptives
Opiates	Lead poisoning
Antihypertensives	Other heavy metals
Propranolol	
Reserpine	
Methyldopa	

Infectious Diseases

Tuberculosis	Hepatitis
Central nervous system	Encephalitis
(CNS) syphilis	Postencephalitis states
Mononucleosis	

Other Medical Conditions
  Acquired Immune Deficiency Syndrome (AIDS)
  Lupus and other collagen-vascular disorders
  Postpartum syndromes
  Postconcussion syndromes
  Chronic subdural hematomas

endogenous depression signifies more than a lack of precipitating event or external cause. He has suggested that endogenous depressions show certain "state" characteristics (i.e., characteristic of acute illness, as opposed to trait, or inborn and persistent), as well as an autonomy that renders the disorder unresponsive to environmental alterations. Furthermore, data support abnormalities in neurophysiology and specific differences in response to organic treatment for the so-called endogenous depressions (18, 19). What is clear and most important is symptom specificity. The presence of particular neurovegetative signs (early morning awakening, weight loss, and psychomotor retardation) all augur a good response to antidepressant medication or electroconvulsive therapy (ECT). Furthermore, in support of this observation, patients with endogenous depression respond to combined treatment with medication and psychotherapy but do not respond to psychotherapy alone. On the other hand, patients with reactive (situational) depression have been shown to respond to either tricyclic medication or psychotherapy alone (20).

The neurotic-psychotic distinction in the nosology of depression bears some consideration. It is of crucial importance to diagnose the presence of psychotic features because of the different treatment requirements for such conditions (i.e., use of antipsychotic medications or ECT rather than antidepressants or psychotherapy alone). The term *neurotic depression* has fallen into disuse and appropriately so. It has come to mean so many different things to so many different people that it has lost its clinical utility (21).

DSM-IIIR has continued to include dysthymia among the Axis I mood disorders. It represents an old condition known previously as neurotic depression. Dysthymia means "ill-humored" and refers to individuals who are habitually gloomy, brooding, and preoccupied with their feelings. Clinically, dysthymia may present as a low-grade depression of at least two years' duration (12, 22). Multicenter collaborative research studies have indicated that one-fourth of patients seen in clinics and university hospitals and diagnosed as having major depression demonstrate a history of dysthymia. Those with both major depression and dysthymia are said to suffer from "double depression" (23, 24). Furthermore, the longer the duration of the chronic low-grade depression, the greater the probability of relapse into major depression and of consequent chronicity (24).

Akiskal's work (25, 26) suggests that one-third of chronic depressions are residual symptomatic states of primary unipolar mood disorder; patients who develop these residual states typically are older and presumably have subaffective disorders. Another third of chronic depressions occur in early life, often the teenage years, and evidence fluctuations over time; these disorders may be conceptualized best as characterological depressions. The final third of chronic depressions are secondary to nonmood disorders, including severe anxiety disorders, somatization disorder, and disabling medical and neurological illnesses. Some diagnostic instruments (e.g., polysomnography) may help in distinguishing characterological subtypes from antidepressant medication-responsive subaffective dysthymias.

DSM-IIIR also provides criteria for the diagnosis of major depression with melancholia. Among the indicators are lack of reactivity to pleasurable stimuli; loss of interest in all, or almost all, activities; diurnal mood variation (AM worse than PM); early morning awakening; and significant anorexia and psychomotor disturbances. Significant evidence to establish this disorder as a separate entity remains to be established. However, those patients with late-onset depressions do appear to differ significantly in their symptom profiles and are more refractory to nonbiological treatments (27).

DIFFERENTIAL DIAGNOSIS

The differential diagnosis of depression requires a thorough knowledge of organic and functional (nonorganic) disorders that can present like depressive syndromes. In other words, secondary depressions must be separated from primary depressions. Failure to distinguish an organic disorder will result not only in the patient's failure to respond to treatment for the ersatz depression but also will allow another disorder to progress without diagnosis and specific treatment. The failure to separate a primary depressive illness from a variety of other functional psychiatric disorders will result in lack of specificity of treatment, with a consequent adverse effect on course and prognosis.

Organic Disorders that Can Mimic Depression

The inpatient psychiatrist initially must rule out any organic disorder that may be masquerading as a depression. It is important not to let the presence of a powerful precipitating event or a past history of depression bias the clinician against considering an organic etiology for the current depressive episode.

Table 1.1 presents a partial list of the organic causes of depression. Careful history taking with additional information from family members, a full review of systems, a complete physical and neurological examination, and appropriate laboratory tests (see Table 1.2 and pages 16–17) will help the clinician rule out an organic disorder.

Psychiatric Disorders that May Be Confused with Depression

A variety of psychiatric disorders may appear to be depressive illness.

Table 1.2. Guidelines for the Laboratory and Radiologic Diagnosis of Depression

Recommended Baseline Laboratory Studies
  Complete blood count with differential
  Electrolytes
  Chemistry panel—including glucose, blood urea nitrigen (BUN)/creatinine (Cr), liver function tests, Ca^{+2} and PO_4
  Serum test for syphilis
  Urine analysis
  Comprehensive serum and/or urine toxic screen, particularly if substance use/abuse is suspected
  TSH and T_4, especially when considering lithium treatment
  EKG—in patients with cardiac disease, on cardiotoxic medication, and/or >40 years old
  β-Human chorionic gonadotropin (β-HCG)—in female patients of child-bearing age
Special laboratory studies
  Serum B_{12} and folate
  Erythrocyte sedimentation rate (ESR)
  Antinuclear antibody (ANA)
  Serum ceruloplasmin
  Tuberculosis skin test
  Lumbar puncture
Radiologic Studies
  Chest film
  Computed tomography (CT) and/or Magnetic Resonance Imaging (MRI)
  Single positron emission computed tomography (SPECT) or positron emission tomography (PET) scans
Diagnostic Studies
  Dexamethasone suppression test (DST)—see text
  Thyrotropin releasing hormone (TRH)-stimulating test—see text
  Electroencephalogram
  Polysomnography—see text

SCHIZOPHRENIA

Patients with schizophrenia often exhibit depressive affect or symptomatology. Further, depressed patients may have psychotic symptoms.

In patients with psychotic depression, the mood disturbance usually precedes the onset of psychotic symptoms. In schizophrenia, psychotic symptoms usually occur first, followed by affective changes. Hence, the mood symptoms are of shorter duration than the psychosis. Premorbid and family histories are very helpful in differentiating patients with schizophrenia from those with delusional depression. Finally, schizophrenia is a diagnosis that is made only when there are persistent psychotic symptoms lasting more than six months, in the absence of significant mood disturbance.

SCHIZOAFFECTIVE DISORDER

This disorder may be a subset of the mood disorders, although the diagnosis has come under considerable question (28). Family history, acute treatment with lithium and/or neuroleptics, and long-term outcome all support considering this syndrome as a mood disorder. However, until greater nosological clarity is obtained, it may be best to avoid this diagnosis.

DYSTHYMIA AND CYCLOTHYMIA

The DSM-IIIR diagnosis of dysthymia is what was previously termed *depressive neurosis* (see "Diagnosis"). Though dysthymia or depressive neurosis resembles a depression, the signs and symptoms are not as severe nor as persistent as those of a depressive episode. Recent studies have shown the utility of antidepressant agents in this disorder, though this remains somewhat controversial (29). Patients with dysthymia can develop a major depressive episode. These cases of dysthymia with a superimposed major depression have been referred to, as noted earlier, as "double depressions" (23, 24).

Cyclothymia is a chronic mood disorder in which the patient demonstrates repetitive episodes of depression and hypomania. Like dysthymia, the periods of depression do not meet criteria for a clinical depression. Hypomania, by definition, is less severe than mania.

PERSONALITY DISORDERS

Personality disorders may present with depressive features. For example, obsessive-compulsive patients can show signs of depression when self-esteem is low or when a loss has occurred. In all cases of personality disorder, the basis for making the diagnosis of a full depressive syndrome is a demonstration of the presence of a constellation of depressive symptoms that have been severe and persistent.

ALCOHOLISM AND SUBSTANCE ABUSE

Depressive symptoms are common among patients who abuse alcohol and other drugs that can depress the central nervous system (e.g., narcotics, tranquilizers, and hypnotics). The diagnosis of primary depression in a patient with alcohol or substance abuse should be strongly considered in the presence of one or more of the following conditions: (*a*) positive family history of depression; (*b*) prior personal history of depression; (*c*) onset of substance abuse after depressive symptoms; and (*d*) worsening of depressive symptoms after weeks of abstinence. Untreated depression, when present, is associated with higher rates of relapse into addictive behaviors (30). The reader should also refer to Chapter 6, "Psychoactive Substance Use Disorders."

UNCOMPLICATED BEREAVEMENT

Persons who have suffered the death of an intimate demonstrate a normal human response called bereavement (31). Bereavement may be indistinguishable in its symptomatology from a depression. Sadness and neurovegetative disturbances are common. Unlike a depression, bereavement does not tend to be associated with feelings of worthlessness and self-reproach. In addition, uncomplicated bereavement is a state that improves over the course of several months.

Bereaved patients who show persistent symptomatology for more than several months or who show severe self-reproach and persistent social disability may have developed a depression superimposed on their bereavement.

EPIDEMIOLOGY

Though alcoholism and phobias are more common in the general population than is depression, primary and secondary unipolar depressions are the most common causes of psychiatric hospitalization. It has been estimated that more than 15% of adults are at risk to develop a clinical depression during the course of their lives (1–3, 32). Some estimates suggest that these figures are low because they are based on research definitions of depression. If dysthymia is included, the risk for depression in the course of a lifetime appears to rise as high as 20–30% (33). Furthermore, only a portion of patients with clinical depression seek out medical or psychiatric care. As a consequence, these figures may be falsely low because of the high number of unreported cases (34).

Incidence

The incidence of a disorder is the number of new cases in a given population in one year. Estimates for first admissions to a psychiatric facility with a diagnosis of mood disorder range from about 10–20 per 100,000. This is an incidence of 0.01–0.02%. Because approximately 10–20% of these cases are manias, the adjusted incidence for depression would be that much less.

Epidemiological findings arising out of multicenter collaborative research on depression suggest that a progressive increase has occurred in the rates of depression in successive birth cohorts through the 20th century. Furthermore, each birth cohort evidenced an earlier age of onset and a decrease in the magnitude of the female-to-male ratio (35).

Prevalence

The period prevalence of a disorder is the total number of cases that exist in a population in a given year.

A cumulative prevalence rate of major depression across the five sites in the Epidemiological Catchment Area (ECA) study averaged 1.5% in the two weeks preceding subject interview. A lifetime prevalence rate of 4.4% was demonstrated in this study (36). It has also been estimated that depression can require hospitalization in 6% of women and 3% of men.

Age, Sex, and Race

Depression may occur at any age. However, evidence from ECA data demonstrated a mean age of onset of 27 years for major depression (36). Admissions to a hospital for depressive disorders, though, seem to peak in the 40–60-year-old age group. Any major psychiatric disorder (excluding dementia and delirium) that presents for the first time in a person's life after the age of 35 is likely to be a depression.

Depressive disorders are at least twice as prevalent in women as they are in men (36). This appears to be true of the range of depressive disorders and is especially true for less severe forms of depression. Weissman and Klerman (37) have demonstrated that the differences in the prevalence of depression in men and women are accurate findings, without methodological error or significant differences in health-seeking behavior. They hypothesize that these differences are multifactorial, with biological influences (either genetic or endocrinological) and psychosocial elements (such as sex discrimination or learned helplessness) acting to render the female more vulnerable to depression.

Differences in the racial distribution of depression have not been established in studies that control sex and social class variables.

Socioeconomic and Marital Status

At one time bipolar disorder was considered a condition of the upper and middle classes (38). However, recent epidemiological research has shown no highly valid or reliable data to indicate that depression is found principally in one socioeconomic stratum.

Several authors have hypothesized that the status disadvantage a married woman experiences is related to her vulnerability to depression (38–40). Their data indicate that married women show higher rates of depression than do married men, and that unmarried women show a lower rate of psychiatric disorder than do unmarried men. Evidence also suggests that the stress of marital separation and/or divorce may be related to increased rates of depressive illness (41).

THEORIES OF ETIOLOGY

Biochemical Hypotheses

Biochemical hypotheses of the etiology of depression have centered on disturbances of central nervous system (CNS) neurotransmitters (42, 43). Monoamines (norepinephrine and serotonin) are the primary neurotransmitters implicated in classical biochemical hypotheses of depressive illness.

Neurotransmitters are chemicals found in the brain that regulate nerve impulse transmission across synapses. The presynaptic neuron releases norepinephrine or serotonin from the neuron into the synaptic cleft. Once in the synaptic junction, the neurotransmitter excites the postsynaptic neuron to fire. The neurotransmitter is then inactivated by a process of reuptake, in which it is taken back into storage vesicles in the presynaptic neuron. The neurotransmitter also may be destroyed within this cell by the action of a monoamine oxidase enzyme.

The original amine hypothesis was derived from clinical research on a number of centrally active medications. Experiments with reserpine demonstrated that norepinephrine and serotonin are depleted by this drug. A monoamine oxidase inhibitor (MAOI), isoniazid, was shown to increase

CNS catecholamines. The tricyclic antidepressants (TCAs) delayed inactivation of neurotransmitters via reuptake blockade. Lithium produced an increase in the reuptake of catecholamines, thereby decreasing the availability of these transmitters. ECT demonstrated an increase in norepinephrine levels.

The original amine hypothesis of depression posits a deficiency of monoamines (norepinephrine and serotonin) in the neural synaptic junction. Antidepressants were thought to alleviate depression by correcting this deficiency, which they achieve by inhibiting uptake or decreasing catabolism once uptake has occurred (44, 45). However, more recent investigations of neurotransmitters in mood disorders have demonstrated findings consistent with *activation* of at least the norepinephrine system. In fact, normal or elevated plasma and/or cerebrospinal fluid (CSF) levels of norepinephrine and its metabolites have been observed in depressed patients (46–48). Moreover, decreases in CSF and plasma 3-methoxy-4-hydroxyphenylglycol (MHPG), a norepinephrine metabolite, have been seen in patients who successfully respond to antidepressant treatment (49, 50). No definitive explanation has been found for the disparate biochemical findings of earlier and more recent studies. It is conceivable that the discrepancy may be secondary to the design and/or methodology of the investigations or to biological differences in subgroups of depressed patients.

Evidence suggests that other neurotransmitter systems may also play a role in depression. Acetylcholine has been posited as an etiologic agent based on data that procholinergic agents can induce depression (51, 52). Decreased CSF and plasma gamma-aminobutyric acid (GABA) levels have been observed in depressed patients (53–55), which has led to speculation about the potential role of GABA in depression. Interestingly, preliminary evidence demonstrates an antidepressant effect of a GABA agonist, progabide (56, 57).

Another focus of research has been on receptor sensitivity as findings point to a decrease in the number of postsynaptic β-adrenergic receptors by almost all antidepressants. The decrease in receptors has been termed *down-regulation;* interestingly, drugs that increase postsynaptic receptors (e.g., reserpine, propranolol) can induce depression (58, 59). Both hypotheses of the etiology of depression may apply, in that disturbances in norepinephrine and serotonin could be etiologic and corrected by antidepressants, but by a process that involves down-regulation of synaptic receptors, perhaps both presynaptically as well as postsynaptically (60, 61).

Research on metabolites of CNS neurotransmitters as well as responsiveness to different TCAs suggests that some depressions are related to catechol (norepinephrine) disturbances while others are related to serotonergic (serotonin) disturbances (44, 45). Of these two different depressive subtypes, the group with deficient catecholamine (norepinephrine) demonstrates low urinary excretion of MHPG. The serotonin-deficient depressive subgroup shows normal or high urinary levels of MHPG and has been shown to have low levels of 5-hydroxyindoleacetic acid (5-HIAA), a metabolite of serotonin. Though there have been claims that low MHPG levels predict response to antidepressants that enhance norepinephrine (e.g., desipramine, imipramine) and that low 5-HIAA levels predict response to serotonergic drugs (e.g., amitriptyline), no consistent evidence for these claims exists (44, 62, 63).

Genetic Hypotheses

Genetic hypotheses on unipolar depression have drawn their data from twin studies, family studies, and adoption studies. The presumed heterogeneity of unipolar major depression has somewhat limited progress in this specific area, in contrast to bipolar disorder which is believed to be genetically more homogeneous. Nevertheless, concordance rates for affective disorder (unipolar and bipolar) in monozygotic twins are estimated to be 75%, whereas concordance for dizygotic twins is 20% (which approximates the morbidity risk among siblings) (64–67).

Furthermore, monozygotic twins reared apart showed a concordance equal to that of monozygotes reared together (68). There are no reports of one twin developing affective disorder and another schizophrenia. Data that separate unipolar from bipolar disorders among twins revealed a concordance of 41% for monozygotic twins with unipolar depression and 13% for dizygotic twins with unipolar depression (67). The degree of difference of concordance rates is similar to that of the combined unipolar/bipolar studies, and dizygotic twins still had a morbidity risk approximating that of siblings.

Family studies of unipolar affective disorder indicate that first-degree relatives have a morbidity risk of approximately 15%. Male first-degree relatives had a risk rate of 11%, compared with 18% for females. Morbidity risk for affective disorder among parents was 13%; among siblings, 15%; and among children, 20% (69–74).

Adoption studies have been developed to try to control for familial factors that are not genetic. Cadoret (75) followed the adopted-away offspring of normal and affectively disordered (unipolar and bipolar) biological parents. Adopted children of affectively disordered biological parents had a risk rate of 38%, and the normal controls had a risk rate of 7%.

Although the mode of transmission of affective disorder remains to be established, these findings strongly support a genetic factor in the etiology of unipolar depression. The data also indicate that unipolar and bipolar disorders are genetically distinct entities and that affective disorders are genetically distinct from schizophrenia.

Other Biological Hypotheses

Several other areas are also under investigation with regard to potential biological hypotheses of major depression. These include neuroendocrinology and circadian rhythms (including sleep physiology). Recent studies related to possible neurohormonal hypotheses have focused on the regulation and functional properties of neurohormones within the hypothalamic-pituitary-adrenal (HPA) and hypothalamic pituitary-thyroid (HPT) axes. Early investigation in this area resulted in the development of the dexamethasone suppression test (DST) and thyrotropin releasing hormone (TRH) stimulation test as possible laboratory tools in the diagnosis of depression. The details of these tests are discussed later in the chapter. Neuroendocrinological investigations of depression were initiated because of the relationship between certain signs of depression (appetite, libido, and sleep disturbances) and the synthesis/release of hypothalamic hormones and their systemic circulation (76). A consistent finding across neuroendocrine studies has been the frequency of elevated cortisol levels among nonpsychotic and psychotic depressed patients (77, 78).

Alterations in the sleep-wake cycle associated with depression and recent findings of possible effects of temperature regulation on mood (11) have resulted in investigations of circadian rhythm disturbances as possible etiologic factors in depression. In fact, sleep deprivation and phase advance treatments have been found to be transiently effective in depressed patients (79). Extensive research has also been done in the area of sleep physiology and its potential relationship to depression. Some consistent abnormalities in sleep electroencephalograms (polysomnograms) among depressed patients are (a) shortened rapid eye movement (REM) latency and (b) increased REM duration and density (i.e., number of rapid eye movements per REM period) (80). Finally, recent work has also been done in the utility of various sleep parameters in the monitoring of antidepressant treatment and in predicting relapse after biological treatment has been stopped (81, 82).

Psychodynamic Hypotheses

Abraham (83) was the first to psychodynamically link grief and melancholy. He stated that normal mourning, or grief, becomes melancholy, or depression, when anger and hostility accompany love for the lost object.

Freud (84), in his famous paper on mourning and melancholia, advanced these ideas. In addition to ambivalent feelings toward the lost object, Freud considered melancholia as a "disturbance of self-regard." The melancholic, unlike the mourner, suffers a loss of self-respect. Furthermore, he described mourning as occurring only in response to a realistically lost object, whereas melancholia could occur in reaction to the unconsciously perceived or imagined loss of an object.

In melancholia, the rage experienced toward the real or imagined loss of the loved object hypothetically is turned upon the self. This "retroflexed rage" (85) is a well-known psychodynamic formulation of melancholy or depression. It helps to explain the self-reproach and loss of self-esteem seen in depression, as well as the melancholic's need for punishment. This theory argues that the aggressive wish is, however, actually meant for the lost object and not the self.

Hostility directed toward the self rather than toward the lost object has epidemiological support in the inverse relationship seen between suicide and homicide (86, 87). Further, one clinical study (88) demonstrated that depressed patients show less expressed anger than do normal controls.

The universality of the retroflexed rage hypothesis is, however, brought into question by the existence of a clearly identified group of "hostile depressives" (89) who show concomitant anger and depression. Furthermore, Weissman et al. (90) demonstrated coexistent hostility and depression in certain patients. Finally, the expression of hostility by depressed patients toward the lost object does not correlate with clinical improvement and may even result in a worsening of the depression (91).

As psychoanalytic theory evolved and the ego became more the locus of study, depression was seen as a disorder of self-esteem (92). Mourning was not truly for the lost object, but for the mourner's loss of self-esteem. The lost person or object would then be understood as symbolic of the individual's lost self-esteem.

Klein's (93) work posits that a capacity for depression exists in all of us. She postulated the "normal depressive position" as the stage of life from 6–12 months. In this stage the infant experiences a fall from the omnipotence of early infancy to the experience of being separate, dependent, and vulnerable. In depression there may be a regression to this former sense of helplessness with a concomitant loss of esteem.

The relationship between separation in early life and depression has been considered. Bowlby (94) posited that an interruption in the normal course of development, by separation or loss, produces "anxious attachment." Spitz (95) studied normal infants after six months of age who had been separated from their mothers and placed in foundling homes. He described a triphasic reaction of protest, despair, and, finally, detachment, which he called *anaclitic depression.*

Brown (96) specifically studied the in-cidence of childhood bereavement (parental death before the age of 15) in depressed patients. Forty-one percent of depressed patients had experienced parental death, in contrast to 16% and 12% in control groups. The loss of mother was significant throughout the first 15 years of life, whereas the loss of father was significant between the ages of five and 15.

A number of studies have tried to clarify the role of separation in acute-onset adult depressive states (97–99). The data allow us to conclude tentatively that though separation events are common precipitants in depressive disorders, separation is not a specific, nor sufficient, cause for depression.

Clinicians have been impressed, over time, that certain personality types appear prone to depression. Obsessive-compulsive and passive dependent personality traits, for example, frequently are found in the premorbid personality evaluation of depressed patients.

Empirical work has, however, brought these clinical impressions into question. Assessment of personality cannot be accurately accomplished when the patient is in a depressed state (100). Though there is modest evidence for obsessive and dependent character constellations in unipolar depressions, the data are strongest for the premorbid trait of introversion (101). There is no evidence that a specific personality constellation (or pathology) exists for subjects who will develop unipolar affective disorder.

Beck's behavioral model of depression (102–104) is built on a cognition of negative expectations. Beck considered hopelessness and helplessness to be central to the experience of depression. His hypothesis is that these affects succeed, not precede, a set of cognitive processes involving a negative self-conception, negative interpretations of one's life events, and a pessimistic view of the future. Helplessness and hopelessness can only ensue from this cognitive set. His cognitive psychotherapy for depression, which has demonstrated efficacy, is aimed at altering cognition. Though cognitive treatment works, it remains to be established that maladaptive attitudes cause depression rather than exist as a symptom of the disorder (105, 106).

The clinician should be well-informed theoretically when meeting the hospitalized depressed patient. Nevertheless, as Klerman has stated repeatedly, anybody may develop a depression: There is no single psychodynamic process, personality type, stressful life event, or developmental experience that is unique to depressive states.

Family and Social Hypotheses

For certain depressed patients, the family is etiologic through the genetic pool. The nuclear family can also contribute to the etiology of depression in ways other than by means of the cell nucleus.

Models of adaptiveness or helplessness are learned. If, as behaviorists suggest, depression is a learned form of helplessness, it would be important to look for models of helplessness within the family. Further, disruptions in the family early in the individual's life, and more specifically, disturbances in the early mother-child relationship, can leave a person vulnerable to depression.

Events in a person's life or social field show a clear relationship to the development of depression (107–110). Major losses, including death, divorce, loss of health, and loss of money, frequently are associated with depression. These stressful life events may, in some persons, be a necessary cause but have not been shown to be a sufficient cause for depression.

In summary, a variety of theories ranging from the biochemical to the psychodynamic have been proposed for understanding the etiology of depression. It is clear that major depression is a complex condition that is caused by a combination of factors. A few investigators have proposed integrative models for the understanding of depression (76, 111, 112).

BIOPSYCHOSOCIAL EVALUATION

Biological Evaluation

A thorough biological evaluation is the first step in the evaluation of any patient who presents with depression. The clinician must feel confident that an organic cause of depression has been ruled out before proceeding with the conventional methods for treating a primary depression. Every psychiatric hospital should have access to the necessary diagnostic resources for this evaluation to occur.

Some of the disorders to be ruled out are listed in Table 1.1.

HISTORY

A detailed history of the patient's *chief complaint* and *present illness* must be obtained. *Past medical and psychiatric illnesses,* including any medications or treatment that the patient has undergone or is currently taking, are essential. A *family history,* with particular emphasis on inheritable medical and psychiatric disorders, is part of the comprehensive history. The person's *habits,* including drug and dietary habits, also must be included.

Furthermore, clinicians should inquire about a history of sexual or physical abuse, for many victims of abuse have depressive symptomatology in association with posttraumatic stress disorder (PTSD). This history is important from diagnostic and therapeutic perspectives.

In taking the history, the physician must be alert to any information regarding recent prescribed or nonprescribed drug ingestion or ingestion of any toxic substance. A history of infection, abnormal neurological activity, or medical treatment of any sort also must be sought.

History taking is done best when the patient's account is augmented by collaborative information from the family and significant others. Any person who has had occasion to witness the patient's behavior or who has pertinent knowledge about the events preceding hospitalization should be contacted.

In the *mental status examination* the clinician must search for any signs of an altered sensorium or prominent cognitive deficits. A mini-mental status may be administered to help document cognitive impairment and to possibly help discriminate between dementia and the pseudodementia of depression. A thorough *review of systems* must be taken. A previous history of depression only suggests only that the current episode is a recurrence. It is unfair to any patient to conclude presumptively, on the basis of past history, that this episode is simply a recurrence. The odds are high that such is the case. Nevertheless, the patient warrants a thorough medical evaluation to rule out the development of an autonomous medical disorder presenting as depression.

PHYSICAL EXAMINATION

A thorough physical examination must be completed to complement the history. Careful attention must be paid to the patient's vital signs and to the neurological examination.

LABORATORY, RADIOLOGIC, AND DIAGNOSTIC STUDIES

Guidelines for the laboratory and radiologic diagnosis of depression are given in Table 1.2.

Neuroendocrine Studies

A disturbance in HPA functioning has been demonstrated in a significant number of patients with primary unipolar depression, as previously mentioned (76). The most specific and documented measure of HPA axis activity is the DST. The DST was one of the first laboratory studies developed to help in the diagnosis of depression.

In recent years, the overall utility of the DST has been investigated extensively (113, 114). The average sensitivity (those with illness who will have a positive test) of the DST is between 40–50% in major depression. For very severe, melancholic depressions, particularly those associated with psychosis, the sensitivity is 60–70%. The specificity of the DST ranges from 70–90% (i.e. the failure to suppress is low in other psychiatric disorders, with a false positive rate generally about 10%). Several factors have contributed to false positive tests, including: (*a*) use of various drugs (e.g., barbiturates, carbamazepine, phenytoin, alcohol, antidepressants); (*b*) recent alcohol withdrawal (3–4 weeks); (*c*) endocrinopathies (e.g., Cushing's syndrome, pregnancy, diabetes mellitus); and (*d*) other medical conditions (e.g., infections, cancer, low body weight—malnutrition/anorexia nervosa, advanced renal or hepatic disease) (113).

The DST may prove to be most useful as a predictor of response. Those patients who have nonsuppression and fail to revert to the suppressed state during treatment are more likely to relapse than are those depressed patients whose DST became normal. For those DST nonsuppressors who fail to revert, continuation on medication appears indicated. Hence, clinicians need to weigh all of the data regarding the clinical utility of the DST and make use of this test wisely. Chapter 13 contains further discussion of this subject (including details of the procedure).

Another neuroendocrine study that has been used in the evaluation of depression is the TRH stimulation test. This has not been used as widely, which may be because of the somewhat complicated and costly nature of the procedure. The overall clinical utility of this test has also been under investigation and remains in question. Discussion of this procedure is also included in Chapter 13.

Sleep Studies

As mentioned earlier, an important research focus in depression has been on sleep physiology. Polysomnography may be of some diagnostic utility in major depression. Consistent findings are (*a*) shortened REM latency and (*b*) increased REM duration and density (80). Investigation continues to examine the role of polysomnography in diagnosis, treatment response, and recurrence of major depression (80–82).

PSYCHOLOGICAL TESTING

Psychological testing can be very helpful in the differential diagnosis of depression. The Bender-Gestalt and WAIS (Wechsler Adult Intelligence Scale) tests can be highly discriminant of organic deficits and can help rule in or out a dementia.

Psychological testing can also inform the clinician about the presence of suicidal ideation and can help assess the patient's impulsivity. A careful assessment of impulsivity gives the clinician further information as to whether patients can be relied upon not to act on their suicidal ideas.

Psychological testing can also uncover the presence of well-guarded psychotic thought processes which, if present, may call for the addition of antipsychotic medication. Finally, psychological testing can offer a profile of the patient's personality formation, both premorbid and current. An understanding of the patient's personality is helpful in devising strategies for allying with the patient and offers prognostic information. Patients with good premorbid functioning and high level personality construction fare better prognostically (see also Chapter 14).

Psychodynamic Evaluation and Formulation

Depression is not specific to any psychosocial stage of development or to any personality configuration. Anyone can develop a depression. For this reason particularly, the psychodynamic evaluation of the hospitalized depressed patient calls for a careful assessment of the patient's underlying psychological structure.

A hierarchical model of development and psychic structure has been offered by Gedo and Goldberg (115). They trace, hierarchize, and show the interaction among the following developmental lines: typical situations of danger; object relations; narcissism; sense of reality; and typical defenses. By examining the person from these perspectives, the clinician can assess the degree of functional organization and formulate whether there is a psychotic core, a narcissistic personality disorder, a neurotic character disorder, or mature adult functioning.

For example, does the patient typically experience danger in the form of moral (good/bad) anxiety; with self and object differentiation and the object a source of gratification; with the reality principle operant and guided by the ego ideal; and with repression the typical defense? If so, a neurotic character structure seems likely. However, if the typical danger is separation, if a grandiose self exists with magical illusions, and if projection and introjection are the typical defenses, a psychotic psychic organization is apt to be operant.

It is beyond the scope of this section or chapter to fully develop and present this model with the complexity and caveats attached to its use. It is a rich model for the psychodynamic assessment of the depressed patient who inherently fails to fit any specific psychosexual stage or developmental niche.

In addition to a developmental, hierarchical model for psychodynamic assessment of the depressed patient, there are aspects of the person's early life and current inner life that bear examination.

Death or early separation from a parent is a common historical event for depressed patients. As noted earlier, this is neither specific nor sufficient cause for a depressive disorder. Family influences extend beyond loss. Depressed patients often come from a family in which low self-esteem and concomitant high expectations exist and are transmitted from one generation to the next (116). Frequently, one child is chosen to bear the parental aspirations and grows to believe that love is contingent on success. At the same time, this child, outwardly loved and protected, is asked to deny his or her dependent yearnings and provide a facade of adequacy and aspirations. The child is urged to work hard and to not complain (deny hostility), without being provided the fundamentals of self-confidence, which entail adequate sources of early love and esteem. In time ". . . self-esteem depends on a combination of support from external objects, maintenance of his own adaptive capacity, and protection from unusual demands or expectations from others. The result is such a fragile balance that recurrent disruptions are inevitable, and life is series of repeated depressions" (116).

Self-esteem and depression are intimately linked. Self-esteem can be considered a self-representation or image of one's *capacity* to obtain gratification for one's needs: Self-esteem is invariably compromised in depression. The ego ideal is what a person wishes to be like; it is an internal collection of goals and aspirations (117). Esteem is high when a person feels close to the ego-ideal and, conversely, diminution of self-confidence and self-esteem accompany falling short of one's ego ideal (or its goals). Failure thereby can herald loss of self-esteem and depressive symptomatology.

In depression-prone people, self-esteem is overly based on continuing approval, admiration, and love from important objects. A disruption or loss (real or imagined) of a sustained relationship will jeopardize sources of esteem and gratification. Depression then may ensue. In this schema, expression of hostility is dangerous, for the patient may destroy the person who is most needed. Furthermore, there is often concomitant guilt over conscious (or unconscious) hostility.

A final and critical area for assessment is that *of suicidal potential*. Suicidality can be assessed along two principal lines: (*a*) the history and mental status examination; and (*b*) a psychodynamic exploration into the motives for suicide and the adequacy of the patient's sustaining environment.

Active inquiry into the patient's suicidality should *never* be omitted from the history and mental status examination of the depressed patient. Inquiry is *not* suggestive; the clinician should not fear introducing an idea that the patient may later act upon. Instead, careful examination of this subject tends to be reassuring to the patient, for it demonstrates that the examiner is willing to hear the patient's most powerful wishes and fears. The patient is asked whether he or she has had thoughts about suicide. If so, a thorough exploration of what these thoughts are, what *method* or *plan* of self-destruction has been considered, whether the *means* to do so (e.g., pills, gun) are available, and whether the patient *intends* to act and *when.* A thorough history of self-destructive behavior and suicidal attempts then should be conducted. As much detail as possible should be obtained in order to assess whether these behaviors were high or low *risk* and whether *rescue* possibilities were high or low.

The history and examination described above are augmented by an empathic reading of the patient's self-destructiveness. However, empathy is often limited in the assessment of the suicidal patient because of the patient's limited capacity to relate and to convey a sense of despair (118).

An understanding of the motives for suicide and their careful assessment through an accurate psychodynamic evaluation and formulation add additional depth and trustworthiness to the suicidal assessment (119–122). The principal *motives* for suicide are murder and escape from pain.

The psychodynamic exploration into these motives will allow the clinician to understand the patient's inner life, with its wishes, drives, and feeling states. However, what is crucial is the capacity of the patient's external world of people and events and internal world of objects and images to provide a sufficient sense of soothing connection with others and of self-worth. Such a capacity, or lack of it, will inform the clinician as to whether the patient may be predisposed to act upon these underlying motives. An *insufficient sustaining external and internal life* will expose the patient to unbearable aloneness and self-contempt and predispose him or her to suicidal action.

Sociocultural Evaluation

An assessment of the home and social environment of the depressed patient is a crucial aspect of the complete patient evaluation.

Social stressors, especially those of loss, are involved in the development of many depressive disorders. In evaluating the patient's social field, the clinician should examine for sources of stress as well as for the patient's resources. Finally, friends and work supports will be important in enabling the patient to return to prior functioning, if these supports are not invested in maintaining the patient's illness. Financial factors also play an important role in how debilitating a depressive illness can become.

BIOLOGICAL TREATMENTS

Psychopharmacological Treatment of Depression

The psychopharmacological treatment of clinical depression is an essential aspect of caring for the hospitalized depressed patient. By the time of psychiatric hospitalization the patient's depressive symptoms have become severe or life-threatening. The patient also may have active suicidal thoughts and behavior. In such cases, environmental and psychosocial interventions generally have had limited or no impact. Moreover, significant medical morbidity and mortality are likely in patients with untreated severe depressions. As a general principle, a patient who requires inpatient care for depression will require medication as part of the overall treatment plan.

During the past 40 years remarkable advances in the biologic treatment of depressive illness have occurred. In fact, 70–90% of patients with major depressive disorder (per DSM-IIIR criteria) will demonstrate marked improvement with a carefully chosen and administered biological therapy regimen. The agent of choice for major depression without psychosis is a TCA. Patients should remain on the initial medication for at least 4–6 weeks. If no clinical response has occurred at six weeks, a variety of alternatives exist. The most simple option is to switch from one TCA to another. However, the clinical utility of this option is controversial and debated. Another alternative is to attempt potentiation of the original TCA with a second agent. Lithium carbonate, L-triiodothyronine (T_3), and estrogen are agents that have been used for TCA augmentation. These potentiation attempts are effective in only a portion of patients (123–130).

Seventy to 80 percent of patients with nonpsychotic major depression will respond to either TCA alone or TCA with lithium, T_3, or estrogen augmentation. For those patients who do not improve with this pharmacologic approach, a variety of other options are available. The more traditional second-line agents are MAOIs. These have been proven to be as effective as TCAs in the treatment of depression but carry a number of serious side effects/complications and dietary restrictions that have limited their use. Additionally, lithium alone, "heterocyclics" (trazodone, maprotiline, amoxapine), and psychostimulants have been found to be useful in some patients with major depression without psychosis. Currently, there are two new and exciting antidepressants, fluoxetine HCl and bupropion HCl, whose efficacy is equal to that of the traditional antidepressants, with fewer side effects (131, 132). The more traditional antidepressants and the new agents are discussed in more detail later in this chapter. Approximately 85% of *non*responders will respond to ECT. These figures are the basis for the estimate that approximately 85% of patients with nonpsychotic major depression will respond to a well-planned somatic treatment program.

Some patients may proceed directly to a second line agent (lithium, MAOI, or new antidepressant) or to ECT at the time of their admission to the hospital. These patients usually have been found to be intolerant of or unresponsive to treatment with tricyclic agents. Some work suggests that patients with a more atypical presentation of their depression (hypersomnia, hyperphagia, and/or rejection sensitivity) may respond better to monoamine oxidase inhibitors than to tricyclics (5, 133, 134). Recent investigations also suggest that mild depressions associated with DST nonsuppression and mood reactivity predict response to MAOIs (135). Finally, for some patients, the immediate use of ECT will be indicated. These are patients for whom antidepressant medication is contraindicated or who present with life-threatening illness. This will be discussed further in the section entitled "Electroconvulsive Therapy."

Patients who present with depression and a history of at least one prior manic episode have a bipolar depression. Though lithium is less likely to provide antidepressant action than is a TCA (50% improvement is reported in one-month trials), there are several important reasons for considering it in this population. First, the use of antidepressants in depressed patients with bipolar disorder puts them at risk of an antidepressant-induced mania or rapid mood cycling during the acute treatment (136). Second, if patients do not develop mania immediately, they are at greater risk for developing rapid cycling of moods during the maintenance phase of treatment (137). Virtually all antidepressants have been demonstrated to have the potential for induction of mania (138). Bupropion HCl is the only agent that has not induced mania in depressed bipolar patients. However, this is a new agent and extensive clinical data are unavailable. Finally, the patient who responds to lithium will be taking a medication that provides acute and prophylactic treatment against recurrences of depression and mania. Lithium may be used concurrently with TCAs and MAOIs in patients with bipolar depression. There have been earlier suggestions that bipolar patients are more responsive to MAOIs than to other antidepressants (139). However, recent clinical evidence suggests that bupropion or the combination of lithium and carbamazepine may be considered as potential first-line treatments for bipolar depression (140). Failure to respond to pharmacological treatment, inability to tolerate these agents, or life-threatening illness indicate the use of ECT in patients with bipolar depression.

Patients with psychotic (delusional) depression require a different treatment approach. These patients do not demonstrate a significant response to standard tricyclic agents alone (141). Antipsychotic medications in combination with antidepressants show better results than does either agent alone (142). A recent study has also demonstrated the potential utility for amoxapine (an antidepressant agent that has an antipsychotic metabolite) for patients with psychotic depression (143). ECT is also extremely effective for psychotic depression. It has a more rapid onset of action and may be better tolerated by some patients, particularly the elderly, than is the combination of medications.

TRICYCLIC ANTIDEPRESSANTS

The tricyclic antidepressants were serendipitously discovered in the mid-1950s by physicians doing research on the phenothiazines. Imipramine was found to have no antipsychotic properties but did result in mood improvement in a number of patients.

The tricyclics exert their biochemical effect in the synaptic cleft of neurons responsible for mood regulation. Their acute mechanism of action is the inhibition of monoamine (norepinephrine and/or serotonin) reuptake. Subsequently there is an alteration of pre- and postsynaptic receptor activity. This leads to a functional increase in monoamines and down-regulation of postsynaptic receptors, which hypothetically produce an improvement in mood. *Guidelines* for the clinical use of tricyclic antidepressants are as follows.

Who? Any patient admitted to the hospital who meets the criteria for nonpsychotic depression with symptoms lasting at least two weeks is a candidate for tricyclic treatment. Patients with psychotic depression tend to require antipsychotics with antidepressants or ECT as first-line somatic treatment. Those patients with an atypical presentation of depression may do better on a MAOI. Elderly patients who are intolerant of tricyclic treatment or whose medical condition contraindicates the use of TCAs may do well with one of the newer antidepressants with fewer side effects, a psychostimulant, or ECT (144).

Contraindications. *Absolute contraindications.*

1. Acute myocardial infarction.
2. Narrow-angle glaucoma. The anticholinergic effects of the TCAs can induce acute glaucoma.

Relative contraindications.

1. Cardiac conduction deficits. Patients with His's bundle conduction defects (e.g., bundle branch block, anterior hemiblock) are sensitive to the conduction effects of most of the tricyclics (145, 146).
2. Congestive heart failure. The anticholinergic effects of the tricyclics induce sinus tachycardia, which can drive a marginally compensated heart into failure. Any patient with a compensated cardiac status must be reviewed carefully before these medications are prescribed. If a tricyclic is to be used, an agent with minimal anticholinergic side effects (like desipramine) is the drug of choice. Table 1.3 lists various side effects of antidepressant agents.
3. An otherwise abnormal EKG or cardiac history. Evidence suggests that the TCAs depress the myocardium in susceptible patients (147). In these cases, the treating psychiatrist, a cardiologist, and the patient should collaborate before tricyclics are used.
4. Pregnancy and lactation. TCAs pass through the placenta and are found in breast milk (148). Collaborative consultation with the patient and an obstetrician are essential before both mother and fetus are affected (149).
5. Seizure disorders. Tricyclics lower seizure thresholds. Safer somatic therapies in depressed patients with seizure disorders include MAOIs and ECT. Alternatively, clinicians may choose to combine anticonvulsant agents with TCAs. However, the concomitant use of these agents may lower TCA blood levels (150).
6. Prostatism. The anticholinergic effects of TCAs can cause urinary retention secondary to increased sphincter tone. An agent with less anticholinergic effect may be indicated.

Table 1.3. Antidepressant Agents

Drug Generic Names	Usual Dosage Range (mg/day)[a]	Neurotransmitter Receptor Activity				Desired Plasma Levels (if applicable)[b]	Common Side Effects
		Norepinephrine	5-Hydroxytryptamine (serotonin)	Muscarinic	Histamine 1		
TCAs							
Amitriptyline	150–300	+	++	+++	++	150–250	Sedation, orthostatic hypotension (OH), dry mouth, elevated heart rate
Imipramine	150–300	++	+	++	+++	150–250	Less sedation, less OH
Nortriptyline	50–150	++	±	++	±	50–150 ("therapeutic window")	
Desipramine	150–300	+++	±	+	0	150–250	Minimal activation, dry mouth, OH
Protriptyline	15–60	+++	±	+++	0	75–250	Moderate activation
MAOIs							
Phenelzine	45–90	N/A	N/A	N/A	N/A	N/A	OH, dry mouth, risk of hypertensive episode, anorgasmia
Isocarboxazid	30–50						
Tranylcypromine	30–50						
Newer Antidepressants							
Amoxapine	150–450	++	+	++	?	Unknown	Potential EPS (extrapyramidal symptoms), tardive dyskinesia
Bupropion	300–450	0	0	0	0	Not available	Insomnia, nausea, agitation, dry mouth
Fluoxetine	20–80	0	++++	0	0	Unknown	Insomnia, nausea, anxiety
Maprotiline	150–225					150–250	Elevated risk of seizures
Trazodone	150–300	+	+++	0/±	0	Unknown	Sedation, OH

Key:
± = minimal, if any effect
+ = mild effect
++ = moderate effect
+++ = marked effect
++++ = very marked effect
[a] May need lower or higher dose depending on clinical condition/physical health/age.
[b] Major active drug and metabolite level combined.

Which one? In addition to the afore-mentioned side effects, which are best avoided, several other factors can help the clinician decide which tricyclic to select (151).

1. A history in the patient or a family member of response to a particular agent suggests the use of that TCA.
2. Side effects may also be desirable. For example, patients with a retarded depression may fare better with a more stimulating and less sedating agent. On the other hand, the treatment of a patient with an agitated depression may be done best with a sedating agent (and avoids the use of a tranquilizing agent in the pharmacotherapeutic regimen).
3. As previously discussed, there is conflicting research evidence as to whether different types of depression are based on differing biogenic amine alterations (44, 45, 62, 63).

   MHPG is the major metabolite of CNS norepinephrine. Low levels of MHPG in the urine of depressed patients may suggest norepinephrine depletion in the brain. Furthermore, a more favorable response to treatment may occur with drugs that act more on the norepinephrine system than on the serotonin system (Table 1.3). More definitive research is needed before these laboratory tests become part of clinical practice.
4. Efforts to correlate the depressed patient's response to dexamethasone (either suppression or nonsuppression) and the efficacy of noradrenergic or serotonergic TCAs have been explored and are discussed earlier in this chapter.

Predictors of response (151–156).
Positive predictors.

1. A history of response to a TCA in the patient or family member.
2. Anorexia and weight loss; middle and late insomnia; psychomotor retardation.

3. Premorbid personality traits of obsessive-compulsiveness.
4. Higher socioeconomic status.
5. A positive response (improved mood and increased activity) to a brief trial on amphetamine. This is associated with a response to an antidepressant. Methylphenidate has demonstrated less of a predictive response (157).

Negative predictors.

1. Hypochondriasis.
2. Multiple previous episodes of depression. "Double depression."
3. Delusions. The treatment of psychotic depression generally requires addition of antipsychotic medication or ECT.
4. "Atypical" depression. MAOIs show some promise in the treatment of this disorder, which generally is refractory to tricyclics.

In addition to these negative predictors of response to the tricyclic treatment of unipolar depression, several other factors are responsible for treatment failure. First, and perhaps foremost, is compliance. An effective treatment alliance with the patient and a schedule of drug administration that reduces complexity will help to enhance compliance.

A second source of treatment problems is the interaction between TCAs and other drugs. The clinician should keep in mind that a variety of prescribed drugs may lower or raise levels of antidepressants. For example, blood levels of tricyclics may be lowered by anticonvulsants (phenytoin, carbamazepine), barbiturates, phenylbutazone, and doxycycline (158). Oral contraceptives, methylphenidate, acetaminophen, chloramphenicol, and MAOIs are among the agents that can raise TCA blood levels (158).

A third factor is the wide interindividual differences in serum tricyclic levels that patients achieve at the same dosage. Some patients on high doses of TCAs may not obtain adequate plasma levels of the drug, while others on low doses may obtain adequate or even toxic levels. Further, some of the secondary amine tricyclics (e.g., nortriptyline and protriptyline) show optimal clinical effect in what has been called a "therapeutic window." This window is a plasma level below and above which the patient will not experience an optimal effect from the medication. A recent report suggests that such a curvilinear relationship may exist for desipramine (159). Standard use of serum tricyclic levels in the hospitalized patient may help diminish this third cause of treatment failure. However, the general utility of plasma TCA levels, except with the aforementioned agents, is a controversial issue (160, 161).

How? Tricyclics are available in oral and parenteral forms. Intramuscular administration of TCAs has not been shown to be more effective and can increase their toxic effects.

There has been some controversy about the quality and equivalency of generic brand tricyclics. Standard brands or generics produced by major pharmaceutical companies attempt to offer the best quality control and reliable drug absorption (162).

How much and how long? Table 1.3 describes the range of doses and serum levels desired for the commonly prescribed antidepressants.

Hospitalized depressed patients in otherwise good health can be started on 50 mg of desipramine or equally potent doses of another TCA, increasing the dosage 25–50 mg/day up to 150–200 mg/day or until adverse effects occur. The initial dose may be lower and upward titration less rapid in a medically compromised and/or elderly patient. A plasma level may be drawn and sent for analysis while the patient is kept at this level or is given further increases. Adjustments in dosage then follow clinical response and plasma level determinations. Though the routine use of serum levels in

outpatient practice is debatable, regular use of levels in an inpatient setting can be quite practical, especially in this era of brief inpatient admissions (161).

A patient who has achieved an optimal serum level and/or is at maximum doses of an agent should remain on that dose for at least 4–6 weeks (163). At least two weeks at an adequate dose and/or level generally are required before any antidepressant effect is noticed. Such antidepressant treatment initially affects sleep, energy, and appetite. Improvement in mood and suicidality typically takes a longer time. In fact, there can be an increased risk of suicide attempts or completed suicide at this point in treatment, because patients continue to feel depressed and hopeless and have energy to act on their self-destructive/suicidal thoughts. If no improvement occurs after six weeks, the decision to continue with the current drug, augment the current medication with another agent, or change to a new antidepressant should be made.

When? Single daily bedtime dosage of a tricyclic increases compliance, aids in any difficulty falling asleep, and generally results in the occurrence of unwelcome side effects (e.g., orthostatic hypotension) while the patient is asleep. No clinical efficacy is lost with once-daily dosing.

Other dosage schedules may be more suitable for specific patients and may minimize some side effects. The physician is wise to include the patient when choosing the medication schedule.

Barbiturates as sleeping medications are best avoided. They are no more effective than other nonbarbiturate sedative-hypnotics, show tolerance, and increase liver microsomal activity with consequent increased TCA metabolism and decreased TCA levels.

Common side effects.

1. Cardiac toxicity.
2. Anticholinergic effects (e.g., dry mouth, urinary retention, and constipation),

which tend to improve with time. The clinician may elect to initiate a procholinergic agent (e.g., bethanechol at 10–30 mg q.d. to t.i.d.) (164).

3. Dizziness (postural hypotension), restlessness (jitteriness), insomnia, tremor.
4. Delirium—anticholinergic CNS toxicity that responds to parenteral physostigmine salicylate (Antilirium), an anticholinesterase inhibitor, at 1–2 mg i.v. slow push every 30–60 minutes or 1–2 mg i.m. every 60 minutes (164).
5. Skin rashes (165).
6. Allergic-obstructive jaundice.

NEWER ANTIDEPRESSANTS

A variety of antidepressants have been introduced in recent years. Anticholinergic side effects, orthostatic hypotension, and cardiotoxicity were among the adverse effects that led to poor tolerance and poor compliance and prompted the investigation and ultimate discovery of new antidepressant agents. Agents offered as alternatives to traditional antidepressants have been amoxapine, maprotiline, trazodone, alprazolam, nomifensine (currently unavailable), fluoxetine, and bupropion.

Amoxapine is a metabolite of the neuroleptic loxapine. Its mode of action is believed to involve uptake inhibition of norepinephrine and blockade of dopamine receptors. The dopamine blockade, as with neuroleptics, may have antipsychotic qualities. In fact, a recent study demonstrated equivalent efficacy of amoxapine and combination of neuroleptic and antidepressant in patients with delusional depression (143). However, a drawback to the use of this agent in this population is the inability to clinically titrate the levels of neuroleptic and antidepressant independently. Furthermore, the occurrence of extrapyramidal symptoms and the potential for development of tardive dyskinesia have limited its clinical use. Moreover, there have been numerous reports of amoxapine-induced seizures from overdosage (150).

Maprotiline has a tetracyclic structure and clinical action similar to standard tricyclics, though it is of a fully separate class of compounds. It appears to be a norepinephrine reuptake inhibitor that resembles desipramine. The utility of maprotiline is limited, though, because of side effects that include skin rashes (3%) and seizure induction, particularly in patients with seizure disorders and in those patients on doses equal to or greater than 225 mg/day (150). The latter adverse effect is common and gives maprotiline little advantage over other standard antidepressant agents.

Trazodone is also chemically distinct from the TCAs. It was introduced as an alternative to more serotonergic agents like amitriptyline; it has diverse mechanisms of action encompassing mixed inhibition of serotonin and norepinephrine reuptake and α-adrenergic blockade. The relatively low anticholinergic side effect profile of trazodone adds to its value. Some patients find the sedative effects intolerable, especially at adequate dose levels. For other patients, the sedation provides significant anxiolytic action. In fact, many clinicians have found trazodone to be most useful as a soporific rather than as a potent antidepressant agent. A potentially serious, albeit relatively uncommon, side effect in male patients receiving trazodone is priapism (166). Clinicians should be aware of this and warn male patients about the possibility of occurrence.

Alprazolam is a triazolobenzodiazepine with properties quite similar to the benzodiazepine diazepam, though 5–10 times more potent. It has clear anxiolytic and antipanic properties. Its capacity to down-regulate receptor sites led to inquiry into its potential as an antidepressant. It has demonstrated some clinical efficacy in depression (167, 168) but remains investigational with regard to this indication. Whether this drug offers more than its predecessor, diazepam, is unclear; like diazepam, it does have the capacity to induce tolerance, disinhibition, dependence, and withdrawal states.

Nomifensine is an isoquinoline antidepressant agent that demonstrated some clinical efficacy when it was released. However, it is no longer available because of significant complications, including hyperthermia, immune hemolytic anemias, and death (169, 170).

Fluoxetine is a bicyclic drug that is a selective serotonin reuptake inhibitor (171). It has demonstrated clinical efficacy equal to that of TCAs without causing the usual bothersome side effects (e.g., anticholinergic or hypotensive effects) (132). Common adverse reactions associated with use of fluoxetine include anxiety, nausea, and insomnia (132). In addition to its utility in depression, clinicians are finding fluoxetine to be helpful in the treatment of obsessive-compulsive disorder and bulimia.

Bupropion is a monocyclic drug that is structurally and pharmacologically different from the TCAs. It seems to function as a weak inhibitor of norepinephrine reuptake and a weak dopamine agonist. Its exact mechanism of action as related to the treatment of depression is unclear (172). Bupropion is a highly activating antidepressant and, while helpful for some anergic patients, generally is less well tolerated by agitated patients. The drug has minimal cardiac (173), anticholinergic, and sedative effects. Commonly reported adverse effects are agitation, nausea, headache, and dry mouth (not secondary to an anticholinergic mechanism) (174). Bupropion has been associated with seizures, particularly in patients with eating disorder or seizure disorder histories (175).

In summary, there is no evidence that the newer antidepressants demonstrate any greater efficacy than do their tricyclic predecessors. However, the different side effect profiles of fluoxetine and bupropion may be better tolerated by patients, arguing for their consideration as first-line drugs, especially in drug-sensitive and/or elderly patient populations. More conservative clinicians may choose to begin treatment with a traditional tricyclic agent. Patients who do not respond to or cannot tolerate traditional agents now have a variety of alternatives that previously did not exist.

MONOAMINE OXIDASE INHIBITORS

The monoamine oxidase inhibitors (MAOIs) were discovered fortuitously approximately 30 years ago during research on antitubercular drugs. After initial enthusiasm, though, clinicians virtually abandoned these drugs because of their association with hypertensive crises. In recent years the MAOIs have regained clinical popularity, primarily for two reasons. First, their risk has been overestimated (176), and second, research has demonstrated their specificity and efficacy in the treatment of atypical depression (133, 134). Moreover, MAOIs have been effective in some depressed patients who are refractory to tricyclic treatment. These agents remain underused, though, and may hold promise for many patients.

Monoamine oxidases are enzymes found within the neuron that metabolize mood-regulating amines. Inhibition of this enzyme by a MAOI results in an increase in CNS biogenic amines. The two more commonly used MAOIs are phenelzine (Nardil) and tranylcypromine (Parnate). Phenelzine is an irreversible inhibitor (a hydrazine) whose action lasts about two weeks after its discontinuation. Its value in the treatment for atypical depression and phobic-anxiety states has been established (133, 134). Patients tend to complain of multiple side effects during treatment with phenelzine, although it shows a lower incidence of hypertensive reactions and is a less activating compound than tranylcypromine. Tranylcypromine is a nonhydrazine MAOI whose action persists for several days after its discontinuation. This drug has a higher incidence of hypertensive reactions and is a highly activating compound that can be helpful with anergic patients (perhaps because of its structural similarity to amphetamine). In fact, investigators recently have reported the autoinduction of increased blood pressure with MAOIs, especially tranylcypromine (177–179). When this occurs, a divided dose regimen (t.i.d. to q.i.d.) has been recommended, which may eliminate this hypertensive reaction; however, such reactions have occurred with single 10-mg doses of tranylcypromine.

Both phenelzine and tranylcypromine can cause hypertensive reactions when the drug interacts with exogenous tyramine and similar sympathomimetic substances. Tyramine is found in a variety of foods that have been produced by putrefaction (e.g., aged cheeses and wines, yogurt, yeast extract, chocolate) and certain medications that contain sympathetic-like compounds (e.g., ephedrine, phenylpropanolamine, L-dopa, amphetamine). Patients must be reliable, allied with treatment, and educated in taking their medication before the physician prescribes a MAOI. Dietary lists are available and can be distributed to patients and families.

Dosages of at least 60 mg/day of phenelzine (about 1 mg/kg) are associated with greater rates of improvement. Divided dosages with a larger portion given at bedtime seem to reduce hypotensive effects that, empirically, correlate with response to phenelzine. Tranylcypromine doses range upward from 20 mg/day, as tolerated.

A pretreatment platelet MAO activity level may be drawn via serum sample. Analysis is available at major laboratories. Clinical improvement is associated with greater than 80% inhibition of the baseline value. Samples for assessment of inhibition can be obtained after 10 days of stabilization on a given dose of phenelzine. Acquisition of platelet MAO inhibition in patients taking tranylcypromine is of little value in that treatment with this agent leads to immediate and complete MAO inhibition.

LITHIUM

Lithium carbonate has been reported to show antidepressant properties in patients with diagnosed bipolar affective disorder (180, 181). A family history of bipolar disorder and the presence of neurovegetative disturbances that are persistent and out of proportion to environmental influences also are associated with an antidepressant response to lithium.

Patients who are refractory to conventional treatment and who demonstrate the historical or clinical features noted above should be considered for a trial on lithium. Lithium carbonate also may be added to tricyclic- or MAOI-treated patients who show minimal response to the antidepressant alone. Some controversy still exists about its actual efficacy, because of conflicting reports on its utility in traditional antidepressant augmentation (123, 124, 129) (see Figures 1.2 and 1.3; see also Chapter 2).

STIMULANTS

Amphetamine (Dexedrine and Benzedrine) and methylphenidate (Ritalin) may be effective in the treatment of a certain population of depressed patients. There have been reports of stimulant efficacy in the treatment of depression in the elderly and/or medically ill patients (182, 183). Additionally, the use of stimulants for treatment of affective and cognitive neuropsychiatric manifestations of Acquired Immune Deficiency Syndrome (AIDS) is rising and has been found to be effective (184). There is less evidence for the effective use of stimulants in primary depression (183).

Stimulants are administered early in the day to avoid problems with insomnia. Five to 10 mg of amphetamine b.i.d. or t.i.d. or 10 mg of methylphenidate b.i.d. or t.i.d. are prescribed as tolerated. If the drug is effective, results are apparent within several

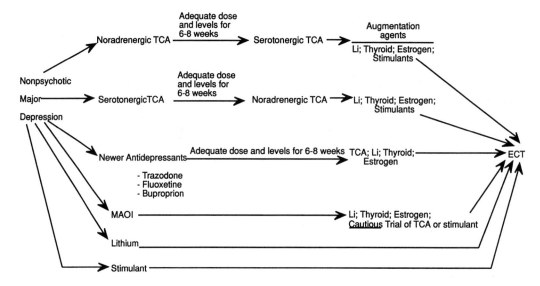

Figure 1.2.   Guidelines for somatic treatment of nonpsychotic major depression.

days, unlike traditional antidepressants, which take weeks. Stimulants may also play a role in the augmentation and/or rapidity of response to TCAs (185). Tolerance does not appear to become a problem in this population.

COMBINED DRUG TREATMENT

Treatment-resistant unipolar depressions, which account for about 15% of cases, have prompted clinicians to search for new methods of treatment. Chronic depression is a severely painful disorder for patients and their intimates. Clinicians are to be encouraged to try less conventional treatments in collaboration with their patients when concerted somatic and psychosocial efforts fail.

As previously discussed, augmentation of TCA or MAOI agents can be done with lithium carbonate. Other potentiating agents include T_3 and estrogen, which may be of particular utility in female patients (125–128). A partial response to a tricyclic may be enhanced with the addition of a stimulant drug or with fluoxetine (186). However, with the fluoxetine-tricyclic combination clinicians need to be mindful of serum tricyclic levels, as toxic levels have been observed (187). Importantly, fluoxe-

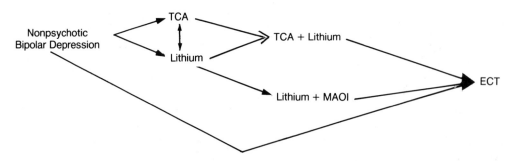

Figure 1.3.   Guidelines for somatic treatment of nonpsychotic bipolar depression.

tine *cannot* be combined with MAOIs, because such a combination can result in a potentially fatal serotonergic syndrome (188). In fact, clinicians *must* have a five-week washout between fluoxetine and MAOI trials.

The use of a MAOI added to an established tricyclic regimen (but not vice versa) may be beneficial in some refractory depressions (189). This should be attempted cautiously in such difficult cases. Tyrosine, an amine precursor, has been reported to show an antidepressant effect (190). Another amine precursor, L-tryptophan, also has been used for potentiation of antidepressants. However, this substance recently was withdrawn from the market because of the increased occurrence of a previously rare syndrome of myalgias associated with eosinophilia (191).

Finally, a number of novel drug combinations and research antidepressants are being studied and employed at various university centers. Treatment-resistant patients and their families can be referred to specialty psychopharmacologists when conventional methods prove unsatisfactory.

Nonpharmacological Somatic Treatment

SLEEP AND LIGHT THERAPY

Potentiation of antidepressant medication has been achieved by advancing the patient's sleep cycle. Simply put, patients sleep from 6:00 PM to 2:00 AM and are not permitted to nap during the day. This advance in the sleep-wake cycle holds promise because of its rapid effect and lack of biological toxicity. Patients are gradually shifted back to their normal cycle (79).

Patients with SADS may benefit from exposure to bright lights before dawn and after dusk. Recent studies have demonstrated consistent efficacy of phototherapy in this subtype of depressed patients (10), making it a simple and relatively nontoxic measure that can be considered for certain patients.

ELECTROCONVULSIVE THERAPY

Electroconvulsive therapy is the most specific and effective of treatments for psychotic, unipolar depression (152, 192) (see Figure 1.4). In addition, 85% of nonpsychotic, unipolar depressives who did not respond to tricyclic treatment will respond to ECT (193). In essence, ECT offers the most breadth and the highest efficacy of all biological treatments for depression.

As a general rule, ECT is reserved for patients who have not responded to adequate trials on antidepressants or who have been unable to tolerate these often-toxic drugs. Elderly and medically ill patients may be treated more safely with ECT than with TCAs and therefore represent possible exceptions to this rule. Severely depressed patients with active suicidal intent or cata-

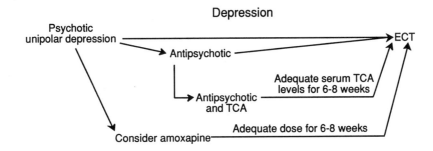

Figure 1.4. Guidelines for somatic treatment of psychotic unipolar depression.

tonically or psychotically depressed patients also may bypass medications, because they may require the more rapid action that ECT provides. In sum, a risk/benefit analysis of the appropriateness of ECT should be made in all cases (194).

ECT increases norepinephrine turnover in the CNS (195). An increased turnover of norepinephrine increases the functional availability of catecholamine and suggests that the mode of action is similar to that of the antidepressant medications.

ECT can be used with remarkable safety in ill, debilitated, elderly, and most tricyclic-intolerant patients when measures are taken to monitor and manage any medical disorder concomitant with the patient's depression. A recent review of the literature has abandoned the concept of absolute contraindications to ECT (194). However, precaution should be taken in cases in which an intracranial space-occupying lesion is present (e.g., tumor, subdural hematoma) and in which a history of recent myocardial infarction exists (196–198).

Mandel et al. (199) reported prediction of response to ECT on the basis of clinical symptomatology. A positive response to ECT has been associated with delusions (somatic or paranoid), sudden onset of symptoms, guilt, mood lability, fluctuating course, and, we would add, a previous response to ECT. Recently, Solan and colleagues (200) looked at psychotic and nonpsychotic depressed patients and did not find the presence of psychosis as generally predictive of response to ECT. They did report a significant difference in response within the psychotic group based on the content of delusions (i.e., those with nihilistic delusions demonstrated better outcome than did those with paranoid delusions). Concomitant personality pathology (especially borderline, hypochondriacal, and dependent features) augurs a poorer response to ECT.

The workup for ECT proceeds along two lines. First, informed consent must be obtained from the patient or guardian (201). Informed consent is the written version of the establishment of a trusting, working alliance with the patient and the patient's family. The second part of the workup is the medical evaluation, which includes:

1. Medical history and review of systems.
2. Physical examination.
3. Complete blood count (CBC), urine analysis, serum test for syphilis, blood urea nitrogen (BUN), glucose, and aspartate aminotransferase (AST).
4. Electrocardiogram (EKG).
5. Chest films.

In addition, the patient's psychotropic medication regimen must be reviewed carefully. Barbiturates should be avoided because they raise seizure threshold. If evening or morning sedation is needed, hydroxyzine or oxazepam may be used. If the patient has been on a tricyclic, the drug should be discontinued as far in advance of ECT as possible. Tricyclics can cause complications with blood pressure during anesthesia and are cardiac depressants. Patients who are receiving neuroleptics should be managed on as low a dose as possible during the course of ECT. However, recent work suggests that concomitant use of neuroleptics with ECT in psychotic patients may improve outcome (202, 203).

ECT can be administered unilaterally or bilaterally. Unilateral, nondominant hemisphere treatment is associated with less post-ECT cognitive difficulties and does not increase the number of treatments needed (204, 205).

Generally, six treatments are given in a series, though some patients may require more to obtain relief. Patients are premedicated with i.m. atropine to reduce secretions and to minimize vagal cardiac dysrhythmias. Methohexital (Brevital), a rapid-acting barbiturate, is given i.v. for anesthesia, and i.v. succinylcholine (Anectine) is used for muscular relaxation.

The electrical stimulus is administered once medication effects are established and oxygenation is achieved via an airway. Many treatment centers try to minimize the dose, which is measured in time and voltage.

Upon completion of the seizure, oxygenation is resumed and the patient is monitored carefully. Most patients are up and about an hour after the treatment is completed. Adverse effects commonly reported with ECT include headache and muscle spasms, which usually improve with treatment of symptoms. Cognitive changes include postictal confusion and anterograde and retrograde amnesia for events surrounding the course of ECT. The amnesia almost always is transient and resolves within 30–60 days after completion of treatment (204).

Considerable misinformation and mystique surround ECT. Patients and their families may be reassured by an open and honest discussion of this procedure with the treating clinician. Several books and videos are available for patient and family information (206, 207). ECT is a safe and highly effective treatment for major depression. All clinicians should be familiar with this treatment and know when to prescribe it, because it holds the remedy for many patients who cannot be treated by other methods.

PSYCHOSOCIAL TREATMENTS

Milieu Management

The salient aspects of the milieu management of the hospitalized, depressed patient are safety, remoralization, (208) and education.

The great preponderance of depressed patients will get better if they do not seriously injure or kill themselves during the course of their illness. Delusionally depressed patients are at significantly higher risk for suicide than are nonpsychotic depressives. Hospitalization of the depressed person often occurs when suicidal ideation or behavior has developed (209–211).

As a consequence, the first responsibility of the hospital staff is to assess the patient's suicidality and establish appropriate safety measures. The patient's possessions are checked for sharp objects or materials that could be used for suicide (e.g., drugs, belt, rope). Many patients will be able to establish a *verbal* (or written) *contract* in which they agree to inform a member of the staff if they experience a compelling impulse toward self-destruction. Patients are told that in hospital (and thereafter) they can learn to talk about, rather than act upon, their impulses.

Those patients who are unable to form this contract may require *constant observation*, where they are always in the company of a staff member or are visible in a ward community space. Severely suicidal patients may require treatment on a closed ward to prevent elopement. Others will require one-to-one supervision to prevent suicidal behavior. The improving depressed patient may gain hope and become less suicidal *or* may acquire the energy to act on the suicidal impulses.

Remoralization is the reexperience of confidence in the self. The depressed patient has lost morale and the hospital can serve to help restore it. The nursing and milieu staff provide the patient with empathic listeners who enable the patient to tolerate the despair. Staff, as well as other patients, offer surcease from the aloneness or guilt that can prompt self-destruction. Ventilation of affects is encouraged in patients at a rate they can tolerate.

The regular rhythm of the ward with its shelter and structure appears to help many depressed patients. Staff also begin to create expectations for dress, self-care, and meal behaviors that had waned prior to admission. Socialization is encouraged but not forced. Structured activities via occupational therapy and patient activity groups enable the depressed patient to reexperience competence. The ward community provides an ambience of belief in each individual's capacity to improve, while gently asserting the person's responsibility to participate in self-care. The depressed patient slowly emerges from the preoccupation with self and rediscovers a healthier self, the world, and morale.

The milieu can also offer the patient an educational experience that can be corrective cognitively as well as emotionally. The depressed patient can learn that depression is a highly treatable disorder that affects large numbers of people. This sense of universality and treatability may be a corrective cognitive experience. Negative self-concepts, maladaptive coping patterns, and indirect or confused communicational styles all become apparent in the ward community. Constructive feedback from patients and staff can foster alternative thinking and behavior. Furthermore, the patient can rediscover that he or she is a person who can care about others and be cared about in turn.

Group therapy, two to three times weekly during the patient's hospital stay, can focus on current stresses and ways of coping with these stresses. Interpersonal and communicational styles also emerge quickly in these groups. Patients can be helped to relearn social skills and to correct relating and communicating difficulties in an atmosphere of group acceptance and support.

Individual Psychotherapy

Individual psychotherapy has a very important place in the treatment of the hospitalized depressed patient. Somatic treatments and psychotherapy complement each other in quite specific ways. Medications or ECT are effective in treating the neurovegetative symptoms (eating, sleeping, motor, and cognitive disturbances), while psychotherapy acts as a specific and effective treatment for the interpersonal and social disturbances that accompany depression (e.g., isolation, dependence, constricted or hostile communication, rumination, and impaired work performance) (106, 212–214). Evidence also indicates that the combination of psychotherapy and pharmacotherapy is more effective than either treatment modality alone and definitely superior to placebo (215).

Arieti (216) has suggested that for some treatment-refractory depressed patients psychotherapy alone is the treatment of choice. He implies that in some cases medications may interfere with the treatment process. Though Arieti's thoughts may apply in some specific cases, it is our view, and that of others (217), that most hospitalized depressed patients require a biological treatment to enable them to form a relationship with a therapist and to have adequate energy and cognitive capacity for psychotherapy.

Inhospital psychotherapy can begin on a daily basis. Meetings may be shorter initially (e.g., 20–30 minutes) if this is all the time the patient can tolerate. As improvement occurs, the time can be increased to 30–50 minutes with the frequency of individual meetings continuing daily or decreasing to 3–4 times per week.

One of three psychotherapeutic approaches may be taken in the treatment of patients with depression. These techniques are: (*a*) psychodynamic; (*b*) cognitive; or (*c*) interpersonal psychotherapies (218). The selection of a specific psychotherapeutic treatment should be based on an individual patient's presentation. All of these approaches have been useful either alone or in combination with medications in different patient populations.

Conventional principles of outpatient exploratory or reconstructive psychotherapy, which entail a nondirective, interpretative therapeutic posture as well as necessary silence, should be eschewed with the hospitalized depressed patient. Nondirective, exploratory psychotherapy unduly stresses the severely depressed person and reinforces the person's unconscious view of unavailable, uncaring caregivers who wish to reject him or her.

Hence, a more psychodynamic approach generally would *not* be the initial psychotherapeutic treatment in the severely depressed patient.

Instead, hospital psychotherapy aims to be supportive and restitutive. The therapist should be active and persistent in inquiry, flexible in scheduling, friendly in demeanor, and interested in contact with relatives (219). Defenses are reinforced, and areas of adaptive functioning are sought and encouraged. Restitutive psychotherapy involves empathic listening, for depressed patients want to share their grief. The therapist must be able to bear the pain with the patient; extra time may be needed for this affect to emerge, especially in view of the depressed patient's psychomotor retardation. The therapist needs to *not* be too warm, or too funny. The depressed patient feels unworthy of excessive warmth and tends to withdraw and feel worse when this is offered. Excessive humor on the part of the therapist denies the patient's grief and is devaluing.

The therapist wishes to convey a sense of hope to the depressed patient. This does not take the form of simple reassurance or universal optimism. The therapist must seek out and understand with the patient the underlying fears and anxieties. For example, the fear that depression is an illness that will last forever was understood in one patient to be a fear of becoming like his mother, who became depressed and remained ill for a lifetime. Only when these underlying concerns are clear can the patient be responded to, reassured, and given hope. In brief, an interpersonal-oriented psychotherapy may be more appropriate for the initial phases of inpatient treatment.

The hospital therapist faces the difficult dilemma of how to be supportive and even protective (in cases of self-destructive behavior) without reinforcing the depressed patient's sense of helplessness. Therapeutic directiveness and permission to be taken care of can stimulate childlike helplessness as well as diminish the patient's self-esteem. Therapeutic efforts to foster autonomy, on the other hand, can be seen by the patient as rejection. In general, acutely depressed patients require dependency gratification and need to be encouraged to accept the care they have previously refused. The therapist can indicate that the patient needs help at this time, while informing the patient that these interventions are only temporary and will change as the patient's needs become clearer and as the capacity for self-care increases.

Aside from establishing clear safety measures to keep depressed patients from self-harm, the clinician should avoid taking responsibility for decisions patients must make. Most important decisions can be deferred until patients have obtained some significant improvement in their depression. Once depression has improved, as it generally does, the clinician can then aide patients in carefully exploring their life dilemmas and determining their own casts of mind.

Dependent needs are pronounced and generally unacceptable to depressed individuals, who also assume that they will not get what they want. Anger, conscious and unconscious, may develop as dependent needs are perceived as being unmet. The depressed patient often seeks nurturance through suffering. This dynamic of deprivation, intense and forbidden dependent needs, and anger over deprivation and anticipated rejection will live itself out in the transference (the historically determined relationship the patient will develop with the therapist). The therapist can never fully satisfy the patient's dependent needs, and anger will soon occupy the therapeutic arena, particularly if the therapist appropriately avoids taking unnecessary control of the patient's life. Anger in the transference should be allowed and should spontaneously lead to anger toward other important people and losses that the patient has experienced. Careful examination and working through in this area allow the clinician to promote patient autonomy and to curtail the helplessness and suffering that is aimed at securing caring. The direct expression of hostility, in therapy or with important others, has not been shown to result universally in clinical improvement (87, 88). The technique just described regards anger as an affect that will naturally accompany (and therefore need not be provoked) the understanding and working through of dependency conflicts, learned helplessness, and the secondary gains of depression. Work of this sort can begin in the hospital, to be continued after discharge in a more explorative and reconstructive manner.

Countertransference feelings can become quite powerful in the treatment of depressed and suicidal patients (220). The therapist who is feeling guilt or anger should suspect covert aggression on the part of the patient. This may occur when the patient is subtly making overwhelming or impossible demands that render the therapist first helpless, then guilty or angry. Boredom and impatience also may be felt in the countertransference, but these feelings are more difficult to work through. The patient has somehow gotten the therapist to reject him or her through boredom and impatience. When this is occurring, the therapist must understand that the patient is unconsciously driving away the very source of nurturance that is so desperately needed. Careful self-inspection, supervision, or con-

sultation may be needed to assist therapists in understanding their part in this process.

As this short-term, restitutive therapy progresses, the therapist and patient begin to make plans for follow-up care. Posthospital psychotherapy in conjunction with appropriate family work and psychopharmacological treatment will improve long-term prognosis. In fact, evidence suggests that continuation of combined psychotherapy and pharmacotherapy has a positive effect on reducing recurrence of depression and enhancing survival time (221–223).

If the patient is to be transferred to another therapist upon discharge, this transfer is best done while the patient is still in the hospital. Two or three meetings for getting acquainted and planning a treatment contract with the outpatient therapist will increase posthospital compliance.

The termination phase of inpatient psychotherapy often is characterized by a looking back on the severe depression and feeling vulnerable to the stresses that did and will continue to exist outside the hospital. Loss of the hospital and the intense contact with the therapist may echo earlier losses and frustrations. Adequate time should be allotted to the termination phase of hospitalization in order to allow the patient time to work through these feelings and to say goodbye to hospital staff and fellow patients.

Family Work

FAMILY EVALUATION AND THERAPY

Most spouses and families of depressed patients welcome contact from the hospital psychiatric social worker or a member of the ward staff. Families often feel left out, unrecognized, and uncared for, because the identified patient generally has been the focus of previous professional contact.

An effective alliance with the patient's spouse or family is critical in several ways. First, additional collaborative history may be essential diagnostically. Second, distortions shaped by the patient's illness can be corrected in the minds of the hospital staff. Contact with the family also allows for a clearer exploration and identification of stressors. Furthermore, an effective alliance with the family will reduce the possibility of their sabotaging treatment for reasons intrinsic to the family's psychopathology or its need to maintain its current equilibrium, which may depend on one person's being ill. Finally, evidence from early studies demonstrates that family intervention positively influences treatment compliance, which correlates with outcome (224). A more recent study has shown that inpatient family work has its greatest effect on the outcome of female patients with affective disorders (225).

The evaluation of the family can be done with once- or twice-weekly meetings for as many meetings as needed. The family can be encouraged to attend any additional family groups that the hospital may offer (e.g., family orientation meetings or a multiple family support group).

Throughout the family contact and therapy the therapist needs to adopt a posture of listening, calming, and educating. Families experience the distress wrought upon them by the depressed person and often are emotionally and financially drained by the time the patient enters the hospital. Many families do not understand depression and can view some symptoms as thoroughly willful. When the family feels heard and empathically responded to, the members can then listen to the therapist educate them about depression.

On the basis of the evaluation, a recommendation for continued family contact or inhospital marital or family therapy is made, when indicated. Indications include marital distress (very common in depression) (226); family psychopathology that rests, at least in part, on the patient's occupying a sick role; or an impasse in the development of the family (e.g., children leaving home) that appears associated with the patient's depression. In brief hospital family therapy, issues and affects are identified, alliances with *all* family members are fostered, and goals for change are negotiated. Plans for follow-up are established, when indicated, and are concretely set in place before discharge to maximize compliance.

GENETIC COUNSELING

Many family members have concerns about the genetic transmission of depression. Parents may worry what they might convey to their children and children may worry about their vulnerability to depression.

If family members do not spontaneously raise these concerns, the clinician ought to mention, in a family meeting, that these are common questions and concerns that families have and thereby encourage their expression.

Genetic factors in the etiology of depression can be reviewed candidly with family members. It is estimated that the risk of developing a depression in first-degree relatives of an affected patient is 15%. A child with one parent with depressive illness is at 26% risk, and a child with both parents affected is at 43% risk. Concordance for dizogytic twins is 13% and is 41% for monozygotic twins (227).

As the clinician explores family concerns and educates its members about the biology of depression, he or she should also emphasize the psychosocial aspects of this disorder and its manageability with early diagnosis and treatment.

CONTROVERSIES IN THE INPATIENT TREATMENT OF DEPRESSION

The Use of ECT

Although ECT has been demonstrated to be a safe and effective treatment for major depression, its use in clinical practice remains controversial. For example, ECT is often underused in medically ill and/or geriatric patients with major depression because of unfounded concerns about its risks. As previously noted in this chapter, ECT is a more rapid and generally safer treatment modality in this population than is pharmacotherapy.

On the other hand, ECT may be overused in the treatment of patients with less clear-cut diagnoses. For example, victims of trauma may exhibit depressed mood, sleep disturbance, isolative behavior, sexual dysfunction, and self-destructive/suicidal ideation or behavior in addition to symptoms characteristic of PTSD (e.g., flashbacks, intrusive phenomena, hypervigilance, and startle response). In the absence of a known trauma history, the clinician might make a diagnosis of chronic major depression, which is apt to resist treatment. When this occurs, such patients undergo complex medication trials and ultimately may be referred for ECT. The use of ECT in this population can divide members of a multidisciplinary treatment team. Some argue that the mood disturbance is secondary to the trauma history and that a primary psychotherapeutic approach (with adjunctive medications) is the best treatment option. Staff may also object to the use of ECT because of the nature of the procedure (i.e., having something done to patients while they are anesthetized), which may recall earlier traumatic experiences. Moreover, some argue that the transient cognitive deficits observed with ECT may interfere with the patient's capacity to make use of individual and milieu psychotherapy.

ECT is a safe and effective treatment that should be considered in the therapeutic regimen for major depression. Clinicians should carefully evaluate patients who present with symptoms of major depression and make use of the best treatment modality (e.g., ECT, medication therapy, individual psychotherapy, group psychotherapy, or a combination) based on the individual patient's clinical picture. A thoughtful approach to clinical care ultimately will result in appropriate use of methods such as ECT and, it is hoped, reduce the current controversy.

Polypharmacy

The recent trend toward polypharmacy (i.e., simultaneous use of more than one antidepressant agent in a given patient) is another controversy in the inpatient care of the depressed patient. Patients with treatment-resistant depression often are placed on complex pharmacotherapeutic regimens in an effort to either produce a response or augment a partial response. Complicated regimens are controversial because of the increased risk of adverse reactions and interactions, the potential for reduced patient compliance, and the increased financial costs.

Some evidence documents the efficacy of various combination treatments. Hence, it is our opinion that such treatment is not unreasonable provided clinicians have thoroughly investigated and discussed alternatives with their patients.

Managed Care

The economic climate of health care and its impact on psychiatric treatment is addressed in Chapter 17. In the last few years, managed care has had a striking impact on inpatient treatment of depressive illness. For example, the need for hospitalization has become based principally on the level of dangerousness to self or others. This criterion can exclude those patients with moderate to severe depression (perhaps an evolving episode) from receiving a comprehensive assessment and an adequate medication trial. Such an assessment and initial treatment may take place on an outpatient basis for those patients with an adequate support system and without significant medical problems. However, patients who lack support or have co-morbid disorders generally cannot receive the services they need outside a hospital.

The rapid turnover of patients associated with managed care creates controversy among staff members (e.g., senior clinicians, nursing staff, and training clinicians) working in the hospital. One aspect of the controversy may relate to adequacy of patient care: whether exclusively somatic treatments may be used in lieu of combined medication and individual/milieu psychotherapeutic treatments (previously described as superior in this population), because the latter may be more time consuming (and therefore more expensive). A rapid turnover of patients on a unit also can be rather disruptive to milieu treatments. For example, such turnover results in a frequently changing composition of milieu groups, which ultimately may reduce the overall efficacy of that treatment. Moreover, as a result of decreased lengths of stay, patients may have to transition to outpatient settings with partly treated conditions. This requires adequate aftercare programs to prevent relapse or complications (e.g., attempted or completed suicide, rehospitalization).

COURSE AND PROGNOSIS

Eighty-five percent or more of patients with unipolar depressions will improve under a specific, carefully chosen biopsychosocial treatment plan. Untreated depressions have been reported to remit spontaneously in 6–9 months (228). Treated depressions can respond in weeks to months. Predictors of recovery from acute symptoms of depression include acute onset, severe illness in those who have no chronic history of depression, and superimposition of an acute episode on a chronic underlying depression (229).

Ten to fifteen percent of depressed patients will have a chronic course. Statistically significant increases in the rate of relapse are associated with underlying chronic depression and three or more previous episodes of affective disorder (230). The multiaxial (biopsychosocial) perspective is helpful in understanding a chronic course.

Depression involves an interplay between biology, person, and environment. Patients with personality disorders whose ego offers fewer resources and poor resilience to depression are apt to have a poorer course and a worse prognosis. Similarly, those patients with limited social resources (family, money, access to medical care) also are apt to demonstrate a poorer course and prognosis.

Weissman et al. (213) have shown that patients treated with a combination of drugs and psychotherapy will have a better prognosis, perhaps because of the interplay between personality and social axes.

Fifty percent of patients who have one episode of depression will have a second, recurrent episode. Patients with two or more episodes show increased risk as the number of episodes increases.

The course and prognosis of depression is, of course, affected by suicide. Bipolar patients show a suicide rate of about 15%. Unipolar patients (including chronic cases) show higher rates (231). In effect, more than 15–20% of patients with depressive disorders will take their own lives. The optimism for treating depression must be tempered with caution, concern, and careful assessment and management of suicidal behavior.

REFERENCES

1. Weissman M, Myers J: *The New Haven Community Survey 1967–1975: Depressive Symptoms and Diagnoses.* Presented to Society for Life History Research in Psychopathology, Fort Worth, Tex., October 1976.

2. Srole L, Langner TS, et al.: *Mental Health in the Metropolis,* New York, McGraw-Hill, 1962.

3. Baldessarini RJ: *Risk rates for depression (letter to the editor)*. Arch Gen Psychiatry, *41*:103–106, 1984.

4. Williams TA, et al.: *Special Report on the Depressive Illnesses*. Washington, D.C., U.S. Department of Health, Education and Welfare, November 1970.

5. Silberman EK, Sullivan JL: Atypical depression. Psychiatr Clin North Am, *7*:535–547, 1984.

6. Aarons SF, Frances AJ, et al.: *Atypical depression: a review of diagnosis and treatment.* Hosp Community Psychiatry, *36*:275–282, 1985.

7. Gelenberg AJ: The catatonic syndrome. Lancet *1*:1339–1341, 1976.

8. McAllister, TW: Overview: pseudodementia, Am J Psychiatry *140*:528–533, 1983.

9. Stoudemire A: Differentiating between depression and dementia. Clinical Advances in the Treatment of Depression, *1*:1–3, 10, 1987.

10. Rosenthal NE, Sack DA, et al.: Seasonal affective disorder. *41*:72–80, 1984.

11. Keller MB: Current concepts in affective disorders. J Clin Psychiatry, *50*:157–162, 1989.

12. American Psychiatric Association: *Diagnostic and Statistical Manual*, ed. 3, (DSM-IIIR), Washington, D.C., American Psychiatric Press, 1984.

13. Robins E, et al.: Primary and secondary affective disorders, in Zubin J, Freyhan FA (eds): *Disorders of Mood*, Baltimore, Johns Hopkins University Press, 1972.

14. Guze SB, et al.: "Secondary" affective disorder: A study of 95 cases. Psychol Med, *1*:426–428, 1971.

15. Akiskal HS, Rosenthal RH, et al.: Differentiation of primary affective illness from situational, somatic and secondary depressions. Arch Gen Psychiatry, *36*:635–643, 1979.

16. Gillespie RD: The clinical differentiation of types of depression. Guy's Hosp Rep, *79*:306–344, 1929.

17. Klerman GL: Clinical phenomenology of depression: Implications for research strategy in the psychobiology of the affective disorders, in Williams TA, et al. (eds): *Recent Advances in the Psychobiology of the Depressive Illnesses*, DHEW Publ. No. (HSM) 70-0953, Washington, D.C., U.S. Government Printing Office, 1972.

18. Klein DF: Endogenomorphic depression. Arch Gen Psychiatry, *31*:447–454, 1974.

19. Nelson JC, Charney DS: Primary affective disorder criteria and the endogenous-reactive distinction. Arch Gen Psychiatry, *37*:787–793, 1980.

20. Prusoff BA, Weissman MM, et al.: Research diagnostic criteria subtypes of depression: Their role as predictors of differential response to psychotherapy and drug treatment. Arch Gen Psychiatry, *37*:796–801, 1980.

21. Klerman GL, et al.: Neurotic depressions: A systematic analysis of multiple criteria and meanings. Am J Psychiatry, *136*:57–61, 1979.

22. Akiskal HS: Dysthymic disorder: Psychopathology of proposed chronic depressive subtypes. Am J Psychiatry, *140*:11–20, 1983.

23. Keller MB, Shapiro RW: "Double depression." Am J Psychiatry, *139*:438–442, 1982.

24. Keller MB, Lavori PW, et al.: "Double depression": two year follow-up. Am J Psychiatry, *140*:689–694, 1983.

25. Akiskal HS: Dysthymic disorder: psychopathology of proposed chronic depressive subtypes. Am J Psychiatry, *140*:11–20, 1983.

26. Akiskal HS: Factors associated with incomplete recovery in primary depressive illness. J Clin Psychiatry, *43*:266–271, 1982.

27. Brown RP, Sweeney JP, et al.: Involutional melancholia revisited. Am J Psychiatry, *141*:24–28, 1984.

28. Pope HG, Lipinski JF, et al.: "Schizoaffective disorder": An invalid diagnosis? A comparison of schizoaffective disorder, schizophrenia and affective disorder. Am J Psychiatry, *137*:921–927, 1980.

29. Kocsis JH, Frances AJ: A critical discussion of DSM-III dysthymic disorder. Am J Psychiatry, *144*:1534–1542, 1987.

30. Hatsukami D, Pickens RW: Posttreatment depression in an alcohol and drug abuse population. Am J Psychiatry, *139*:1563–1566, 1982.

31. Lindemann E: Symptomatology and management of acute grief. Am J Psychiatry, *101*:141–148, 1944.

32. Boyd JH, Weissman MM: Epidemiology of affective disorders: A re-examination and future directions. Arch Gen Psychiatry, *38*:1039–1046, 1981.

33. Essen-Moller E, Hagnell O: The frequency and risk of depression within a rural population group in Scandinavia. Acta Psychiatr Scand (Suppl 162), 37:28–32, 1961.

34. Klerman GL, Barrett JE: The affective disorders: Clinical and epidemiological aspects, in Gershow S., Shobsin B (eds): *Lithium: Its Role in Psychiatric Treatment and Research,* New York, Plenum Press, 1973.

35. Klerman GL, Lavori PW, et al.: Birth-cohort trends in rates of major depressive disorder among relatives of patients with affective disorder. Arch Gen Psychiatry, 42:689–693, 1985.

36. Weissman MM, Leaf PJ, Tischler GL, et al.: Affective disorders in five United States communities. Psychol Med, 18:141–153, 1988.

37. Weissman MM, Klerman GL: Sex differences and the epidemiology of depression. Arch Gen Psychiatry, 34:98–111, 1977.

38. Faris RE, Dunham HW: *Mental Disorders in Urban Areas,* Chicago, University of Chicago Press, 1939.

39. Radloff L: Sex differences in depression. The effects of occupation and marital status. Sex Roles, 1:249–269, 1975.

40. Weissman MM, Paykel ES: *The Depressed Woman: A Study of Social Relationships,* Chicago, University of Chicago Press, 1974.

41. Kiecolt-Glaser JK, Glaser R: Psychosocial moderators of immune function. Ann Behav Med, 9:16–20, 1987.

42. Goodwin FK, Bunney WE: A psychobiological approach to affective illness. Psychiatric Ann, 3:19, 1973.

43. Schildkraut JT: The catecholamine hypothesis of affective disorders: A review of supporting evidence. Am J Psychiatry, 122:509–522, 1965.

44. Maas JW: Biogenic amines and depression. Biochemical and pharmacological separation of two types of depression. Arch Gen Psychiatry, 32:1357–1361, 1975.

45. Baldessarini RJ: Biogenic amine hypotheses in affective disorders. Arch Gen Psychiatry, 32:1087–1093, 1975.

46. Siever LJ, Davis KL: Overview: toward a dysregulation hypothesis of depression. Am J Psychiatry, 142:1017–1031, 1985.

47. Lake CR, Pickar D, Ziegler MG, et al.: High plasma norepinephrine levels in patients with major affective disorder. Am J Psychiatry, 139:1315–1318, 1982.

48. Koslow JH, Maas JW, Bauder CL, et al.: CSF and urinary biogenic amines and metabolites in depression and mania: A controlled, univariate analysis. Arch Gen Psychiatry, 42:1181–1185, 1985.

49. Linnoila M, Karoum F, Calil HM, et al.: Alteration of norepinephrine metabolism with desipramine and zimelidine in depressed patients. Arch Gen Psychiatry, 39:1025–1028, 1982.

50. Nyback HV, Walters JR, Aghajanian GK, et al.: Tricyclic Antidepressants: effects on the firing rate of brain noradrenergic neurons. Eur J Pharmacol, 32:302–312, 1975.

51. Janowsky DS, Risch SC, Parker D, et al.: Increased vulnerability to cholinergic stimulation in affective disorder patients. Psychopharmacol Bull, 16:29–31, 1980.

52. Snyder SH: Cholinergic mechanisms in affective disorders. N Engl J Med, 311:254–255, 1984.

53. Berrettini WH, Nurnberger JI, Hare TA, et al.: Plasma and CSF GABA in affective illness. Br J Psychiatry, 141:483–487, 1982.

54. Gold BI, Bowers MJ Jr, Roth RH, et al.: GABA levels in CSF of patients with psychiatric disorders. Am J Psychiatry, 137:362–364, 1980.

55. Petty F, Schlesser MA: Plasma GABA in affective illness: A preliminary investigation. J Affective Disord, 3:339–343, 1981.

56. Morselli PL, Bossi L, Henry JF, et al.: On the therapeutic action of SL 76-002, a new GABA-mimetic agent: preliminary observations in neuropsychiatric disorders. Brain Res Bull, 5 (Suppl 2):411–414, 1980.

57. Thaker GK, Moran M, Tamminga CA: GABA-mimetics: A new class of anti-depressant agents. Arch Gen Psychiatry, 47:287–288, 1990.

58. Sulser F: Mode of action of antidepressant drugs. J Clin Psychiatry, 44(5):14–20, 1983.

59. Richelson E: The newer antidepressants: Structures, pharmacokinetics, pharmacodynamics, and proposed mechanisms of action. Psychopharmacol Bull, 20(2):213–223, 1984.

60. Charney DS, Heninger GR, Sternberg DE: The effect of mianserin on alpha-2 ad-

renergic receptor function in depressed patients. Br J Psychiatry, 144:407–416, 1984.

61. Hyttel J: Experimental pharmacology of selective 5-HT reuptake inhibitors. Clin Neuropharmacol, 7(Suppl 1):866–867, 1984.

62. Koslow SH, Maas JW, et al.: CSF and urinary biogenic amines and metabolites in depression and mania. Arch Gen Psychiatry, 40:999–1010, 1983.

63. Muscettola G, Potter WZ, et al.: Urinary MHPG and major affective disorders. Arch Gen Psychiatry, 41:337–342, 1984.

64. Rosanoff AJ, Handy LM, Plesset IR: The etiology of manic-depressive syndromes with special reference to their occurrence to twins. Am J Psychiatry, 91:725–762, 1935.

65. Kallmann FJ: Genetic principles in manic-depressive psychosis, in Hoch P, Zubin J (eds): Depression, New York, Grune & Stratton, 1954.

66. Allen MG, Cohen S, Pollin W, et al.: Affective illness in veteran twins: A diagnostic review. Am J Psychiatry, 131:1234–1239, 1974.

67. Bertelsen A, Harvald B, Hange M: A Danish twin study of manic-depressive disorders. Br J Psychiatry, 130:330–351, 1977.

68. Price JS: The genetics of depressive behaviour, in Coppen A, Walk A (eds): Recent Developments in Affective Disorders: A Symposium, Kent, England, Royal Medico-Psychological Association, 1968.

69. Perris C: A study of bipolar (manic-depressive) and unipolar recurrent depressive psychoses. Acta Psychiatr Scand Suppl, 194:1–189, 1966.

70. Gershon E, Mark A, Cohen N, et al.: Transmitted factors in the morbid risk of affective disorders: A controlled study. J Psychiatr Res, 12:283–299, 1975.

71. James NM, Chapman CJ: A genetic study of bipolar affective disorder. Br J Psychiatry, 126:449–456, 1975.

72. Trzebiatowska-Trzeciak O: Genetical analysis of unipolar and bipolar endogenous affective psychoses. Br J Psychiatry, 131:478–485, 1977.

73. Tsuang MT, Winokur G, Crowe R: Morbidity risks of schizophrenia and affective disorders among first-degree relatives of patients with schizophrenia, mania, depression, and surgical conditions. Br J Psychiatry, 137:497–504, 1980.

74. Winokur G, Cadoret R, Dorzab J, et al.: Depressive disease: A genetic study. Arch Gen Psychiatry, 24:135–144, 1971.

75. Cadoret RJ: Evidence for genetic inheritance of primary affective disorder in adoptees. Am J Psychiatry, 135:463–466, 1978.

76. Gold PW, Goodwin FK, Chrousos GP: Clinical and biochemical manifestations of depression: relation to the neurobiology of stress. N Engl J Med, 319:413–420, 1988.

77. Gold PW, Chrousos GP, Kellner C, et al.: Psychiatric implications of basic and clinical studies with corticotropin releasing factor. Am J Psychiatry, 141:619–627, 1984.

78. Gold PW, Loriaux DL, Roy A, et al.: Responses to CRH in the hypercortisolism of depression and Cushing's disease: Pathophysiologic and diagnostic implications. N Engl J Med, 314:1329–35, 1986.

79. Sack DA, Nurnberger J, et al.: Potentiation of antidepressant medications by phase advance of the sleep-wake cycle. Am J Psychiatry, 142:606–608, 1985.

80. Reynolds CF, Kupfer DJ: Sleep research in affective illness: State of the art circa 1987. Sleep, 10:199–215, 1987.

81. Grunhaus L, Tiongco D, Roehrich H, et al.: Serial monitoring of antidepressant response to electroconvulsive therapy with sleep EEG recordings and dexamethasone suppression tests. Biol Psychiatry, 20:805–808, 1985.

82. Rush JA, Erman MK, Giles DE, et al.: Polysomnographic findings in recently drug-free and clinically remitted depressed patients. Arch Gen Psychiatry, 43:878–884, 1986.

83. Abraham K: Notes on the psychoanalytical investigation and treatment of manic-depressive insanity and allied conditions, in: The Selected Papers of Karl Abraham, London, Hogarth Press, 1927.

84. Freud S: Mourning and melancholia, in Strachey J (ed): Standard Edition, vol. 14, London, Hogarth Press (1917), 1958.

85. Fenichel O: Depression and mania, in: The Psychoanalytic Theory of Neurosis, New York, Norton, 1945.

86. Kendell R: Relationship between aggression and depression: Epidemiological implications of a hypothesis. Arch Gen Psychiatry, 22:308–318, 1970.

87. Henry A, Short J: Suicide and Homicide, Chicago, Free Press of Glencoe, Ill., 1954.

88. Friedman A: Hostility factors and clinical improvement in depressed patients. Arch Gen Psychiatry, *23*:524–537, 1970.

89. Paykel E: Classification of depressed patients: A cluster analysis derived grouping. Br J Psychiatry, *118*:275–288, 1971.

90. Weissman M, Fox K, et al.: Hostility and depression associated with suicide attempts. Am J Psychiatry, *130*:450–455, 1973.

91. Klerman G, Gershon E: Imipramine effects upon hostility in depression. J Nerv Ment Dis, *150*:127–132, 1970.

92. Bibring E: The mechanism of depression, in Greenacre P (ed): *Affective Disorders*, New York, International Universities Press, 1953.

93. Klein M: A contribution to the psychogenesis of manic-depressive states, in *Contributions to Psychoanalysis*, pp. 228–310, London, Hogarth Press, 1945.

94. Bowlby J: The process of mourning. Int J Psychoanal, *42*:317–340, 1961.

95. Spitz RA: Anaclitic depression, in: *The Psychoanalytic Study of the Child*, vol. 2, New York, International Universities Press, 1946.

96. Brown F: Depression and childhood bereavement. J Ment Sci, *107*:754–777, 1961.

97. Leff M, Roatch J, et al.: Environmental factors preceding the onset of severe depressions. Psychiatry, *33*:293–311, 1970.

98. Paykel E, Myers J, et al.: Life events and depression. Arch Gen Psychiatry, *21*:753–760, 1970.

99. Clayton P, Halikas J, et al.: The depression of widowhood. Br J Psychiatry, *120*:71–77, 1972.

100. Hirschfeld RMA, Klerman GL, et al.: Assessing personality: Affects of the depressive state on trait measurement. Am J Psychiatry, *140*:695–699, 1983.

101. Akiskal HS, Hirschfeld RMA, et al.: The relationship of personality to affective disorders. Arch Gen Psychiatry, *40*:801–810, 1983.

102. Beck AT: Depressive neurosis, in Arieti S, Brody EB (eds): *American Handbook of Psychiatry*, pp. 61–90, ed. 2, vol. 3, New York, Basic Books, 1974.

103. Rush AJ, Beck AT, et al.: Comparative efficacy of cognitive therapy and pharmacotherapy in the treatment of depressed outpatients. Cognit Ther Res, *1*:17–37, 1977.

104. Kovacs M, Beck AT: Maladaptive cognitive structures in depression. Am J Psychiatry, *135*:525–533, 1978.

105. Silverman JS, Silverman JA, et al.: Do maladaptive attitudes cause depression? Arch Gen Psychiatry, *41*:28–30, 1984.

106. Simons AD, Garfield SL, et al.: The process of change in cognitive therapy and pharmacotherapy for depression. Arch Gen Psychiatry, *41*:45–51, 1984.

107. Ilfeld FW: Current social stressors and symptoms of depression. Am J Psychiatry, *134*:161–166, 1977.

108. Lloyd C: Life events and depressive disorder reviewed. II. Events as precipitating factors. Arch Gen Psychiatry, *37*:541–548, 1980.

109. Paykel ES: Life stress, depression, and attempted suicide. J Hum Stress, *2*:3–12, 1976.

110. Fava GA, Munari F, Pavan L, et al.: Life events and depression: A replication. J Affect Dis, *3*:159–165, 1981.

111. Gold PW, Goodwin FK, Chrousos GP: Clinical and biochemical manifestations of depression. N Engl J Med, *319*:348–353, 1988.

112. Ehlers CL, Frank E, Kupfer DJ: Social zeitgebers and biological rhythms. Arch Gen Psychiatry, *45*:948–952, 1988.

113. APA Task Force on Laboratory Tests in Psychiatry: The dexamethasone suppression test: An overview of its current status in psychiatry. Am J Psychiatry, *144*:1253–1262, 1987.

114. Arana GW, Baldessarini RJ, Ornsteen M: The dexamethasone suppression test for diagnosis and prognosis in psychiatry. Arch Gen Psychiatry, *42*:1193–1204, 1985.

115. Gedo JE, Goldberg A: *Models of the Mind: A Psychoanalytic Theory*, chaps. 6, 7, 11, and 12, Chicago, University of Chicago Press, 1973.

116. MacKinnon RA, Michels R: *The Psychiatric Interview in Clinical Practice*, pp. 174–229, Philadelphia, W. B. Saunders Co., 1971.

117. Sederer LI: Heiress to an empty throne: Ego-ideal problems in contemporary women. Contemp Psychoanal, *12*:240–251, 1976.

118. Buie DH: Empathy: Its nature and limitations, Presented at the Annual Fall Meeting of the American Psychoanalytic Association, New York, December 1979.

119. Havens L: The anatomy of a suicide. N Engl J Med, *272*:401–406, 1965.

120. Havens L: Recognition of suicidal risks through the psychological examination. N Engl J Med, 276:210–215, 1967.

121. Maltsberger JJ, Buie DH: The devices of suicide. Int Rev Psychoanal, 7:61–72, 1980.

122. Buie DH, Maltsberger JJ: *The practical formulation of suicide risk.* Cambridge, Mass., Firefly Press, 1983.

123. Heninger GR, Charney DS, et al.: Lithium carbonate augmentation of antidepressant treatment. Arch Gen Psychiatry, 40:1335–1342, 1983.

124. Montigny C, Cournoyes G, et al.: Lithium carbonate addition in tricyclic antidepressant resistant unipolar depression. Arch Gen Psychiatry, 40:1327–1334, 1983.

125. Goodwin FK, Prange AJ: Potentiation of antidepressant effects by L-triiodo thyronine in tricyclic nonresponders. Am J Psychiatry, 139:34–38, 1982.

126. Schwarcz G, Halaris A, et al.: Normal thyroid function in desipramine nonresponders converted to responders by the addition of L-triiodothyronine. Am J Psychiatry, 141:1614–1616, 1984.

127. Gelenberg A (ed): For the treatment-resistant depressed woman: estrogen? Biological Therapies in Psychiatry, 12:1 and 4, 1989.

128. Gelenberg A (ed): Estrogen for treatment-resistant depression: unimpressive results. Biological Therapies in Psychiatry, 8:42, 1985.

129. Gelenberg A (ed): Adjuncts and adjuncts. Biological Therapies in Psychiatry, 12:43, 1989.

130. Gelenberg A (ed): T$_3$ for treatment-resistant depression: Negative findings. Biological Therapies in Psychiatry, 9:43, 1986.

131. Feighner JP, Boyer WF, Herbstein J: New antidepressants. Psychiatry Letter, 6:1–4, 1988.

132. Cooper GL: The safety of fluoxetine: An update. Br J Psychiatry, 153 (Suppl 3):77–86, 1988.

133. Quitkin FM, Stewart JW, McGrath PJ, et al.: Phenelzine versus imipramine in the treatment of probable atypical depression: defining syndrome boundaries of selective MAOI responders. Am J Psychiatry, 145:306–311, 1988.

134. Liebowitz MR, Quitkin FM, Stewart JW, et al.: Antidepressant specificity in atypical depression. Arch Gen Psychiatry, 45:129–137, 1988.

135. Davidson J, Lipper S, Pelton S, et al.: The response of depressed inpatients to isocarboxazid. J Clin Psychopharmacol, 8:100–107, 1988.

136. Wehr TA, Goodwin FK: Do antidepressants cause mania? Psychopharmacol Bull, 23:61–65, 1987.

137. Wehr TA, Goodwin FK: Rapid-cycling in manic-depressives induced by tricyclic antidepressants. Arch Gen Psychiatry, 36:555–559, 1979.

138. Wehr TA, Goodwin FK: Can antidepressants cause mania and worsen course of affective illness? Am J Psychiatry, 144:1403–1411, 1987.

139. Prieu RF, Kupfer DJ, et al.: Drug treatment in the prevention of recurrences in unipolar and bipolar affective disorders. Arch Gen Psychiatry, 41:1096–1104, 1984.

140. Kramlinger KG, Post RM: The addition of lithium to carbamazepine. Arch Gen Psychiatry, 46:794–800, 1989.

141. Chan CH, Janicak PG, Davis JM, et al.: Response of psychotic and nonpsychotic depressed patients to tricyclic antidepressants. J Clin Psychiatry, 48:197–200, 1987.

142. Spiker DG, Weiss JC, et al.: The pharmacological treatment of delusional depression. Am J Psychiatry, 142:430–436, 1985.

143. Anton RF, Burch EA: Amoxapine versus amitriptyline-perphenazine in the treatment of psychotic depression, in American College of Neuropharmacology Abstracts of Panels and Posters, p. 196, 1989.

144. Katon W, Raskind M: Treatment of depression in the medically ill elderly with methylphenidate. Am J Psychiatry, 137:963–965, 1980.

145. Stoudemire A, Atkinson P: Use of cyclic antidepressants in patients with cardiac conduction disturbances. Gen Hosp Psychiatry, 10:389–397, 1988.

146. Roose SP, Glassman AH, Giardina EGV, et al.: Tricyclic antidepressants in depressed patients with cardiac conduction disturbances. Arch Gen Psychiatry, 44:273–275, 1987.

147. Lindy DC, Glassman AH, Roose SP: Cardiovascular effects of tricyclic antidepressants, Psychiatry Letter, 6:5–9, 1988.

148. Nurnberg HG, Prudic J: Guidelines for treatment of psychosis during pregnancy. Hosp Community Psychiatry, 35:67–71, 1984.

149. Calabrese JR, Gulledge AD: Psychotropics during pregnancy and lactation: A review. Psychosomatics, 26:413–426, 1985.

150. Markowitz JC, Brown RP: Seizures with neuroleptics and antidepressants. Gen Hosp Psychiatry, 9:135–141, 1987.

151. Stern SL, Rush AJ, et al.: Toward a rational pharmacotherapy of depression. Am J Psychiatry, 137:545–552, 1980.

152. Bielski RJ, Friedel RO: Prediction of tricyclic antidepressant response: A critical review. Arch Gen Psychiatry, 33:1479–1489, 1976.

153. Amsterdam J, Brunswick D, et al.: The clinical application of tricyclic antidepressant pharmacokinetics and plasma levels. Am J Psychiatry, 137:653–662, 1980.

154. Van Kammen DP, Murphy DL: Prediction of imipramine antidepressant response by a one-day-d-amphetamine trial. Am J Psychiatry, 135:1179–1184, 1978.

155. Fawcett J, Siomopoulos V: Dextroamphetamine response as a possible predictor of improvement with tricyclic therapy in depression. Arch Gen Psychiatry, 25:247–255, 1971.

156. Maas JW, Koslow SH, et al.: Pretreatment neurotransmitter metabolite levels and response to tricyclic antidepressant drugs. Am J Psychiatry, 141:1159–1171, 1984.

157. Little KY: Amphetamine, but not methylphenidate predicts antidepressant efficacy. J Clin Psychopharmacol, 8:177–183, 1988.

158. Glassman R, Salzman C: Interactions between psychotropics and other drugs: An update. Hosp Community Psychiatry, 38:236–242, 887, 1987.

159. Coryell W, Turner R, Sherman A: Desipramine plasma levels and clinical response: evidence for a curvilinear relationship. J Clin Psychopharmacol, 7:138–142, 1987.

160. Boyer WF, Lake CR: Initial severity and diagnosis influence the relationship of tricyclic plasma levels to response: A statistical review. J Clin Psychopharmacol, 7:67–71, 1987.

161. Task Force on the Use of Laboratory Tests in Psychiatry. Tricyclic antidepressants—blood level measurements and clinical outcome. Am J Psychiatry, 142:155–162, 1985.

162. Rosenbaum JF, Votolato NA, deVito RA, et al.: Generic drugs: A roundtable discussion. J Clin Psychiatry Monograph Series, 7:2–12, 22–26, 1989.

163. Quitkin FM, Rabkin JG, et al.: Duration of antidepressant drug treatment: What is an adequate trial? Arch Gen Psychiatry, 41:238–245, 1984.

164. Pollack MH, Rosenbaum JF: Management of antidepressant-induced side effects: A practical guide for the clinician. J Clin Psychiatry, 48:3–8, 1987.

165. Warnock JK, Knesevich JW: Adverse cutaneous reactions to antidepressants. Am J Psychiatry, 145:425–430, 1988.

166. Warner MD, Peabody CA, Whiteford HA, et al.: Trazodone and priapism. J Clin Psychiatry, 48:244–245, 1987.

167. Gelenberg A: Alprazolam: Is it an antidepressant? Biol Ther Psychiatry, 7:1, 1984.

168. Fawcett J, Edwards JH, Kravitz HM, et al.: Alprazolam: An antidepressant? Alprazolam, desipramine and an alprazolam-desipramine combination in the treatment of adult depressed outpatients. J Clin Psychopharmacol, 7:295–310, 1987.

169. Cole JO: Where are those new antidepressants we were promised? Arch Gen Psychiatry, 45:193–194, 1988.

170. Sokl RJ, Hewitt S, Booker DJ, et al.: Fatal immune hemolysis associated with nomifensine. Br J Psychiatry, 291:311–312, 1985.

171. Stark P, Fuller RW, Wong DT: The pharmacologic profile of fluoxetine. J Clin Psychiatry, 46:7–13, 1985.

172. Dufresne RL, Weber SS, Becker RE: Bupropion hydrochloride. Drug Intell Clin Pharmacol, 18:957–964, 1984.

173. Roose SP, Glassman AH, Giardina EGV, et al.: Cardiovascular effects of imipramine and bupropion in depressed patients with congestive heart failure. J Clin Psychopharmacol, 7:247–251, 1987.

174. Bryant SG, Guernsey BG, Ingrim NB: Review of bupropion. Clin Pharm, 2:525–537, 1983.

175. Davidson J: Seizures and bupropion: A review. J Clin Psychiatry, 50:256–261, 1989.

176. Davis JM: A review of the new antidepressant medications, in Davis JM, Maas JW (eds): The Affective Disorders, Washington, D.C., Am Psychiatric Association, 1983.

177. Fallon B, Foote B, Walsh BT, et al.: "Spontaneous" hypertensive episodes with MAOIs. J Clin Psychiatry, 49:163–165, 1988.

178. Linet LS: Mysterious MAOI hyper-

tensive episodes. J Clin Psychiatry, 47:563–565, 1986.

179. Keck PE, Pope HG Jr, Nierenberg AA: Autoinduction of hypertensive reactions by tranylcypromine? J Clin Psychopharmacol, 9:48–51, 1989.

180. Mendels J: Lithium in the treatment of depression. Am J Psychiatry, 133:373–378, 1976.

181. Doyal LE, Morton WA: The clinical usefulness of lithium as an antidepressant. Hosp Community Psychiatry, 35:685–691, 1984.

182. Wharton RN, Perel JM, et al.: A potential clinical use for methylphenidate with tricyclic antidepressants. Am J Psychiatry, 127:1619–1625, 1971.

183. Sate SL, Nelson JC: Stimulants in the treatment of depression: A critical overview. J Clin Psychiatry, 50:241–249, 1989.

184. Fernandez F, Levy J, Galizzi H: Response of HIV-related depression to psychostimulants: case reports. Hosp Community Psychiatry, 39:628–631.

185. Gelenberg A (ed): Treating treatment-resistant depression: antidepressants + stimulants? Biological Therapies in Psychiatry, 8:1–2, 1985.

186. Weilburg JB, Rosenbaum JF, Beiderman J, et al.: Fluoxetine added to non-MAOI antidepressants converts nonresponders to responders. J Clin Psychiatry, 50:447–449, 1989.

187. Aranow RB, Hudson JI, Pope HG, Jr, et al.: Elevated antidepressant plasma levels after addition of fluoxetine. Am J Psychiatry, 146:911–913, 1989.

188. Sternbach H: Danger of MAOI therapy after fluoxetine withdrawal. Lancet, 2:850–851, 1988.

189. White K, Pistole T, et al.: Combined MAOI-TCA treatment. Am J Psychiatry, 137:1422–1425, 1980.

190. Gelenberg AJ, Wojcik JD, et al.: Tyrosine for the treatment of depression. Am J Psychiatry, 137:622–623, 1980.

191. Hertzman PA, Blevins WL, Mayer J, et al.: Association of the eosinophilia-myalgia syndrome with the ingestion of tryptophan. N Engl J Med, 322:869–873, 1990.

192. Glassman AH, Kantor SJ, et al.: Depression, delusion and drug response. Am J Psychiatry, 132:716–719, 1975.

193. Crowe RR: Electroconvulsive therapy: A current perspective: N Engl J Med, 311:163–167, 1984.

194. Weiner R, Fink M, Hammersley DW, et al.: APA announces development of guidelines for effective use of electroconvulsive therapy. Hosp Community Psychiatry, 41:208–209.

195. Schildkraut JJ, Draskoczy P: Effects of electroconvulsive shock on norepinephrine turnover and metabolism: Basic and clinical studies, in Fink M, Kety S, et al. (eds): Psychobiology of Convulsive Therapy, Washington, D.C., V.H. Winston & Sons, 1974.

196. Maltbie AA, Wingfield MS, Volow MR, et al.: Electroconvulsive therapy in the presence of brain tumor. Case reports and an evaluation of risk. J Nerv Ment Dis, 168:400–405, 1980.

197. Fried D, Mann JJ: Electroconvulsive treatment of a patient with known intracranial tumor. Biol Psychiatry, 23:176–180, 1988.

198. Greenberg LB, Mofson R, Fink M: Prospective electroconvulsive therapy in a delusional depressed patient with a frontal meningioma. A case report. Br J Psychiatry, 153:105–107, 1988.

199. Mandel MR, Welch CA, et al.: Prediction of response to ECT in tricyclic-intolerant or tricyclic-resistant depressed patients. McLean Hosp J, 2:203–209, 1977.

200. Solan WJ, Khan A, Avery DH, et al.: Psychotic and nonpsychotic depression: Comparison of response to ECT. J Clin Psychiatry, 49:97–99, 1988.

201. Culver CM, Ferrell RB, et al.: ECT and special problems of informed consent. Am J Psychiatry, 137:586–591, 1980.

202. Friedel RO: The combined use of neuroleptics and ECT in drug-resistant schizophrenic patients. Psychopharmacol Bull, 22:928–930, 1986.

203. Gujavarty K, Greenberg LB, Fink M: Electroconvulsive therapy and neuroleptic medication in therapy-resistant positive symptom psychosis. Convulsive Therapy, 3:111–120, 1987.

204. Weiner RD, Rogers HJ, Davidson JR, et al.: Effects of electroconvulsive therapy upon brain electrical activity. Ann NY Acad Sci, 462:270–281, 1986.

205. Sackheim HA, Portnoy A, Neeley P,

et al.: Cognitive consequences of low-dosage electroconvulsive therapy. Ann NY Acad Sci, 462:326–340, 1986.

206. Endler NS: *Holiday of Darkness,* New York, Wiley-Interscience, 1982.

207. Fink M: *Informed ECT for Patients and Their Families.* Lake Bluff, Ill. Somatics, Inc., 25-minute video (VHS/Beta), 1986.

208. Frank J., Hoehn-Saric R, et al.: *Effective Ingredients of Successful Psychotherapy,* New York, Brunner/Mazel, 1978.

209. Roose SP, Glassman AH, et al.: Depression, delusions and suicide. Am J Psychiatry, 140:1159–1162, 1983.

210. Cotton PG, Drake RE, et al.: Dealing with suicide on a psychiatric inpatient unit. Hosp Community Psychiatry, 34:55–59, 1983.

211. Schoonover SC: Intensive care for suicidal patients, in Bassuk EL, Schoonover SC (eds): *Lifelines: Clinical Perspectives on Suicide,* pp. 137–152, New York, Plenum, 1982.

212. Klerman GL, DiMascio A, et al.: Treatment of depression by drugs and psychotherapy. Am J Psychiatry, 131:186–191, 1974.

213. Weissman MM, Prusoff BA, et al.: The efficacy of drugs and psychotherapy in the treatment of acute depressive episodes. Am J Psychiatry, 136:555–558, 1979.

214. Weissman MM, Klerman GL, et al.: Treatment effects on the social adjustment of depressed patients. Arch Gen Psychiatry, 30:771–778, 1974.

215. Conte HR, Plutchik R, Wild KV, et al.: Combined psychotherapy and pharmacotherapy for depression: A systematic analysis of the evidence. Arch Gen Psychiatry, 43:471–479, 1986.

216. Arieti S: Psychotherapy of severe depression. Am J Psychiatry, 134:864–868, 1971.

217. Rounsaville BJ, Klerman GL, et al.: Do psychotherapy and pharmacotherapy for depression conflict? Arch Gen Psychiatry, 38:24–29, 1981.

218. Karasu TB: Toward a clinical model of psychotherapy for depression. I: Systematic comparison of three psychotherapies. Am J Psychiatry, 147:133–147, 1990.

219. Klerman GL: Depression in the medically ill. Psychiatr Clin North Am, 4(2):301–317, 1981.

220. Maltsberger JT, Buie DH: Countertransference hate in the treatment of suicidal patients. Arch Gen Psychiatry, 30:625–633, 1974.

221. Simons AD, Murphy GE, Levine JL, et al.: Cognitive therapy and pharmacotherapy for depression: Sustained improvement over one year. Arch Gen Psychiatry, 43:43–48, 1986.

222. Frank E, Kupfer DJ, Perel JM: Early recurrence in unipolar depression. Arch Gen Psychiatry, 46:397–400, 1989.

223. Kupfer DJ, Frank E, Perel JM: The advantage of early treatment intervention in recurrent depression. Arch Gen Psychiatry, 46:771–775, 1989.

224. Glick ID, Clarkin JF, Spencer JH, et al.: A controlled evaluation of inpatient family intervention: I. Preliminary results of the six-month follow-up. Arch Gen Psychiatry, 42:882–886, 1985.

225. Haas GL, Glick ID, Clarkin JF, et al.: Inpatient family intervention: A randomized clinical trial: II. Results at Hospital Discharge. Arch Gen Psychiatry, 45:217–224, 1988.

226. Friedman AS: Interaction of drug therapy with marital therapy in depressive patients. Arch Gen Psychiatry, 32:619–637, 1975.

227. Tsuang MT: Genetic counseling for psychiatric patients and their families. Am J Psychiatry, 135:1465–1475, 1978.

228. Robins E, Guze SB: Classification in affective disorders, in Williams TA, Katz MM, et al. (eds): *Recent Advances in the Psychobiology of the Depressive Illnesses,* Washington, D.C., U.S. Government Printing Office, 1972.

229. Keller MB, Shapiro RW, et al.: Recovery in major depressive disorder. Arch Gen Psychiatry, 39:905–910, 1982.

230. Keller MB, Shapiro RW, et al.: Relapse in major depressive disorder. Arch Gen Psychiatry, 39:911–915, 1982.

231. Miles CP: Conditions predisposing to suicide: A review. J Nerv Ment Dis, 164:231–246, 1977.

2

Mania

Robert B. Aranow, MD
Lloyd I. Sederer, MD

Mania is a syndrome with multiple etiologies. Recent research has produced important improvements in its diagnosis, treatment, and prevention. Features of mania include disturbances of mood characterized by elevated, irritable, or expansive mood; hyperactivity; pressured speech; flight of ideas; distractibility; poor judgment; and, often, psychosis (1, 2).

Because of a recent distinction in the nosology of mania (3), it is now considered either primary or secondary in nature. Primary mania is an affective or mood disorder. Secondary mania occurs secondary to a variety of organic disorders (e.g., drug intake, infection, neoplasm, epilepsy, or metabolic disturbances).

CASE EXAMPLE: *Primary mania.* Mr. A., a 23-year-old college student, indicated that although this was his first psychiatric contact, he had a history of mood problems dating back to about age 17. Since then the patient reported an annual mood cycle characterized by periods of social withdrawal, increased sleep, weight gain, and general feelings of sadness, during the fall and winter. In contrast, during the late spring and summer he experienced periods of elation, increased energy and activity, and a decreased need to sleep. The summer before his admission to the hospital the patient reported feeling quite elated with little need for sleep. He began working three jobs simultaneously; one involved a somewhat shaky business scheme in which he resold half-fare airline coupons. Mr. A. also attempted to purchase the apartment house where he lived, as an investment.

As Mr. A.'s business endeavors began to fail, he became increasingly irritable and disorganized. He reported that during the week before admission he did not sleep at all and believed he was hearing special messages from the radio. Finally, he became extremely suspicious of other people and, on the night of admission, he became combative when friends approached him.

His friends were able to usher him to an emergency ward; his thoughts were severely disorganized and he continued to be combative. He required treatment with i.m. (intramuscular) haloperidol and the use of mechanical restraints. From the emergency ward the patient was involuntarily hospitalized on a locked inpatient unit.

DIAGNOSIS AND DIFFERENTIAL DIAGNOSIS

Primary mania is the manic syndrome found in patients with a manic or bipolar type mood disorder (see Figure 1.1., page 5). The revised third edition of the *Diagnostic and Statistical Manual of Mental Disorders* of the American Psychiatric Association (DSM IIIR) offers the following diagnostic criteria for a manic episode (italics added):

A. A distinct period of abnormally and persistently *elevated,* expansive, or irritable *mood.*

B. During the period of mood disturbance, at least three of the following symptoms have persisted (four if the mood is only irritable) and have been present to a significant degree:
1. inflated self-esteem or *grandiosity*
2. *decreased* need for *sleep,* e.g., feels rested after only three hours of sleep
3. more talkative than usual or pressure to keep talking *(pressured speech)*
4. *flight of ideas* or subjective experience that thoughts are racing
5. *distractibility,* i.e., attention too easily drawn to unimportant or irrelevant external stimuli
6. *increase* in goal-directed *activity* (either socially, at work or school, or sexually) or psychomotor agitation
7. *excessive* involvement in *pleasurable* activities which have a high potential for painful consequences; e.g., the person engages in unrestrained buying sprees, sexual indiscretions, or foolish business investments

C. Mood disturbance sufficiently severe to cause a *marked impairment* in occupational functioning or in usual social activities or relationships with others, or to necessitate hospitalization to prevent harm to self or others.

D. No periods of delusions or hallucinations lasting two weeks or more, in the absence of prominent mood symptoms (i.e. before the mood symptoms developed or after they have remitted).

E. Not superimposed on Schizophrenia, Schizophreniform Disorder, Delusional Disorder, or Psychotic Disorder NOS.

F. It cannot be established that an organic factor initiated and maintained the disturbance. *Note:* Somatic antidepressant treatment (e.g., medication, electroconvulsive therapy [ECT]) that apparently precipitates a mood disturbance should not be considered an etiologic organic factor.

A patient exhibiting a single episode meeting the above criteria would be accorded the DSM-IIIR diagnosis: *Bipolar Disorder, manic,* whether the patient has a history of depressive episodes or not.

Historically, this syndrome has been termed *manic-depression* and is termed *manic-depressive psychosis, manic type* by the ICD-9-CM (International Classification of Diseases) diagnostic system developed by the World Health Organization and used in much of the rest of the world.

Stages of Mania

Carlson and Goodwin (4) offer an analysis of the sequences of a manic episode. In their study of 20 primary mania patients, they observed three stages of mania characterized predominantly by mood (see Table 2.1.).

All patients entered stage I, characterized by increased speech and physical activ-

Table 2.1.

Stage	Mood	Thoughts	Behavior
I.	Euphoria	*Coherent* Grandiose Racing	*In Control:* Increased activity and speech, hyper-religious, hyper-sexual
II.	Anger Irritability Depression	*Delusional* Paranoid	*Explosive:* Hyperactive, assaultive
III.	Severe panic	*Incoherent* Hallucinations	*Frenzied:* bizarre, disoriented Flight of ideas

ity; labile, euphoric, and often irritable mood; and cognitive features such as grandiosity and tangentiality, although thoughts remained coherent.

The intermediary stage II was also found in all patients in their study. In this stage, speech was more pressured and physical activity increased. Mood became increasingly dysphoric. Irritability progressed to general hostility followed by explosive and combative episodes. Racing thoughts of the initial phase transformed into flight of ideas. Grandiosity reached delusional proportions.

Seventy percent of the patients entered stage III, a dysphoric panic characterized by bizarre behavior and incoherent thought processes. Delusions and hallucinations were present and some patients experienced disorientation. Carlson and Goodwin noted that this sequence was consistently present in *both* directions in all patients; the rate of acceleration from stage I to stages II and III varied from several hours to several days.

When viewed alone, stages II and III can be confused diagnostically with schizophrenia (5). A reliable recent history of sudden onset consistent with stages I and II, in addition to a past history of affective disorder in patients or their family, can be helpful in distinguishing acute mania from schizophrenia.

Hypomania is a related term which DSM-IIIR defines as a distinct period meeting criteria A and B, *without* causing marked *impairment* or requiring hospitalization (e.g., without C). Hypomania can be regarded as one degree below stage I mania. Delusions are never present. Individuals with episodes of hypomania, who suffer from major depression and lack a history of manic syndrome, are described as suffering from *bipolar II* disorder. In the DSM-III-R these symptoms would fall under the more general category of bipolar disorder NOS. Some consider individuals with a bipolar II

pattern (e.g. depression and hypomania) to be more likely to progress to bipolar disorder (referred to as bipolar I) than individuals with unipolar depression alone. In contrast to unipolar depression, it is not clear whether bipolar II individuals are also more likely to develop mania (see below) when treated with antidepressants (6).

Rapid cycling occurs when a patient suffers four or more episodes of mania and/or major depression within one year (1). This pattern of bipolar disorder is often relatively more difficult to treat and more disabling.

Differential Diagnosis of Primary Mania:

1. Organic mental disorders of secondary mania (see following section).
2. Schizophrenia. As discussed in Chapter 3, the diagnosis of schizophrenia is made longitudinally following at least six months of signs of illness. Acute manic-like episodes should never be initially diagnosed as schizophrenia, regardless of how severe or bizarre (7, 8).
3. Schizoaffective disorder. Controversy exists about the diagnosis of schizoaffective disorder and how it may differ from mood and schizophrenic disorders (9, 10).
4. Personality disorders. Cyclothymic personality disorders may present in an aggravated state that resembles mania. In these cases, a diagnosis of bipolar disorder NOS would be in order.
5. Delirium. Acute, stage-III type mania can show the disorientation, emotional lability, bizarre hallucinations, and delusions typical of delirium. This form of mania, termed *acute delirious mania*, can mimic delirium.
6. Dementia. Manic pseudodementia is a syndrome of reversible cognitive impairment. In elderly bipolar patients this manic presentation may be mistaken for dementia (11–13).

Secondary Mania

Secondary mania is a manic syndrome of organic etiology with clinical features indistinguishable from primary mania (3). The clinician is wise to consider the diagnosis of secondary mania in patients who present with manic symptomatology without a past or family history of mood disorder or who are over 40.

Differential Diagnosis of 2° Mania

1. Drug ingestion
   a. Steroids (glucocorticoid and anabolic)
   b. Stimulants
      Amphetamine ("ice," "speed")
      Cocaine ("crack")
      Methylphenidate
      Sympathomimetics (decongestants)
   c. L-dopa
   d. Phencyclidine ("angel dust") (14)
2. Toxin Ingestion
   Bromine
3. Medication withdrawal
   Reserpine (15)
4. Metabolic Disturbances
   Postoperative states
   Hemodialysis
   Thyrotoxicosis (15)
5. Infection
   General paresis, neurosyphilis (16)
   Postencephalitic mania
   Q-fever ("query"-fever)
   Influenza
6. Neoplasm
   Central nervous system (CNS) Tumors
7. Epilepsy
8. Multiple Sclerosis (17)
9. Vascular Lesions of the CNS

CASE EXAMPLE: *Secondary Mania.* Glaser (18) has described the case of a 41-year-old woman who developed manic symptoms following intramuscular cortisone for treatment of severe rheumatoid arthritis. The patient received 300 mg of cortisone on day 1, 200 mg on day 2 and day 3, and then 100 mg thereafter for nine days. On day 2, the patient's arthritic symptoms began to improve, and on the third day the patient developed a clinical picture of pressured speech, elation, and jocularity. Over the next few days the patient became increasingly elated, irritable, unable to sleep, and hostile. By the 12th day, the patient manifested stage-III mania and was delusional and assaultive. The patient had a clear sensorium throughout the course of her mania.

She was admitted to a psychiatric unit. After receiving four electroconvulsive treatments, her manic symptomatology cleared completely. A review of the patient's personal and psychiatric history revealed no prominent psychopathology.

EPIDEMIOLOGY

The data presented below pertain only to primary manic or bipolar disorders. Prevalence and incidence and rates for secondary mania are not available.

Incidence

The incidence of a disorder is the number of new cases in a given population during the course of one year. On the basis of epidemiological data collected in Scandinavia and the U.S., for bipolar illness exclusively, incidence is estimated to be 0.009–0.015% for men and 0.007–0.03% for women (19).

Prevalence

The DSM-III-R reports that the percentage of the adult population that has suffered from bipolar disorder is estimated between 0.4% and 1.2%. The "period prevalence" or total number of cases that exist in a population in any given year for bipolar disorder is estimated to be in the range of 0.1–0.8 per thousand per year (20).

Age, Sex, and Socioeconomic Status

The age of onset for bipolar disorder is generally in the 20s. Recent data indicate that bipolar disorder, unlike unipolar depression, appears equally common in women and men (1). A number of reports indicate a link between bipolar disorder, on the one hand, and educational, occupational, and social achievement and higher levels of creativity, on the other (21–24).

Families

Among first-degree relatives of afflicted patients the risk of developing bipolar disorder is about 10 times that found in the general population. The prevalence of affective illness in relatives of patients diagnosed with mood disorder of any type (unipolar or bipolar) is estimated at 10–25% for the first-degree relatives of diagnosed patients. However, studies indicate the prevalence is more pronounced in relatives of patients with bipolar disorder than in relatives of patients with unipolar disorder (20, 25–28).

Twin studies support the high rate of mood disorder found in the relatives of manic patients. Twin studies show a concordance rate for bipolar disorder of 68% for monozygotic twins and 23% for same-sex dizygotic twins.

THEORIES OF ETIOLOGY

Biological Hypotheses

Recent and persuasive evidence of genetic predisposition to bipolar disorder and the relative effectiveness of treatment medication have led to an increasing acceptance of a medical model for the syndrome. The biochemical understanding of mood disorders has focused primarily on the biogenic amines, a group of chemical transmitters active in certain selective sections of the CNS. The biogenic amines discussed most frequently are norepinephrine, dopamine, and serotonin.

Hypotheses suggest that mania is characterized by increased function of biogenic amines, particularly norepinephrine (29, 30). Supporting data are derived from indirect evidence obtained from drug effects. We know that mania can be precipitated by drugs that enhance central nervous system amine transmission and suppressed by drugs that decrease amine transmission. For example, lithium can decrease the amount of norepinephrine available at receptor sites, with subsequent clinical improvement. Furthermore, dopamine-stimulating (e.g., cocaine, L-dopa) and blocking agents (e.g., neuroleptics) respectively induce and mute mania in some patients (31–33).

Levels of norepinephrine's cerebrospinal fluid metabolite, 3-methoxy-4-hydroxyphenylglycol (MHPG), have been abnormal across several studies, unlike the metabolites of dopamine and serotonin. MHPG is also the only metabolite that has been correlated with manic symptomatology (34).

Finally, the clinical states associated with biogenic amine changes may reflect a disturbance in the balance between different brain transmitters. For example, physostigmine (an acetylcholine precursor) suppresses manic symptoms in some patients with clinical mania (35). Such findings may result from direct increase in brain cholinergic activity or, more likely, an alteration in the balance among brain neurotransmitter systems (36, 37).

Psychosocial stress is often implicated as a precipitating factor in manic episodes (38, 39). Post proposes a biological model that explains the tendency for cycle length to decrease as the numbers of episodes increases (see Course and Prognosis below)

(40). He postulates a pattern of stress-induced sensitization and kindling, analogous in some ways to seizure activity, to explain how repetition of life stressors eventually precipitate full-blown manic episodes at progressively lower thresholds. Such a mechanism would make episodes progressively easier to evoke and therefore decreasingly dependent on external factors. It might also explain the efficacy of certain anticonvulsant agents (see below) in the prophylaxis of bipolar disorder.

Wehr (41) has demonstrated that sleep deprivation has antidepressant properties that trigger manic symptoms in bipolar patients. He speculates that travel, certain medications, and emotional reactions to stress as well as to joyful experiences can induce insomnia and may therefore trigger a manic spiral. He notes that the best treatments for acute mania have primarily sedative effects and that minimization of sleep disturbance may be a major aspect of resolving mania. Patients and families should be advised that careful avoidance of sleep disruption may be an effective strategy in the prevention of recurrent mania.

Recently, two biological markers appear trait specific and, therefore, independent of clinical state. Lewy et al. have demonstrated that in response to light the nighttime plasma melatonin levels of manic and euthymic bipolar patients appear to decrease twice as much as normal (42). Sitaram et al. described heightened sensitivity (independent of clinical state) to rapid eye movement (REM) induction due to arecoline, a muscarinic cholinergic agonist in patients with major affective disorder (43).

In summary, research in the areas of biochemical neurotransmitters point to the importance of biogenic amines, especially norepinephrine, in clinical states of mania. It remains uncertain whether amines are the primary etiologic factors or whether mania reflects a disturbed balance of general neurotransmitter activity. Research into the biology of mania has generated a number of increasingly sophisticated models of the syndrome. This is an era of accelerating progress in our biological understanding of this disorder.

Genetic Hypothesis

As noted earlier, the lifetime risk of developing affective illness for first-degree relatives of patients with mood disorders ranges from 10–25% (16, 24–27). This contrasts with a risk of only 1–2% in the general population. This greater than 10-fold magnitude of risk for morbidity among first-degree relatives supports a dominant gene theory of genetic transmission.

The concordance rates for bipolar mood disorders are 68% for monozygotic twins and 23% for same-sex dizygotic twins. These figures also support a significant genetic contribution and represent a pattern consistent with an autosomal dominant gene with incomplete penetrance.

Studies of different bipolar family pedigrees indicate linkage to a number of different chromosome loci. The diversity of these results indicates that inheritance may be non-Mendelian because of genetic heterogeneity and incomplete penetrance (susceptibility is not always manifested as illness). The complexity of the current data indicates the possibility of interactions among several genes and genetic-environmental interactions (44).

Coryell et al. (21) demonstrate that first-degree relatives of bipolar patients exhibit a higher rate of academic and social success than first-degree relatives of unipolar patients. In view of the relatively high incidence of this largely genetically determined disorder, some speculate that certain "bipolar genes" may actually have conferred an evolutionary advantage to family members and therefore were "selected" (45). Bipolar disorder may result from dysregulation of the abilities conferred by these genes.

In summary, genetic factors in bipolar affective disorder are indisputable. Morbidity risk in first-degree relatives and twin studies indicate genetic contribution to etiology. The mode of genetic transmission remains uncertain.

Psychodynamic Hypotheses

In the early 20th century, psychoanalytic theories predominated in American psychiatry. Almost all individual psychopathology was thought to result from the interaction between drives or early, often repressed, experiences of emotional trauma and the individual's pathological, inadequate, or overwhelmed mechanisms of defense. Optimism existed about the potential for psychoanalytic treatment to cure a range of psychiatric disorders.

Karl Abraham (46) hypothesized that in mania the superego merges with the ego, thereby endowing the ego with excess libidinal energy and narcissism. This psychodynamic construction contrasted with his notion of depression in which the superego is excessively punitive and critical of the ego.

Observing the *bipolarity* of the illness, the literature generally described mania as a defense against melancholia (47). The importance of denial as the basic defense mechanism in mania and hypomania has been repeatedly described (48).

In 1953, Rochlin (49) posited a theory of mood lability based on shifts between an intense but denied identification with a seductive, masochistic mother who is devalued and aggressive, and sadistic masculine wishes. These wishes strengthen the denial of identifying with the mother and repress passive and masochistic longings. Depression was associated with identifying with the devalued, weak mother, and elation was associated with a denial of this hated iden-

tification through aggressiveness, sadistic impulses, and wishes. The emphasis of this work was in the vicissitudes of mood, which can lead to states of clinical disorder.

In 1978, MacVane et al. (50) studied the psychological functioning of patients in remission from bipolar affective disorder and did not find the presence of the dependent character features and conventional, conformist behaviors reported by others (51). His work cast doubt on the previously held psychodynamic views of bipolar patients. Central to MacVane's work was that all patients studied were well-stabilized on lithium.

In summary, psychodynamic contributions to mania have focused on aspects of denial as a basic defense mechanism. Biological treatment has called much of this extensive literature into question. More research in this area is needed.

THE BIOPSYCHOSOCIAL EVALUATION

The Biological Evaluation

The inpatient unit must have ready access to diagnostic facilities for the biological assessment of mania. The clinicians's first task is to separate out 2° mania from 1° mania.

History

Mania in a patient 40 years or older with a negative psychiatric and family history of affective disorder should be considered 2° mania until proven otherwise. In taking the history, the physician must be alert to any recent ingestion of prescribed or nonprescribed drugs, exposure to toxic substances, a history of infection, or any abnormal neurological activity.

In addition, the physician must take a detailed history of the present illness and past medical and psychiatric illnesses, including any current or past medication or treatment; a family history, with particular emphasis on inheritable disorders and psychiatric syndromes; drug and dietary habits; and a thorough review of systems.

History-taking is best done with collaboration from the family, significant others, and anyone else who has witnessed the patient's behavior or has pertinent knowledge about events before hospitalization.

As noted in the above section on the stages of mania, a reliable history about the sequence and timing of symptoms leading up to presentation helps make an accurate diagnosis.

Physical Examination

The physician must pay particular attention to the patient's vital signs and the neurological examination, inspecting carefully for any focal signs or evidence of an altered sensorium.

Laboratory Studies

1. Routine Studies. Complete blood count (CBC), urine analysis, serum test for syphilis, blood glucose, sodium (Na), potassium (K), chlorine (Cl), carbon dioxide (CO_2), calcium (Ca), phosphate (PO_4), creatinine, blood urea nitrogen (BUN), alkaline phosphatase, serum glutamic-oxaloacetic transaminase (SGOT), bilirubin-T/D (total/direct), and thyroxine (T_4).

2. Special Studies. Toxic screening of the urine and/or blood for any suspected drug or toxin (including stimulants, steroids, antidepressants, L-dopa, and bromine). Pregnancy test. Blood culture lumbar puncture and testing for the presence of human immunodeficiency virus (HIV) (with patient consent) may be indicated to rule out organic causes.

Radiological Studies

Studies to rule out organic causes such as a Skull series, computerized tomography (CT) scan or magnetic resonance imaging (MRI), single photon emission tomography (SPECT) or positron emission tomography (PET) scan may be indicated by suggestive findings.

Additional Diagnostic Studies

Electrocardiogram (EKG); urine specific gravity following a 12-hour fast for baseline urine concentrating ability, especially if lithium therapy is under consideration, electroencephalogram (EEG) (with awake and sleep tracings).

The thyrotropin-releasing hormone (TRH) test, in which the magnitude of the release of thyroid-stimulating hormone (TSH) is measured after the infusion of TRH, has been reported as a biological marker in distinguishing mania from schizophrenia. This is not yet part of a standard workup for mania (52–54).

Psychological testing can be helpful, especially once the mania has subsided, to determine the presence of any persistent disorder or evidence of organic impairment.

Baseline Thyroid Studies for Workup and (Before) Lithium Therapy

T_4 and TSH are usually adequate for routine screening.

Psychodynamic Evaluation

The psychodynamic evaluation begins with a careful developmental history that includes prenatal, preschool, latency, and adolescent information, elaborated by a work, military, play, marital, and sexual history.

An examination of the patient's ego functioning can be helpful. Knowledge about past and present functioning, defensive style—especially the use of denial—object relations, and capacity for adaptation and pleasure, helps the clinician to know the patient as a person. Understanding how the patient may have experienced events leading up to presentation and what defenses he or she may use helps the clinician to explain the patient's illness in a way that will best suit the patient's character style.

Sociocultural and Family Evaluation

The sociocultural evaluation focuses on information about the patient's social class and ethnic and religious background. How home, community, and work have shaped the patient's belief system should emerge from this evaluation.

Particular attention should be paid to current life events that may have precipitated the patient's disorder. How the patient's family, friends, and colleagues have responded to these stressors and to the patient is important.

The patient's value system about medical care and the patient's mode of entry into the care-giving system will often be critical to the clinician's ability to develop a working alliance with the patient.

Mania is a destructive process for both patients and their families. In mania, relations with family members, friends, and professional associates are often severely disturbed. In addition, errors in judgment during the manic illness can create catastrophic legal and financial difficulties. Employment may be jeopardized or even lost.

Discussing the impact of the manic episode on the patient's family and professional and social world is a critical part of inpatient assessment. Such a discussion may provide the opportunity to begin rebuilding a world severely disrupted by the patient's illness.

HOSPITAL TREATMENT

Hospital Treatment of Primary Mania

PSYCHOPHARMACOLOGICAL MANAGEMENT

Psychopharmacological management is the mainstay of treating the acutely manic patient. Although lithium is the most specific antimanic agent, clinical improvement generally does not take place until 7–10 days after treatment is initiated. Most patients with suspected mania therefore will first be prescribed antipsychotic and/or sedative medications. Lithium may then be started if the diagnosis of mania is confirmed.

Under conventional treatment, neuroleptics are used to treat acute mania before lithium's clinical effects develop. As therapeutic levels of lithium begin to develop, the need for antipsychotic medications diminishes, and the clinician can then lower the dose of antipsychotic and anxiolytic medications accordingly. Some patients may be able to discontinue antipsychotic or anxiolytic medications completely and be treated with lithium alone for the latter part of their hospitalization. Other patients will require combined lithium and neuroleptic treatment. This combination is generally safe, though reports of toxicity and persistent organic dysfunction call for judicious use and careful monitoring of this combined drug regimen. The hospitalized manic patient is especially prone to severe side effects and toxicity within 1–2 weeks after starting lithium. During this time the patient is generally taking higher doses of neuroleptic which may interact with the then-substantial action of lithium. Many patients tolerate a decrease in neuroleptic as adequate lithium levels are obtained, minimizing side effects (55–57).

1. Antipsychotics. Antipsychotic medications are highly effective in treating target symptoms of hyperactivity, anxiety, hostility, delusions, hallucinations, insomnia, and negativism. Antipsychotic medications are generally the first-line treatment of the acute manic state. The patient can be started on a protocol for antipsychotic medications outlined in Chapter 3. Though antipsychotics are effective in reducing many of the symptoms of mania, they are *not specifically antimanic.*

If the clinician decides to begin the patient on lithium, the clinician will notice that the patient will begin to show a reduced need for antipsychotic medication after 5–10 days of treatment. An early sign of excess antipsychotic medication is sedation, particularly in the morning. As the patient begins to obtain the therapeutic effect of lithium, the antipsychotic medication may then be reduced slowly. During the reduction, the clinician should monitor the patient for a breakthrough of manic symptomatology. If there is no breakthrough, the antipsychotic medication can be decreased and eventually discontinued. A relatively rapid decrease of neuroleptic medication (over a period of 1–3 weeks) reduces the risks of side effects.

However, some patients may require treatment with both antipsychotic medication and lithium throughout hospitalization. As neuroleptics induce a wide range of uncomfortable and potentially serious side effects, every effort must be made to place these patients on the lowest amount of antipsychotic medication necessary to manage their behavior and symptoms. Recent evidence suggests that during long-term treatment patients with affective disorder may be significantly more susceptible to developing tardive dyskinesia than schizophrenic patients (58, 59). The patient may be discharged on an antipsychotic medication with follow-up aimed at having the patient on the lowest dose of medication needed for effective treatment. The risks and benefits of neuroleptic treatment should be discussed with the patient (and family, when indicated) once the patient has been stabilized on medications.

Because of the long half-life of neuroleptic anti-manic effects, discontinuing neuroleptics shortly before discharge may place the patient at increased risk of relapse following discharge. As powerful external pressures force hospitals to shorten inpatient lengths-of-stay, it is often prudent to keep the patient on a low dose of antipsychotic medication upon discharge. This may reduce the risk of relapse during the often-stressful initial transition back to regular functioning and also enable the outpatient clinician to view the patient on a stable dose of medication. It is often difficult for a newly assigned outpatient clinician to judge whether a patient's increasing anxiety immediately following discharge reflects the natural stresses of transition home or is actually the early stages of psychotic relapse resulting from recent neuroleptic discontinuation.

2. Sedatives. During acute mania, PRN supplemental sedative medication is often necessary to reduce agitation. Traditionally, neuroleptics have been used for sedation. Recently, the use of sedative medication has significantly reduced the need for neuroleptics during the acute phase of mania, thereby reducing the risk of a number of uncomfortable and potentially serious side effects (60). Anxiolytics generally produce sedation with fewer and more predictable side effects than neuroleptics. In addition, recent evidence indicates that patients with affective disorders who take neuroleptics are at higher risk for the development of tardive and acute dystonias (58, 59).

Lorazepam in hourly doses of 0.5–2 mg, up to 10 mg per day in medically healthy patients, can help manage agitation during the acute phase of mania. Lorazepam's relatively short half-life makes it easy to adjust doses according to the needs of the moment.

Long-term adjunctive treatment with clonazepam (see anticonvulsants below) in place of neuroleptics may also be more effective in a subgroup of bipolar patients (60). Anxiolytics have not demonstrated antipsychotic effects. If a patient remains agitated despite the addition of lithium and requires anxiolytics for an extended period, lithium may not be effective for that patient. Alternative antimanic treatments (and neuroleptics) should be considered. If regular doses of anxiolytics are used for a significant period, care should be taken to minimize the risk of withdrawal.

Recent experience (61) indicates that acutely manic patients who respond to lithium respond well when treated without neuroleptics. These patients often do well on lithium and a sedative. Sedative and lithium treatment without neuroleptics may soon evolve into a first-line treatment for acute mania.

3. **Lithium.** Lithium is a cation and a unique chemical agent for the treatment of acute mania as well as for the prophylactic treatment of bipolar affective disorders (62–64).

a. *Indications:* Lithium is a mood stabilizer with antidepressant and antimanic properties. To date it is the best-studied and most effective antimanic agent known. In a two-year double-blind study, the relapse rate for lithium-treated patients was 25%, in contrast to 61% of patients taking placebo (65).

It is beyond the scope of this chapter to fully discuss maintenance treatment. The reader is referred elsewhere for a review of lithium maintenance and prophylaxis (66–68).

Barring specific contraindications, lithium is the *drug of choice* for the treatment of 1° mania.

b. *Preliminary Evaluation Studies and Contraindications to Lithium Treatment:* The patient's thyroid, renal, electrolyte, and cardiac status are important aspects of the preliminary evaluation. Abnormalities in any of these systems is a possible contraindication to lithium use. Medical consultation is necessary if lithium is to be used in the presence of significant abnormalities.

Lithium, which has serious teratogenic effects, particularly on the developing heart, should be avoided during pregnancy, especially in the first trimester. Its risks should be carefully discussed with women of child-bearing age who consider its use. Contraception, pregnancy monitoring, and options in the event of subsequent accidental or planned pregnancy should be fully discussed before starting treatment (69, 70).

In addition, the patient's general physical status and reliability should be assessed. Lithium treatment requires daily administration and careful blood monitoring. Its use can result in severe toxicity or death when taken in excessive amounts, either accidentally or intentionally.

c. *Administration:* Lithium carbonate is available in capsules or tablets in slow-release or regular forms. It is also available in liquid form as lithium citrate. Lithium is never administered by injection. It is absorbed readily in the gut and metabolized almost completely by the kidney.

The half-life of lithium ranges from about 18–36 hours, depending on individual renal function. As a rule, the elderly excrete lithium more slowly than the young. Therefore, older people tend to require lower doses because for them the drug has a longer half-life.

Lithium can be administered in divided or single daily doses. Recent evidence indicates that single daily doses may significantly lower the risk of glomerulosclerosis, renal interstitial fibrosis, and polyuria (71–73). Once-a-day dosing is easier to remember and, when given at night, may allow level-dependent side effects to dissipate during sleep. In order to avoid excessive level-dependent side effects when first starting lithium, it is often best to administer two doses—one in the morning and one in the evening—until therapeutic levels are attained. Administration can gradually move toward one evening dose while side effects are monitored. Administration at night requires less total daily lithium; levels should be monitored during transition to a single dose schedule. Patients unable to tolerate their full dose at night may need to continue divided doses (in some cases up to four doses per day).

Administering the drug with or just after meals and in slow-release forms can reduce gastrointestinal irritation. Diarrhea appears to be more common with slow-release forms and least common with the liquid.

In acute mania the clinician seeks to obtain a 12-hour serum lithium level of around 1.0 milliequivalent per liter (meq/l). Blood levels are drawn in the morning, approximately 12 hours after the previous evening's dose. No morning dose of medication is provided until blood is drawn. During the first week of hospitalization, blood levels may be drawn every other day to observe the effects of the dosage and to monitor entrance into the therapeutic range. Once the patient has entered this range and remained stable, blood levels may be drawn once or twice per week according to clinical needs. After several weeks, the patient may go to a less frequent schedule of blood levels, e.g., once a week, then once every other week, then once a month.

The patient is generally begun on 600–900 mg/day of lithium. The dose is then increased every few days with guidelines drawn from serum lithium levels.

Once the mania has subsided, recent data indicate that lithium levels between 0.8–1.0 meq/l have a significantly lower incidence of relapse than levels between 0.4–0.6 meq/l (74, 75). This maintenance level of lithium is indicated for the inpatient's postmanic phase and for posthospital prophylaxis. Some patients do well at a lower blood level; others require higher levels. The *patient's clinical status*, not his blood level, should determine the proper dose of lithium.

d. *Side Effects:* Intoxication from lithium occurs when the dose exceeds clinical needs. Some patients, especially the elderly, demonstrate lithium toxicity at relatively low dosages. The signs and symptoms of lithium toxicity are *nausea, vomiting, diarrhea, tremor, muscular weakness, ataxia,* and *drowsiness.* More severe intoxication may involve muscle hyper-irritability with increased deep-tendon reflexes, twitching, fasciculation, and nystagmus. The patient's mental status changes as intoxication increases; initial confusion may progress to stupor and then coma. Seizures may occur with severe intoxication.

The first step in the management of toxicity is to discontinue the lithium treatment. Frequently, if intoxication is discovered early, this alone will be adequate. In more severe cases, medical consultation is indicated, and the use of gastric lavage, fluid-loading, and careful electrolyte balance may be needed.

Cardiovascular side effects of lithium include EKG changes (T-wave flattening or inversion), hypotension, and arrhythmias.

Renal side effects of lithium include diabetes insipidus with polyuria and polydipsia. Lithium-induced diabetes insipidus generally responds to reducing the lithium dose or administering a thiazide diuretic (which may cause marked increase in serum lithium and decrease in serum potassium; careful monitoring is necessary when diuretics are used). Amiloride, a potassium-sparing diuretic that acts on the collecting tubule, is also effective in ameliorating lithium-induced polyuria (76, 77).

Recent extensive studies indicate that the risk of serious renal impairment such as interstitial fibrosis due to lithium therapy is far less common than previously thought. Evidence indicates that renal failure caused by lithium therapy is rare (68). Possible renal changes should be discussed with the patient and creatinine levels should be checked every 3–6 months (78).

Lithium also has effects on the *thyroid*. Approximately 5% of lithium-treated patients develop hypothyroidism; 3% develop a benign, diffuse, nontoxic goiter (79). Evidence indicates that when lithium does produce overt hypothyroidism, subtle, preexisting autoimmune thyroiditis was often present (80). Thyroid function tests should be checked at least twice a year.

Weight gain, a common complaint for a subgroup of patients, can be a strong disincentive to compliance. In a longitudinal study, weight gain occurred within the first 12 months of lithium treatment and averaged four kg. Weight remained stable thereafter (81).

Tremor is a common and often troublesome side effect. A lower dose of lithium may alleviate the tremor. β-adrenergic blockers such as propranolol are often very helpful. Metoprolol, a lipophilic centrally active cardioselective B_1 blocker, may be used for patients who cannot take propranolol because of bronchospasm (83, 84).

Dermatologic changes with lithium treatment include dry skin, folliculitis, exacerbation of acne vulgaris, and ulcerations.

e. *Caveats:* Keep in mind that toxicity from antipsychotic agents and lithium may increase if the two drugs are combined (55, 56). A clinician should pay particular attention to the effects of this drug combination several days to one week into lithium treatment when the patient is approaching the therapeutic range of lithium and still taking high doses of antipsychotic medications.

approaching the therapeutic range of lithium and still taking high doses of antipsychotic medications.

Some patients may show lithium intoxication while in normal serum level range. Serum lithium level should be used as a guide only. The patient's *clinical state* is the determining factor in adjusting dosage.

A number of conditions and medications can alter the kinetics of lithium and thereby change the serum concentration. Dehydration (due to hot weather, diarrhea, etc.), low serum potassium and diuretics can unexpectedly elevate previously stable levels. Serum lithium and electrolyte levels should be monitored carefully when a patient is taking other medications (85, 86). Ibuprofen (Motrin) is a commonly used drug which raises mean lithium levels 15% (87). Older patients, especially those with impaired renal functioning, excrete lithium more slowly and are more susceptible to lithium toxicity.

Alcohol and sedatives are frequently used by bipolar patients trying to modulate their dysphoric moods. Clinicians should be alert to signs of nonprescribed drug use on admission and to any symptoms of withdrawal from CNS depressants while the patient is in the hospital.

Evidence indicates that an abrupt discontinuation of lithium therapy may produce withdrawal mania. A gradual withdrawal may be clinically safer (88).

4. Barbiturates. Highly agitated patients taking high doses of antipsychotic medication and beginning lithium therapy may benefit from a bedtime dose of 120–180 mg of sodium amytal.

5. Anticonvulsants Anticonvulsants can be a substitute for, or an adjunct to, lithium treatment.

a. *Carbamazepine* (Tegretol), an anticonvulsant with a molecular structure similar to imipramine, is currently viewed as the leading alternative to lithium. Initial studies indicate that carbamazepine has antimanic and antidepressant effects and may work synergistically with lithium when response to lithium is incomplete. Controlled studies have demonstrated carbamazepine's effectiveness as a prophylactic agent in 72% of 81 patients studied (40). Patients with rapid-cycling bipolar disorder appear to respond well to carbamazepine (89).

Carbamazepine has a number of potentially serious side effects and requires careful monitoring of blood counts, liver functions, and serum levels. A benign transient elevation in liver enzymes occurs in some patients (89). Agranulocytosis is a potentially life-threatening side effect with an incidence of one in 20,000–40,000 patients. Baseline laboratory tests should include CBC, platelet count, creatinine, and liver function. CBC should be monitored regularly (weekly during the first two months is considered conservative). Patients should be warned to stop the medication, notify their clinician, and have a CBC performed in the event of fever, infection, or petechiae. Skin reactions, from rash to Stevens-Johnson syndrome can occur (90). Ataxia, diplopia, dizziness, dysarthria, nausea, and vomiting are not uncommon dose-related side effects. Carbamazepine has potentially serious interactions with a number of other medications. When carbamazepine is taken concurrently with neuroleptics and other anticonvulsant medications, hepatic enzyme induction can result in the need for markedly higher doses to attain similar clinical effects and blood levels. Carbamazepine is also teratogenic and should not be given during pregnancy (see cautions related to lithium above) (91).

Despite the list of complications above, carbamazepine is generally well-tolerated and often effective when used with reasonable caution. More research is needed to further establish which patterns of illness respond well to carbamazepine and what serum levels are appropriate.

b. *Valproate* (Depakote, Depakene, Valproic Acid) is an anticonvulsant that should be considered when lithium or carbamazepine are ineffective or cannot be tolerated. In a placebo-controlled study of 36 bipolar patients who had failed to respond to or were intolerant of lithium, McElroy et al. (92) found valproate significantly superior to placebo in treating acute mania. Several open trials, both alone and in combination with lithium, have indicated moderate to good acute and prophylactic antimanic effects (93, 94). Further data are needed to confirm and determine degree of effectiveness.

c. *Clonazepam*, a potent long-acting benzodiazepine, anticonvulsant, and serotonin agonist, is the least toxic of the currently available antimanic agents. As an anticonvulsant, it is most effective in petit mal and myoclonic seizures. It can be useful in treating acute mania, significantly reducing the need for neuroleptics (see sedatives above). Chouinard reports success in using clonazepam alone (without neuroleptics) during the first week of treatment for acute mania, starting lithium during the second week (95).

Long-term prophylactic use of clonazepam as a mood-stabilizing agent in cases of inadequate response to lithium has met with mixed results. It can be considered when alternatives have failed (96).

6. Novel Agents. A variety of other agents, including verapamil, clonidine, and clorgyline, have been reported effective for some cases of mania. They can be considered when other efforts have failed (97–100).

ECT

Electroconvulsive therapy has long been recognized as a clinically effective treatment for mania (101, 102).

Patients who are intolerant of antipsychotics or lithium should be considered for ECT. For patients with severe excitement bordering on frenzy, associated combativeness, and for whom it is difficult to administer adequate doses of medication, ECT can be considered as a first line of treatment for mania. In these severely manic patients, some of whose illnesses are known to run fatal courses, ECT may be the most sensible treatment because of its rapid action, high effectiveness, and safety.

MILIEU MANAGEMENT

Manic patients' poor judgment, severe denial, grandiosity, euphoria, and hyperactivity frequently preclude their voluntary admission. Many manic patients therefore refuse treatment and are hospitalized involuntarily, particularly if their symptoms include danger to themselves or others.

However, some manic patients will seek voluntary admission, especially when pressured by friends, family, and work associates. For these patients, a clear understanding of what limits they must place on their own behavior is a critical part of the initial milieu management. Threatening, combative, or sexually provocative behaviors and alcohol or drug abuse must be limited for the benefit of the individual patient and the rest of the patient community.

Preventing articulate, argumentative,

and often coherent manic patients from pursuing extravagant, careless, or sexual goals can be difficult for the clinician. It is helpful to keep in mind that, following recovery, bipolar patients are often mortified to discover the outrageous transgressions they have pursued during mania. During the period when their judgment is impaired, it must be explained that these behaviors are symptoms of the illness and cannot be tolerated. Firm, consistent, and carefully explained limit-setting is essential to clinical management and to the prevention of dangerous acting-out (103).

Decreasing stimulation by restricting visitors and providing periods of time alone are part of the milieu treatment of the manic patient. Many of the milieu management techniques for the acutely psychotic patient apply to the acutely manic patient. These are outlined in Chapter 3.

Janowsky et al. (104, 105) have described common interpersonal maneuvers of the manic patient. These include: (*a*) manipulating the self-esteem of others; (*b*) making individual and group conflict overt; (*c*) projecting responsibility; (*d*) progressively testing limits; and (*e*) alienating family members. Understanding these interpersonal maneuvers enables ward staff to control their anger and anticipate the manic patient's behavior. Patients may attempt to divide staff members or attack or flatter them, deny and/or project personal responsibility, and test limits constantly.

A manic patient generally has great impact on the rest of the ward community. Agitation and irritability in any patient tends to raise the general level of anxiety in the community. In addition, manic patients may threaten legal action against the ward or attempt to call a variety of authorities in an effort to deny their mania.

The community meeting is an important forum for ward patients and staff. Staff can allay ward anxiety by explaining the nature of the manic patient's symptomatology and enlisting other patients in the treatment plan for the manic patient.

INDIVIDUAL PSYCHOTHERAPY

ALLIANCE BUILDING IN THE MANIC PHASE

Explorative psychotherapy with the acutely manic patient is an exercise in futility. All the clinician can hope for during this phase is to obtain a comprehensive history and begin to develop an alliance with the patient through empathic support, firm limit-setting, and effective chemotherapy.

THE POSTMANIC PHASE

When bipolar patients are manic or euthymic they tend to deny their illness and show little affinity for treatment. To them the euphoria of the moment is real and its loss can feel devastating.

As mania subsides and painful reality emerges, patients may minimize their illness, reject medication, wish to flee the hospital, and not participate in plans for outpatient follow-up.

The degree of denial observed in otherwise coherent and often insightful manic patients should not be underestimated. Pope et al. (106) speculate that this may not be "denial"; there may actually be a biological basis for the inability to recognize illness during acute mania, much like the "anosognosia" or ignorance of illness observed in some neurological conditions.

At the point when mania is abating and dysphoric affect is emerging, the clinician may be most successful in establishing a psychotherapeutic alliance. Knowing how the patient has dealt with past adverse news can help at the time when the patient is first able to realize that he or she has serious, potentially psychotic and lifelong illness. At this time, if the clinician can assist patients in not resorting to denial or flight and aid them in bearing dysphoric affect, psychotherapy can begin.

Initial psychotherapeutic work should aim to help patients recognize the existence of their illness and the feelings this creates. Incorporating the existence of a mental illness into their self-image can be devastating without supportive help. Individual and group therapy with other bipolar patients can help maintain self-esteem and minimize denial.

In helping to foster a sense of control over the illness, it is useful to review carefully the events and symptoms that preceded decompensation. If stressful events may have precipitated the manic episode, the patient should be encouraged to be on the lookout for similar situations.

As Kraeplin initially observed, for a given patient the particular symptoms of an attack of mania were remarkably similar, episode to episode (107). Recent data indicate that for an individual bipolar patient the symptoms and duration of successive prodromes of the same polarity are remarkably consistent (108). A careful history of the early symptoms of mania leading up to the episode should be identified using any sources available to the patient: roommates, family, coworkers, etc. If there has been more than one episode, patterns should be sought. A series of subtle changes in sleep, energy, mood, and behavior (see hypomania above) can often be identified. Once these are defined, if that is possible, it is helpful to get patients to agree to allow their clinician and significant others to help them monitor for any similar early signs of relapse. Permission by the patient to allow significant others to communicate relevant observations directly to the clinician may be essential in identifying an early episode at a time when denial often prevents patients from recognizing or reporting their own symptoms. Early treatment often prevents further decompensation and hospitalization.

As treatment progresses, the clinician can help the patient to repair and reestablish personal and professional relationships. As the patient's history may show, important relationships are often damaged during the manic episode.

Finally, the patient can be counseled on the nature and course of bipolar illness. The clinician should constantly work on developing an alliance with the patient by emphasizing the disorders treatability through medication and psychotherapy (109), and the importance of early intervention.

FAMILY WORK

FAMILY COUNSELING

Single or recurrent episodes of mania are highly disruptive to the patient's family. The clinician should try to help the family see the mania as a treatable illness. This can alter an often angry and limited perspective in which the patient's symptomatic behavior is interpreted as willful, hostile, irresponsible, or weak.

Marital instability is often characteristic for bipolar patients. Fifty-seven percent of bipolar patients' marriages end in divorce while only 8% of unipolar patients suffer a similar fate (110). Spouses of unipolar patients tend to feel sympathy for their suffering, anger toward their dependency, and guilt for somehow contributing to the depression; little doubt exists that the marriage will continue. In contrast, spouses of bipolar patients are frequently motivated to seek divorce.

Spouses of bipolar patients are frequently the principal object of the patient's anger and seen as villains, opponents, and "bad parents." Furthermore, the spouse may be deeply wounded by the manic individual's infidelity. Spouses also generally find themselves answering complaints from the patient's social and professional community (104).

Supportive, empathic meetings between a social worker or unit staff member and family members can begin without the patient. An alliance with the family can be established around treatment for the manic patient. During these meetings the family worker can discuss the impact of the manic episode on the family and make personality assessments of individual family members.

Once the manic patient's symptomatology is under control, family meetings can include the patient. During these meetings, general family evaluation can begin. The clinician should pay particular attention to the way the family manages affective and power issues.

As the patient improves and hospitalization is ending, the family can seek short-term family therapy. Mental illness and well-being, dependence and independence, mood fluctuations, and caretaking roles can be addressed (111).

GENETIC COUNSELING

Genetic counseling for psychiatric patients and their families is a relatively new and valuable service.

Tsuang (112) provides an overview of the subject and an excellent description of the stages of counseling. As noted earlier, the risk of developing bipolar disorder for first-degree relatives of patients with the illness is nearly 20-fold higher than normal. Furthermore, it has been estimated that siblings of the patient with bipolar disorder have a 26% risk of becoming ill if one parent has a history of affective disorder and 43% risk when both parents do (113).

An understanding of the patient and family members is essential for providing information at a level they can understand and at a pace they can accept.

Hospital Treatment of Secondary Mania

When manic symptomatology is secondary in nature, the clinician's task is to diagnose the underlying cause and correct the organic disturbance. Frequently, the correction of the underlying course may take considerable time or be impossible. Furthermore, it may be essential to correct the manic symptomatology in order to proceed with the diagnostic evaluation.

When secondary manic symptomatology needs to be corrected by psychopharmacological management, the same form of treatment used for primary mania is applicable (3, 18, 114–124). Unless contraindications are present, the patient may be started on a neuroleptic medication and lithium added if the response to the neuroleptic is unsatisfactory. Also, ECT has been used effectively in cases of secondary mania.

CONTROVERSIES IN TREATMENT

Despite recent major developments in the diagnosis and treatment of mania, old controversies remain and new controversies will continue to emerge.

As research continues, the utility of distinguishing bipolar II patterns of illness from both unipolar depression and bipolar I will, it is hoped, become clear. Schizoaffective disorder is a diagnosis whose value is widely debated. Outcome studies will help clarify whether these categorical distinctions are helpful in determining optimal treatment.

The role of external mental and physical stress in precipitating manic and depressive episodes is unclear. Further research is needed to evaluate the "kindling" model of bipolar disorder. This model indicates that efforts should be made to prevent the cycle of sensitization to stress that increases patient vulnerability to relapse.
Whether environmental manipulation or medication can prevent "kindling" is not clear. When a recently manic individual with a high-stress, exciting job asks how much he or she has to cut back late hours and international travel, it is difficult to assess the costs and benefits of such changes.

Whether certain character styles are more susceptible to stress and hence to mania is unclear. Whether psychotherapy can bring about changes that help prophylactically to reduce susceptibility, and the relative effectiveness of insight-oriented, cognitive, or behavioral techniques, are important questions.

When lithium works, it is not known how long to continue it as a prophylactic agent if the patient remains symptom free, especially if the patient suffers uncomfortable side effects. If a patient does have occasional episodes of "breakthrough" mania, how does the clinician decide whether, and to what degree, lithium is helping? Furthermore, the prophylactic use of anticonvulsants remains controversial and in need of extensive verification.

A significant number of patients do not fully respond to lithium. Until recently, the single most effective option was to add neuroleptic medication to the lithium regimen (with significant risk of producing tardive dyskinesia). With increasing numbers of alternative antimanic regimens available, it is often difficult to know how many different medication trials (involving different side effects, risks, and often requiring several weeks each) to ask a patient to tolerate before deciding to stay with and accept a partial response.

Decades ago, ECT was used extensively, often involuntarily and without current levels of safety. These practices contributed to a stigma perpetuated by caricatures in the media. Despite its safety record and documented effectiveness in the treatment of acute mania, the use of ECT remains stigmatized. As a result, ECT is probably underused.

The degree to which the use of antidepressants in treating bipolar depression causes mania or induces rapid cycling is also not clear (131). Certain antidepressants are believed to be more likely to induce mania than others. Unfortunately, there is little data and wide disagreement about which antidepressants are safest.

COURSE AND PROGNOSIS

A number of recent studies have attempted to document the *natural course* of bipolar disorder. These studies contain a number of confounding factors that preclude a definite view of how treatment affects course and outcome.

Estimates of the percentage of bipolar patients whose illness begins with a manic episode average just above 50% (125). Tohen et al. (126) studied 24 first-episode manic patients upon presentation to the hospital, six months after presentation, and four years later. The average length of the first (treated) episode was 42.5 days, the median was 49 days, and the range was from 17–129 days.

During the first six months, five (21%) patients all relapsed into depression. The probability of remaining in remission for six months was found to be 66% for patients with psychotic features and 88% for patients without. The overall probability for all first-episode patients remaining in remission for one year was 58% and over four years, 42%. The majority of relapses occurred during the first year. No significant differences were found between those who relapsed and those who did not, in terms of age of onset, use of psychotropic medication, or family history of affective illness. Sixteen (67%) had a family history of affective illness or alcoholism in at least one first-degree relative.

Four years after the first episode, 23 (96%) rated their overall satisfaction with various areas of functioning in their lives as fair to very good, despite the illness. Investigators rated patient's global social adjustment as fair to very good for 20 (83.3%) and poor to very poor for four (16.7%). After four years, 11 (46%) were not taking any

psychotropic medication. Twelve of the 13 still on medication were taking lithium, either alone (seven or 29%), in combination with a neuroleptic agent (three or 12.5%), or in combination with an antidepressant (two or 8%). First-episode patients such as those analyzed in this study are likely to have the best prognosis and do not make up the majority of psychiatric admissions for mania.

Keller (127) analyzed 155 patients diagnosed with bipolar disorder and divided them into three groups: patients with manic symptoms only, at time of entry; patients with depressed symptoms only; or patients with a combination of depressed and manic symptoms. He found that those who were manic only recovered at a faster rate than did the others. Median times for recovery on medication were: five weeks after entry for manics, nine weeks for depressives, and 14 weeks for the mixed and cycling patients. He concluded that mixed and cycling patients have a far more pernicious course than do those with purely manic episodes.

In a review of the literature, Goodwin et al. (125) note that cycle length decreases with increasing numbers of episodes. Furthermore, the frequency of episodes increases with the total duration of the illness (and therefore with patient age). Many studies also indicate that the age at which the patient first experiences the illness correlates with the subsequent frequency of the episodes. Zis et al. (128) analyzed 105 patients and calculated that the probability of the second episode of bipolar disorder following the first within 24 months was 20% for those in their 20s at onset, 50% for those in their 30s, and 80% for those over 40. Perris (129) reported that 62% of the patients whose first episode was manic went on to have a predominantly manic course, whereas 25% had a predominantly depressive course. The converse was true for those whose illness first presented with a depression.

With the advent of effective treatments, mortality rates appear to have declined. In an early study (1933), Derby documented that 22% of hospitalized manic patients died; 40% of these deaths were from exhaustion (130). Suicide, an unfortunately common outcome in bipolar disorder, has a lifetime prevalence estimated between 10–15% (125).

REFERENCES

1. American Psychiatric Association: Diagnostic and Statistical Manual of Mental Disorders, ed. 3, (DSM-IIIR). Washington, D.C., American Psychiatric Association, 1987.

2. Winokur G, et al.: *Manic Depressive Illness,* St. Louis, C.V. Mosby, 1969.

3. Krauthammer C, Klerman GL: Secondary mania. Arch Gen Psychiatry, *35:*1333–1339, 1978.

4. Carlson GA, Goodwin FK: The stages of mania. Arch Gen Psychiatry, *28:*221–228, 1973.

5. Abrams R, Taylor MA: Importance of schizophrenic symptoms in the diagnosis of mania. Am J Psychiatry, *138:*658–661, 1981.

6. Quitkin FM, Kane J, Rifkin A, et al.: Prophylactic lithium carbonate with and without imipramine for bipolar I patients: A double-blind study. Arch Gen Psychiatry, *38:*902–907, 1981.

7. Pope HG, Lipinski JF: Diagnosis in schizophrenia and manic-depressive illness. Arch Gen Psychiatry, *35:*811–828, 1978.

8. Pope HG: Distinguishing bipolar disorder from schizophrenia in clinical practice: guidelines and case reports. Hosp Community Psychiatry, *34:*322–325, 1983.

9. Pope HG, Lipinski JF, et al.: Schizoaffective disorder: An invalid diagnosis? Am J Psychiatry, *137:*921–927, 1980.

10. Brockington IF, Hillier VF, et al.: Definitions of mania: Concordance and prediction of outcome. Am J Psychiatry, *140:*435–439, 1983.

11. Bond TC: Recognition of acute delirious mania. Arch Gen Psychiatry, *37:*553–554, 1980.

12. Chiles JA, Cohen DP: Pseudodementia and mania. J Nerv Ment Dis, *167:*357–358, 1979.

13. Cowdry RW, Goodwin FK: Dementia of bipolar illness: Diagnosis and response to lithium. Am J Psychiatry, *138:*1118–1119, 1981.

14. Slavney PR, et al.: Phencyclidine abuse and symptomatic mania. Biol Psychiatry, *12:*697–699, 1977.

15. Staseik C, Zetin M: Organic manic disorders. Psychosomatics, *26:*394–402, 1985.

16. Mapelli G, Bellelli TP: Secondary mania (letter to the editor). Arch Gen Psychiatry, *39:*743, 1982.

17. Mapelli G, Ramelli E: Manic syndrome associated with multiple sclerosis: Secondary Mania? Acta Psychiatr Belg, *81:*337–349, 1981.

18. Glaser GH: Psychotic reactions induced by corticotropin (ACTH) and cortisone. Psychosom Med, *15:*280–291, 1953.

19. Boyd JH, Weissman MM: Epidemiology of affective disorders. Arch Gen Psychiatry, *38:*1039–1046, 1981.

20. Krauthammer C, Klerman GL: The epidemiology of mania, in Shopsin B (ed), *Manic Illness,* pp. 11–28, New York, Raven Press, 1979.

21. Coryell W, Endicott J, Keller M, et al.: Bipolar affective disorder and high achievement: A familial association. Am J Psychiatry, *146:*983–988, 1989.

22. Faris REL, Dunham HW: *Mental Disorders in Urban Areas: An Ecological Study of Schizophrenia and Other Psychoses,* Chicago, University of Chicago Press, 1939.

23. Maltzberg B: Mental disease in relation to economic status. J Nerv Ment Dis, *123:*256, 1956.

24. Woodruff RA, et al.: Manic depressive illness and social achievement. Acta Psychiatr Scand, *47:*237–249, 1971.

25. Reich T, et al.: Family history studies: V. The genetics of mania. Am J Psychiatry, *125:*1358–1369, 1969.

26. Johnson GFS, Leeman MM: Analysis of familial factors in bipolar affective illness. Arch Gen Psychiatry, *34:*1074–1083, 1977.

27. Weissman MM, Gershon ES, et al.: Psychiatric disorders in the relatives of probands with affective disorders. Arch Gen Psychiatry, *41:*13–21, 1984.

28. Gershon ES, Hamovit J, et al.: A fam-

ily study of schizoaffective, bipolar I, bipolar II, unipolar, and normal control probands. Arch Gen Psychiatry, 39:1157–1167, 1982.

29. Annitto W, Shopsin B: Neuropharmacology, in Shopsin B (ed): *Manic Illness*, pp. 128–149, New York, Raven Press, 1979.

30. Schildkraut JJ: The catecholamine hypothesis of affective disorders. Am J Psychiatry, 122:509–522, 1965.

31. Schildkraut JJ: The effects of lithium on biogenic amines, in Gershon S, Shopsin B (eds): *Lithium: Its Role in Psychiatric Research and Treatment*, New York, Plenum Press, 1973.

32. Gerner RH, et al.: A dopaminergic mechanism in mania. Am J Psychiatry, 133:1177–1180, 1976.

33. Jouvent R, Lecrubier Y, et al.: Antimanic effect of clonidine. Am J Psychiatry, 137:1275–1276, 1980.

34. Swann AC, Secunda S, et al.: CSF monoamine metabolites in mania. Am J Psychiatry, 140:396–400, 1983.

35. Davis KL, et al.: Physostigmine in mania. Arch Gen Psychiatry, 35:119–122, 1978.

36. Nadi NS, Nurnberger JI, et al.: Muscarinic cholinergic receptors in skin fibroblasts in familial affective disorder. N Engl J Med, 311:225–230, 1984.

37. Snyder SS: Cholingeric mechanisms in affective disorders. N Engl J Med, 311:254–255, 1984.

38. Ambelas A: Psychologically stressful events in the precipitation of manic episodes. Br J Psychiatry, 135:15–21, 1979.

39. Ezquiaga E, Guitierrez JLA, Lopez AG: Psychosocial factors and episode number in depression. J Affective Disord, 12:135–138, 1989.

40. Post RM, Weiss SR: Sensitization, kindling and anticonvulsants in mania. J Clin Psychiatry, (Suppl 12) 50:23–30, 1989.

41. Wehr TA: Sleep loss: A preventable cause of mania and other excited states. J Clin Psychiatry, (Suppl 12) 50:8–16, 1989.

42. Lewy AJ, Nurnberger JI, Wehr TA, et al.: Supersensitivity to light: Possible trait marker for manic-depressive illness. Am J Psychiatry, 142:725–727, 1985.

43. Sitaram N, Dube S, Keshavan M, et al.: The association of supersensitive cholinergic REM-induction and affective illness with pedigrees. J Psychiatr Res, 21:487–497, 1987.

44. Gershon ES: Recent developments in the genetics of manic-depressive illness. J Clin Psychiatry, (Suppl 12) 50:4–7, 1989.

45. Wilson, DR: A deductive approach to the evolutionary epidemiology of bipolar disorder. Proceedings of the first meeting of the Evolution and Human Behavioral Society, Ann Arbor, Mi., 1988.

46. Abraham K: *Selected Papers on Psycho-Analysis*, London, Hogarth Press, 1950.

47. Lewin B: *The Psychoanalysis of Elation*, New York, W.W. Norton, 1950.

48. Deutsch H: The psychology of manic-depressive states, with particular reference to chronic hypomania, in *Neurosis and Character Types*, pp.203–217, New York, International University Press, 1965.

49. Rochlin G: Disorder of depression and elations. J Am Psychoanal Assoc, 1:438–457, 1953.

50. MacVane JR, et al.: Psychological functioning of bipolar manic-depressives in remission. Arch Gen Psychiatry, 35:1351–1354, 1978.

51. Cohen MB, Baker G, Cohen RA, et al.: An intensive study of 12 cases of manic-depressive psychosis. Psychiatry, 17:103–137, 1954.

52. Extein I, Pottash ALC, et al.: Differentiating mania from schizophrenia by the TRH test. Am J Psychiatry, 137:981–982, 1980.

53. Extein I, Pottash ALC, et al.: Using the protirelin test to distinguish mania from schizophrenia. Arch Gen Psychiatry, 39:77–81, 1982.

54. Amsterdam JD, Winokur A, et al.: A neuro-endocrine test battery in bipolar patients and health subjects. Arch Gen Psychiatry, 40:515–521, 1983.

55. Coffey EC, Ross DR: Treatment of lithium neuroleptic neurotoxicity during lithium maintenance. Am J Psychiatry, 137:736–737, 1980.

56. Spring G, Frankel M: New data on lithium and haldol incompatibility. Am J Psychiatry, 138:818–821, 1981.

57. Gelenberg A (ed): *Biological Therapies in Psychiatry Newsletter*, Massachusetts General Hospital, vol. 7, no. 6, 1984.

58. Kane JM, Woerner M, Borenstein M, et al.: Integrating incidence and prevalence of

tardive dyskinesia. Psychopharmacol Bull, 22:254–258, 1986.

59. Nasrallah HA, Churchill CM, Hamdan-Allan GA: Higher frequency of neuroleptic induced dystonia in mania than in schizophrenia. Am J Psychiatry, 145:1455–1456, 1988.

60. Sachs GS, Rosenbaum JF, Jones LJ: Adjunctive clonazepam for maintenance treatment of bipolar affective disorder. J Clin Psychopharm, 10:42–47, 1990.

61. Choinard G: Clonazepam in acute and maintenance treatment of bipolar affective disorder. J Clin Psychiatry, (Suppl 10) 48:29–36, 1987.

62. Baldessarini RJ: *Chemotherapy in Psychiatry,* pp. 57–75, Cambridge, Harvard University Press, 1977.

63. Gershon S, Shopsin B: *Lithium: Its Role in Psychiatric Research and Treatment,* New York, Plenum Press, 1973.

64. Davis, JM: Overview: Maintenance therapy in psychiatry, II. Affective disorders. Am J Psychiatry, 133:1–13, 1976.

65. Prein RF, Caffey EM, Klett CJ: Factors associated with lithium responses in the prophylatic treatment of bipolar manic-depressive illness. Arch Gen Psychiatry, 31:189–192, 1974.

66. Prien RF, Kupfer DJ, et al.: Drug therapy in the prevention of recurrences in unipolar and bipolar affective disorders. Arch Gen Psychiatry, 41:1096–1104, 1984.

67. Prien RF: NIMH Report: Five center study clarifies use of lithium, imipramine for recurrent affective disorders. Hosp Community Psychiatry, 35:1097–1098, 1984.

68. Schou M: Lithium prophylaxis; Myths and realities. Am J Psychiatry, 146:573–576, 1989.

69. Gelenberg A (ed): Lithium during pregnancy: Risks of cardiovascular malformations, in *Biological Therapies in Psychiatry Newsletter,* Massachusetts General Hospital, vol. 4, No. 1, 1981.

70. Nurnberg HG, Prudie J: Guidelines for treatment of psychosis during pregnancy. Hosp Community Psychiatry, 35:67–71, 1984.

71. Hetmar O, Brun C, Clemmensen L, et al.: Lithium: Long-term effects on the kidney. II. Structural changes. J Psychiatr Res 21:279–288, 1987.

72. Hetmar O, Clemmensen L, Ladefoged J, et al.: Lithium: Long-term effects on the kidney. III. Prospective study. Acta Psychiatr Scand 75:251–258, 1987.

73. Plenge P, Mellrup T: Lithium and the kidney: Is one daily dose better than two? Compr Psychiatry 27:336–342, 1986.

74. Gelenberg AJ, Carroll JA, Baudhuin MG, et al.: The meaning of serum lithium levels in maintenance therapy of mood disorders: A review of the literature. J Clin Psychiatry, (Suppl 12), 50:17–22, 1989.

75. Gelenberg AJ, Kane JM, Keller MB, et al.: Comparison of standard and low serum levels of lithium for maintenance treatment of bipolar disorder. N Engl J Med, 321:1489–1493, 1989.

76. Ramsey TA, Cox M: Lithium and the kidney: A review. Am J Psychiatry, 139:443–449, 1982.

77. Battle DC, von Riotte AB, et al.: Amelioration of polyuria by amiloride in patients receiving long-term lithium therapy. N Engl J Med, 312:408–414, 1985.

78. Gelenberg AJ, Wojcik JD, Falk WE: Effects of lithium on the kidney. Acta Psychiatr Scan, 75:29–34, 1987.

79. Hicks R: Thyroid and the psychiatrist. Biological Therapies in Psychiatry (MGH Newsletter), 1:1,2,7, 1978.

80. Calabrese JR, Gulledge AD, Hahn K, et al.: Autoimmune thyroiditis in manic-depressive patients treated with lithium. Am J Psychiatry, 142:1318–1321, 1985.

81. Vestergard P, Schou M: Prospective studies on a lithium cohort, 3: Tremor, weight gain, diarrhea, psychological complaints. Acta Psychiatr Scan, 78:434–441, 1988.

82. Prakash R: A review of the hematologic side effects of lithium. Hosp Community Psychiatry, 36:127–128, 1985.

83. Ebadi, M: Management of tremor by beta adrenergic blocking agents. Gen Pharmacol, 11:257–260, 1980.

84. Gaby NS, Lefkowitz DS, et al.: Treatment of lithium tremor with metoprolol. Am J Psychiatry, 140:593–595, 1983.

85. Jefferson JW, Greist JH: *Primer of Lithium Therapy,* p. 109–118, Baltimore, Williams & Wilkins, 1977.

86. Perry PJ, Calloway RA, et al.: The-

ophylline-precipitated alterations of lithium clearance. Acta Psychiatr Scand, *69*:528–537, 1984.

87. *Physician's Desk Reference*, p. 2239, Oradell, N.J., Medical Economics Company, Inc., 1990.

88. Mander AJ, Loudon JB: Rapid recurrence of mania following abrupt discontinuation of lithium. Lancet 2:15–17, 1988.

89. Post RM: Clinical perspectives on the use of carbamezepine in manic-depressive illness. Fair Oaks Hospital Psychiatry Letter, *3*:4, 1985.

90. Falk WE: Carbamezepine (tegretol) for manic-depressive illness: An update. Biological Therapies in Psychiatry (MGH newsletter), *8*:1,2,24, 1985.

91. Jones KL, Lacro RV, Johnson KA, et al.: Pattern of malformation in the children of women treated with carbamazepine during pregnancy. N Engl Med, *320*:1661–1666, 1989.

92. McElroy SL, Pope HG Jr, Keck PE Jr, Hudson JI: Valproate treatment of acute mania: A placebo-controlled study. Presented at the American Psychiatric Association Annual Meeting, New York, May, 1990.

93. Prein RF, Gelenberg AJ: Alternatives to lithium for preventive treatment of bipolar disorder. Am J Psychiatry, *146*:840–848, 1989.

94. McElroy SL, Keck PE, Pope HG: Sodium valproate: Its use in primary psychiatric disorders. J Clin Psychopharmacol, *7*:16–24, 1987.

95. Chouinard G: The use of benzodiazepines in the treatment of manic-depressive illness. J Clin Psychiatry, (Suppl 11), *49*:15–19, 1988.

96. Aaronson TA, Shukla S, Hirschowitz J: Clonazepam treatment of five lithium-refractory patients with bipolar disorder. Am J Psychiatry, *146*:77–80, 1989.

97. Giannini AJ, Extein I, et al.: Clonidine in mania. Drug Dev Res, *3*:101–103, 1983.

98. Znbenko GS, Cohen BM, et al.: Clonidine in the treatment of mania and mixed bipolar disorder. Am J Psychiatry, *141*:1617–1618, 1984.

99. Giannini AJ, Houser WL, et al.: Antimanic effects of verapamil. Am J Psychiatry, *141*:1602–1603, 1984.

100. Potter WZ, Murphy DL, et al.: Clorgyline. Arch Gen Psychiatry, *39*:505–510, 1982.

101. McCabe MS: ECT in the treatment of mania: A controlled study. Am J Psychiatry, *133*:688–691, 1976.

102. Weiner RD: The psychiatric use of electrically induced seizures. Am J Psychiatry, *136*:1507–1517, 1979.

103. Gunderson JG: Management of manic states: The problem of fire setting. Psychiatry, *37*:137–146, 1974.

104. Janowsky DS, Leff M, et al.: Playing the manic game. Arch Gen Psychiatry, *22*:252–261, 1970.

105. Janowsky DS, El-Yousef MK, et al.: Interpersonal maneuvers of manic patients. Am J Psychiatry, *131*:250–255, 1974.

106. Pope HG, Lipinski JF, Cohen BM: Psychotherapy of bipolar patients. Unpublished manuscript, 1987.

107. Kraeplin I: *Manic-Depressive Insanity and Paranoia*. Edinburgh, E. & S. Livingstone, 1921.

108. Molnar G, Feeney MG, Fava GA: Duration and symptoms of bipolar prodomes. Am J Psychiatry, *145*:1576–1578, 1988.

109. Jamison KR, Goodwin FK: Psychotherapeutic issues in bipolar illness., in Grinspoon L (ed): *Psychiatry Update: Volume II*, pp. 319–337, Washington, D.C., 1983.

110. De-Nour AK: Psychosocial aspects of the management of mania, in Belmaker RH, Van Praag HM (eds): *Mania: An Evolving Concept*, pp. 349–365, New York, Spectrum Publications, 1980.

111. Mayo JA, O'Connell RA, et al.: Families of manic-depressive patients: Effect of treatment. Am J Psychiatry, *136*:1535–1539, 1979.

112. Tsuang MT: Genetic counseling for psychiatric patients and their families. Am J Psychiatry, *135*:1465–1475, 1978.

113. Winokur G, Clayton P: Family history studies: Two types of affective disorders separated according to genetic and clinical factors, in Wortis J (ed): *Recent Advances in Biological Psychiatry*, Vol. 9, New York, Plenum Publishing Corp., 1967.

114. Rosenbaum AH, Barry MJ: Positive therapeutic response to lithium in hypomania secondary to organic brain syndrome. Am J Psychiatry, *132*:1072–1073, 1975.

115. Goolker P, Schein J: Psychic effects of ACTH and cortisone. Psychosom Med, 15:589–597, 1953.

116. Carney MW: Five cases of bromism. Lancet, 2:523–524, 1971.

117. Jefferson JW: Questioning a diagnosis. Am J Psychiatry, 133:1208–1209, 1976.

118. Weisert KN, Hendrie HC: Secondary mania? A case report. Am J Psychiatry, 134:929–930, 1977.

119. Oppler W: Manic psychosis in a case of parasagittal meningioma. Arch Neurol Psychiatry, 64:417–430, 1950.

120. Steinberg D, Hirsch SR, et al.: Influenza infection causing manic psychosis. Br J Psychiatry, 124:140–143, 1974.

121. Kane CS, Taylor TW: Mania associated with the use of INH and cocaine. Am J Psychiatry, 119:1098–1099, 1963.

122. Ryback RS, Schwab RS: Manic response to levodopa therapy: Report of a case. N Engl J Med, 285:788–789, 1971.

123. France RD, Krishnan KR: Alprazolam-induced manic reaction (letter to the editor). Am J Psychiatry, 141:1127–1128, 1984.

124. Price LH, Charney DS, et al.: Three cases of manic symptoms following yohimbine administration. Am J Psychiatry, 141:1267–1268, 1984.

125. Goodwin FK, Jamison KR: The natural course of manic-depressive illness, in Post RM, Ballenger JC (eds): Neurobiology of Mood Disorders, pp. 20–37, Baltimore, Williams & Wilkins, 1984.

126. Tohen N, Waternaux CM, Tsuang MT, Hunt AT: Four-year follow-up of twenty-four first-episode manic patients. J Affective Disorders, in Press.

127. Keller MB: The course of manic-depressive illness. J Clin Psychiatry, (Suppl 11), 49:4–6, 1988.

128. Zis AP, Grof P, Goodwin FK: The natural course of affective disorders: Implications for lithium prophylaxis, in Cooper et al.: Lithium: Controversies and Unresolved Issues, pp. 381–398, Amsterdam, Excerpta Medica, 1979.

129. Perris C: Study of bipolar (manic-depressive) and unipolar recurrent depressive psychosis. Acta Psychiatra Scand, (Suppl 194), 42:68–82, 1966.

130. Derby IM: Manic-depressive "exhaustion" deaths. Psychiatr Q, 7:435–449, 1933.

131. Wehr TA, Goodwin FK: Can antidepressants cause mania and worsen the course of affective illness? Am J Psychiatry, 144:1403–1411, 1987.

Schizophrenic Disorders

Lloyd I. Sederer, MD

DEFINITION

Schizophrenia is not a unitary disorder. Varied clinical presentations, natural histories, family histories, and responses to treatment lead us to believe that a spectrum of pathology exists which we can term schizophrenic disorders.

Though there is considerable controversy in the field about the essential features of the schizophrenic disorders, the third edition of the *Diagnostic and Statistical Manual of Mental Disorders* (DSM-IIIR) (1) details the current state of thinking in this area. The features that distinguish schizophrenia* include the absence of any organic or affective disorder that may have existed before or concurrent with the schizophrenic disorder, a characteristic acute symptom complex and a deterioration in functioning over time (see Diagnosis, page 71), and a tendency toward onset early in adult life and a proclivity toward chronicity.

---

*In this chapter schizophrenia and schizophrenic disorders will be used interchangeably with the understanding that both terms convey a spectrum of disorders.

CASE EXAMPLE: This was the first psychiatric hospitalization for Ms. A., a 23-year-old unemployed, white, single female admitted to the hospital with the chief complaint of "nervousness."

The patient maintained that she had been "sick all of my life." On more specific questioning she indicated that her problems dated back to the ninth grade. At that time she began to suspect that she was not normal; she became suspicious of other people, withdrew from friends and family, and began to develop a "dream world" in which she imagined becoming an actress. She became increasingly preoccupied in her fantasy world while listening to music and spending hours grooming herself in front of a mirror.

Although she did poorly for the remainder of high school, she did graduate and began to work in a factory doing simple assembly work. She continued to live at home. Her work was considered marginal and her isolation continued.

At age 20, Ms. A. was laid off from work. Thereafter, she became more isolated and withdrawn and began to think that she was really two people—someone who was attractive, social, and active and someone who was "deranged." She became obsessed with the idea that someone else existed who was either identical to her or could be created by surgery. She fantasized that eggs found in her menses could be recycled in such a way as to produce clones of herself. Her suspiciousness increased and she began to experience the words "no children" inserted into her thoughts.

In the course of the next year, Ms. A. continued her isolation at home, doing little and relying heavily on her family. She developed an additional preoccupation that her face had changed its appearance. She began to worry that her nose would begin to grow if she touched it.

Several weeks before admission the patient became particularly despondent about her life and planned suicide, mixing together bleach and toilet bowl cleaner which she thought would create a gas that would poison her. Her mother discovered this plan and arranged for psychiatric consultation.

DIAGNOSIS

Demence Precoce (dementia praecox), a term denoting early dementia, was introduced by Morel in 1852 (2). Morel described a clinical case in which thought disorder (dementia) occurred in an adolescent boy. By the end of the 19th century Kraepelin proposed that the term dementia praecox refer to those psychotic patients whose disorder is of early onset and which proceeds along a chronic and deteriorating course (3). Kraepelin, inspired by Koch's principles of etiology and pathogenesis, sought to separate dementia praecox from "circular insanity" (manic-depressive illness) and to establish that discrete mental disorders exist with different causes, courses, and prognoses.

Less than two decades after Kraepelin, Bleuler introduced the term schizophrenia, literally split soul, in order to portray a very different view of this disorder (4). Bleuler stressed that in schizophrenia mental functions (e.g., will, cognition, and affect) were split and that disparate feelings could not be integrated. From his experience with a large hospital population which he systematically and longitudinally studied, he also argued that not all cases of "dementia praecox" take a pernicious and deteriorating course.

Bleuler's diagnostic criteria have been characterized as the "four A's." His work continues to have conceptual utility.

1. *Autism:* A tendency to withdraw from reality into idiosyncratic fantasy.
2. *Association:* A loosening of thoughts or associations.
3. *Affect:* Affects or feelings tend to be split off or inappropriate to the situation at hand.
4. *Ambivalence:* Profoundly mixed or contradictory feelings or attitudes tend to preoccupy the patient, sometimes to the point of immobility.

For Bleuler, symptoms of hallucinations, delusions, catatonic stupor, and negativism were of secondary importance.

Schneider approached the diagnosis of schizophrenia from a phenomenological perspective in which particular internal experiences were the hallmark of schizophrenia (5). In his view, schizophrenia was characterized by "first-rank" symptoms which were pathognomonic of the disorder. Though considerable evidence refutes the diagnostic certainty of his criteria, their subjective and clinical utility are quite valuable (6–10).

1.   Audible thoughts: Patients experience hallucinatory voices that echo or speak their thoughts aloud.

2.   Voices debating or disagreeing: Patients experience hallucinatory voices engaged in debate or argument, frequently about themselves.

3.   Voices commentating: Patients experience hallucinatory voices that comment on their actions.

4.   Somatic passivity: Patients believe that sensations are imposed upon their bodies by an outside force.

5.   Thought withdrawal: Patients experience their thoughts as withdrawn or taken out of their minds by an outside force.

6.   Thought insertion: Patients experience thoughts as put into their minds by an outside force.

7. *Thought broadcasting:* Patients experience their thoughts as being disseminated to the world around them.

8. *"Made" feelings:* Patients experience their feelings as not their own but imposed upon them.

9. *"Made" impulses:* Patients experience, and generally act upon, a compelling impulse which they believe is not their own.

10. *"Made" acts:* Patients experience their actions and will to be under the control of an outside force.

11. *Delusional perception:* Patients take a percept in their environment (e.g., a person or event) and ascribe idiosyncratic value to it. The perception is then developed into a delusion.

The current consensus, as offered by the DSM-IIIR of the American Psychiatric Association, is Kraepelinian in its tone. DSM-IIIR describes schizophrenic disorders as generally occurring in adolescence or early adulthood and resulting in chronic deterioration in multiple areas of life functioning.

DSM-IIIR creates a diagnostic framework for schizophrenia built on three legs:

(*a*) observable, describable symptoms such as delusions and hallucinations; associative and affective disturbances; and behavioral abnormalities; (*b*) deterioration in functioning in school, work, interpersonal relations or self-care; (*c*) duration of at least six months. Prodromal and residual symptoms are also identified. DSM-IIIR (and the soon to be DSM-IV) enables us to more specifically diagnose this disorder which has suffered from diagnostic trends and cultural biases. As diagnostic reliability improves so will our capacity to conduct outcome-oriented treatment research and more accurately project course and prognosis.

DIFFERENTIAL DIAGNOSIS

Organic Disorders

Table 3.1 outlines the organic differential diagnosis of schizophrenia. If any of these conditions is suspected, further evaluation is essential. Consultations with internal medicine, neurology, and infectious disease should be obtained according to the disorder suspected.

Table 3.1. Organic Differential Diagnosis of Schizophrenia

Toxins—Exogenous	*Infections*	*Nutritional Deficiencies*
Amphetamines	Viral encephalitis: herpes	Niacine: pellagra
Cocaine	Meningitis; viral or bacterial	Thiamine: Wernicke-Korsakoff's
Psychomimetics	Meningitus; lues	syndrome
LSD (lysergic acid diethylamide)	SBE (subacute bacterial endocarditis)	*Vascular Abnormalities*
PCP[17] (phencyclidine)	*Metabolic—Endocrine*	Collagen disorders
Mescaline	Thyroid	Aneurysm
Alcohol	Hyperthyroidism	Intracranial hemorrhage
Alcoholic hallucinosis	Hypothyroidism	*Cerebral Hypoxia*
Alcohol withdrawal states,	Adrenal disease	Secondary to severe anemia
including DTs (delirium	Addison's disease	Secondary to decreased
tremens)	Cushing's disease	cardiac output
Barbiturates	Porphyria	*Miscellaneous*
Barbiturate intoxication	Electrolyte imbalances	Complex partial seizures:
Barbiturate withdrawal	*Space-Occupying Lesions*	temporal lobe epilepsy
Steroids	Tumors	Wilson's disease
Anticholinergics	Primary tumors	Huntington's chorea
	Metastases, e.g., lung, breast	Normal pressure hydrocephalus
	Subdural hematoma	
	Brain abscess	

Functional Disorders

Affective Disorders

1. Mania (see Chapter 2).
2. Delusional (psychotic) depression.

In an affective disorder the patient's symptoms meet the criteria for an affective disorder and either precede or are concurrent with the psychotic symptomatology.

Because there appear to be no pathognomonic signs of schizophrenia, the patient must be assessed longitudinally. The diagnosis of schizophrenia should be deferred until symptoms are present for six months.

Schizoaffective Disorder

There has been controversy about the validity of this diagnosis (11, 12). Until nosological clarity is improved, it is best to avoid the diagnosis of schizoaffective disorder, when possible. If affective symptomatology is present, the patient should be considered for trials on the variety of biological treatments known to be effective in affective disorders (e.g., a combined tricyclic and neuroleptic regimen, lithium, or electroconvulsive therapy [ECT]).

Delusional Disorder

Formerly known as paranoia, delusional disorder is a syndrome in which a persistent delusion preoccupies the patient. Delusions may be persecuting, jealous, erotic, grandiose, or somatic. The syndrome occurs without evidence of an affective disorder, an organic brain syndrome, and without the characteristic acute symptoms of schizophrenia (e.g., hallucinations, bizarre delusions, loose or incoherent thought processes, disorganized behavior) (13).

Schizophreniform Psychosis

Schizophreniform psychoses are *brief* psychotic episodes whose symptoms are indistinguishable from those of schizophrenia. When the syndrome is of less than six months duration, it is considered a schizophreniform psychosis (14, 15).

Personality Disorders

Paranoid personality: Paranoid individuals are unusually mistrustful and suspicious, emotionally constricted, and hypersensitive. They do not, however, evidence psychotic symptomatology.

Schizotypal personality: This relatively new diagnostic term was introduced in the DSM-III, though the concept it refers to is not new. In the past, these patients were referred to as latent, borderline, or ambulatory schizophrenics (16). Schizotypal individuals show a variety of oddities in their thinking, behavior, perceptions, and speech. They are peculiar in demeanor and often show social anxiety and isolation as well as a limited capacity for relatedness. Thinking may be magical and ideas of reference may occur.

Though many of these features suggest schizophrenia, schizotypal patients do not meet the criteria for schizophrenia. They fall short of demonstrating the severe and persistent signs of schizophrenia.

Borderline Personality with Psychosis: Borderline patients may show transient disturbances in reality testing and may have brief psychotic episodes. The presence of other symptomatology (see Chapter 4) and the transiency of the psychotic process easily distinguishes these patients over time.

EPIDEMIOLOGY

Incidence

The incidence of a disorder is the number of new cases in a given population during the course of one year. The World Health Organization (WHO) cross-cultural study of schizophrenia revealed a range from .15–.42 cases per thousand, or .015–0.4% of the population (17). Not a great variation in incidence was found in the seven disparate research sites. Several reports in this country describe an incidence of schizophrenia of .05% (18–20). This translates into greater than 100,000 new cases of schizophrenia in the U.S. each year.

Lifetime Prevalence

The National Institute of Mental Health (NIMH) Epidemiologic Catchment Area (ECA) study reported the total lifetime prevalence for schizophrenia to range from 1.0–1.9% (21, 22). The ECA figures are higher than the 1.0% prevalence estimates that have been generally accepted (23). If schizophreniform disorders are added to those estimates another 0.1–0.3% of the population is affected, bringing estimates of schizophrenic-spectrum patients to number almost several million in the United States.

Age, Sex, Race

The onset of schizophrenia is typically in adolescence or young adulthood. Schizophrenia is most prevalent in persons aged 15–50, though late-onset is not as uncommon as previously described (21, 22, 24). Men and women are equally affected though onset is often earlier in men. Schizophrenic disorders were thought to be more common in nonwhites than whites but recent work calls this distinction into question (25).

Socioeconomic Status

The prevalence of schizophrenia is highest in lower socioeconomic levels of society. Controversy exists whether this is related to "social causation" or "drift." In the former, the increased stresses of lower socioeconomic living are attributed to fostering schizophrenia. The latter hypothesis argues that social factors do not pertain etiologically but that, instead, schizophrenics drift toward the lower echelons of society (20, 26, 27).

Families

In families where there is one schizophrenic parent, 12% of the children are likely to develop schizophrenia. In families with two schizophrenic parents, 35–45% of the children are likely to develop schizophrenia (23).

THEORIES OF ETIOLOGY

Genetic

A genetic role in the etiology of schizophrenia, particularly the chronic expression of the disorder, is clear. Evidence for this conclusion derives from twin studies, family pedigree studies, and investigations of adoptees.

Studies of twins reveal a significantly higher concordance of schizophrenia in monozygotic than dizygotic twins. Concordance is 40–50% in monozygotic twins in contrast to 9–10% concordance in dizygotic twins (28, 29). As noted earlier, the incidence of schizophrenia in the general population is approximately 0.05%, whereas the incidence in parents of schizophrenics is 5% and in siblings, about 10%.

In a joint project between Danish and American investigators, Kety et al. (30) studied the relatives of schizophrenic patients who were adoptees. More specifically, they studied the prevalence and types of mental illness in the biological and adoptive relatives of adoptees who become schizophrenic. The study findings demonstrated that 13.9% of those genetically related to the schizophrenic index cases received a diagnosis in the schizophrenic spectrum. This finding compares to 2.7% of the adoptive relatives of the schizophrenic index cases who were found to have schizophrenic spectrum disorders. These differences, if accurate, (31–35) are highly significant statistically and strongly support the operation of genetic factors in schizophrenia.

Kety's findings support genetic transmission in schizophrenia, though they may not be finally conclusive. In utero influences, trauma at birth, and very early mothering influences might account for the same findings. However, a significant percentage of schizophrenic disorders was found in the paternal half siblings of schizophrenics with whom they shared no prenatal or postnatal environment.

In a pedigree study of seven English and Icelandic families made possible by advances in genetic research, a specific dominant allele locus on chromosome 5 was identified as predisposing individuals to schizophrenia (35). However, contrary evidence has also been reported, leaving many more questions about where and how the gene pool exerts its actions (26, 37).

In summary, incidence studies in the general population, twin studies, and prevalence studies in adoptive relatives all support the hypothesis that genetic factors operate in the transmission of schizophrenia. However, the evidence is not adequate to support a conclusion that a genetic etiology is a sufficient cause of schizophrenia. A polygenic model appears likely in which biologic liability to illness increases as the individual approaches the upper end of a curve (representing genetic loading). Therefore, risk to relatives of an affected proband would be highest in first-degree relatives and decrease as relatives became more distant. The polygenic model would also conform to the evidence that risk of schizophrenia also confers risk for schizophrenic spectrum disorders (e.g., schizoaffective disorder and schizotypal personality) (38). By inference, such a model also points to the importance of environmental factors in the development of schizophrenia, which is consistent with a (genetic) diathesis-stress model of schizophrenia.

Biochemical Hypotheses

Abnormalities in dopamine have been the dominant biochemical theory of schizophrenic psychoses. The dopamine hypothesis grew out of psychopharmacological findings on the action of drugs that either improve or mimic schizophrenia. The antipsychotic agents with their dopamine blockade, the paranoid psychosis of amphetamine toxicity, and the fact that amphetamine, (39) methylphenidate, and L-dopa can all induce psychotic episodes in schizophrenic patients provided inferential support to the hypothesis that schizophrenia is an hyperdopaminergic condition that principally affects the mesolimbic and mesocortical regions of the brain (39–41).

The advent of Positron Emission Tomography (PET) and postmortem brain investigations have added more direct evidence of the role of dopamine in schizophrenia (42). In particular, schizophrenic patients may demonstrate hyperactivity of D2 receptors (43, 44). However, excess dopamine activity may not be what is influencing behavior in chronic schizophrenics with negative symptoms; reduced dopamine activity or even cholinergic hyperactivity may be implicated for that disorder (45, 46).

Though dopamine has had center stage for inquiry and theory, other neurotransmitters may also be implicated in the biochemistry of schizophrenia (47). Serotonin, acetylcholine, norepinephrine, and gamma-aminobutyric acid (GABA) as well as neuropeptides may play a part in the pathophysiology of the disorder. No single factor has been clearly established though treatment is empirically aimed at muting dopamine activity, especially in the mesolimbic pathways of the central nervous system (CNS).

Neuropathological Hypotheses

Computerized axial tomography (CT) scanning prompted a renaissance of interest in neuropathological and neuroanatomic theories of schizophrenia. Subsequent technical advancements in imaging (e.g., magnetic resonance imaging [MRI], positron emission tomography [PET], single photon emission tomography [SPECT]) have enabled researchers to monitor cerebral blood flow and disclose brain physiology and chemistry. Accumulating evidence now supports the view that some patients with schizophrenia have larger cerebral ventricles and/or evidence of cortical atrophy when compared to same-age normal controls and the siblings of affected individuals. Poor premorbid history, cognitive impairment, negative symptoms, and poor response to treatment have been correlated with abnormal neuroanatomical findings (48–52).

Cerebral blood flow studies report deficits in frontal lobe perfusion in schizophrenic patients, especially when engaged in a task requiring frontal lobe activity. PET, which can assay and visualize neuronal metabolism, further supports frontal deficits in schizophrenia (42, 53–55).

Brain electrical activity mapping (BEAM) performed on schizophrenic patients has shown increased frontal and left parietal frequencies. Nuclear magnetic resonance (NMR), a technique that allows for mapping specific brain nuclides, may yield knowledge in the years to come (56).

Neurostructural and neurophysiological research into schizophrenia has only begun. The techniques available offer considerable promise in advancing our understandings of schizophrenia and shaping our biological treatments.

Perceptual-Cognitive Hypotheses

Consistent with abnormal neuroanatomic and neuropathological findings are reports of cognitive impairment in schizophrenia. Though more research needs to accumulate, important data suggest a dementing process influences schizophrenic cognition (57, 58).

Perceptual theorists suggest that schizophrenic withdrawal and apathy is a defensive maneuver against a flooding of perceptions that the schizophrenic cannot receive and adequately assimilate (59). The primary disturbance has been described as an inability to filter out, or "gate," extraneous percepts from meaningful stimuli. A diminished or limited capacity for sensory gating may be a trait deficit of schizophrenia (60, 61).

Lidz (62) regards the schizophrenic's deficiencies in category formation as instrumental to cognitive dysfunction. Category formation, he hypothesizes, is the cognitive process by which extraneous percepts and associations are filtered out. The schizophrenic's limited (and egocentric) capacity to form categories and filter properly render him vulnerable to perceptual overload and cognitive dysfunction.

Psychodynamic Hypotheses

Ego Disturbances

Early psychoanalytic theory espoused the primacy of drives. As the theory matured, recognition of and respect for the ego developed. Hartmann, in particular, described the capacity of the ego to sustain itself in the face of drives, to organize adaptive responses, and to maintain dimensions of its functioning that are conflict free (62). Hartmann broadened early defense/conflict notions of schizophrenia to include ego defects. He regarded the ego of schizophrenic patients to have an inborn deficit which would be overwhelmed by internal drive demands, particularly aggressive needs.

Ego psychology has been generally eclipsed by object-relations theory and the work of the British object-relations school (especially Klein, Fairbairn, Guntrip and Winnicott) (63). Melanie Klein was a forerunner of this theoretical movement and her ideas underly many of her successors. Klein (64) hypothesized that a constitutional (biological) defect in very early ego functions (which include the capacity to regulate and control drives, relate to objects in the environment, understand and respond to the external reality, and function cognitively) renders children vulnerable to disturbances in the relationship with their mother. A disturbance in any of these ego functions, particularly a drive disturbance with consequent intense hostility and aggression in the infant, may produce distortions in the mother-infant relationship and promote the development of a personality which will be highly vulnerable to disorganization.

Less constitutionally predisposed theorists also attribute schizophrenia to disturbances in the mother-infant relationship. Margaret Mahler (65, 66) has postulated the importance of the separation-individuation phase of childhood development as crucial in the pathogenesis of schizophrenia. The psychological task for children at this developmental stage is achieving a sense of self separate from their mother, with clear self-boundaries and a capacity to appreciate the separateness and constancy of other persons in their environment. Mahler suggested that the schizophrenic person never achieves a sense of object constancy. An impaired ego leaves the schizophrenic adult especially sensitive to stress, particularly loss. When stressed, the schizophrenic regresses in ego functions. More specifically, the schizophrenic, when stressed, no longer can employ higher ego defenses which maintain boundaries and reality as well as integrate feelings and drives. Stress induces a regression and more primitive defenses compromising reality are employed. The typical defenses in schizophrenic psychosis are delusional denial, projection, and severe distortion.

Interpersonal Disturbances

Harry Stack Sullivan's (67, 68) theoretical writings and clinical practice perhaps stand at the heart of the interpersonal

schools. Sullivan helped extricate psychoanalytic thinking from its intrapsychic locus and relocate it to the interpersonal sphere. Sullivan believed that mental illness arises from a failure in interpersonal relationships. He maintained that psychiatric illness or well-being was the product of continuous interaction from birth onward between the individual and important others in the environment.

Sullivan considered the schizophrenic patient as a human being who had been robbed, early in life, of crucial opportunities for interpersonal learning and gratification. Built into this conception is the premise that the development of a real and corrective human relationship with the schizophrenic patient could improve the patient's attempts at establishing a more secure and gratifying interpersonal world.

Family Hypotheses

The families of schizophrenic patients have been examined for their communication patterns, psychopathology, and relationship structures.

Though it is unlikely that disturbed and disordered *communication* in a family is sufficient cause for schizophrenia, an interactive effect between a genetic diathesis and familial influences may help explain the pathogenesis of the disorder (69–73). It is important to recognize that the view that difficulties within the family may be a product of a subclinically disordered child is as valid as the view that the family may have generated the child's illness.

A now dated but significant early theory of communication in schizophrenic families is that of "double binds." (70). In a double bind, contradictory messages are given to a recipient who is unable to escape from the transaction. For example, the mother of a schizophrenic patient arrived on the ward to visit. Upon her arrival, the patient warmly put his arms around her. She visibly stiffened and he withdrew his embrace. Mother then said, "Don't be so embarrassed about showing your feelings." Double-bind theory is based on observing a pattern of behavior or interaction. It does not aim to portray mothers as villainous or as "schizophrenogenic." If this pattern is established within a family, the entire sequence of the double bind may not be needed to induce an experience of confusion and panic in the schizophrenic patient.

Lidz (69, 74) has reported that the parents of schizophrenics employ defective language and categories which, in turn, transmit irrationality to the child. In his view the parents sacrifice language and categorization in order to maintain their distorted and egocentric view of the family and the world. These parents are said to be in tenuous emotional balance and must therefore distort their perceptions in a profoundly egocentric manner in order to avoid deeper distress and disorganization. The children thus inhabit a family in which they must distort or invalidate their perceptions (to conform to those of their parents) or be rejected. Lidz emphasized that severe parental egocentricity precludes their capacity to separate and distinguish their feelings and perceptions from those of the child (and others). Examples include parental intrusiveness into the child's life without consideration for the child's needs or feelings, a belief that the child cannot function in any way without the parent(s), and the use of the child to provide meaning and purpose for the parent(s). Lidz hypothesized that the boundary disturbances that follow are central to the origin and characteristics of the schizophrenic thought disorder.

Wynne and Singer (71, 75, 76) have described thought disorder in which distortion, diffusion, and confusion prevail in families. Their work offers important examples of the *psychopathological signs and symptoms* seen in schizophrenic families. Schizophrenic families, they maintained, are "pseudomutual"; that is, characterized by a compelling need to believe that all the members share the same needs and expectations. Unclear messages, contradictions, denial of what is said or perfectly obvious, and fragmented and amorphous communications making focus difficult are all examples of how the pseudomutual family disturbs thought and communication. These maneuvers maintain the illusion that divergence or individuality do not exist within the family.

Cognitive disturbances in schizophrenic families also include difficulties in family members sharing a focus of attention and bringing subjects to a close. The tendency is towards disruptive and unusual verbal behavior that does not allow communication to proceed in a rational, goal-directed fashion. Families of schizophrenic patients may also show many other symptoms of schizophrenia, namely, loose associations, idiosyncratic thinking, paranoia, and ambivalence.

Family *structure* is the way the family organizes and ranks its relationships. Schizophrenic families may show markedly rigid, chaotic, or disturbed structures and relationships. The parents of female schizophrenic patients have been described by Lidz (69) as "schismatic." In the parents' marriages overt strife exists between the parents, who exhibit "emotional divorce" (albeit not actual). Such parents may invite the child to join as an ally in this battle of mutual derogation. The mother's preexisting low self-esteem and doubt about her mothering is repeatedly intensified by the father who regards women with contempt. The mother conveys a sense of meaninglessness about her life and cannot feel gratified by a daughter because of the mother's unhappiness in being a woman. Though perhaps well functioning out of the home because of his rigid organization, the father is as disturbed as the mother. The father is generally deeply insecure in his masculinity and needs his wife to comply passively with whatever he needs to maintain his self-esteem. Disagreement or difference on the wife's part is seen as hostility and insubordination. Since the mother cannot meet the father's needs for unwavering and unrealistic admiration, he turns to the daughter in a manner that approximates an incestuous relationship. The female child is torn between both parents and compromises her needs and development as she repeatedly changes alliances and constantly fends off rejection from both parents.

The families of male schizophrenics in Lidz's work tend to show "marital skew." The mother is highly intrusive in her son's life without regard for him as a separate person with separate feelings and needs. Empty and unfulfilled as a woman, the mother conveys that life would be meaningless without her son. The boy eventually believes that his mother cannot live without him and (because he has developed so rudimentary a belief in himself) that he is unable to live without her. This is true symbiosis. The father in these families is passive, inept, and subject to constant derision. The boy cannot turn to his father to escape identification and symbiosis with the mother. As a result, severe boundary and gender disturbances ensue.

From these theories we could infer that parental or family system pathology is causal (and potentially blameworthy) in the development of schizophrenia. Such a conclusion today would be erroneous. Parents and their children are in dynamic equilibrium and influence each other. Although disturbances exist in the functioning of families, these may be epiphenomena of the disease process rather than etiopathogenic influences. More recent work has focused on disturbances in families as they influence the course of the disorder. These are the "expressed emotion" and psychoeducation models of the family of schizophrenic patients. Because of its central role in assessment and treatment, this material will be addressed in the respective sections that follow.

THE BIOPSYCHOSOCIAL EVALUATION

The biopsychosocial evaluation integrates biological, psychodynamic, and social factors with understanding, evaluating, and treating psychiatric disorders. In general, schizophrenia presents to the inpatient clinician as acute psychosis. The workup for the acutely psychotic patient will be described below in its biological, psychodynamic, and social and family aspects.

The Biological Evaluation

(See also Differential Diagnosis Section, page 84)

History

A detailed history includes the present illness; past medical and psychiatric illnesses, including any past or current medications or treatments; family history, with particular emphasis on inheritable disorders and psychiatric syndromes in the family; habits, including drug and dietary; a thorough review of systems, with particular attention to history of trauma or any recent changes in any of the organ systems; and a thorough *mental status examination.*

History taking is best done from the patient with collaborative information obtained from family and significant others who have witnessed the patient's behavior and the progressive development of the illness.

The Physical Examination

Particular attention must be paid to the patient's vital signs and pupils, the presence of nuchal pain and rigidity, the presence of diaphoresis, and the neurological examination.

Laboratory Studies

Routine admission tests can include a complete blood count (CBC), urinalysis, toxic screen, serum test for syphilis, blood glucose, sodium (Na), potassium (K), chlorine (Cl), carbon dioxide (CO_2), calcium (Ca), phosphate (PO_4), creatinine, blood urea nitrogen (BUN), alkaline phosphatase, serum glutamic-oxaloacetic transaminase (SGOT), bilirubin-total/direct (T/D), thyroxine (FT_4), and free thyroxine (FT_4). Additional studies may be warranted for selected patients, based on specific signs, symptoms or abnormal laboratory findings. These include blood cultures, zinc, magnesium, bromine, ceruloplasm, ammonia (NH_3), erythrocyte sedimentation rate (ESR), vitamin B_{12}, folic acid, arterial blood gases, electrocardiogram (EKG), lumbar puncture, human immunodeficiency virus (HIV) testing and screens for anabolic steroids.

Electroencephalogram (EEG) assessment (including sleep-deprivation studies) may be indicated wherever cerebral dysrhythmias are suspected as a part of the differential diagnosis or as contributing to the patient's instability. BEAM studies are advancing the diagnostic information of the traditional EEG.

Imaging

The era of brain imaging is upon us with its remarkable advances in technology (42). The routine use of CT scans and MRI for patients with schizophrenic illness is not yet established. Even the use of these tests for patients with first episodes of psychosis has not been established (77–79). However, CT and MRI examination may be crucial in assessing particular patients and should be used as available tools in the biological workup of psychotic patients.

Treatment Tests

1. I.V. glucose for hypoglycemia
2. I.V. physostigmine salicylate for anticholinergic delirium
3. I.V. thiamine for Wernicke's encephalopathy

Psychodynamic Evaluation and Formulation

Cognition and Affect

Regardless of whether the clinician adheres to DSM-IIIR, Bleuler, or Schneider, a careful descriptive assessment of the patient is essential. This assessment includes the patient's cognitive, perceptual, and affective functioning and symptomatology.

The cognitive disorder of schizophrenia may present with disturbances in the *flow of thought;* by the experience of *thought control or possession;* with disturbances in the *content of thought;* and by a *formal thought disorder* (80). Thought *flow* may show rate disturbances in which thinking is slow or rapid, with the latter more characteristic of excited psychotic states. Thought flow can also be disordered by disturbances of the train (or continuity) of thinking. Common examples of discontinuity found in schizophrenia are thought blocking, tangentiality, and perseveration.

Schizophrenic patients frequently exhibit *thought control or possession.* They report that their thoughts (or mind) are controlled by alien forces, that thoughts are put into or taken out of their mind, and that they are "made to do" a variety of behaviors. These are all examples of thought control. Delusions are the characteristic disturbance in the *content of thought* found in schizophrenia. Delusions, or fixed idiosyncratic beliefs that conform to the schizophrenic's reality (and to no one else's) may be persecutory, grandiose, or somatic.

Formal disturbances of thought include logical errors, impaired abstracting ability, and incoherence. Logical errors frequently arise from egocentricity or idiosyncratic premises. Concrete interpretations of reality (e.g., "How is it that you came to the hospital? By car.") reflect impaired abstraction and are quite common to schizophrenia. Incoherence is often the result of disordered associations which Bleuler described.

Perceptual disturbances in schizophrenia occur in the form of hallucinations. Auditory hallucinations include voices conversing about oneself, hearing one's thoughts aloud, or hearing an ongoing commentary about one's actions. Visual hallucinations may also occur; their presence in the absence of auditory hallucinations should prompt the clinician to search for an organic etiology. Tactile, olfactory, and gustatory hallucinations should arouse questions of organicity, though they may be found in schizophrenia especially when auditory hallucinations are present.

Affective disturbances in schizophrenia are characteristically a blunted, flat, or inappropriate affect—an affect not appropriate to the social situation or topic of discussion. Examples include giggling when discussing the death of a family member or smiling during an intensely hostile family meeting. As a rule these inappropriate affects become understandable as the patient's inner life becomes apparent. The affect that was so inappropriate to the immediate external context may be quite appropriate to the patient's inner thoughts, hallucinations, or delusions. Anhedonia, or the absence of pleasure, frequently inhibits many aspects of the schizophrenic's life.

Core Conflicts

Problems with psychological separateness and identity are central to the schizophrenic's dilemma. A defective sense of self and disturbed boundaries make it difficult for schizophrenics to *differentiate* themselves from others. They view themselves as either potentially merged with another or as distinct but helpless, terrified, and abandoned. As the clinician attempts to form a therapeutic relationship he or she will arouse the patient's fear of fusion; yet if the clinician is too distant the patient will continue to feel estranged and terrified. This same dilemma existed before admission; if

this delicate balance was disturbed (e.g., with a family member(s), therapist, friend, or lover), what precipitated hospital admission may be revealed.

Schizophrenics' limited ego capacities and disturbed boundary and communicational skills render them vulnerable and *dependent*. Though clearly dependent, schizophrenics fear the intimacy of a relationship that provides for their needs. They also tend to deny this helplessness to maintain an already compromised sense of self-esteem. This dilemma may have characterized the prodrome to hospitalization and needs to be carefully understood, particularly since this situation may replicate itself in the hospital.

Anger and *aggression* are particularly difficult for the schizophrenic because of boundary disturbances and weak repressive capacities. Anger may therefore threaten self, other, and world, and threaten to explode into unrestrained rage. Healthy assertion and aggression may be denied with consequent passivity and apathy (81).

History and Formulation

The psychosocial history of the schizophrenic patient is no different from that of any psychiatric patient, though additional collaborative information may be needed. Early development must be understood with particular emphasis on the patient's place in the family and relationships with family members and peers. Separations and other important stresses should be noted. The patient's educational, social, and occupational efforts are central to understanding the patient's strengths, weaknesses, and prognosis. Sexual and marital history will need to be explored tactfully, as tolerated by the patient. Past psychiatric treatment, with special attention to the patient's relationship with the therapist, also needs careful exploration.

Premorbid functioning (the patient's adaptive capacities before the onset of the illness) can be assessed by examining (*a*) the patient's functioning in relationships, work, and play and (*b*) the patient's personality style and employed characteristic defenses. The clinician seeks to understand the patient's highest level of functioning and to understand whether deterioration was sudden or insidious. Furthermore, the history seeks to clarify whether the patient was schizoid, obsessional, depressed, or hysterical, or showed some other premorbid personality style. Closely linked to this is information regarding the patient's principal defensive operations (e.g., withdrawal, reaction formation, intellectualization, denial, depression, somatization, acting-out) (82).

The case formulation lends meaning to the patient's decompensation by depicting stresses in the patient's life that were related to the onset of psychosis. Detail is sought in order to understand carefully what happened to the patient, with whom, when, and where. These stressors are best understood and explained in terms of the core conflicts and dilemmas of schizophrenics and their limited capacities to respond. The formulation can also chronicle the regression from premorbid functioning to acute (or chronic symptomatology). This regression can be described in terms of behavior, symptomatology, and ego defenses (e.g., from work to unemployment, from withdrawal to delusional preoccupation, from intellectualization to denial, distortion, and projection).

Social and Family Evaluation

An assessment of the home and social environment of the schizophrenic patient is a crucial aspect of the complete patient evaluation.

Family studies (73, 74, 83–90) have demonstrated that schizophrenics who return to home environments that include a relative who is critical, hostile, or emotionally over-involved tend to have a high relapse rate. This contrasts with those schizophrenics who can return to a more ac-cepting and emotionally neutral environment. The WHO studies that demonstrate a better outcome for schizophrenics in traditional, nonwestern societies where families are more tolerant support this view (91). On the other hand, a social environment that allows for marked isolation and absence of stimulation will also foster regression and social withdrawal and promote relapse.

In addition to evaluating the emotional tone and degree of environmental stimulation of the family, the clinician should examine family structure. In some families there is a pathological need for an ill person for the homeostasis of the family. More precisely, the clinician should examine for secondary (or conscious) gain from illness for the patient and other family members. Carefully reviewing the schizophrenic's relationship to the mother and father and scrutinizing the mother-father relationship are additional aspects of the family evaluation. These relationships are examined for enmeshment (over-involvement) of the schizophrenic with one parent; this is one mode families can employ to detour conflict away from the parents or avoid intimacy problems within the couple. In order for schizophrenic patients to develop appropriate autonomy, they must be willing to differentiate and separate from their families and families must be willing to let this happen.

HOSPITAL TREATMENT

Concurrent Drug and Alcohol Abuse

The prevalence of substance abuse among severely mentally ill young adults (most of whom are schizophrenics) has been reported to exceed 50% (92–97). All too often clinicians who work with schizophrenic patients miss the co-morbid diagnosis of chemical dependence.

Young chronically mentally ill patients reported that they employed alcohol and drugs in order to relieve social anxiety and alter the negative symptoms of schizophrenia (95). Clinically, drug use and abuse had a clear adverse affect on daily functioning, especially on maintaining housing, obtaining food, and managing finances. Rehospitalization rates and suicidal behavior are also higher in the drug abusing schizophrenic patient. Even minimal amounts of alcohol abuse destabilizes this fragile population (96).

Inpatient units may want to include urine and blood toxic screens in the admission laboratory exam to aid discovery of concurrent substance disorder. In view of the severely destabilizing effects of alcohol and drug abuse on the treatment, course, and prognosis of schizophrenia, obtaining and maintaining abstinence must be a priority in treatment. Clinicians can expect "double denial" in this patient population; denial is integral to both disorders. A 12-Step Recovery model can be a recognized part of or an available resource to the inpatient unit. Staff will need to be familiar with addiction treatment and actively integrate it into the conceptual framework of the unit (98). Conversely, any recovery group that works with schizophrenic patients must understand that these patients require medication and that their medication is different from addictive substances (e.g., lithium is not librium). Furthermore, because schizophrenic patients often have difficulty in groups (especially confrontational groups) a recovery program must conform to schizophrenic patients' needs for structure, affective moderation, and distance and privacy.

PSYCHOPHARMACOLOGICAL MANAGEMENT

Under special circumstances such as on a research unit with ample staff and a commitment to nondrug treatment, it may be possible to treat the acute psychosis of schizophrenia without medications (99). As a rule, however, it is standard practice to treat this psychosis psychopharmacologically (100). Neuroleptic (or antipsychotic) medications are the drugs of choice but not the sole pharmacological strategy. Effectively engaging the patient in an "exclusively" somatic treatment will require a thoughtful psychosocial assessment and the development of a therapeutic alliance that will enhance medication compliance.

Neuroleptic (Antipsychotic) Agents

Data suggest that all commercially available antipsychotic agents are clinically and equally effective, with the possible exception of clozapine (see below).

The neuroleptic medications have proved unquestionably the most effective treatment in remedying the symptoms of acute psychosis of schizophrenia (100, 101). Furthermore, antipsychotic medications have shown high effectiveness in treating particular target symptoms. These include hallucinations, acute delusions, combativeness, anxiety, hostility, hyperactivity, negativism, insomnia, and poor general self-care. Though findings do not indicate beneficial effects of neuroleptics on negative symptoms (blunted affect, withdrawal, amotivation, poverty of speech and thought), evidence suggests some patients have improved (102).

A target symptom approach allows for clear outcome criteria for the medication regimen and is the basis of the increasingly popular strategy of using more than one class of medications (e.g., neuroleptic and anxiolytic, neuroleptic and lithium). The treatment of schizophrenia or any psychiatric disorder should provide systematic trials of medication of adequate dose (not too high or too low) and duration. Through such trials the clinician, patient, and family can judge which medication(s) provides optimal benefit weighed against unwelcome side effects. Systematic trials require the *systematic discontinuation* of medications; patients should not remain unnecessarily on medications and thereby accumulate interactive and excessive side effects from multiple drugs.

Choice of agent. All neuroleptic agents are effective when given in adequate dosages. (See dosage section.) Physicians need to acquaint themselves with several neuroleptic medications in different classes in order to have use of a variety of agents. In choosing a medication, the following *guidelines* apply:

1. The patient's history may be helpful. If a patient responded favorably to a drug in the past, this would support its use once again. If the patient was allergic to or responded adversely to a drug in the past, this would relatively or absolutely contraindicate its reuse.
2. Psychiatrists choose medications which they know. In the course of training or clinical practice a physician ought to become familiar with the phenothiazines (chlorpromazine, thioridazine, trifluoperazine, perphenazine, fluphenazine); a butyrophenone (haloperidol); a thioxanthene (thiothixene); a dibenzoxapine (loxapine); and a dihydroindolone (molindone). In addition, the prescribing psychiatrist should be aware of new medications, new findings, (103) drug combinations, and alternate strategies of administration (104, 105) as potential avenues for nonresponsive patients. Although all psychiatrists need not provide these treatments themselves, they should know of their existence and how patients can receive tertiary care if they require it.
3. A particular neuroleptic may be chosen for its specific side effects. When sedation is preferable, one of the more sedating agents such as chlorpromazine may

be selected. When anticholinergic side effects must be avoided, an agent with very low anticholinergic properties such as haloperidol would be indicated. *High-potency neuroleptics (e.g., haloperidol, fluphenazine, trifluoperazine, thiothixene) are generally minimally hypotensive, sedating, and anticholinergic; they are, however, highly extrapyramidal. *Low-potency neuroleptics (chlorpromazine, thioridazine) tend to have fewer extrapyramidal problems, but often induce hypotension, sedation, and anticholinergic symptomatology. Perphenazine, loxapine, and molindone fall somewhere in between the high- and low-potency agents.

Route of administration. Neuroleptic medications can be given orally or intramuscularly. Oral medications are available in elixir and tablets. Elixir is more rapidly absorbed than tablets and presents less possibility of "cheeking." Intramuscular (i.m.) administration can be employed when symptoms must be treated rapidly as in the case of a combative patient. Parenteral administration should also be considered when there is doubt about gastrointestinal absorption.

Caffeine, found in coffee, tea, and caffeinated beverages, can bind or precipitate out neuroleptic medications and stimulate microsomal activity in the liver (thereby increasing the catabolism of antipsychotic agents) (106–109). As a consequence, the ingestion of caffeine in combination with a neuroleptic medication may significantly interfere with the absorption and half-life of the drug and potentially limit clinical improvement. Though it is debatable whether the interference stems from caffeine or tan-

---

*High and low potency refer to the number of milligrams needed for clinical effect. All agents are potent; the terms refer to whether the dose required will be in the range of 2–60 mg (high potency) or 400–3000 mg (low potency).

nic acid, clinicians may want to eliminate caffeinated beverages from the kitchen area of the hospital and inform patients about this interaction.

Dosage. At least 300 mg of chlorpromazine or its equivalent in another neuroleptic are generally necessary for antipsychotic effect. One hundred milligrams of chlorpromazine is roughly equal to 100 mg of thioridazine and to 5 mg of trifluoperazine, haloperidol, thiothixene, and fluphenazine. Table 3.2 provides a list of the commonly used antipsychotics and their equivalent dosages.

It is advisable to document a *dose-response curve* in the neuroleptic treatment of an acute psychotic episode. The effect on the target symptoms and the side effects the patient experiences are monitored at varying doses of medication in order to choose the most effective dose for the patient. Figure 3.1 provides an example of a dose response curve. Evidence from ongoing treatment and dosage studies suggests that the optimal range of dose is narrow and high doses of medication are generally not necessary or effective (47, 110, 111).

Neuroleptic blood levels. Unlike lithium and tricyclic antidepressant levels, optimum neuroleptic blood levels are in the infancy of their development. The need clearly exists to provide the lowest possible therapeutic dose (and thereby limit exposure and consequent risk of tardive dyskinesia) and to minimize side effects. Difficulties in developing valid and accurate measurements are related to the presence of metabolites and cross-reactivity among metabolites, the parent compound, and any other psychoactive agent the patient may be taking. Emerging studies show that plasma levels of neuroleptics vary enormously among patients and that there probably is a therapeutic window for haloperidol. If upper and lower limits of effectiveness for haloperidol exist (i.e. a therapeutic window) clinicians will want to keep in mind that a dosage decrease may be helpful for some patients (112–114).

As our technology develops, blood levels may add to treatment planning. Currently, however, their utility is quite limited. They may be of value in assessing compliance and determining the interaction of other drugs on neuroleptic levels (e.g., carbamazepine and haloperidol).

Schedule of administration. Upon admission to an inpatient unit in recent years, acutely psychotic patients have often been managed by a medication regimen of *rapid neuroleptization* in which doses of antipsychotic medication are administered every half hour or hour until there is evidence of "lysing" of the psychotic episode or until sedation sets in. However, recent studies have demonstrated that patients receiving rapid, and higher, dosage schedules did no better clinically than patients who received standard doses and routine administration (e.g., 3 times a day [t.i.d.]). Furthermore, no evidence exists that those receiving rapid neuroleptization had briefer hospital stays (115–117). Patients receiving rapid neuroleptization did show a higher incidence of extrapyramidal disorders, thereby requiring greater amounts of antiparkinson agents, and were exposed to

Table 3.2. Equivalent Oral Dosages of Antipsychotic Medications Compared to 100 mg of Chlorpromazine (Thorazine)

Drug	(Trade Name)	Dose (mg)
Haloperidol	(Haldol)	2–5
Trifluoperazine	(Stelazine)	5
Perphenazine	(Trilafon)	10
Thioridazine	(Mellaril)	100
Fluphenazine	(Prolixin)	2–5
Thiothixene	(Navane)	5
Loxapine	(Loxitane)	15
Molindone	(Moban)	10
Mesoridazine	(Serentil)	50
Acetophenazine	(Tindal)	20
Clozapine	(Clozaril)	50
Pimozide	(Orap)	2–5

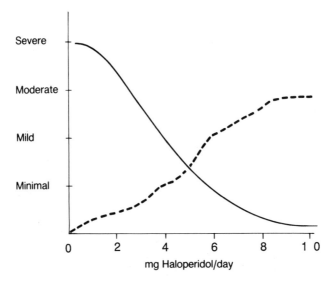

Figure 3.1.   Dose-response curve. *Dashed line,* side effects; *solid line,* degree of symptomatology.

higher doses of antipsychotic medication during the course of hospitalization.

These studies suggest the judicious use of neuroleptics when clinically feasible. Recompensation from psychosis is a process that cannot be condensed into hours. Kept on conservative neuroleptic regimens, acutely psychotic patients will restitute from days to weeks to a nonpsychotic state, thereby avoiding excessive exposure to neuroleptics and their adverse effects.

In general, 300–600 mg/day of chlorpromazine, or its equivalent (see Table 3.2) in other neuroleptics like trifluoperazine, haloperidol, or perphenazine, will be effective for the antipsychotic treatment of acute psychosis. Adjunctive benzodiazepines have become increasingly used to provide additional tranquilization without increasing the patient's exposure to neuroleptics. Lorazepam (1–2 mg p.o.) or oxazepam (10–20 mg p.o.) can be written as p.r.n. (as the occasion arises) or maintenance orders and administered up to several times per day, especially in the first few days of hospitalization. The concurrent use of anxiolytics provides for *rapid tranquilization* which is different from

rapid neuroleptization (118). Many patients require this level of intervention for their safety and comfort. When initiated, the clinician must recognize that this is a brief intervention; there is no evidence that the longer term prescription of anxiolytics is effective.

ADVERSE EFFECTS:

Extrapyramidal Syndromes.

1. Acute dystonia. This generally occurs within the first few days of treatment. It is more common in younger patients, especially males. Acute dystonic reactions are characterized by sudden marked and often subjectively frightening tonic contractions of the muscles of the tongue, neck, back (opisthotonus), mouth, or eyes (oculogyric crisis).

Acute dystonic reactions can be treated effectively with i.m. benztropine (Cogentin), 1 or 2 mg, or diphenhydramine (Benadryl), 25 or 50 mg i.m. or i.v. The patient should then be placed on a maintenance dose of the agent chosen (e.g., benztropine, 1 mg twice a day [b.i.d.], or amantadine, 100–300 mg/day, which may reduce confusional side effects [119]).

2. Drug-induced parkinsonism. This is a common side effect from antipsychotic medication. It tends to appear within the first few weeks of treatment. The features of drug-induced parkinsonism include bradykinesia (slowed movements), rigidity, and tremor. Marked (expressionless) faces, stooped posture, drooling, and gait disturbances are also common. So-called "postpsychotic depressions" are often bradykinesic parkinsonian states which are highly treatable if diagnosed.

Treatment is with oral antiparkinson agents, e.g., benztropine (Cogentin), 1–4 mg/day; diphenhydramine (Benadryl), 25–100 mg/day; or amantadine (Symmetrel), 100–300 mg/day, all in divided dosages. Antiparkinson agents can often be reduced or discontinued after several weeks. The patient is then observed to see if parkinsonism returns.

3. Akathisia. Akathisia is a neuroleptic-induced syndrome of motor restlessness and subjective inability to sit still or, in more severe cases, a feeling of marked anxiety and dysphoria (120, 121). Akathisia is easily confused with worsening psychosis and mistakenly prompts the use of additional neuroleptic medication, thereby escalating the problem. Furthermore, a variety of impulsive and bizarre behaviors have been associated with the dysphoria of akathisia, including suicide attempts (122–124).

Psychotic patients with somatic preoccupations or delusions are especially vulnerable to interpreting akathisia as a form of external influence. Patients (especially young men) who rely on the experience of body well-being and activity as a defensive style are apt to have these adaptations undermined by the akathisic experience (125–127). Finally, "the consumer has a point" (127): schizophrenic patients who have a dysphoric response to a neuroleptic do poorly with further medication treatment and frequently are noncompliant. These dysphoric responses were highly correlated with the diagnosis of akathisia.

Treatment of akathisia begins with considering a decrease in dose or change of neuroleptic. Antiparkinson agents provide little relief from akathisia. Benzodiazepines (diazepam, 2–5 mg p.o., b.i.d.–t.i.d., or lorazepam, 1 mg p.o., b.i.d.–t.i.d.) can be helpful and, as noted earlier, can reduce the need for antipsychotic medication. Propanolol has proven to be quite beneficial within days with a dosage range of 20–80 mg/day, given in divided doses (128–129). Caution about the interaction between propanolol and neuroleptics is indicated, in view of one clear instance of hypotension and cardiopulmonary arrest when this beta blocker was administered concurrently with haloperidol (130). Nadolol, another beta blocker, and clonidine, a central noradrenergic blocker, have shown effectiveness (131, 132).

4. Neuroleptic-induced catatonia. A gradual development of catatonia in patients on high-potency neuroleptic drugs may be a result of the drug itself (133). If present, neuroleptic-induced catatonia must be diagnosed in order not to be mistaken for a worsening of the patient's psychotic symptomatology. Treatment involves changing the neuroleptic medication or adding amantadine (Symmetrel) 100 mg p.o., t.i.d.

5. Tardive dyskinesia. Tardive dyskinesia is a late-onset, abnormal movement disorder that occurs in a substantial proportion of patients treated with maintenance neuroleptic medication. A cumulative effect seems apparent, with an estimated incidence of 3–4% for each year of treatment and a higher incidence in the elderly population (where it may be associated with akinesia early in treatment) (134–136).

The syndrome of tardive dyskinesia is often heralded by fasciculations of the tongue. Later manifestations include involuntary, persistent movements of the tongue, lips, and facial muscles (lingual-buccal-facial dyskinesia). More severe cases can demonstrate choreoathetoid (spasmodic and/or writhing) movements of any or all portions of the upper and lower extremities and truncal and diaphragmatic dyskinesias.

Tardive dyskinesia must be looked for in all patients on neuroleptic medication and carefully reviewed as a possible side effect with patients when they are in a nonpsychotic state. No effective treatment has yet been developed for this complex and all too common disorder (137, 138). Fortunately, only a small percentage of cases are severe and once established, the disorder may not be progressive, even with continued neuroleptic treatment (139).

OTHER ADVERSE EFFECTS

Neuroleptic Malignant Syndrome

The neuroleptic malignant syndrome is a quartet of muscular rigidity, fever, autonomic dysfunction, and disturbances of mental status (140, 141). Incidence is estimated at approximately 1%, with the disorder generally associated with high-potency neuroleptics. Young men and patients with organic brain disease are reported to be at higher risk. The pathophysiology of this disorder is unknown. What is known is that this syndrome can come on rather explosively (1–2 days) and can cause death (142). Early recognition is therefore essential.

Treatment of the neuroleptic malignant syndrome involves immediately stopping the neuroleptic. A differential diagnosis of other possible explanations for the patient's symptoms must be explored while respiratory, renal, and cardiovascular functioning are monitored and treated accordingly. Though some patients with this disorder may respond to drug discontinuation and supportive measures, (143) dantrolene sodium and bromocriptine, each alone or in combination, may be vital in refractory cases (140, 144–146).

Anticholinergic Effects

These include dry mouth, blurry vision, urinary retention, and slowing of the bowel. Patients with "narrow angle" glaucoma should not be prescribed neuroleptic agents without ophthalmological consultation.

Cardiovascular Side Effects

Orthostatic hypotension is commonly found with the low-potency agents (e.g., chlorpromazine and thioridazine).

Hypothalamic Effects

Changes in appetite and libido, breast enlargement, and galactorrhea are the more common hypothalamic effects.

Jaundice

Jaundice is generally the allergic, cholestatic type that is benign and responds to withdrawal of medication.

Agranulocytosis

Agranulocytosis is a rare, potentially fatal, side effect of neuroleptic medication. It is an allergic, nondose-related phenomenon for which the clinician must always be on the alert. Patients who show fever, sore throat, or signs of some infectious process should have an immediate white blood count to rule out agranulocytosis.

Seizures

Neuroleptic medications can lower seizure threshold, especially in high-risk patients. Haloperidol, fluphenazine and molindone may be less likely to induce seizures than other agents (147).

Mental Status Changes

Very little has been said or written about adverse *psychological* effects of neuroleptics on schizophrenic patients. Nevertheless, patients frequently note disagreeable changes in their mental state which add to their psychic discomfort and may cause them to discontinue medication.

Nevins (148) observes that changes may occur in ego defensive activities, in needed psychotic restitutive symptoms, and in body image. For example, defensive denial or motor activity may be altered by medication allowing for the emergence of painful inner feelings of grief and passivity; autistic and psychotically driven autoerotic activities may cease and allow expression of repressed sexual and dependent wishes and fears; psychotic omniscience may give way to severe depression and self-derogation; and the peripheral and central effects of neuroleptics (e.g., dry mouth, sedation, rigidity) may be interpreted psychotically as brain damage or punishment from God.

Neuroleptics and Pregnancy and Lactation

Neuroleptic agents pass through the placenta and have been detected in breast milk. Every effort must be made not to expose the fetus or newborn to medication of any sort, including antipsychotic agents. When neuroleptics appear essential, risk/benefit concerns must be addressed with the patient and family and informed consent obtained (149).

Clozapine

An important advance in the pharmacotherapy of psychoses is clozapine, a dibenzodiazepine that is structurally related to the neuroleptic loxapine but different in several significant ways. Unlike other agents, clozapine has greater serotonergic, adrenergic, and histaminergic blocking action than dopamine blockade. Clozapine also selectively blocks dopamine in cortical and limbic regions, relatively sparing the nigrostriatal and tuberoinfundibular areas of the brain, presumably resulting in the drug's clinical advantage.

As many as 30% of medication-resistant schizophrenic patients may respond to clozapine (150–152). Patients with both positive and negative symptoms have been reported to improve. Patients who have been unable to tolerate neuroleptics because of severe drug-induced parkinsonism, akathisia, dystonias, or tardive dyskinesia are also candidates for clozapine.

Because of the drug's 1–2% risk of agranulocytosis, careful white-cell monitoring is needed. With early detection of this immunological side effect patients can recover but can never be re-exposed to the drug. All patients receiving clozapine must be enrolled in the Clozaril Patient Management System (CPMS) through which their white counts are tracked by a nationally available home health-care company. Seizures have also been a troublesome part of the side-effect profile, though low to moderate dosage (300–500 mg/day) significantly reduces the risk of seizures. Additional side effects include hypersalivation, drowsiness, hypotension, and hyperthermia.

Clozapine appears to be well-tolerated with other medications. Care must be taken with other drugs that can cause the side effects noted above. A small proportion of patients who will respond, will do so in six weeks; others may require as many as nine months. Informed consent is routine in patient preparation for a clozapine trial.

Anxiolytic Agents

Anxiolytic (antianxiety agents or minor tranquilizers) are growing in value in the treatment of acute psychosis (153–154). Anxiolytics (e.g., lorazepam, alprazolam, diazepam, oxazepam) are useful for treating akathisia and can be used concurrently with neuroleptics for the symptoms of acute psychosis (see Antipsychotic Agents, page 83).

˙Lithium

Lithium is known to be effective in the acute and maintenance treatment of affective disorders. Neuroleptic medications remain the drugs of choice for treating the acute psychosis of schizophrenia. However, in cases where a considerable affective component may be suspected or excitement seems a primary target symptom, lithium as a single agent or an adjunct to neuroleptic medication should be considered (155).

Carbamazepine

Carbamazepine (Tegretol) has been shown to be helpful in schizophrenic patients with abnormal EEGs (156). This anticonvulsant has not been demonstrably helpful as an adjunct or alternate to neuroleptics in patients with normal EEG function. Furthermore, carbamazepine can reduce neuroleptic blood levels, thereby diminishing a potentially effective treatment.

Antidepressants

The concurrent use of antidepressants in patients with schizophrenic illness is debatable. Clearly, schizophrenic patients can become depressed. However, major depression can be mistakenly diagnosed (when the patient is suffering from drug-induced akinesia, negative symptoms, or demoralization). The side effects of antidepressants can exacerbate effects patients are already experiencing from other medications. And acutely psychotic patients may have their psychotic symptoms exacerbated by antidepressants (157).

Propanolol

Propanolol (Inderal) is a β-adrenergic blocker commonly used in treating cardiovascular disorders (158–159). Clinical trials from some years ago showed propanolol to be helpful as an *adjunct* to antipsychotic medications in treatment-resistant, chronically psychotic, schizophrenic patients. This may have been the result of increasing plasma concentrations of the neuroleptic the patient was receiving rather than the direct action of propanolol (160). These findings have not been well-replicated. However, propanolol and nadolol are effective in managing akathisia (see Adverse Effects, pages 87) (161).

Calcium Channel Blockers

Verapamil, nifedipine, and diltiazem are available calcium channel blockers useful for a variety of cardiovascular disorders, asthma, Raynaud's disease, and vascular headaches. They have not been demonstrated to be useful in schizophrenia though they may help diminish the symptoms of tardive dyskinesia (162–163).

Barbiturates

Barbiturates were routinely used before the era of neuroleptic medication. They are still helpful as potent sedating agents for highly agitated patients. A dose of 120–180 mg of sodium amytal prescribed at bedtime can be an adjunct in treating the acutely psychotic patient who has already received adequate antipsychotic and anxiolytic medication.

ELECTROCONVULSIVE THERAPY (ECT)

ECT is never the first-line treatment for the acute psychosis of schizophrenia unless a life-threatening catatonia exists or the patient cannot tolerate any neuroleptic medication. In general, lack of response to a variety of medications should lead to a search for toxic psychosocial factors rather than an immediate prescription of a course of ECT. For patients in which this search is unsuccessful, ECT may prove to be beneficial if adequate medication trials have been completed. Catatonic and affective symptoms are more responsive than apathy, autism, and delusional preoccupation (164, 165).

MILIEU MANAGEMENT

Milieu treatment has traditionally been based on a belief that interpersonal and group processes can be designed to yield corrective emotional experiences. Through the therapeutic use of staff, structure, and group activities, patients could develop behaviors and ego capacities and achieve rehabilitation. These views are best illustrated by the therapeutic community efforts that emerged after World War II (166, 167). The theory and technology of the early therapeutic communities has now become dated: decreases in length of stay, markedly heterogeneous inpatient populations, and advances in our knowledge of how a powerful milieu can harm as well as heal have dramatically altered the nature of inpatient milieu treatment (168, 169).

Though some authors have questioned whether the milieu is of any value once "gross neglect" has been corrected, such a dim view of the value of the milieu is not sustained by carefully examining this treatment modality (170–173). Milieus that provide high patient/staff ratios in small units, cultivate patient responsibility, consider psychosis to have meaning, and believe in the power of the milieu are indeed effective. The central questions today may be those of clarifying which environment best suits which patient (treatment specificity) and what are the beneficial and the adverse elements of the milieu. Furthermore, hospital settings will be challenged to refashion their milieu to suit short stays and to offer crisis intervention, pharmacological treatment, and aftercare planning. As hospital treatment programs reshape to changing patterns of care, certain lessons from

the care of schizophrenic patients bear noting.

What appears especially unbearable to schizophrenic patients is an overstimulating environment (174–177). Explanations of why such a milieu may be toxic vary: overload in schizophrenics who have a basic defect in processing input (178); the essential need for separateness, distance, privacy, and even isolation in psychotic patients (179–181); and the organism's need to protect itself from overwhelming external stimulation (182). For many patients, not only will a less intense milieu prevent negative reactions, it may also be valuable in permitting the recompensation process to occur.

Overstimulation can occur through a highly peopled or activity-filled environment. Multiple meetings, groups, lively and provocative discussions, affective exploration, and placing high value on interaction are the ingredients of modern milieu treatment; they are also what can be deleterious to the patient who requires privacy, quiet, and isolation. Similarly, milieus that invite self-disclosure, place particular emphasis on "here and now" communication, and encourage open expression of anger and aggression can be toxic to the psychotic patient (183–185). Confrontation may be the most deleterious form of overstimulation for it can simultaneously excite the patient and unravel needed defenses.

Milieus that persist in advocating principles of democracy, egalitarianism, role blurring, and absent hierarchies are apt to be quite confusing to psychotic patients who require structure, clarity, accountability, and firm authority (168, 183, 184, 186, 187). Especially problematic are units in which the therapeutic milieu, in attending to "stylish" ideologies that enhance the working milieu of the staff, may conflict with the needs of these especially vulnerable patients (188–190).

The difficulties schizophrenic patients experience in group therapy parallel those of the milieu. Interestingly, group therapy for schizophrenic patients began in a format that was responsive to the special needs of psychotic patients. More than 60 years ago, Lazell met with schizophrenics in groups which provided information through lectures (191). His approach avoided what subsequently was discovered to be especially toxic to schizophrenic patients, namely, excessive uncovering, insight-oriented exploration, and self-disclosure (192–195). Group therapy for schizophrenic patients can be beneficial if the group experience avoids these pitfalls and, instead, attends to what we have come to understand about these patients. Therapists must be active, provide structure whenever needed, and offer liberal support and practical advice. Reality testing must be done whenever needed, social skills enhanced, and specific problems (and solutions) identified. Above all, self-esteem must be protected. Homogeneous, or "level," groups appear to be more effective than mixed groups; expectations are then similar for the members and success can be achieved by all (196–197). Groups can be constructed specifically to provide inpatient psychoeducation for both schizophrenic patients and their families (198). In such groups an illness model of schizophrenia is presented and coping and management strategies are taught.

Important advances in milieu care are also emerging from the field of psychosocial rehabilitation (199, 200). However, social-skills training and vocational preparation and rehabilitation can begin only in a hospital. Integrating the acute facility with long-term ambulatory rehabilitation will be central to planning for comprehensive systems of care in the 1990s.

INDIVIDUAL PSYCHOTHERAPY

The effective long-term psychotherapy of schizophrenia deeply depends on the quality of the therapist. Genuineness, accurate empathy, and warmth are the human qualities associated with successful outcome in the psychotherapy of schizophrenia (201–203).

Schwartz (202, 204) has likened the psychotherapy of schizophrenia to an heroic endeavor for therapist and patient alike. The schizophrenic's inner disorganization, turmoil, and profound psychic deprivation make constriction, withdrawal, and autistic preoccupation a powerfully seductive alternative to the pain and risks of psychotherapeutic engagement. The growth of a separate self for the schizophrenic, the essential task of psychotherapy, requires facing the bleakness and anguish of his past, the emptiness of his present, and the grief of being a separate person. The therapist, in turn, must provide inscrutable honesty, unwavering will, and unusual capacity to bear difficult and frightening feelings in order to allow and encourage the patient onto the rigorous and awesome path of evolving a separate self. Schwartz urges the therapist not to be put off by patients' wishes to see their therapists as special, endowed, even immortal. Heroic images of the therapist will permit and guide the genesis of patients' personal, unique, and valued images of themselves as separate people who can stand on their own without fear of dissolution of self or other.

Paradoxically, while engaged in this heroic pursuit, therapists are asked to maintain an attitude that their patient is simply another human being in pain with whom they are about to enter a relationship (67–68). Furthermore, Fromm-Reichmann (205–206) cautions therapists against trying to cure the schizophrenic patient. Such heroism, humanity, and humility are indeed a remarkable combination when found in the same person.

The psychotherapy of schizophrenia must be *antiregressive* (207–208). The patient's decompensation and regression in ego functioning was in response to events, feelings, and thoughts which he or she could not bear. Short of death, psychosis is the ultimate form of withdrawal. The therapy process cannot condone avoidance, for that sacrifices reality, relatedness, and self-esteem. The therapist wishes to ally with the patient's frail ego in examining the life events and inner realities that prompted flight into psychosis. Explorations into the precipitants of the decompensation and the nature of the patient's current relationships should occur only in the framework of an active, supportive, antiregressive stance by the therapist.

In the most developed empirical study to date, moderately ill, young, hospitalized schizophrenic patients were randomly assigned to intensive or supportive psychotherapy (209, 210). Intensive psychotherapy focused on the treatment relationship, transference, and the past. Supportive treatment focused on adjustment in the present. Those in intensive treatments were seen at least three times a week by experienced analysts. Those in supportive psychotherapy were seen weekly. Both groups received state-of-the-art psychopharmacology. The results of this study support the central importance of providing reality-based, antiregressive, and adaptation-oriented psychotherapy. Those schizophrenic patients seen in intensive psychotherapy remained in the hospital longer and were less likely to return to functioning at home or at a job. Furthermore, intensively treated patients showed a very high dropout rate (greater than 50% within six months), despite the use of senior clinicians. It appears likely that this dropout group suffered serious, negative outcomes (211).

In an antiregressive psychotherapy, primary process (unconscious) productions and transference distortions about the therapist are met with reality explanations and a return to the therapeutic task of understanding why the patient finds his or her life so intolerable. All the patient's efforts to be adaptive and reality bound, however rudimentary, should be respected and encouraged.

As the therapy proceeds, therapists can strive to understand their patients in a manner that lends coherence to the patient's psychotic productions. As therapists come to understand the unconscious avoidance aims and methods of the psychotic productions, they can enable patients to begin to experience thoughts and feelings as belonging to them rather than others (in the form of delusional and hallucinatory projections). Delusions and hallucinations should never be confronted. They will soften as the underlying need for them diminishes.

Schizophrenic patients' accounts of the illness and its demands and agonies lends important support to the provision of psychotherapy (212, 213). Patients have described the confusion (cognitive and identity), altered perceptions, and attention deficits of schizophrenia and the utility of psychotherapy in coping with these problems. Furthermore, it is through the medium of psychotherapy that hope, motivation, and human striving is maintained over the course of a long, often debilitating, illness.

When engaged in providing psychotherapy to schizophrenic patients, the clinician must remember how frightening this process can be (214, 215). Schizophrenic patients have a terror of close contact with others, which renders them remarkably limited in their capacity to articulate feelings and ideas. Furthermore, patients frequently are afraid of the power of their feelings which they may imagine as having the capacity to destroy them or the therapist. These fears must be addressed as they emerge, without negating them. Therapists can state that they realize that the patient has these fears and that the therapy will help the patient understand them and be less afraid. Lidz (216) has emphasized that the absence of options for action—the absence of exits—finalizes the patient's entrance into a schizophrenic regression. As a consequence, the therapist must always allow the patient choice and an exit. For some patients this may entail an open door while for others it may be permission to forestall talking until they are ready. Flexibility in meeting time (e.g., 15 minutes) and place (e.g., day room or patio) is critical to working effectively with the psychotic patient whose mental state permits only limited attention and calls for a subjectively safe milieu.

As the therapy examines aspects of the patient's life and family relations, themes of loss and grief will develop (217). The patient's rage or sexual fantasies may emerge in the psychotherapy. If those latter areas of conversion are initiated by the patient, they can be gently explored. As a rule, however, matters of sex and rage generally can wait until the ego has recompensated and can better manage the attendant affect. Concurrent work with family members is often essential during therapy in order to enlist their alliance, preclude their sabotaging treatment, and enable them to grow and thereby allow the patient to grow.

As patients improve and their egos recompensate, they begin to see why they had considered life intolerable. Grief and conflict can be borne, at least for brief moments, without psychotic defensive disorganization. A reality-based perspective allows patients to see what they can do for themselves and recognize that they are not as isolated and helpless as they had believed. This is the foundation for patients' renewed self-esteem and for their efforts at modest, but realizable, life goals.

The transition out of the hospital is particularly difficult for the schizophrenic patient. Whenever possible, the therapist should continue with the patient after discharge. Continuity of psychotherapeutic care is a vital handhold for a person whose inner world is deeply fragmented and whose real and imagined losses are already staggering in magnitude.

THE FAMILY

Family Evaluation and Therapy

The critical importance of the family in the schizophrenic patient's life cannot be overemphasized. For this reason, all families of hospitalized schizophrenic patients must be evaluated by a member of the inpatient staff. This evaluation provides collaborative information on the schizophrenic patient's illness and informs the hospital staff about the resources available through the family.

Furthermore, unless an effective alliance is established with the family, therapeutic efforts will lack an essential ingredient for their success. The family is vital in supporting the schizophrenic patient through years of acute and chronic illness. Families enter the mental health system already burdened by their own guilt and shame; we do not need to add to their suffering. Families should be approached as partners with the hospital and other caregivers in a long-term system of care.

The current direction of family treatment for schizophrenia began in Britain more than 20 years ago. Social psychiatry researchers discovered that hospitalized patients who returned to their families had higher rates of readmission than those patients who were discharged to hostels and boarding homes. In the sample of patients who returned to family living, the highest risk for recurrence of psychosis was found in excessively emotionally involved families (218). Subsequent work refined the family factors involved in poor outcome: families high in "expressed emotion" (EE), that is, overinvolved, critical, and overtly hostile interactions, were those that evidenced the poorest outcome for schizophrenic patients. Patients from high-EE families relapsed at a rate of 56%, compared to 21% of patients from low-EE families. More than 35 hours per week of contact by schizophrenic patients with high-EE family members appeared to be especially harmful. The role of antipsychotic medications was also studied and the results are quite striking. Patients who had high contact with high-EE families and no medication had a relapse rate of 92%; this rate dropped to 53% when these patients received neuroleptic medication. Patients who had low contact with high-EE families evidenced a 42% relapse rate when unmedicated, which dropped to 15% when medicated with antipsychotic agents. For schizophrenic patients of high-EE families, reducing contact with their families and prescribing antipsychotic medication was critical in averting relapse (87, 219–222).

The British work has been replicated in the United States, thereby ending any debate about validity of these findings in English-speaking countries (73, 223–226). The impact of the family on the course of the schizophrenia and the implications for treatment have been established for British and American patients, at the very least.

On the basis of this data, family treatment approaches have evolved which substantiate that decreasing family contact in high-EE families or teaching patients and families better methods of coping or changing negative attitudes of key family members will result in improved posthospital functioning for schizophrenic patients (227, 228).

For families of hospitalized schizophrenic patients, educating the family and important others about the nature, course, and management of schizophrenia is essential. Family work can also involve training in effective problem-solving, particularly concerning stressful life events. Family training may also include transforming overinvolvement to concern and generalized criticism to specific dissatisfactions (73, 229–231). Family intervention cannot cure

schizophrenia. However, careful pharmacotherapy, family therapy, social skills training, occupational rehabilitation, alternative housing, and practical, reality-based psychotherapy can dramatically alter the course of the disorder. Families need to understand this and be engaged as allies in a potentially lifelong endeavor. Only when families do not respond or persistently resist the treatment approaches outlined above should more intensive interventions be employed (e.g., strategic and systemic family therapies) (230, 232).

Informative and supportive texts for the families and friends of schizophrenic patients have been written (233–235). These books can serve as adjuncts to the direct care provided to families.

Genetic Counseling

As noted earlier, family, twin, and adoption studies all point to the presence of environmental and genetic factors in the transmission of schizophrenia.

Biological children of schizophrenics, adopted and raised in a separate environment, show a high prevalence of schizophrenia and other psychiatric disorders, including personality disorders and mental retardation. Adoptees from families without a history of schizophrenia, raised by schizophrenic parents, showed only a 4.8% rate of schizophrenia, compared with a rate of 19.7% among adopted-away biological offspring of schizophrenic parents. These findings support a genetic predisposition to schizophrenia. They also suggest that schizophrenia in a parent does not promote its development in a child if that child is not genetically predisposed (236).

The risk for schizophrenia in the general population is roughly 1%. The risk rate for schizophrenia in first-degree relatives of schizophrenics is approximately 10%, whereas the risk for more distant relatives is only about 3%. These risk figures are estimates for the more severe form of schizophrenia that we have been discussing in this chapter, with features of early onset, history of recurrence, and tendency towards chronicity.

CONTROVERSIES IN THE INPATIENT TREATMENT OF SCHIZOPHRENIC PATIENTS

HOSPITAL LEVEL OF CARE

Questions of whether, when, and for how long schizophrenic patients should be hospitalized pervade clinical and fiscal considerations for this population. Clearly, the great predominance of schizophrenic patients do not require lengthy or enduring asylum *if* deinstitutionalized, community care is available (237). However, a small minority may not be able to exist effectively without 24-hour care (238).

For most schizophrenics, the inpatient facility is only one element in a comprehensive system of care. Ambulatory treatments (medications, case management, partial hospital, individual and group therapy), rehabilitation and sheltered workshops, community residences and supervised apartments are among the services needed by chronic patients.

The inpatient clinician must understand the chronicity of this illness and recognize that the goal of inpatient treatment cannot be cure. Inpatient treatment is necessary when safety is uncertain, supports have collapsed, and outpatient treatment has failed or cannot provide the necessary intensity of care. Hospital care must be directed at specific interventions that enable the patient to recompensate adequately to return to (or develop) a community-based system of care.

CIVIL LIBERTIES

Psychiatrists frequently wrestle with the moral and ethical dilemmas of commitment and involuntary treatment. Court activity in this area has been robust over the past 20 years. Clinicians can find themselves in remarkable binds, such as having the responsibility of a committed patient without the authority to treat (because of the right to refuse treatment) or having the potential liability for a patient's dangerousness when prediction is hardly possible.

Despite our litigious times, nothing can replace sound clinical judgments. There are times when patients cannot be responsible for themselves because of mental illness. At those times, we are professionally responsible for implementing potentially effective treatments within the due processes of our state and federal laws.

At times the dilemma does not derive from the legal system. Instead, countertransference difficulties of assuming control over another person's life are at the core of our conflict. The values we place on patient autonomy, self-responsibility, and freedom coupled with our training in the importance of neutrality and anonymity are part of what can handcuff us. When our denial of the gravity of a patient's illness keeps us from actively intervening, we can further abrogate our role as responsible clinicians in the long-term care of the chronically mentally ill.

PSYCHOSOCIAL TREATMENTS

Psychotherapy of psychosis has a long and honored tradition. Many of the great clinicians of this century devoted their careers, writings, and teachings to this endeavor. As somatic therapies and community mental health developed, the value and the role of psychotherapy changed.

While evidence is clear that medication and family intervention can reduce relapse in schizophrenic patients, the effectiveness of psychotherapy is less clear. Emotionally evocative and confrontational therapies that focus on the transference and genetic reconstruction are frequently beyond the capacities of a schizophrenic patient, especially during the psychotic phase of the illness. Practical and active psychotherapies are better tolerated and provide a core therapeutic relationship around which a variety of therapeutic services can be organized. Someone must reach and ally with the schizophrenic patient. Like anyone in distress, schizophrenic patients seek a person with whom and a setting in which they can understand and come to terms with their illness. Herein seems to lie a critical place for the psychotherapy of the schizophrenic patient.

Future research is needed to define which mode of psychotherapy (e.g., practical-directive, explorative-evocative, individual, group, family) best suits which patient, and when, during the course of the patient's illness, a specific treatment modality would be most useful. A paradigm for individual and illness-stage specific treatment has yet to be developed.

PSYCHOPHARMACOLOGICAL TREATMENTS

Medications cannot cure schizophrenia. However, they are vital in curtailing the symptoms of acute psychosis and essential (for most schizophrenics) in preventing relapse. The importance of neuroleptics only underscores the troubling adverse effects and unwelcome side effects they so commonly produce.

Until new agents are developed that produce better side-effect profiles and do not cause tardive dyskinesia, we are left to balance benefit and risk. With the exception of emergency situations, our best sources of information and alliance in the complex process of prescription are our patients and their families. Whenever possible, low-dose or intermittent neuroleptic treatment (targeting symptoms) should be tried. Augmenting-agents and nonneuroleptic drugs can also be considered if they add to effectiveness or reduce side effects. Above all, systematic trials, developed in collaboration with patients under informed consent and with benefits and risks weighed and documented, will best serve our patients and offer clinicians a solid basis for risk-management.

THE SUBSTANCE ABUSING SCHIZOPHRENIC PATIENT

As discussed earlier (see page 82), substance abuse among schizophrenic patients, especially the young, is alarmingly prevalent. Psychiatric treatment facilities will need to improve in identifying these dual-diagnosis patients. Routine admission urine and blood toxicology may be useful because of the degree of denial that often exists. Psychiatric units will need to integrate addictions treatment with medical and dynamic interventions. Unless this occurs, the schizophrenic patient's course of treatment will suffer because of the profoundly destabilizing effects of alcohol and drug abuse.

COURSE, PROGNOSIS, AND PROFESSIONAL EXPECTATIONS

The grim diagnosis of dementia praecox is no longer with us. We even have reason to believe after some years of acute illness, many schizophrenic patients can stabilize and reconstruct their lives. Yet the toll of this illness must not be underestimated, nor can we naively minimize the functional limitations that are a part of chronic schizophrenia (239).

Schizophrenia as an illness confronts clinicians with the devastating effects of chronic psychosis and, consequently, the limitations of our treatments. Facing such painful realities may, at times, be as difficult for providers of care as it is for patients. We sometimes manage this difficulty by having unrealistic expectations of our schizophrenic patients or avoiding them altogether. We can also confront the impairments, dependencies, and chronicity of the disease and respond accordingly. Only then can we and our patients overcome a sense of inadequacy and hopelessness and begin to experience the gratification of the hard work of rehabilitation and of a life rebuilt from the chaos of this disorder.

COURSE AND PROGNOSIS

Schizophrenia typically begins insidiously in early adult life. Most schizophrenic patients show premorbid features of shyness, social withdrawal, awkwardness, and an inability to form close relationships. The onset of schizophrenia is uncommon (but not rare) after age 40 (24).

Positive prognostic signs in schizophrenia include the presence of a supportive family, particularly a spouse; a family history of an affective disorder; and a premorbid history of good social relations and school performance. Poor prognosis is suggested by an insidious onset, a family history of schizophrenia, and a restricted or blunted affect (240–245). Though high EE may be correlated with relapse, no clear evidence suggests that expressed emotion is causal in the disorder. It is possible the stress of illness upon the family can evoke a dysfunctional response which may then aggravate the patient's course and prognosis (87, 243).

Some schizophrenic patients are at high risk for suicide. Care must be taken to identify those patients and provide early intervention and protective hospital care (246, 247). Depressive symptoms frequently antecede suicide in schizophrenic patients, though a major depressive episode may not be apparent. Hopelessness, more than any other depressive symptom, may be the best clinical marker of evolving suicidal potential (244).

Hogarty et al. (248, 249) examined relapse in schizophrenic patients for a two-year period following hospitalization. They found that patients treated with placebo had 80% relapse rates compared with 48% of those treated with neuroleptic medication. Patients treated with a problem-solv-

ing, interpersonal, and rehabilitative form of psychotherapy in addition to neuroleptics showed a further decrease in rate of relapse, though this was only apparent after six months of treatment. Glick and Hargreave's two-year follow-up studies on hospitalized schizophrenic patients demonstrated that longer-term hospital stays (90–120 days) resulted in a better course than shorter stays (21–28 days) for patients with good prehospital functioning. This finding was more pronounced for female patients. In the clinicians' opinion longer-term hospitalization resulted in greater compliance with long-term, posthospital treatment (medications and psychotherapy) and consequently reduced psychiatric morbidity (250). Whether the gains of longer-term hospitalization could be achieved by partial hospital and aftercare services coupled with intensive family work is an important research question.

Longitudinal studies on the course of schizophrenia demonstrate varied findings. Whereas some studies disclose poor levels of adjustment in the great majority of cases, (251, 252) other work suggests a more sanguine outcome. Evidence is accumulating that considerable heterogeneity of outcome exists and that many schizophrenic patients can show improvement even after years of psychotic symptomatology (253, 254). The view that the predominant outcome of schizophrenia is of a deteriorated, chronically ill person appears to be in error. In fact, over time many schizophrenic patients can recompensate to a relatively symptom-free and productive life.

REFERENCES

1. American Psychiatric Association: *Diagnostic and Statistical Manual*, ed. 3, (DSM-IIIR), Washington, D.C., American Psychiatric Association, APA Task Force on Nomenclature, 1987.

2. Morel BA: Etudes Cliniques: Traite Theorique et Pratique des Maladies Mentales, Paris, Masson, 1952.

3. Kraepelin E: *Dementia Praecox,* London, Livingston, 1918.

4. Bleuler E: Dementia Praecox oder die gruppe der Schizophenien, in Aschoffenburg (ed): *Handbuch der Psychiatrie,* Leipzig, 1911 (Trans. J Zinkin, 1960, New York).

5. Schneider K: *Clinical Psychopathology,* (Hamilton MW trans), New York, Grune & Stratton, 1959.

6. Pope HG, Lipinski JF: Diagnosis in schizophrenia and manic-depressive illness. Arch Gen Psychiatry, *35:*811–823, 1978.

7. Fish F: The concept of schizophrenia. Br J Med Psychol, *39:*269–273, 1966.

8. Silverstein ML, Harron M: First-rank symptoms in the post-acute schizophrenic: A follow-up study. Am J Psychiatry, *135:*1481–1486, 1978.

9. Harron M, Quinlan D: Is disordered thinking unique to schizophrenia? Arch Gen Psychiatry, *34:*15–21, 1977.

10. Koehler K: First rank symptoms of schizophrenia: Questions concerning clinical boundaries. Br J Psychiatry, *134:*226–248, 1979.

11. Pope HG, Lipinski JF, et al.: Schizoaffective disorder: An invalid diagnosis? Am J Psychiatry, *137:*981–982, 1980.

12. Levitt JJ, Tsuang MT: The heterogenicity of schizoaffective disorder: implications for treatment. Am J Psychiatry, *145:*926–936, 1988.

13. Kendler KS: Demography of paranoid psychosis. Arch Gen Psychiatry, *39:*890–902, 1982.

14. Fogelson DL, Cohen BM, et al.: A study of DSM-III schizophreniform disorder. Am J Psychiatry, *139:*1281–1285, 1982.

15. Coryell W, Tsuang MT: DSM-III schizophreniform disorder. Arch Gen Psychiatry, *39:*66–69, 1982.

16. Zilboorg G: The problem of ambulatory schizophrenias. Am J Psychiatry, *113:*519–525, 1956.

17. World Health Organization: Schizophrenia: An international follow up study. Chichester, UK, John Wiley & Sons, 1979.

18. Dunham HW: Community and schizophrenia: An epidemiologic analysis, Detroit, Wayne State University Press, 1965.

19. Warthen FJ, Klee GD, Bahn AK, et al.: Diagnosed schizophrenia in Maryland, Washington, D.C., Am Psychiatric Assn, 1967. (APA Research Report No. 22)

20. Kohn ML: Social class and schizophrenia: A critical review, in Rosenthal D, Kety SS (eds): *The Transmission of Schizophrenia.* Oxford, Pergamon Press, 1968.

21. Regier DA, Myers JK, Kramer M, et al.: The NIMH epidemiologic catchment area program. Arch Gen Psychiatry, *41:*934–941, 1984.

22. Robbins LN, Helzer JE, Weissman MM, et al.: Lifetime prevalence of specific psychiatric disorders in three sites. Arch Gen Psychiatry, *41:*949–958, 1984.

23. Babigian HN: Schizophrenia: in Kaplan HI, Sadock BJ (eds): *Comprehensive Textbook of Psychiatry,* ed. 4, Baltimore, Williams & Wilkins, 1985, p. 643.

24. Harris MJ, Collum CM, Jeste OV: Clinical prescription of late onset schizophrenia. J Clin Psychiatry, *49:*356–360, 1988.

25. Mukherjee S, Shukla S, Woodle J, et al.: Misdiagnosis of schizophrenia in bipolar patients: A multiethnic comparison. Am J Psychiatry, *140:*1571–1574, 1983.

26. Faris REL, Dunham HW: *Mental Disorders in Urban Areas,* Chicago, University of Chicago Press, 1939.

27. Goodman AB, Siegel C, et al.: The relationship between socioeconomic class and prevalence of schizophrenia, alcoholism, and affective disorders treated by inpatient care in a suburban area. Am J Psychiatry, *140:*166–170, 1983.

28. Kety SS: Genetic and biochemical aspects of schizophrenia, in Nichol A (ed): *Harvard Guide to Modern Psychiatry,* Cambridge, Belknap Press, 1978.

29. Gottesman II, Shields J: *Schizophrenia and Genetics: A Twin Study Vantage Point,* New York, Academic Press, 1972.

30. Kety SS, et al.: Mental illness in the biological and adoptive families of adopted individuals who have become schizophrenic, in Fieve R, et al. (eds): *Genetic Research in Psychiatry,* Baltimore, Johns Hopkins University Press, 1975.

31. Lidz T, Blatt S, et al.: Critique of the Danish-American studies of the adopted-away

offspring of schizophrenic parents. Am J Psychiatry, *138*:1063–1068, 1981.

32. Lidz R, Blatt S: Critique of the Danish-American studies of the biological and adoptive relatives of adoptees who became schizophrenic. Am J Psychiatry, *140*:426–434, 1983.

33. Baron M, Gruen R, et al.: Modern research criteria and the genetics of schizophrenia. Am J Psychiatry, *142*:697–701, 1985.

34. Abrams R, Taylor MA: The genetics of schizophrenia: A reassessment using modern criteria. Am J Psychiatry, *140*:171–175, 1983.

35. Sherrington R, Brynjjolfson J, Petrusson H, et al.: Localization of a susceptibility locus for schizophrenia on chromosome 5. Nature, *336*:164–167, 1988.

36. Dworkin RH, Lenzenweger MF, Moldin SO, et al.: A multidimensional approach to the genetics of schizophrenia. Am J Psychiatry, *145*:1077–1083, 1988.

37. Pardes H, Kaufmann CA, Pincus HA, et al.: Genetics and psychiatry. Am J Psychiatry, *146*:435–443, 1989.

38. Kendler KS, Gruenberg AM: An independent analysis of the Danish adoption study of schizophrenia. Arch Gen Psychiatry, *41*:555–564, 1984.

39. Snyder SH: Amphetamine psychosis: A "model" schizophrenia mediated by catecholamines. Am J Psychiatry, *130*:61–67, 1973.

40. Garver DL, Schlemmer RF, et al.: A schizophreniform behavioral psychosis mediated by dopamine. Am J Psychiatry, *132*:33–38, 1975.

41. Meltzer HY, Stahl SM: The dopamine hypothesis of schizophrenia: A review. Schizophr Bull, *2*:19–76, 1976.

42. Andreasen NC: *Brain imaging: Applications in psychiatry,* Washington DC, American Psychiatric Press, 1989.

43. Owen F, Cross AJ, et al.: Increased dopamine receptivity in schizophrenia. Lancet *2*:223–225, 1978.

44. Farde L, Ehrin E, Ericksson E, et al.: Substituted benzamides as ligands for visualization of dopamine receptor binding. Proc Natl Acad Sci USA, *81*:3863–3867, 1985.

45. Karoum F, Karson CN, Bigelow LB, et al.: Preliminary evidence of reduced combined output of dopamine and its metabolites in chronic schizophrenia. Arch Gen Psychiatry, *44*:604–607, 1987.

46. Tandon R, Greden JF: Cholinergic hyperactivity and negative schizophrenic symptoms. Arch Gen Psychiatry, *46*:745–753, 1989.

47. Cohen BM: Neuroleptic drugs in the treatment of acute psychosis: How much do we really know? in Casey DE, Christensen AV (eds): *Psychopharmacology: Current Trends,* pp. 47–61, New York, Springer-Verlay, 1988.

48. Weinberger DL, Wagner RL, et al.: Neuropathological studies in schizophrenia: A selective review. Schizophr Bull, *9*:193–212, 1983.

49. Illowsky BP, Juliano DM, Bigelow LB, et al.: Stability of CT scan findings in schizophrenias. J Neurol Neurosurg Psychiatry, *51*:209–213, 1988.

50. Cohen BM, Buonanno F, Keck PE, et al.: Comparison of MRI and CT scans in a group of psychiatric patients. Am J Psychiatry, *145*:1084–1088, 1988.

51. McCorley RW, Faux SF, Shertow M, et al.: CT abnormalities in schizophrenia, Arch Gen Psychiatry, *46*:698–708, 1989.

52. Weinberger DR: Implications of normal brain development for the pathogenesis of schizophrenia. Arch Gen Psychiatry, *44*:660–669, 1987.

53. Wolkin A, Jaeger J, et al.: Persistence of cerebral metabolic abnormalities in chronic schizophrenics as determined by positron emission tomography. Am J Psychiatry, *142*:564–571, 1985.

54. Volkow ND, Brodie JD, Wolf AP, et al.: Brain metabolism in schizophrenia before and after acute neuroleptic administration. J Neurol Neurosurg Psych, *49*:1199–1202, 1986.

55. Farde L: PET studies of patients treated with antipsychotic drugs. Psych Annals, *19*:530–535, 1989.

56. Morhisa JM, Duffy FH, et al.: Brain electrical activity mapping in schizophrenic patients. Arch Gen Psychiatry, *40*:719–728, 1983.

57. Taylor MA, Abrams R: Cognitive impairment in schizophrenia. Am J Psychiatry, *141*:196–201, 1984.

58. Grove WR, Andreasen NC: Language and thinking in psychosis: Is there an input abnormality? Arch Gen Psychiatry, *42*:26–32, 1985.

59. McReynolds P: Anxiety, perception and schizophrenia, in Jackson DD (ed): *The Eti-*

ology of Schizophrenia, New York, Basic Books, 1960.

60. Freedman R, Adler LE, Gerhardt MW, et al.: Neurobiological studies of sensory gating in schizophrenia. Schizophr Bull, *13:*669–678, 1987.

61. Baker N, Adler LE, Franks RD, et al.: Neurophysiological assessment of sensory gating in psychiatric inpatients. Biol Psychiatry, *22:*603–617, 1987.

62. Hartmann H: Ego psychology and the problem of adaptation. New York, International University Press, 1958.

63. Greenberg JR, Mitchell SA: Object relations in psychoanalytic theory. Cambridge, Harvard University Press, 1983.

64. Klein M: The significance of early anxiety situations in the development of the ego, in *The Psychoanalysis of Children,* ed. 3, (Strachey A, trans), London, Hogarth Press, 1948.

65. Mahler MS, Furer M: Observations in research regarding the symbiotic syndrome of infantile psychosis. Psychoanal Q, *29:*317, 1960.

66. Mahler MS: *On Human Symbiosis and the Vicissitudes of Individuation,* New York, International Universities Press, 1978.

67. Sullivan HS: *The Interpersonal Theory of Psychiatry,* New York, Norton, 1953.

68. Sullivan HS: *Schizophrenia as a Modern Process,* New York, Norton, 1963.

69. Lidz T: *The Origins and Treatment of Schizophrenic Disorders,* New York, Basic Books, 1973.

70. Bateson G, et al.: Towards a theory of schizophrenia. Behav Sci, *1:*251–264, 1956.

71. Wynne LC, et al,: Pseudomutuality in the family relations of schizophrenics. Psychiatry, *21:*205–220, 1958

72. Wynne LC, Singer M, et al.: Communications of the adoptive parents of schizophrenics, in Jorsted J, Ugelstad G (eds): *Schizophrenia 75,* Oslo, Universitatforlaget, 1976.

73. Doane JA, Falloon IRH, et al.: Parental affective style and the treatment of schizophrenia. Arch Gen Psychiatry, *42:*34–42, 1985.

74. Lidz T: A developmental theory, in Shershow JC (ed) *Schizophrenia: Science and Practice,* pp. 69–95, Cambridge, Harvard University Press, 1978.

75. Wynne LC, Singer M: Thought disorder and family relations of schizophrenics: A

research strategy. Arch Gen Psychiatry, *9:*191–198, 1963.

76. Wynne LC, Singer M: Thought.disorder and family relations of schizophrenics. A classification of forms of thinking. Arch Gen Psychiatry, *9:*159–206, 1963.

77. Goodstein RK: Guide to CAT scanning in hospital psychiatry. Gen Hosp Psychiatry, *7:*367–376, 1985.

78. Battaglia J, Spector IC: Utility of the CAT scan in a first psychotic episode. Gen Hosp Psychiatry, *10:*398–401, 1988.

79. Weinberger DR: Brain disease and psychiatric illness; When should a psychiatrist order a CAT scan? Am J Psychiatry, *141:*1521–1527, 1984.

80. Manschreck TC, Keller MB: Disturbances of thinking, in Lazare A (ed): *Outpatient Psychiatry: Diagnosis and Treatment,* pp 265–270, Baltimore, Williams & Wilkins, 1979.

81. MacKinnon RA, Michels R: The psychiatric interview, in *Clinical Practice,* pp. 230–258, Philadelphia, W.B. Saunders Co., 1971.

82. Vaillant G: *Adaptation to Life,* pp. 75–90, Boston, Little, Brown & Co., 1977.

81. Brown GW, et al.: Influence of family life on the course of schizophrenic disorders: A replication. Br J Psychiatry, *121:*241–258, 1972.

84. Vaughn CE, Leff JP: The influence of family and social factors on the course of psychiatric illness. Br J Psychiatry, *129:*125–137, 1976.

85. Vaughn CE, Snyder KS, et al.: Family factors in schizophrenic relapse. Arch Gen Psychiatry, *41:*1169–1177, 1984.

86. Koenigsberg HW, Hardley R: Expressed emotion: From predictive index to clinical construct, Am J Psychiatry, *143:*1361–1373, 1986.

87. Kanter J, Lamb HR, Loeper C: Expressed emotion in families: A critical review. Hosp Community Psychiatry, *38:*374–380, 1987.

88. Falloon IRH, Boyd JL, McGill CW, et al.: Family management in the prevention of morbidity of schizophrenia. Arch Gen Psychiatry. *42:*887–896, 1985.

89. Leff J: Family factors in schizophrenia. Psych Annals, *19:*542–547, 1989.

90. Hogarty GE, Anderson CM, Reiss DJ, et al.: Family psychoeducation, social skills training and maintenance chemotherapy treatment in

the aftercare treatment of schizophrenia. Arch Gen Psychiatry, 43:633–642, 1986.

91. Sartorius N, Jablensky A, Korten A, et al.: Early manifestations and first-contact incidence of schizophrenia in different cultures. Psychol Med, 16:909–928, 1986.

92. Ananth J, Vandewater S, Kamal M, et al.: Missed diagnosis of substance abuse in psychiatric patients. Hosp Community Psychiatry, 40:297–299, 1989.

93. Miller FT, Tanenbaum JH: Drug abuse in schizophrenia. Hosp Community Psychiatry, 40:847–849, 1989.

94. Miller FT, Busch F, Tanenbaum JH: Drug abuse in schizophrenia and bipolar disorder. Am J Drug Alcohol Abuse, 15:291–295, 1989.

95. Caton CLM, Gralnick A, Bender S, et al.: Young chronic patients and substance abuse. Hosp Community Psychiatry, 40:1037–1040, 1989.

96. Drake RE, Wallach MA: Substance abuse among the chronic mentally ill. Hosp Community Psychiatry, 40:1041–1046, 1989.

97. Sederer LI: Multiproblem patients: Mental disorders and substance abuse, in Milkman HB, Sederer LI (eds): *Treatment Choices in Alcoholism and Substance Abuse,* pp. 163–181, Lexington, Mass., Lexington Press, 1990.

98. Minkoff K: An integrated treatment model for dual diagnosis of psychosis and addiction. Hosp Community Psychiatry, 40:1031–1036, 1989.

99. Carpenter WT, et al.: The treatment of acute schizophrenia without drugs: An investigation of some current assumptions. Am J Psychiatry, 134:14–20, 1977.

100. Kane JM: The current status of neuroleptic therapy. J Clin Psychiatry, 50:322–328, 1989.

101. May PRA: *Treatment of Schizophrenia,* New York, Science House, 1968.

102. Brier A, Wolkowitz OM, Aoran AR, et al.: Neuroleptic responsivity of negative and positive symptoms in schizophrenia. Am J Psychiatry, 144:1549–1555, 1987.

103. Feinberg SS, Kay SR, Elijovich LR, et al.: Pimozide treatment of the negative schizophrenic syndrome. J Clin Psychiatry, 49:235–238, 1988.

104. Carpenter W: Early, targeted pharmacotherapeutic intervention in schizophrenia. J Clin Psychiatry, 47:23–29, 1986.

105. Carpenter WJ, Heinrichs DW, Hanlon TE: A comparative trial of psychopharmacologic strategies in schizophrenia. Am J Psychiatry, 144:1466–1470, 1987.

106. Kulhanek F, Linde OK, et al.: Precipitation of antipsychotic drugs in interaction with coffee or tea (letter to the editor). Lancet 2:1130, 1979.

107. Hirsch SR: Precipitation of antipsychotic drugs in interaction with coffee or tea (letter to the editor). Lancet, 2:1130, 1979.

108. Bowen S, Taylor KM, et al.: Effect of coffee and tea on blood vessels and efficacy of antipsychotic drugs, (letter to the editor), Lancet, 1:1217–1218, 1981.

109. Kulhanek F, Linde OK: Coffee and tea influence pharmacokinetics of antipsychotic drugs (letter to the editor). Lancet, 2:359–360, 1981.

110. Baldessarini RJ, Cohen BM, Teicher MH: Significance of neuroleptic dose and plasma level in the pharmacological treatment of psychoses. Arch Gen Psychiatry, 45:79–91, 1988.

111. Kec PE, Cohen BM, Baldessarini RJ, et al.: Time course of antipsychotic effects of neuroleptic drugs. Am J Psychiatry, 146:1289–1292, 1989.

112. Gelenberg A: Haloperidol levels: A therapeutic window? Biol Ther Psychiatry 7:36, 1984.

113. Simpson GM, Yadalam K: Blood levels of neuroleptics: State of the art. J Clin Psychiatry, 46 (5, sec.2):22–28, 1985.

114. Shostak M, Perel JM, Stiller RL, et al.: Plasma haloperidol and clinical responses. J Clin Psychopharmacol, 7:394–400, 1987.

115. Neborsky R, Janowsky D, et al.: Rapid treatment of acute psychotic symptoms with high- and low-dose haloperidol. Arch Gen Psychiatry, 38:195–199, 1981.

116. Van Putten T, Marder SR, Mintz J: A controlled study of different dose levels of haloperidol in newly admitted schizophrenics. Arch Gen Psychiatry, 47:754–758, 1990.

117. Rifkin A, Dodd SR, Karajgi BM: The effect of dose of Haldol and outcome of acute schizophrenia. Paper presentation, American

Psychological Association annual meeting, San Francisco, 1989.

118. Dubin WR: Rapid tranquilization: Antipsychotics or benzodiazepines. J Clin Psychiatry, 49:5–12, 1988.

119. McEvoy JP, McCue M, Freter S: Replacement of chronically administered anticholinergic drugs by amantadine in outpatient management of chronic schizophrenia. Clin Ther, 9:429–433, 1987.

120. Van Putten T: The many faces of akathisia. Compr Psychiatry, 16:43–47, 1975.

121. Ratey JJ, Salzman C: Recognizing and managing akathisis. Hosp Community Psychiatry, 35:975–977, 1984.

122. Keckich WA: Neuroleptics: Violence as a manifestation of akathisia. JAMA, 240:2185, 1978.

123. Shear MK, Frances A, et al.: Suicide associated with akathisia and depot fluphenazine treatment. J Clin Psychopharmacol, 3:235–236, 1983.

124. Drake RE, Ehrlich J: Suicide attempts associated with akathisia. Am J Psychiatry, 142:499–501, 1985.

125. Anderson BG, Reker D, et al.: Prolonged adverse effects of haloperidol in normal subjects. N Engl J Med. 305:643–644, 1981.

126. Kendler KS: A medical student's experience with akathisia. Am J Psychiatry, 133:454–455, 1976.

127. Van Putten T, May PR, et al.: Response to antipsychotic medication: The doctor's and the consumer's view. Am J Psychiatry, 141:16–19, 1984.

128. Lipinski JF, Zubenko GS, et al.: Propanolol in the treatment of neuroleptic-induced akathasia. Am J Psychiatry, 141:412–415, 1984.

129. Dupuis B, Catteau J, Duman SP, et al.: Comparison of propanolol, sotalol, and betaxolol in the treatment of neuroleptic-induced akathisia. Am J Psychiatry, 144:802–805, 1987.

130. Alexander HE Jr, McCarty K, et al.: Hypotension and cardiopulmonary arrest associated with concurrent haloperidol and propanolol therapy. JAMA, 252:87–88, 1984.

131. Ratey JJ, Sorgi P, et al.: Nadolol as a treatment for akathisia. Am J Psychiatry 142:640–642, 1985.

132. Zubenko GS, Cohen BM, et al.: Use of clonidine in treating neuroleptic-induced akathasia. Psychiatry Res, 13:253–259, 1985.

133. Gelenberg AJ, Mandel MR: Catatonic reactions to high potency neuroleptic drugs. Arch Gen Psychiatry, 34:947–950, 1977.

134. Granacher RP: Differential diagnosis of tardive dyskinesia: An overview. Am J Psychiatry, 138:1288–1297, 1981.

135. Wolf ME, Mosnaim AD: Tardive dyskinesia: Biological mechanisms and clinical aspects, Washington, D.C., American Psychiatric Press, 1988.

136. Gardos G, Cole JO, Salomon M, et al.: Clinical forms of severe tardive dyskinesia. Am J Psychiatry, 144:895–902, 1987.

137. Jeste DV, Wyatt RJ: Prevention and management of tardive dyskinesia. J Clin Psychiatry, 46:14–18, 1985.

138. Kane JM (ed): Drug maintenance strategies in schizophrenia. Washington, D.C., American Psychiatric Association, 1984.

139. Casey DE: Tardive dyskinesia: What is the natural history? International Drug Therapy Newsletter, 18:13–16, 1983.

140. Lazarus A, Mann SC, Caroff SN: The neuroleptic malignant syndrome and related conditions. Washington, D.C., American Psychiatric Press, 1989.

141. Levinson DF, Simpson GM: Neuroleptic-induced extrapyramidal symptoms with fever. Arch Gen Psychiatry, 43:839–848, 1986.

142. Shalev A, Hermosh H, Munitz H: Mortality from neuroleptic malignant syndrome. J Clin Psychiatry, 50:18–25, 1989.

143. Misiaszek JJ, Potter RL: Atypical neuroleptic malignant syndrome responsive to conservative management. Psychosomatics, 26:62–66, 1985.

144. Coons DJ, Hillman FJ, et al.: Treatment of neuroleptic malignant syndrome with dantrolene sodium: A case report. Am J Psychiatry, 139:944–945, 1982.

145. Zubencko G, Pope HG: Management of a case of neuroleptic malignant syndrome with bromocriptine. Am J Psychiatry, 140:1619–1620, 1983.

146. Lazakus A: Treating neuroleptic malignant syndrome (letter to the editor). Am J Psychiatry, 141:1014–1015, 1984.

147. Markowitz JC, Brown RP: Seizures

with neuroleptics and antidepressants, Gen Hosp Psychiatry, 9:135–141, 1987.

148. Nevins DP: Adverse response to neuroleptics in schizophrenia. Int J Psychoanal Psychother, 6:227–241, 1977.

149. Cohen LS: Psychotropic drug use in pregnancy. Hosp Community Psychiatry, 40:566–567, 1989.

150. Kane J, Honigfield G, Singer J, et al.: Clozapine for the treatment-resistant schizophrenic, Arch Gen Psychiatry, 45:789–796, 1988.

151. Marder SR, Van Putten T: Who should receive Clozapine? Arch Gen Psychiatry, 45:865–867, 1988.

152. Lieberman JA, Kane JM, Johns CA: Clozapine: Guidelines for clinical management. J Clin Psychiatry, 50:329–338, 1989.

153. Salzman C: Use of benzodiazepines to control disruptive behavior in inpatients. J Clin Psychiatry, 49:13–15, 1988.

154. Donyon R, Angrist B, Peselow E, et al.: Neuroleptic augmentation with Alprazolam. Am J Psychiatry, 146:231–234, 1989.

155. Alexander PE: Antipsychotic effects of lithium in schizophrenia. Am J Psychiatry, 136:283–287, 1979.

156. Neppe VM: Carbamazepine as adjunctive treatment in nonepileptic chronic inpatients with EEG temporal lobe abnormalities. J Clin Psychiatry, 44:326–331, 1983.

157. Kramer MS, Vogel WH, DiJohnson C, et al.: Antidepressants in "depressed" schizophrenic inpatients. Arch Gen Psychiatry, 46:922–928, 1989.

158. Hanssen T, Heyden T, et al.: Propanolol in schizophrenia. Arch Gen Psychiatry, 37:685–690, 1980.

159. Yorkston NJ, Gruzelier JH, et al.: Propanolol as an adjunct to the treatment of schizophrenia. Lancet, 2:575–578, 1977.

160. Peet M, Bethell MS, et al.: Propanolol in schizophrenia: I. Comparison of propanolol, chlorpromazine, and placebo. Br J Psychiatry, 139:105–111, 1981.

161. Lader M: β-adrenoceptor antagonists in neuropsychiatry. J Clin Psychiatry, 49:213–223, 1988.

162. Pollack MH, Rosenbaum JF, Hyman JE: Calcium channel blockers in Psychiatry. Psychosomatics, 28:356–369, 1987.

163. Reiter S, Adler L, Angrist B, et al.: Effects of Verapamil on tardive dyskinesia and psychosis in schizophrenic patients. J Clin Psychiatry, 50:26–27, 1989.

164. Greenblatt M: Efficacy of ECT in affective and schizophrenic illness. Am J Psychiatry, 134:1001–1005, 1977.

165. Salzman C: The use of ECT in the treatment of schizophrenia. Am J Psychiatry, 137:1032–1041, 1980.

166. Jones M: The concept of a therapeutic community. Am J Psychiatry, 112:647–650, 1956.

167. Cummings J, Cummings E: Ego and milieu. New York, Atherton, 1962.

168. Sederer LI: Inpatient psychiatry: What place the milieu? (editorial). Am J Psychiatry, 141:673–674, 1984.

169. Kahn EM, White EM: Adapting milieu approaches to acute inpatient care for schizophrenic patients. Hosp Community Psychiatry, 40:609–614, 1989.

170. Van Putten T, May PR: Milieu therapies of the schizophrenias, in West LJ, Fluin ED (eds): Treatment of Schizophrenia: Progress and Prospects, p. 239, New York, Grune & Stratton, 1976.

171. May PR, Tuma HA, et al.: Schizophrenia: A followup study of the results of five forms of treatment. Arch Gen Psychiatry, 38:776–784, 1981.

172. Gunderson JG: A reevaluation of milieu therapy for nonchronic schizophrenic patients. Schizophr Bull, 6:64–69, 1980.

173. Gunderson JG: If and when milieu therapy is therapeutic for schizophrenics, in Gunderson JG, Will O, Mosher EL (eds): Principles and Practice of Milieu Therapy, New York, Jason Aronson, 1983.

174. Van Putten T: Milieu therapy: Contraindications? Arch Gen Psychiatry, 29:640–643, 1973.

175. Eissler KR: Psychiatric ward management of the acute schizophrenic patient. J Nerv Ment Dis, 105:397–402, 1947.

176. McReynolds P: Anxiety perception and schizophrenia, in Jackson DD (ed): The Etiology of Schizophrenia, pp. 248–292, New York, Basic Books, 1960.

177. Spotnitz H: The need for insulation

in the schizophrenic personality. Psychoanal Q, 49:3–25, 1962.

178. McGhie A: Psychological studies of schizophrenia. Br J Med Psychol, 39:281–288, 1966.

179. Stierlin H: Individual therapy of schizophrenics and hospital structure, in Burton A (ed): *Psychotherapy of the Psychoses,* pp. 329–348. New York, Basic Books, 1961.

180. Will OA: Human relatedness and the schizophrenic reaction. Psychiatry, 22:205–223, 1959.

181. Bouvet M: Technical variation and the concept of distance. Int J Psychoanal, 39:211–221, 1958.

182. Freud S: *Beyond the Pleasure Principle,* standard ed, vol 18, London, Hogarth Press, 1920.

183. Johnson JM, Parker KE: Some antitherapeutic effects of a therapeutic community. Hosp Community Psychiatry, 34:70–71, 1983.

184. Spadoni AF, Jackson JA: Milieu therapy in schizophrenia: A negative result. Arch Gen Psychiatry, 34:1047–1052, 1977.

185. Klass DB, Grune GA, et al.: Ward treatment milieu and post-hospital functioning. Arch Gen Psychiatry, 34:1047–1052, 1977.

186. Kernberg OF: The therapeutic community. A re-evaluation. J Natl Assoc Private Psychiatr Hosp, 12:46–55, 1981.

187. Raskin DE: Problems in the therapeutic community. Am J Psychiatry, 128:492–493, 1971.

188. Fischer A, Weinstein MR: Mental hospitals, prestige, and the image of enlightenment. Arch Gen Psychiatry, 25:41–48, 1971.

189. Shershow JC: Disestablishing a therapeutic community. Curr Concepts Psychiatry, 3:8–11, 1977.

190. Islam A, Turner DL: The therapeutic community: A critical reappraisal. Hosp Community Psychiatry, 33:651–653, 1982.

191. Lazell EW: The group treatment of dementia praecox. Psychoanal Rev, 8:168–179, 1921.

192. Kanas N, Rogers M, et al.: The effectiveness of group psychotherapy during the first three weeks of hospitalization: A controlled study. J Nerv Ment Dis, 168:487–492, 1980.

193. Pattison EM, Brissenden E, et al.: As-sessing special effects of inpatient group psychotherapy. Int J Group Psychother, 17:283–297, 1967.

194. Strassberg DS, Roback HD, et al.: Self-disclosure in group therapy with schizophrenics. Arch Gen Psychiatry, 32:1259–1261, 1975.

195. Weiner MF: Outcome of psychoanalytically oriented group psychotherapy. Group, 8:3–12, 1984.

196. Yalom ID: *Inpatient Group Psychotherapy,* New York, Basic Books, 1983.

197. Maves PA, Schulz JW: Inpatient group treatment on short-term acute care units. Hosp Community Psychiatry, 36:69–73, 1985.

198. Greenberg L, Fine SB, Cohen C: An interdisciplinary psychoeducational program for schizophrenic patients and their families in an acute care setting. Hosp Community Psychiatry, 39:277–282, 1988.

199. Liberman RP: Psychiatric rehabilitation of chronic mental patients, Washington, D.C., American Psychiatric Press, 1987.

200. Paul GL, Lentz RJ: *The psychosocial treatment of the chronic mental patient.* Cambridge, Harvard University Press, 1977.

201. Rogers CR: *The Therapeutic Relationship and Its Impact,* Madison, University of Wisconsin Press, 1967.

202. Schwartz DP: Psychotherapy, in Shershow JC (ed): *Schizophrenia,* Cambridge, Harvard University Press, 1978.

203. McGlashan TH: Intensive individual psychotherapy of schizophrenia: A review of techniques. Arch Gen Psychiatry, 40:909–920, 1983.

204. Schwartz DP: Schizophrenia: Individual psychotherapy, in Kaplan HI, Sadock BJ (eds): *Comprehensive Textbook of Psychiatry,* ed. 5, pp. 806–815, Baltimore, Williams & Wilkins, 1984.

205. Fromm-Reichmann F: *Principles of Intensive Psychotherapy,* Chicago, University of Chicago Press, 1950.

206. Fromm-Reichmann F: Notes on the development of treatment of schizophrenia by psychoanalytic psychotherapy. Psychiatry, 11:262–273, 1948.

207. Engle RP, Semrad EV: Brief hospitalization, the recompensation process, in Abroms

GM, Greenfield NS (eds): *The New Hospital Psychiatry*, New York, Academic Press, 1971.

208. Drake RE, Sederer LI: Inpatient psychotherapy of chronic schizophrenia: Avoiding regression. Hosp Community Psychiatry, 27:897–901, 1986.

209. Stanton AH, Gunderson JG, Knapp PH, et al.: Effects of psychotherapy in schizophrenia: I. Design and implementation of a controlled study. Schizophr Bull 10:520–563, 1984.

210. Gunderson JG, Frank AF, Katz HM, et al.: Effects of psychotherapy in schizophrenia. II. Comparative outcome of two forms of treatment. Schizophr Bull 10:564–598, 1984.

211. Katz HM, Frank A, Gunderson JG, et al.: Psychotherapy of schizophrenia: What happens to treatment dropouts? J Nerv Ment Dis, 126:109–140, 1958.

212. Hatfield AB: Patients' accounts of stress and coping in schizophrenia. Hosp Community Psychiatry, 40:1141–1145, 1989.

213. Anonymous: A Recovering Patient: "Can We Talk?": The schizophrenic patient in psychotherapy. Am J Psychiatry, 143:68–70, 1986.

214. Will AO: Psychotherapeutics and the schizophrenic reaction. J Nerv Ment Dis, 126:109–140, 1958.

215. Havens L: Explorations in the uses of language in psychotherapy: Counterprojective statements. Contemp Psychoanal, 16:53–67, 1980.

216. Lidz TS, Fleck S, et al.: *Schizophrenia and the Family*, New York, International Universities Press, 1965.

217. Semrad EV: *Teaching Psychotherapy of Psychotic Patients*, New York, Grune & Stratton, 1969.

218. Brown GW, Monck EM, Carstairs GM, et al.: Influence on family life on the course of schizophrenic illness. Br J Prev Soc Med, 16:55–68, 1962.

219. Brown GW, Rutter ML: The measurement of family activities and relationships. Hum Relations, 19:241–263, 1966.

220. Brown GW, Birley JLT, Wing JK: Influence of family life on the course of schizophrenic disorders; a replication. Br J Psychiatry, 121:241–258, 1972.

221. Vaughn CE, Leff JP: The influence of family and social factors on the course of psychiatric illness: A comparison of schizophrenic and depressed neurotic patients. Br J Psychiatry, 129:125–137, 1976.

222. Leff JP, Vaughn CE: The role of maintenance therapy and relative expressed emotion in relapse of schizophrenia: A two-year follow-up. Br J Psychiatry, 139:102–104, 1981.

223. Vaughn CE, Snyder KS, Freeman W, et al.: Family factors in schizophrenic relapse: A replication. Schizophr Bull, 8:425–426, 1982.

224. Vaughn CE, Snyder KS, et al.: Family factors in schizophrenic relapse: Replication in California of British research on expressed emotion. Arch Gen Psychiatry, 41:1169–1177, 1984.

225. Karno M, Jenkins JH, de la Selva A, et al.: Expressed emotion and schizophrenic outcome among Mexican-American families. J Nerv Ment Dis, 1975:143–151, 1987.

226. Moline RA, Singh S, Morris A, et al.: Family expressed emotion and relapse in schizophrenia in 24 urban American patients. Am J Psychiatry, 142:1078–1081, 1985.

227. Snyder KS, Liberman RP: Family assessment and intervention with schizophrenics at risk for relapse, in *New Directions for Mental Health Services, No. 12, New Developments in Interventions with Families of Schizophrenics*, pp. 49–59, San Francisco, Jossey-Bass, 1981.

228. Falloon IRH, Boyd JL, McGill CW: *Family care of schizophrenia: A problem solving approach to mental illness*, New York, Guilford Press, 1984.

229. Tarrier N, Barrowclough C, Vaughn C, et al.: The community management of schizophrenia: A controlled trial of a behavioral intervention with families to reduce relapse. Br J Psychiatry, 153:532–542, 1988.

230. McFarlane WR: *Family therapy in schizophrenia*, New York, Guilford Press, 1983.

231. Leff JL: Family factors in schizophrenia. Psych Annals, 19:542–547, 1989.

232. McFarlane WR, Beels CC: A decision-free model for integrating family therapies for schizophrenia, in McFarlane WR (ed): *Family Therapy in Schizophrenia*, pp. 325–335, New York, Guilford Press, 1983.

233. Arieti S: *Understanding and Helping the Schizophrenic: A Guide for Family and Friends*, New York, Basic Books, 1979.

234. Torry EF: Surviving schizophrenia: A family manual, New York, Harper & Row, 1983.

235. Shore D (ed): Schizophrenia: Questions and Answers. Rockville, MD Schizophrenia Research Branch, National Institute of Mental Health, 1986. (U.S. Department of Health and Human Services Publication No. 86-1457).

236. Tsuang MT: Genetic counseling for psychiatric patients and their families. Am J Psychiatry, 135:1465–1475, 1978.

237. Gudeman JE, Shore MF: Beyond Deinstitutionalization. N Engl J Med, 311:832–836, 1984.

238. Lamb HR, Peele R: The need for continuing asylum and sanctuary. Hosp Community Psychiatry, 35:798–802, 1984.

239. Lamb HR: Some reflections on treating schizophrenics. Arch Gen Psychiatry, 43:1007–1011, 1986.

240. Keefe RSE, Mohs RC, Losonczy MF, et al.: Premorbid sociosexual functioning and long-term outcome in schizophrenia. Am J Psychiatry, 146:206–211, 1989.

241. Kay SR, Maw MS: The positive-negative distraction in drug-free schizophrenic patients. Arch Gen Psychiatry, 46:711–718, 1989.

242. McGlashan TH: The prediction of outcome in chronic schizophrenia. Arch Gen Psychiatry, 43:167–176, 1986.

243. Parker G, Johnston P, Hayward L: Parental "experienced emotion" as a predictor of schizophrenic relapse. Arch Gen Psychiatry, 45:806–813, 1988.

244. Drake RE, Cotton PG: Depression, hopelessness, and suicide in chronic schizophrenia. Br J Psychiatry, 148:554–559, 1986.

245. Prudo R, Blum HM: Five-year outcome and prognosis in schizophrenia: A report from the London Field Research Center of the International Pilot Study of Schizophrenia. Br J Psychiatry, 150:345–351, 1987.

246. Drake RE, Gates C, et al.: Suicide among schizophrenics: Who is at risk? J Nerv Ment Dis, 172:613–617, 1984.

247. Herz MI: Recognizing and preventing relapse in patients with schizophrenia. Hosp Community Psychiatry, 35:344–349, 1984.

248. Hogarty GE, Goldberg SC, et al.: Drug and sociotherapy in the aftercare of schizophrenic patients, II. Arch Gen Psychiatry, 31:609–618, 1974.

249. Hogarty GE, Goldberg SC, et al.: Drug and sociotherapy in the aftercare of schizophrenic patients, III. Arch Gen Psychiatry, 31:609–618, 1974.

250. Glick ID, Hargreaves WA: Psychiatric Hospital Treatment for the 1980s: A Controlled Study of Short vs. Long Hospitalization, Lexington, Mass, Lexington Books, D.C. Heath & Co., 1979.

251. Harron M, et al.: Is modern-day schizophrenic outcome still negative? Am J Psychiatry, 135:1156–1162, 1978.

252. McGlashan TH: The Chestnut-Lodge follow-up study. Arch Gen Psychiatry, 41:586–601, 1984.

253. Bleuler M: The course, outcome, and prognosis of schizophrenic psychoses, in Flach, F (ed): The Schizophrenias, pp. 1–21, New York, W.W. Norton, 1988.

254. Harding CM, Zubin J, Strauss JJ: Chronicity in schizophrenia: Fact, partial fact, or artifact? Hosp Community Psychiatry, 38:477–486, 1987.

4

Borderline Character Disorder

Lloyd I. Sederer, MD
Jane Thorbeck, EdD

DEFINITION

Character-disordered patients of all types (including borderline characters) show disturbed, inflexible patterns of relating to themselves and others that are established by adolescence or earlier. These patients manifest impaired functioning in their relationships, work, and play, and they experience personal distress (1–5).

The term *borderline* first appeared in the psychoanalytic and psychiatric literature in the 1930s, though its antecedents can be traced to a decade earlier (6–8). The term referred then to patients in whom a psychoneurotic condition masked a psychosis or to those with a tendency to react negatively to therapy and become dramatically regressed or suicidal.

Today the terms *borderline character disorder* and *borderline personality organization* represent patients who present with a specific pathological personality organization. The character of these patients shows *specific traits* and is *not* merely a transitory state between neurosis and psychosis (3). In fact, because *persistent instability* is characteristic of borderline patients, they have

been described as being "stably unstable" (3).

Under highly structured, supportive conditions borderline characters may appear to be asymptomatic and functioning at a neurotic level. However, when stressed they *regress* and demonstrate clear disturbances in their capacity to contain and manage feelings and impulses. This may happen in response to disappointment, loss, or absence of routine and structure; under the influence of drugs or alcohol; or during a psychotherapeutic transference storm. This basic vulnerability to regression renders the borderline patient unstable. Mood, behavior, self-image, cognition, and interpersonal relationships are all subject to this instability, and symptoms may appear in any or all of these areas.

CASE EXAMPLE: Ms. O. was a 19-year old college freshman who presented for her first psychiatric admission with the chief complaint of "I've been depressed since Thursday."

A more careful history revealed that the patient complained of feeling "all speeded up," with difficulty falling asleep and some early morning awakening in the 2–3 weeks before admission. The patient reported that "it might be fun to die" and had intermittent suicidal ideation with thoughts of jumping out of a window of a moving train. Further, during this period the patient had two transient experiences in which she thought a person on the television was talking to her. These symptoms began rather precipitously following a breakup with a boyfriend whom she had known only briefly. This relationship ended after the patient posed in the nude for a film that was being made by a male friend of her boyfriend.

The patient reported feeling depressed for much of her lifetime with intermittent feelings of being "dead inside." She had an extensive history throughout her adolescence of heterosexual relationships characterized by superficiality and promiscuity. She reported having difficulty maintaining relationships because, as she put it, "when you get to know someone you find out they are as screwed up as you are." The patient had a history of amyl nitrate, Percodan, and marijuana abuse.

On admission, the patient was surrounded by several family members, all of whom appeared anxious and exasperated. In the interview, the patient showed labile affect with periods of crying, anger, and thinly veiled seductiveness. She was not psychotic at the time of interview nor did she show a prominent neurovegetative depression. Suicidal ideation was described and the patient requested hospitalization in order to "work on my self-image." In view of the patient's suicidal ideation and precipitous decompensation, she was admitted for crisis intervention, diagnostic evaluation, and short-term hospital treatment.

ETIOLOGICAL CONSIDERATIONS

Biological Hypotheses

Numerous authors have hypothesized an affectively disordered component to borderline pathology (9–18). Evidence of an affective disorder playing an etiological role in borderline pathology is supported by the presence of depressive symptomatology, significant increases in the prevalence of affect disorders in relatives of borderline patients, epidemiological lifetime prevalence rates of depression in borderline patients, similarities in electroencephalogram (EEG) sleep between borderline and affectively disordered patients, and response to medications that target dysthymic symptoms. Gunderson and Elliot (14) propose that the observed concurrence of borderline and affective disorders occurs despite their heterogeneity. They hypothesize that individuals who develop either disorder start with a biophysiological limitation or vulnerability that increases their risk of psychological impairment in early childhood development. The observed overlap is then due to a convergence of innate and early environmental factors that combine to produce depression, chronic dysphoria, and borderline behavior.

Heterogeneity of biological influences is likely for borderline pathogenesis. Andrulonis et al. (19–21), studying a long-term inpatient population of patients with marked functional impairment and past treatment failures, identified three subcategories of borderline disorders, distinct from one another and from a schizophrenic control group. The first group had no history of past or current symptoms of major or minimal brain dysfunction. This group had a history of acting-out behaviors, drug and alcohol abuse, depression, and a family history of affective disorder; these patients were predominantly female with the onset of their disorder occurring in adolescence. A second group had a history of significant head trauma, epilepsy, or encephalitis. A third group had a history of past or current documented severe hyperactivity, distractibility, and/or learning disabilities. The second and third groups were often males with early developmental problems and symptoms of episodic dyscontrol, adult minimal brain disorder, or limbic abnormalities. These latter two groups were considered organically brain disordered. From these findings, Andrulonis et al. posit a nonorganic borderline group who respond to a relationship-based, insight-oriented psychotherapy, a stable and structured living environment, and perhaps the adjunctive use of neuroleptics, antidepressants, or lithium. On the basis of the second and third groups, the authors also posit an organically dysfunctional dimension to some borderline patients, often male, who require structure and consistency in their relationships and environment, special education and vocational training, directive family therapy, and perhaps stimulants or anticonvulsants.

One model to explain the genetic diathesis in borderline pathology has been advanced by Meissner (22). He organizes borderline character types along a spectrum on the basis of the presence or absence of psychosis or mood disorder. For example, latent schizophrenia would represent the psychotic end of the borderline spectrum; hysteroid dysphoria would represent the affectively disordered end of the spectrum; and the "as if" personality would represent a borderline patient without features of psychosis or mood disorder. In his model, Meissner demonstrates the interplay between genetics and environment. According to Meissner, schizophrenic biological factors play a role in the more psychotically disabled characters, and an affective diathesis plays a role in the more mood-disordered characters. Treatment planning, including choice of medication, course, and prognosis, derive from accurate diagnosis along this character spectrum.

Psychodynamic and Developmental Hypotheses

Recent theoretical investigations into the pathogenesis of borderline personality derive from trauma theory (23, 24). Certain clinical findings are characteristic of both borderline pathology and chronic posttraumatic stress disorder (PTSD): affect dysregulation and intolerance; hyperactivity and irritability; chronic dysphoria and depression; subjective "deadness and emptiness"; risktaking, impulsive and self-destructive

behaviors; and substance use and abuse. Investigators therefore have been prompted to hypothesize that childhood physical and sexual abuse are instrumental in the genesis of borderline pathology (25–27). Empirical evidence to support this hypothesis, especially in women (who primarily carry the diagnosis of borderline character), is accumulating (28–31). We will return to this subject in the section on psychotherapy. The importance of chronic familial trauma in the understanding, prevention, and treatment of borderline patients will occupy clinical inquiry and discussion in the years to come.

More established and perhaps more familiar hypotheses on the pathogenesis of borderline character derive especially from the object relations theorists, including Mahler, Winnicott, Adler, and Kernberg.

In work based on child observation, Margaret Mahler (32) has described the second to the fifth months in the infant's life as the *symbiotic phase* of development. In this phase the infant's dependence is absolute and the child requires near total empathic understanding from the mother (33).

Borderline patients have had an adequate experience in the symbiotic phase and encounter their difficulties in the next phase of development, the *separation-individuation phase*. This phase spans from five months to three years in the child's life. It is the time when the child begins to develop muscular and psychological autonomy. Successful maturation through the development tasks of separation and individuation requires what Winnicott has called a "good enough mother" (33–35). This mother is able to contain the prominent pregenital, aggressive impulses of the child by nonpunitive, nonanxious, and firm limit setting. She does so without curtailing her love and understanding. According to Adler (36), this mother has a basic confidence in her own goodness. Believing in herself, she is able to frustrate the child (when this is appropriate) without fearing the child's anger. Her empathic qualities enable her to complement this frustration with understanding. In turn, the child learns to tolerate physical and emotional frustration and separation from the mother through gradually developing a comforting internal image of her.

In summary, the "good enough mother" provides a "holding environment" (33, 37) in which she empathetically, reliably, and firmly contains the child through the separation-individuation process. Successful mastery of this period establishes the child's capacity for ambivalence, object constancy, and tolerance of separation without serious regression.

Kernberg (4, 38) provides a different perspective on early development. He suggested that borderline patients demonstrate excessive aggression early in childhood as an outgrowth of either constitutional predisposition or persistent frustration of the child. The child's early experience with his mother does not allow him to develop an image of a mother who can tolerate powerful, negative feelings toward her. As a consequence, the ability to integrate positive and negative aspects of mother, and in turn the self, does not develop. In the absence of this integration, known as ambivalence, the child must dissociate good and bad, for they cannot be tolerated simultaneously in regard to the self or others. This dissociation is called splitting (see section entitled "Ego Operations, Character Diagnosis, and the Psychodynamic Formulation"). Splitting weakens the ego, for it must compromise reality. This weakened ego poorly tolerates anxiety and frustration and shows a vulnerability to further regression. In addition, this limited ego has a diminished capacity for object constancy and therefore cannot sustain a stable, trusting relationship with another which would mitigate the desperate fear of aloneness.

Family Hypotheses

Families of borderline patients have been regularly studied with a range of findings of variable validity and reliability.

Early parental losses or abrupt and traumatic separations from parents are significant in the histories of borderline patients (39, 40). The borderline patient's frequent and persistent use of transitional objects has been hypothesized as deriving from these early familial disruptions (41). The presence of significant psychopathology in both mothers and fathers of borderline patients has been demonstrated across socioeconomic lines (42, 43). Parents of borderline patients are given to neglect. Maternal depression and unpredictability are not offset by paternal involvement and stability. The prevalence of addictive disorders, incest, domestic violence, and other Axis II disorders are prominent in the families of borderline patients. (The role of parental abuse in the development of borderline symptomatology has been addressed in the section on dynamic and developmental contributions to this disorder.)

Shapiro and Zinner offer a family or systems perspective on borderline psychopathology (44–46). In their studies on adolescent borderlines they draw upon the developmental and object-relations perspective of Winnicott, Mahler, and Kernberg. These authors have found that neither parent need be borderline. Instead they postulate that the family system as a whole functions in a regressed manner under the pressure of a shared unconscious fantasy that angry or hostile feelings can destroy a loved object. Believing in this fantasy, the family then employs the defense of splitting in order to protect their attachment to the loved object.

Shapiro and Zinner maintain that the parents of the borderline patient suffer from marked conflict in regard to autonomy and dependency issues. When a specific, unconsciously chosen child reaches adolescence, that child reactivates critical separation issues that were never mastered by the child or the parents. This specific child's *dependent* wishes and needs are experienced by the rest of the family as *devouring demands* from which they withdraw. Theoretically, dependent wishes are seen as so devouring because they represent the denied and otherwise unrecognized dependent needs of the parents, needs which the parents themselves never had met.

The specific adolescent's efforts at *autonomy* are experienced by the family as a form of *hateful abandonment.* This adolescent is viewed by the family as wanting to separate because he hates and wishes to reject the family. Regressive splitting of "good and bad" feelings occurs because the family cannot function at a mature level of ambivalence. In this regressed state, the family tries to limit the adolescent's strivings for autonomy.

Masterson (47, 48) has also studied the borderline adolescent. He hypothesizes that the essence of the borderline dilemma is the conflict between natural autonomous growth and fear of parental abandonment. Masterson maintains that the mother (and father) suffers from a borderline syndrome. His observations suggest that mother rewards the child's regressive clinging and withdraws libidinal support in response to the child's independent efforts. In effect, according to Masterson, the borderline parents of the borderline adolescent are still tied to their respective mothers from whom they were unable to separate. The parents' developmental failure renders them incapable of facilitating the child's mastery of the separation-individuation phase of development. When separation issues are intensified by an adolescent child, these parents experience a renascence of internal conflict which they then act out with this child.

Family hypotheses on the genesis of borderline pathology are intriguing and frequently therapeutically useful. However, these contributions are new, sometimes conflicting, and the data are of variable statistical strength. The etiology of borderline disorders is multifactorial and a singular focus on the family is shortsighted. Biological contributions and the role of temperament need further development. Furthermore, the families of schizophrenic patients have suffered for too long under the concept of the "schizophrenogenic mother/family," adding to the family's burden and impairing our capacity to ally with, educate, and support adaptive efforts by a family. Until more is known about the etiology of borderline disorders, we must take care not to repeat this mistake with families of borderline patients, thereby fostering guilt and defensiveness, and alienating those closest to our patients.

DIAGNOSIS AND DIFFERENTIAL DIAGNOSIS

The diagnosis and differential diagnosis of the borderline patient can be approached from two major perspectives. The first is a *symptomatic* perspective in which constellations of symptoms provide a basis for nosology. The second perspective is *developmental and psychodynamic* and builds a nosology based on maturational processes and a psychology of the mind. Neither perspective need exclude the other.

Symptomatic Diagnosis and Differential Diagnosis

SYMPTOMATIC DIAGNOSIS

Borderline characters typically show features of the following symptomatic picture: (1, 2, 5, 49, 50)

1. Affective instability with rapid mood shifts to anxiety, irritability, or depression.

2. Unstable and intense interpersonal relationships.
3. Difficulty in being alone and chronic feelings of boredom and emptiness.
4. Impulse disorders, addictions, and self-injurious behavior with the chronic, repetitive emergence of impulses in the service of gratifying instinctual needs.
5. Transient psychotic experiences.
6. Polymorphous (multiple, at times coexisting, sexual deviations) perverse sexual trends.

SYMPTOMATIC DIFFERENTIAL DIAGNOSIS

The symptomatic differential diagnosis (1, 5, 22, 51–55) of the borderline patient includes the following.

Schizophrenia. As noted in Chapter 3, schizophrenia is a longitudinal diagnosis that requires greater than six months of thought, volitional, and affective disturbances. Affect in schizophrenia tends to be flat, while borderline affect is unstable, intense, and often angry. Schizophrenics tend to be socially isolated, unlike borderline patients who show compulsive and intense social behavior.

Major Depressive Episode. A major depressive episode is marked by neurovegetative signs (appetite, sleep, and psychomotor disturbances) that have persisted for at least several weeks (see Chapter 1). Borderline patients regularly suffer from a co-morbid depressive disorder (56–59). The trait disorder of character pathology generally cannot stabilize under the adverse influence of a concurrent state disorder like depression.

Histrionic Personality Disorder. Histrionic patients show exaggerated expressiveness and are given to impulsive behavior. These symptoms, however, are more marked in conflicted areas (e.g., sexuality) in the histrionic person, whereas the borderline patient shows more generalized and diffuse affective and impulsive dyscontrol.

Sexuality tends to be inhibited in the histrionic, promiscuous and polymorphous in the borderline. Cognitively, histrionics may be diffuse and impressionistic but without the reality disturbances that the borderline individual may evidence.

Narcissistic Character Disorder. Narcissistic characters (1, 60–62) suffer from a disturbance in self-regard. They are manifestly grandiose in their self-importance and are preoccupied with fantasies of greatness, power, and privilege. In their interpersonal relationships they are exploitative, idealizing or devaluing, and entitled. Unlike the borderline, they generally do not regress to transient psychotic states or severe panic.

Drug and Alcohol Use and Abuse. Frequently, borderline patients have a history of continuous use or regular abuse of alcohol and drugs. Very often these substances were a part of the admission drama in which the patient overdosed or acted in an impulsive and self-destructive way, while in an intoxicated state.

Diagnostic dilemmas and treatment controversies pervade the clinical arena of substance-abusing borderline patients. Over time, the abuse of intoxicants can induce personality regressions and unleash a variety of impulsive and self-destructive behaviors consistent with borderline pathology (63). Conversely, borderline characters can turn to psychoactive substances to mute affective instability and to ameliorate dysphoria. Furthermore, chemical dependency and borderline pathology can and do coexist. Finally, chronic abuse of central nervous system intoxicants (especially alcohol, sedatives, and benzodiazepines) or an autonomous affective disorder can produce a depressive symptom picture in a borderline patient who may then rely further on drugs of abuse to self-medicate the depression.

Alcohol and drug abuse obscure an accurate diagnosis of an affective disorder. Furthermore, the predominance of depressive symptoms in chemically abusing patients are often organic affective disorders that will remit with abstinence. For these reasons we recommend that the first step in diagnosing and treating drug-using borderline patients be the attainment of abstinence (64). In some cases, particularly with sustained abstinence, the putative diagnosis of borderline disorder will no longer be accurate as character organization substantially improves without the dissolution effects of addiction. In all cases of borderline patients with co-morbid substance abuse (with or without affective disorder), recovery from a transient character regression and a developmental progression beyond the pronounced limitations of a borderline ego require abstinence.

Patients cannot adequately proceed, biologically or psychologically, on a path of character development or remission from depression if they continue regularly to abuse psychoactive drugs. Biologically, drugs of abuse have a direct and deleterious effect on the brain (especially the limbic system). They also interfere with the pharmacokinetics of any prescribed mood-altering drug. Psychologically, regular use of drugs impairs ego function, represents denial of illness, and may result in life-endangering behaviors.

If the patient cannot abstain because of denial and the compulsive drive of addiction, then referral for treatment of substance abuse would be in order. This can begin in the hospital and continue on an outpatient basis. A period of at least 1–3 months is often (though not always) needed for biology and psychology to reconstitute to a nondependent state; in this state, mood disorder and character pathology can be accurately assessed.

EGO OPERATIONS, CHARACTER DIAGNOSIS, AND THE PSYCHODYNAMIC FORMULATION

The Defensive Operations of the Ego

Borderline patients are driven by powerful pregenital aggressive impulses and possess an internal world of all good and all bad object images. Their chaotic, intense, and ever-changing lives behaviorally represent the ego's adaptive efforts to master these impulses and comply with these images through the defenses of splitting, projective identification, idealization, and devaluation.

Borderline patients' inability simultaneously to maintain loving and hating aspects of their self-image or image of others is the core dilemma for the borderline ego. The need to preserve a sense of the good and loving in the presence of feelings of the bad and hating is managed by the defense of splitting.

Splitting is the defense of keeping consciously separate from each other feelings and perceptions that are opposite or contradictory. In other words, positive and negative feelings and percepts are alternately, but never concomitantly, in consciousness. Splitting is different from *denial*, in which whole percepts are disavowed or denied and generally substituted by wish-fulfilling fantasies. Denial severely compromises reality and is seen in the psychotic disorders. Splitting is also different from repression in which an intolerable affect or idea is temporarily expelled from consciousness. Repression underlies neurotic defensive operation. Splitting is the defense that characterizes the borderline patient's efforts to preserve a relationship characterized by marked neglect, abuse, or manipulation, yet needed for emotional survival. Splitting also underlies the borderline defenses of projective identification, primitive idealization, omnipotence, and devaluation.

Through the defense of *projective identification,* an unacceptable part of the patient's self (e.g., an impulse or a judgment about the self) is dissociated (split) from consciousness and attributed to someone else. An identification with the other then occurs because that person now has the projected qualities of the self; the patient then behaves in response to this projection. For example, if an aggressive impulse is projected, it is then easily recognized (unconsciously identified with) and responded to with distrust or retaliation. Projective identification is a primitive defense since the impulse or percept is not effectively mastered. The ego is weakened by the processes of splitting and projective identification, and the patient is left to respond to or control the recipient of his projections. Nevertheless, projective identification must also be understood as the borderline patient's *effort at a relationship,* however flawed and disturbing. Through projective identification borderline patients evoke feelings in the recipient that are like their own: they have made someone else feel like they do. For therapists, projective identification allows for empathy because they can experience how their patient is feeling.

Primitive idealization is the tendency to see someone else as totally good. Bad aspects of that person are dissociated and may be taken on by the self or attributed to others. *Omnipotence* is the conviction that the self is all powerful (through a process of identification with a magically idealized other). *Devaluation* is the tendency to see someone else as totally bad. It is the complementary defense of idealization.

Character Diagnosis

Character diagnosis, unlike descriptive diagnosis, is rooted in developmental and ego-defensive considerations. Kernberg has written extensively in the area of character pathology and differential diagnosis (2, 4, 65, 66). Although we will attempt to summarize some of his work here, we urge the reader to read the primary source material. Our aim is to provide a framework for understanding character-disordered patients along a *continuum of psychopathology.* It provides a tool for differentiating borderline patients from other character-disordered patients and for understanding individual patient regressions and progressions as they occur over the course of time and in psychotherapy.

Kernberg approaches the classification of character pathology from the perspectives of the *defensive operations of the ego, superego* development, instinctual development,* and the nature of the person's *internalized object relationships†.* He has offered a classification of levels of organization (higher, intermediate, and lower) of character pathology. This continuum confines itself to character pathology. In doing so it omits psychosis, which would occur before the more disturbed end of the spectrum, and neurosis and normality, which would represent the next and final steps of development after higher-level character pathology. Obsessional and hysterical characters are good examples of higher-level characters, while borderline patients, in particular, exemplify the lower end of the character continuum. *Table 4.1* summarizes this classification, further detailed below.

The *defensive operations of the ego* form a continuum in which higher level characters employ repression as the major defense

---

*The superego is a theoretical construct which describes the mental functions of morality, conscience, and guilt. The superego can be punitive, critical, and evoke guilt. It can also be loving and rewarding through a component known as the ego ideal.

†Internalized object relationships are the introjections and identifications of the emotionally valued people in the person's life that form the basis of the ego's identity.

Table 4.1. Continuum of Character Pathology[4,65]

Higher	Intermediate	Lower
Superego—well-integrated but severe. *Ego*—well-intergrated; ego identity with stable self-concept and stable representational world. Defensive operations—repression primary; little or no instinctual infiltration into defensive character traits, which are primarily inhibitory and sublimatory. Adaptation—somewhat constricted due to neurotic defenses but *not* seriously impaired. Object relationships—deep and capable of experiencing guilt, mourning, and wide range of affects. *Instincts*—sexual and aggressive drives are partially inhibited; genital phase and oedipal conflicts predominate; no pathological condensation of genital level strivings with pregenital aggressiveness. *Examples*—obsessive-compulsive characters; most hysterical characters; depressive-masochistic characters.	*Superego*—punitive, rigid, and less integrated; decreased capacity for guilt; paranoid trends. *Ego*—subject to contradictory demands of superego, i.e., be great, powerful, and attractive and morally perfect. Defensive operations—repression still primary, but some dissociation and defensive splitting occurs in limited areas; character traits are partially infiltrated by instinctual strivings (e.g., structured impulsivity). Adaptation—variable; subject to mood swings, distrust. Object relationships—capacity for involvements with others is possible but characterized by conflict. *Instincts*—genital level reached but pregenital (especially oral) conflicts emerge as major regressive trend; aggressive nature of pregenital conflicts is muted. *Examples*—many narcissistic characters; passive-aggressive characters; sadomasochistic characters; hysteroid characters (lower level hysterics).	*Superego*—minimally integrated; tendency to project aspects of primitive, punitive superego; severely impaired capacity for guilt and concern. *Ego*—synthetic function seriously impaired; identity diffusion results from lack of stable self-concept and experience of stable external world; ego weakness with poor anxiety tolerance and impulse dyscontrol. Defensive operations—splitting is primary with related projective identification, omnipotence, and devaluation; character defenses are typically impulsive and instinctually infiltrated. Adaptation—generally paranoid secondary to projected superego aspects and projective identification; severely limited conflict-free ego and adaptive capacities; repetitive failures in work, play, and relationships. Object relationships—object constancy not fully reached; relationships tend to be intensely dependent or threatening; unintegrated good and bad internal images and past object relationships. *Instincts*—excessive pregenital aggression fosters a condensation of pregenital and genital conflicts; polymorphous perverse drives infiltrate all relationships. *Examples*—borderline characters; antisocial characters; many narcissistic characters; prepsychotic characters (schizoid and paranoid).

with the related defenses of intellectualization, rationalization, undoing, and higher levels of projection. Instinctual wishes are sublimated and do not appear in their original and primitive form in higher-level characters. Intermediate-level characters also employ repression but the defensive barrier is weak, and the impulse is partially expressed in behavior (e.g., passive-aggressiveness). Intermediate-level characters use splitting as the predominant defense with the related mechanisms of projective identification, omnipotence, idealization, and devaluation. Impulses (e.g., agressive and sexual) frequently break through these limited defenses.

The *superego development* of lower-level characters is severely limited by a weak, impaired ego and its use of defensive splitting. Idealized notions of the self and others create unreachable expectations of power and greatness while a punitive superego insists on fearful obedience. Higher-level characters have developed a stable ego identity with a capable repressive barrier which excludes unacceptable instincts and impulses from consciousness. Furthermore, the punitive superego is modified by its integration with more realistic and caring parental introjects in the form of the ego ideal.

The instinctual development of higher-level characters reveals adequately inhibited aggression, genital primacy, and oedipal-level conflicts. Intermediate-level characters have reached a genital level of organization but regress repeatedly to pregenital levels, particularly to oral (or dependent) fixation points. Lower-level characters evidence marked pregenital aggressiveness which is said to pervade all their functioning.

The internalized object relationships of lower-level characters (such as borderline and schizoid personalities) are severely disturbed. In the absence of object constancy and with splitting as a primary defense, their internal images are alternately all good and all bad. As a consequence, neither self nor others can be perceived as benign, whole, or constant. Intermediate-level characters have developed a stable, integrated sense of self and others, but in a highly conflicted manner. Higher-level characters possess a stable sense of self and experience a relatively limited degree of conflict.

Psychodynamic Formulation

The inpatient psychodynamic formulation attempts to address what kind of internal vulnerability has been stressed by the current misfortunes of the patient's life to sufficiently destabilize him and require hos-

pitalization. The formulation often includes a genetic reconstruction (in this case, early familial and developmental) of familial influences; a character construction; and an hypothesis about what the clinician can expect in the transference and countertransference. A variety of models for the dynamic formulation exist, each with varying utility depending on the patient and the theoretical perspective of the clinician (67, 68).

Borderline patients who enter the hospital generally have experienced a real or anticipated object loss or disappointment in the degree of holding or containment their sustaining world provides. This loss powerfully reverberates with an inner experience (shaped by early loss, unpredictability, or outright abuse by caretaking figures) of panicky dread of aloneness, even annihilation. Desperate manipulation and self-destructive behaviors can ensue as the patient seeks to gain some measure of control and channel intense, aggressive drives and dependent needs. In these cases the transference can contain elements of urgent idealization and attachment or projection and severe devaluation admixed with fears of victimization. Clinicians may experience an aversion to the intensity of the object relation and also feel as if their efforts to help are inadequate or sadistic.

When possible, the formulation should attempt to examine and answer questions regarding the patient's capacity to use a dynamically orientated psychotherapy. A more developed formulation will usefully inform consultation to an ongoing therapy and treatment planning. The capacity to use a dynamic therapy is related to the patient's capacity for alliance; ego competencies of intelligence and object orientation; established superego responses of guilt and concern; a motivation for change (not only gratification); and a capacity to internalize the therapist and hence restructure the internal object world (22, 69).

EPIDEMIOLOGY

Accurate incidence, prevalence, and socioeconomic data on borderline psychopathology are not available. Estimates are of 2–4% prevalence in the general population. Prevalence estimates for psychiatric patient populations, inpatient and outpatient, range from 15–25% (70). On inpatient units, borderline patients represent the most common personality-disorder diagnosis.

Women are diagnosed twice as frequently as men as having borderline-personality disorder. Although the disorder is well recognized in the United States and Europe, no evidence demonstrates its universality across all cultures.

HOSPITAL TREATMENT

The effective hospital treatment of the borderline patient is one of the major challenges in contemporary hospital psychiatry. Borderline patients require special management strategies in order to *minimize the difficulties* they experience in the hospital. Primary among these difficulties is a negative response to treatment, with pronounced, rapid *regression* and *acting out* of deviant and dangerous behavior.

Indications for hospitalization of the borderline patient include a life-threatening crisis; a transient psychotic episode; a relapse into drug abuse; persistent depressive symptomatology; or an impasse or severe transference reaction in outpatient psychotherapy. Diagnostic uncertainty regarding a concurrent affective or psychotic disorder would also be an indication for acute hospitalization. Intermediate (2–6 months) and long-term hospitalization will be discussed in the Controversies Section.

The following hospital treatment guidelines are based on an understanding of the vicissitudes of the borderline patient's early life and the vulnerabilities that grow out of this period. These guidelines have also been fashioned on the education anvil of empirical experience and treatment failures (71–73).

Preadmission Contact

As a general rule, it is advisable for the unit's admitting officer (often a physician) and a member of the unit staff (often a nurse) to meet and develop a treatment plan with the borderline patient before admission. From the start, doctor and nurse, admissions officer, and ward staff present themselves to the patient in a unified manner. The *splitting and distortion* that tend to occur if the patient meets one clinician for admission evaluation and another upon arrival on the unit are thereby minimized.

Furthermore, the preadmission meeting is designed to limit the borderline patient's defensive use of *primitive idealization*. The defensive use of primitive idealization in the borderline patient creates a mythic vision of the hospital and its staff as an all-good, all-caring, and all-correcting experience. Unless primitive idealization is identified and defused from the start, the patient is likely to experience a major disappointment, with regression and probable acting out soon after admission.

At the preadmission meeting the following issues may be negotiated with the patient.

GOALS FOR HOSPITALIZATION

Typically, borderline patients present with diffuse or global goals for hospitalization which, of course, can never be achieved. Discrete goals set during the preadmission meeting help prevent an interminable and directionless hospitalization.

Examples of hospital goals include ending life-threatening suicidal or homicidal ideation; evaluating for and beginning individual, outpatient psychotherapy; evaluating and treating transient, psychotic states or persistent, depressive symptomatology; evaluating and initiating medications; evaluating alternate living arrangements, including a halfway house or a new home; and consulting with a patient and therapist who are experiencing a prolonged outpatient therapeutic impasse or a crisis in therapy. It helps to write out the goals developed, though we have reservations about calling this a "contract." The term contract can be legalistic and adversarial and blind us from appreciating that the agreement is not exactly between two equal partners. Clearly, although goals and an agreement are sought, the clinician must recognize that the patient has a limited capacity for fulfilling the obligations of the contract.

TIME FRAME OF HOSPITALIZATION

Borderline patients tend to regress in the hospital, especially after several weeks on a unit. The preadmission meeting negotiates a time frame for hospitalization, generally *10–21 days*, within which the patient is expected to realize the goals of hospitalization. A time frame helps to preclude an experience of the hospital as timeless (like the unconscious). It allows the patient a rational time for achieving certain goals without encountering the dependency problems that an extended hospitalization fosters.

BEHAVIORAL LIMITS (WARD RULES)

The ward rules, basically behavioral limits, are explained to the patient during the preadmission meeting. The sanctions for rule breaking (which include restriction of privileges, warning, transfer, and discharge) are mentioned to the patient, *emphasizing the need to maintain the patient's physical safety*. The ward rules should address the following:

1. *Violence toward the Self or Others.* Violence toward the self or others will not be condoned. Before admission to an open unit patients make a commitment to verbally inform staff of, rather than act upon, any impulse to hurt themselves or anyone else. Locked containment, seclusion, and observed status are necessary alternatives for those patients who cannot control destructive impulses.
2. *Drugs.* The presence and/or use of nonprescribed drugs (legal or illegal) is strictly forbidden.
3. *Sexual Activity with Others.* Sexual activity with patients or visitors is not permitted.
4. *Ward Treatment Program.* During the preadmission meeting the hospital staff explains to the patient the nature of the unit and the treatments it provides. At this meeting the staff asks the patient to make a commitment to participate in the hospital treatment program of individual evaluation, group therapy, milieu therapy, medications when indicated, case conferences and consultations that relate to his care, and family meetings as indicated. It is often helpful to tell patients that they are *entitled to* a full treatment program.

The preadmission meeting and treatment plan can do more than minimize defensive splitting, primitive idealization, regression, and acting out. It is also an opportunity for *alliance building* with a borderline patient. The meeting is an opportunity to ally with the healthy part of the patient's ego and create a sense of hopeful expectation. When regressions occur, as they almost inevitably do, the working alliance can then be resurrected around the preadmission plan with its goals, time frame, and agreement about permissible and nonpermissible behaviors on the unit.

Frequently, *family work* will be integral to the patient's recompensation. In some cases the families of borderline patients will only agree to evaluation when there is a crisis. Insisting on family participation before admission while the crisis is alive may, in some cases, be the only time to effectively establish family participation in the patient's hospital treatment.

Managing Regressions

Time spent in developing preadmission plans and ward behavior rules will help reduce the incidence of regressions but will not prevent them. Borderline patients will predictably revert to earlier levels of defensive organization as a central aspect of their psychological construction.

For certain borderline patients in long-term treatment, regressions may have utility (36). In our view, however, regressive states in short-term hospital care are disruptive, dangerous, and not beneficial to psychotherapeutic work. The following comments apply to the work of relatively short (weeks–months) inpatient care.

Borderline regressions call for an increase in activity by the therapist and unit staff. Clear limits must be set on destructive behaviors and expectations about functioning in the community must be created. Reality testing is generally impaired in regressive states. Staff should expect that patients' capacities to test reality have diminished and work with patients to improve their understanding of their environment and correct distortions that have developed in their minds. The therapeutic alliance is also invariably fractured in the regressive episode. The restoration of the alliance occupies a priority treatment goal. Without such an alliance there is no common ground on which to proceed. Finally, regressive states in patients can and do induce regressive states in staff through the process of projective identification. Unit staff must be alert to countertransference feelings, mobilized at these times, which distort how we experience the patient and causes us to regard the patient as someone who is hateful, hopeless, or worthless. We earn our wages at these times as we labor (and ask patients to labor) to understand and alter our countertransference difficulties.

Psychopharmacological Management

Borderline patients enter the hospital in acute distress superimposed upon chronic feelings of dysphoria, lability, depression, and anergia as well as a variety of impulsive and self-destructive or suicidal behaviors. Some may evidence impaired reality testing and psychotic symptomatology. For many of these patients the judicious use of medications will allow for some degree of subjective relief and behavioral stabilization and may complement and enable psychosocial approaches to their care. No medications are without side effects and risks. In this patient population, risks also include self-destructiveness from indiscriminate abuse and overdose of prescribed medications. A careful, well-documented assessment of the risk/benefit formula by the prescribing doctor, in conjunction with the patient (and family, when appropriate), should precede the administration of any but emergency medications.

Pharmacological treatment begins with a diagnostic assessment to identify any concurrent or co-morbid psychiatric disorder and target symptoms apt to respond to medication (9–15, 19–21, 64, 74).

MANAGING A DRUG WITHDRAWAL STATE

Psychoactive substance use, abuse, and dependence are remarkably common co-morbid conditions in borderline patients (59, 64, 75). Sedatives of the central nervous system (CNS) (alcohol and hypnotics) and tranquilizers are preferred drugs of abuse in borderline characters and, importantly, can produce withdrawal states. If the history obtained from the patient, friends, or family is positive for substance abuse, or the patient shows signs or symptoms of a withdrawal state, the clinician must begin treatment for withdrawal. The reader is referred elsewhere for the diagnosis and treatment of alcohol, barbituate, and hypnotic withdrawal states (see Chapters 6 and 7).

ANXIOLYTIC (ANTIANXIETY) AGENTS

Borderline patients often complain and manifest signs of marked anxiety. Many such patients will have used and abused benzodiazepines as one of their preferred self-medication agents. Furthermore, many borderline patients report feeling better on such agents (76, 77). However, the effect of benzodiazepines in these patients is a complex phenomenon. Benzodiazepines can produce states of marked disinhibition with serious self-destructive behavior in this patient population (76, 78). Furthermore, this class of drugs has abusive and addictive potential, thereby adding to its risk.

Though short- and mid-range acting benzodiazepines may offer some subjective feeling of improvement, they carry substantial potential adverse effects. Therefore, their use is generally not indicated. The role of longer-acting benzodiazepines such as clonazepam is a clinical alternative worth considering, though no good studies of its effectiveness and problems are currently available.

ANTIDEPRESSANTS

1.   Tricyclic Antidepressants. Tricyclic antidepressants (TCAs) may be used for a borderline patient who shows criteria for a major depressive episode that has lasted for at least several weeks (see Chapter 1). Though distinct depressive episodes with a constellation of neurovegetative signs that last for several weeks are possible in borderline patients, what the clinician generally encounters is the mood lability of the borderline patient. Tricyclic antidepressants have a role in the treatment of depressive disorders and are highly effective in managing the neurovegetative target symptoms of depression. Their effectiveness, in borderline patients with co-morbid depressions, is limited and evidence suggests that those who do not respond may become worse on TCAs (demonstrating impulsive, self-destructive, and assaultive behavior and self-referential thinking) (79). Tricyclic antidepressants generally are not helpful in managing characterological mood lability (17).

2.   Fluoxetine. This activating, serotonin-uptake inhibitor is now in general use for a wide range of depressive and other disorders. Some borderline patients with depression may do well with this agent. It is important to monitor this drug for its adverse effect of increased anxiety and dysphoria, for it can destabilize a fragile borderline patient and potentially aggravate suicidal behavior (80).

3.   Monoamine Oxidase Inhibitors. Klein and Davis have noted the value of monoamine oxidase inhibitors (MAOI) in patients they regard as having "hysteroid dysphoria" (16, 81). These patients are characterized by repeated dysphoric states, rejection sensitivity, impulse dyscontrol, and a tendency toward substance abuse. Phenelzine (Nardil) has been used effectively in these patients. Dosages of 45 mg or more per day appear to reduce their emotional lability and, consequently, the disordered impulsive behaviors that occur during dysphoric states. Prolonged maintenance treatment appears necessary since discontinuing medication is reported to result in recurrence of symptomatology.

Tranylcypromine (Parnate) also is effective in certain borderline patients, even those without diagnosable major depression (74). Mood disturbances and impulsivity are target symptoms for this medication. Desired responses can include diminished anxiety and rage, improved mood, and a capacity to experience pleasure.

MOOD STABILIZERS

1.   Lithium Salts. Rifkin et al. have recommended the use of lithium in patients they term as having "emotionally unstable character disorders" (17). Rifkin bases this recommendation on the hypothesis that this disorder is an affective illness characterized by depressive and hypomanic swings that last no longer than a few days at a time.

The clinical features of the "emotionally unstable character disorder" are found in some borderline patients. Therefore, lithium carbonate can be considered an alternative treatment for this disorder. Lithium must be used cautiously because of its possible cardiac and long-term renal effects and the risk of serious toxicity and death from overdose (See Chapter 2).

2. Carbamazepine. Carbamazepine (Tegretol) has a demonstrable effect on reducing impulsive behavior in borderline patients (74, 78). Carbamazepine can attenuate the frequency and magnitude of behavior dyscontrol. However, in one study, three of 17 borderline patients treated with this agent developed major depression with melancholia (82). All three untoward effects occurred in patients with a history of depression. Carbamazepine may also induce aplastic anemia, agranulocytosis and hepatitis. In prescribing this drug, the physician is well advised to explicitly document consent and rigorously monitor side effects, particularly since carbamazepine does not have Federal Food and Drug Administration approval for this disorder.

3. Neuroleptics. Borderline patients who experience episodic psychotic states; evidence affective lability with a prominence of anger, anxiety, and/or depression; or have a history of self-destructive behavior (including suicidal efforts, drug abuse, and sexual promiscuity) have responded to treatment with low-dose, high-potency neuroleptic medication (83, 84). High-potency rather than low-potency neuroleptics are preferable because they are not sedating, which appears to help considerably with compliance.

Trifluperazine (Stelazine), fluphen-azine (Prolixin), haloperidol (Haldol), thiothixene (Navane), and perphenazine (Trilafon) are all effective, high-potency agents. Thioridazine (Mellaril) has also been reported to be helpful (85). *Titrating the correct dosage* appears to be a critical aspect of the effective neuroleptic treatment of these patients. *Small doses* of these *high-potency* neuroleptics are generally all that are necessary. The patient may be started on 1 or 2 mg of any of the high-potency medications and built up to a range of 2–10 mg per day. The clinician should document a dose-response curve in which diminution of symptomatology is measured against the dosage and adverse effects of the neuroleptic. Psychotic symptoms, paranoid ideation, and anxiety, depression, and hostility may all improve on neuroleptic medication (79, 86). Though benefits are clear to clinicians, patients often do not feel subjectively better. Such subjective complaints (and consequent noncompliance) are often symptomatic of akathisia which may complicate treatment.

Individual Psychotherapy

Individual psychotherapy for borderline patients in hospitals has traditionally been based on lengths of stay of at least several months (87, 88). An important challenge to today's clinician is understanding what can and cannot be provided through this treatment modality in a several-week admission of a borderline patient. In our view, the work of brief hospitalization of a borderline patient is, principally: crisis intervention, diagnostic assessment, pharmacological and environmental manipulation, initiation of psychotherapy, and consultation to ongoing care. Therefore, the role of individual psychotherapy must precisely relate to and enable these other interventions.

Individual psychotherapy begins along two simultaneous lines. The first is formulation (see page 117) developed to help answer the question, "Why is the patient in this hospital now?" Second, through this inquiry the therapist seeks to initiate a working or "helping" alliance (89–91). Optimally, the therapist invites partnership, provides empathy and respect, and enhances the patient's experience of control through understanding.

As we have detailed elsewhere (92), individual therapy can vary markedly. A supportive psychotherapy aims to contain affects and impulses; strengthen defenses against anxiety and panic; support human ties; restore shattered self-esteem and morale; and provide hope (93, 94). This form of therapy is technically different from an uncovering or evocative psychotherapy. In the latter, affects and impulses are mobilized; defenses examined and perhaps confronted; conflicts highlighted; and historical and transference phenomena are sought and deliberated.

With few exceptions, the hospitalized borderline patient can benefit from a brief, supportive, and adaptationally oriented psychotherapy. Assessing the patient, therapist, and the unit is best done before initiating a more evocative treatment, especially when confinement may only be a few weeks (92). There are patients for whom the latter will be indicated and needed for stabilization; for example, patients working through a transference storm or impasse or needing extra support in confronting traumatic memories. In these cases, a clear and documented formulation and psychotherapy treatment plan will help in clinically mastering a difficult process and obtaining the support of skeptical colleagues and external review organizations.

Brief psychotherapy of borderline patients may not evidence its effectiveness initially. As Waldinger and Gunderson have reported (95), repetitive, brief treatments may occur before patients can establish themselves in an ongoing and effective treatment. For the clinician who will attempt an insight-orientated, affectively evocative psychotherapy, certain technical considerations may prove helpful. Pine has challenged the distinction between supportive and insightful therapies. Instead, he asks what are the optimal techniques for the treatment of fragile personalities (96). He stresses that given the proper support, the mutative work of insight and interpretation in fact can be done with patients with compromised psychological structure. According to Pine, patients must evidence some degree of reliable defensive organization to protect them against overwhelming affective states and must have a modicum of trust and alliance to maintain a view that the therapist does not seek to humiliate, hurt, or abandon them. If the patient has these capacities, the therapist can provide a dynamic therapy in the context of considerable "holding" (33, 34). The therapist must increase the patient's degree of activity in the treatment process (i.e., create an active partnership in hard work); avoid open-ended and vague questions; and approach affectively disorganizing material with warning and during times of emotional quiescence and readiness. As Pine put it, "strike when the iron is cold."

During therapeutic encounters with borderline patients, the clinician can anticipate a steady exodus of projective constructions from the patient. Any effective engagement with the primitive patient will require the therapist to be open to these projections rather than seeking to avert them. To some theorists, the crucial element in fostering intrapsychic change occurs through a process during which the therapist receives projections (especially projective identifications), "metabolizes" them, and then verbally returns them to the patient in a form altered by the higher defensive organization of the therapist (97, 98). For example, when patients project unbearable experiences of helplessness and self-loathing, therapists must allow themselves to personally experience these same affects in order to "metabolize" or detoxify them through their own capacity to modulate raw and intense affective states. Therapists can then return the altered experience to the patient, as, in this instance, perhaps, a sense of realistic limitation and self-doubt. Humor, especially irony and humility, can be important elements in the success of this complex interpersonal process.

For patients who have had traumatic early histories, psychotherapy may wittingly or unwittingly confront their recrudescence. Considerable controversy exists as to whether the acutely decompensated patient has the ego capacity to tolerate and work through traumatic memories. Yet there are times when this must be done and times when the support of the hospital is needed for their successful resolution. Whether to direct therapeutic work to the traumatic memories is a matter of clinical judgment. To acknowledge their reality and their power and help the patient develop alternatives to their painful expression will be essential in allying with the patient and enabling a compromised ego to mature.

The difficulty inherent in working with this patient population is no more apparent than in the frequency by which we all err in the process (92). Countertransference problems, especially, provoke a variety of technical errors. These errors tend to occur in five areas:

1. *Empathy.* Confusing sympathy and empathy is a source of common technical error in psychotherapeutic work with the borderline patient. In spite of almost intolerable levels of distress, the borderline patient cannot tolerate much in the way of warmth, comfort, kindness, or intimacy. It follows that the patient cannot tolerate an overly sympathetic therapist. Sympathy is not empathy. This is a lesson the borderline patient will drive home. An empathetic therapist is atuned to what the patient needs and what the patient can tolerate. Overly warm or sympathetic behavior with

patients already fighting for affective modulation and interpersonal distance can be dangerous. A prominent sympathetic display can frighten the patient and stimulate rapid withdrawal, regression, and acting out.

2. *Transference.* The borderline patient's proclivity toward intense and rapidly shifting transferences, often of psychotic proportions and frequently beyond alliance and interpretation, makes cultivating the transference akin to wearing red in the bullring. For the therapist to be silent or concentrate on the patient-therapist relationship during the acute phase of the patient's disorder fosters regression in the transference followed by increased acting out.

This position of eschewing a central focus on the therapist-patient dyad, and the transferences therein, seems contrary to Kernberg's position on the centrality of interpreting transference in the treatment technique he calls expressive psychotherapy (expressive therapy is differentiated from supportive therapy and traditional psychoanalysis (87). However, Kernberg's recommendations are for outpatient work or extended inpatient work which is different from short-term hospital treatment of regressed borderline patients that involves weeks, not months or years.

3. *Confrontation.* Confrontation is an especially seductive therapeutic tack; these patients quickly encourage us to surmise that no less a club than confrontation will mitigate their avoidant and irresponsible tendencies (87, 99–102). Short of confronting imminent life-threatening impulses which do not bow to everyday exploration, the technique of confrontation may do harm in a variety of ways. Especially provocative (and evocative of brewing transference feelings) is confronting the patient's rage.

Borderline patients are also well-known for their entitlement. Their expectation of special status and their readily observable stance—"Why haven't you done something for me lately?''—are familiar. Confronting this position of entitlement neglects an understanding that borderline patients cannot occupy a psychological middle ground. To confront away overvaluation of the self is to leave the patient with its opposite, namely, devaluation of the self. Confronting entitlement may abruptly bring borderline patients into affective sight of their profound worthlessness and self-loathing. Stripping these patients of the thin, though entitled, robe of self-esteem is to expose them to their most malevolent introjects.

4. _Interpretation and Management._ Interpretation is the psychotherapeutic technique of rendering the patient's unconscious conscious. Interpretation is accomplished by explaining to the patient the feelings, wishes, impulses, and conflicts that exist out of awareness. Using interpretations, especially the tendency of therapists to be openly, that is vocally, intuitive, even if correct in their formulations, is yet another source of adverse consequence in working with borderline patients.

CASE EXAMPLE: A staff member informed a patient how his recent drug taking and fugue states were related to difficulties in the outpatient therapy. In fact, the staff member went on to say, these symptoms were an effort to run away from intense, even cannibalistic, longings for the therapist. On the unit, the patient became more passive and inactive; he reported he felt he could do very little without "checking it out with his therapist."

An interpretation offered in this manner is essentially therapeutic intolerance on the therapist's part. The patient generally feels intruded upon, because the interpretation preempts the patient's willingness to reassess his position vis-à-vis himself and other people. When tempted to offer such bits of deft psychology, therapists may be trying to soothe themselves. Desperate behaviors and the patient's primitive feelings (such as hate and murderous rage) are a major test of skill and patience. At these times one is vulnerable to a need to do something, to replace badness with goodness, hatred with brotherly love. It is indeed difficult to stand by and witness the savage and painful nature of some patients' lives.

One can also feel tempted to compensate for the patient's early privations and try to give or replenish, in the form of words and understanding, what the patient did not receive in early life. At such moments, well-chosen words are like sedatives: they quiet people down, they do not help to heal the wounds. They help professionals to feel potent at a time when they would otherwise feel the limits of their role (102).

At times, management of a patient's activities, or lack of them, may serve the same purpose.

CASE EXAMPLE: A woman in her thirties was given a great deal of fine advice about how to go about managing her home and finances. The more the staff said, the less she did. Before long, many staff were angry with her for not following through on all that they had said.

Therapeutic maneuvers, be they interpretation of unconscious processes or management of everyday life, may neglect the patient in two ways. First, in soothing the patient's distress the therapist fails to provide the patient with an opportunity to speak, without demand for change, about that which is most hateful and grievous in him. No one else is likely to provide this form of inquiry so essential to healing the split ego. Second, when therapists behave with omniscience and omnipotence they invite magical fantasies on the part of their patients. Therapists must tolerate autonomy and initiative on the patient's part, through the struggle of trial, effort, failure, and eventual mastery.

5. _Pain._ One infrequently challenged therapeutic assumption is that patients seek to be disentangled from their pain. Working by this assumption would have us encourage, cajole, and otherwise influence borderline patients to rid their lives of the pain begotten by their bodies, their environment, or their families and friends. Pain may be, however, a very particular experience for borderline patients whose early life and object experiences were not of the pleasurable sort that allows normal development to consolidate around trust and love (103–105).

For borderline patients, early life was inconsistent and painful. For some, pain becomes a symbolic affect that represents the nature of (and perpetuation of) the relationship with the mother. For these patients the attachment to pain is equivalent to their continued attachment to the primary object, namely, mother. Attachment to and identification with pain, pain as mother, is a far cry better than a barren inner world, devoid of human representation. For these patients, pain as the bad mother is better than no mother at all.

The inpatient therapist will find these patients exceedingly difficult. Short of life-threatening behavior, painful behaviors and attachments cannot be managed away by containment or strict limits. What can be hoped for is the diminution of these destructive behaviors in the course of a long-term outpatient psychotherapy.

PSYCHOTHERAPY CONSULTATION

Perhaps more often than not a borderline patient enters the inpatient setting already under the care of, and frequently upon referral from, an outpatient therapist. At such times the inpatient clinician and the unit staff automatically are put into the position of consultant to the outpatient caregiver. Even if the unit's primary evaluator is a junior resident, he or she has the task of examining and evaluating the outpatient treatment and, in particular, the ongoing psychotherapy. When a unit recognizes this responsibility and responds to it, a crucial service can be provided to the patient and to the therapist (106–108).

Hospitalization of a borderline patient in ongoing outpatient therapy does *not* signal treatment failure. An effective psychotherapy may mobilize feelings and drives that render patients at risk to themselves or require that they have the emotionally sustaining environment of a hospital to contain and limit a precipitous regression. Difficulties in therapy may also occur. They may reside in the patient's limitations or in the therapist's countertransference or in technical difficulties.

Consulting effectively with the referring therapist is a delicate procedure; the therapist may be threatened with feeling exposed. The difficulties he is having or, worse, a failure on his part may become apparent. The therapist should be encouraged to continue his meetings during hospitalization in order to counter the patient's fear of abandonment and allow the consultation to explore the ongoing treatment process.

Consultation is best done after the unit's treatment team has had an opportunity to fully evaluate and then review the individual patient, family, environmental situation, nature of the current crisis, and the ongoing psychotherapy. The availability of a senior consultant at a case conference will allow the staff to present its formulation and recommendations for critical review before presenting this material to the referring therapist.

Frequently, the dilution of transference and the containing power of the hospitalization will be adequate to resolve the crisis that prompted admission and allow outpatient care to resume. In these instances the unit has been supportive to the referring therapist and can encourage his ongoing treatment of a difficult patient. At other times consultation may enable the therapist to deepen or redirect the therapy in a manner more beneficial to the patient. If countertransference issues are the impediment, these can be explored supportively with the therapist in order to permit him access to feelings of which he may have been unaware. In some cases termination or transfer is indicated and can be managed while the patient has the benefit of the holding environment of the inpatient unit. Clearly, when consultation is offered, it is provided in a sensitive manner that recognizes the difficulties we all experience in working with borderline patients.

Milieu Management

The milieu management of the borderline patient has two aspects: the patient and the unit staff. Any unit which intends to regularly admit and treat borderline patients must attend to the treatment issues for the patient and provide ample and capable supervision and support for the staff.

Though the comments that follow are based on treating patients with lengths of stay of several weeks to several months, the principles underlying them are applicable to shorter and longer stays.

THE PATIENT

The essence of the milieu management of the hospitalized borderline patient is the capacity to ensure physical safety without compromising empathy.

The physical *safety* of the patient and other patients and staff on the ward must always be the *first priority* of the milieu. Clear, consistent, and firm limits that contain the patient's regression and aggression must be established. All milieu decisions are then organized on the basis of these limits, derived from a fundamental *concern* for the patient's safety and well-being. It is this concern that allows for continuous *empathy* which is integral to allying with the borderline patient and without which the healing process cannot occur. Empathy is not sympathy. Empathy is the capacity of a person or group to experience and resonate with the affective state of another. It is an identification with another person without a loss of boundaries (109–111).

Abroms (112), has listed priorities for setting limits. Although the milieu priorities

he recommends apply particularly to borderline patients, they are applicable to all types of patients. They are as follows:

1. Destructive behavior
2. Disorganized behavior
3. Deviant behavior—rule-breaking behavior or acting out
4. Withdrawn behavior
5. Dependent behavior

The following *procedural guidelines* allow for effective limit setting and make the process understandable to patients: (113)

1. Set few limits
2. Clearly define limits
3. The limits explained to the patient should not differ from the limits written in the order book
4. Limits should be realistic
5. Enforce limits promptly—failure to enforce limits promptly condones the pathological behavior and promotes further acting out
6. Give sound reasons for limits

Borderline patients will probably test the limits that the staff establish. It is important to recognize that this early *limit testing* represents patients' effort to discover *whether the staff care enough to contain them* and *whether the staff has the capacity to do so.* Typically, limit testing occurs at a time when the patient is experiencing stress. It is also essential for the therapist and staff to be aware of the nature of the patient's distress and developmental vulnerabilities in order to maintain an empathic stance while firmly setting needed limits.

It is generally a mistake to wait for large infractions of the ward rules before responding. An *early response* to rule infractions allows for working with the patient while an alliance may still be present. Early intervention may also preclude further escalation of the pathological behavior. If a patient breaks a ward rule, immediate limit setting can be done by the available staff on the unit. Members of the staff, particularly those assigned to the patient, may then make time to meet to *review the incident.* The patient's history, the acuteness or chronicity of the behavior, presence or absence of psychosis, the psychodynamics of the act, gravity of the act, and the degree of therapeutic alliance must all be reviewed. On the basis of this review, an individually oriented treatment plan can be made.

When the staff has developed a plan for intervention, it must be explained to patients in language they can understand. Whenever possible, staff should describe behaviors alternate to those pathologically expressed in the incident.

The treatment plan developed must aim to contain the patient's pathology in a nonpunitive manner while maximally facilitating the patient's return to the tasks and goals of hospitalization. Often ward restriction and observation may be adequate to accomplish these ends. At times the judicious use of medication may enable the patient to control unbearable affects and impulses, thereby permitting the patient to remain in treatment. On occasion, the need to provide safety for patients and for those around them may demand that restraint or seclusion be ordered. In most instances we can hope for but not expect a full or immediate resolution of the regressive symptoms. We can, however, expect steady and visible progress toward that end. Frequently patients will later report that the staff's firmly containing their aggression was, despite their verbal protests, welcome.

Some patients will require transfer to a locked unit which has a capacity for managing destructive behavior. Staff must take time to help patients understand why transfer is necessary and inform patients that once their violent impulses are under control they can be reevaluated for return to an open unit. Similarly, for some patients, a breach of ward rules will mark the end of their capacity to maintain a working treatment alliance. They would then be discharged, if considered safe to leave the hospital. Staff can use the discharge process therapeutically to help the patient understand what has happened and why.

At times it will be important to *inform* a member of the *patient's family* of the incident. At other times it may be advisable to meet with the family, particularly if the family has played an instrumental role in the genesis of the rule-breaking behavior.

Some units have a readmission policy in which discharged patients are not allowed readmission for a specific period of time (e.g., 1–2 months). Alternatively, an evaluation of the circumstances surrounding discharge and the postdischarge course, rather than an established policy, may allow for greater fairness and better patient care. Evaluation would explore whether the work of the previous admission was completed and, if not, why, and who might bear responsibility (e.g., patient, family, staff). Why the posthospital regression occurred would also be considered in order to answer whether the unit can be helpful. Finally, questions surrounding whether the patient could be better managed by outpatient or partial hospital care would also be addressed. Through the mechanism of an evaluation for readmission the door can be left open for the patient (and outpatient therapist), thereby allowing for clinically appropriate readmission whenever this becomes necessary (114, 115).

Managing Suicidal Behavior

Suicidal behavior has been reported to range from 3–8.5% of borderline patients with a mean age of 27 (116–118). Because borderline patients tend to improve over time (at least to become less impulsive and chaotic), their long range survival is highly dependent on managing their suicidal behavior during their high-risk years.

Completed and attempted suicides in

borderline patients are more prevalent in those who have a concurrent affective disorder and/or substance abuse (117, 119). These findings underline the crucial importance of identifying and actively treating any co-morbid disorder found in this patient population. Two important studies that examined completed suicides in borderline inpatients (and those within a month after discharge) identified staff countertransference problems. The studies identified rejection of the patient and repressive attitudes, including mandating patient discharge in the face of patient's explicit wishes to remain hospitalized, as significant risk factors of suicidal behavior (120, 121).

These findings stress the vital role treating clinicians can play in diminishing the rate of a mortal outcome in these patients. Yet, paradoxically, we as clinicians cannot prevent borderline patients from taking their lives, especially over a sustained period of time. Suicidal behavior in the course of an ongoing treatment must be recognized as a breakdown in the therapeutic alliance. Furthermore, threat of suicide undermines ongoing therapy. Patients and their families must understand that beyond acute interventions aimed at providing temporary safety (such as a brief hospitalization), only patients can bear responsibility for their existence (87, 122).

The unlocked, voluntary psychiatric unit repeatedly confronts the problem of how to manage emergent suicidal ideas and impulses in hospitalized borderline patients. The gravity of this problem and its recurrent and time-consuming nature require special milieu attention.

The milieu management of suicidal ideas and impulses begins with the critical *separation of idea from action.* From the beginning of hospitalization the patient is helped to understand that the unit staff accept and welcome patients' talking about those feelings and ideas that disturb them and threaten their well-being. Simulta-

neously, the staff must inform patients that suicidal behavior cannot be tolerated. If patients can come to staff to express and begin to understand their suicidal ideation, then patients can safely be treated in an unlocked unit. However, if patients cannot behaviorally contain their self-destructive impulses (e.g., if the patient continues to burn himself with a cigarette) then the first priority of the milieu, namely, patient safety, cannot be met. The patient then requires transfer to a locked unit where behavioral containment can be provided.

A further distinction that merits attention is that between *idea and threat.* Staff can respond to a suicidal idea (or impulse) through a variety of psychotherapeutic, milieu, and pharmacological interventions if the patient knows this idea will not be acted upon. If, however, the patient cannot state unequivocally that he can control his impulses, then staff experience this patient as a suicidal threat. As long as staff must attend to the threat of suicidal behavior they are subject to patient manipulation. Furthermore, their energies are marshalled around security measures which render the staff unable to attend to helping the patient understand and tolerate grief and pain. For these reasons, patients who become suicidal threats also require transfer to a locked unit. Once suicidal activity or threat has abated, the patient can be evaluated for return to the unlocked unit.

With this foundation established, and idea distinguished from action and threat, the milieu can be highly effective in attenuating a patient's distress and consequent suicidal ideation. Psychoactive medications may play an important role, as discussed earlier in this chapter. Refuge within the shelter and support of a ward community, away from the stresses that had overwhelmed the patient, can also be palliative.

Further intervention relies on a thorough formulation of the patient's motives for suicidal behavior and the environmental reinforcers of such action (123–125). Manipulative suicidal attempts defined as low-risk, high-rescue behaviors with a coercive interpersonal aim, are extremely common in borderline patients (Gunderson reported a rate of 75% in a hospitalized sample (126). Manipulative behavior may be quite different in its motives than true suicide attempts; to add to the confusion, they may coexist. Furthermore, an increase in severity or frequency of manipulative suicidal behavior may predict a life-threatening attempt (127).

The wish to murder the self or another (carried out through the self), escape from pain, and reunion fantasies with a lost love object are common motives for suicide. Suicidal ideas and threats that empower patients, enabling them to transform their experience of themselves from helpless victim to powerful controller, are powerfully reinforcing. Disruptions in the patient's sustaining world (be they losses of family, friends, neighbors, pets, living quarters) are common and powerful destabilizing phenomena for the borderline patient. Dysphoria, despair, and unbearable aloneness can ensure and prompt self-destructive and potentially lethal behavior.

Finally, many patients with chronic suicidal ideation will hold onto these ideas, as we see psychotic patients hold onto their delusions. Unit staff will need to see that this attachment satisfies a basic comforting need and represents a psychologically familiar and adaptive act on the patient's part. We can understand this type of suicidal ideation to serve the patient, as would a transitional object. When this is the case, we are wise not to try to disentangle patients from their suicidal ideation.

THE STAFF

The staff of an inpatient unit has the complex and demanding therapeutic task of providing the patient with continuing concern and emotional availability while withstanding angry and devaluing onslaughts and labile and primitive affects. In addition, staff must set limits and promptly, firmly, and consistently maintain them.

As the staff devotes itself to this endeavor, the patient is engaged in a set of verbal tactics and psychological defensive processes that invite staff to retaliate or withdraw (72, 102, 125, 128–130). The patient may move about the unit making invidious comparisons among staff members as he repeatedly shifts attachments and alliances: today's favored staff member is apt to become the target of tomorrow's hostility. Legitimate authority is repeatedly assaulted by statements that suggest that if the staff really cared about the patient, they would not be so rigid about rules. Fair staff expectations of cooperation become special favors in which the patient considers himself to be doing something for the staff for which he should be especially rewarded.

Through the defensive process of splitting, some staff members are idealized while others are seen as cruel and malevolent. Because of the borderline patient's sensitivity to minor frustration, staff who are briefly idealized will soon become the focus of angry projections. The borderline patient's use of projective identification causes him to disown an aspect of himself and attribute it to a staff member, identify with it, and respond accordingly. Because these patients are particularly adept at sensing unconscious processes in those about them, their projections will frequently resonate with unconscious feelings in the staff. In keeping with the completed process of projective identification, if, for example, the projected impulse is rage, as it often is, the patient responds with defensive fear, anger, or devaluation to staff rage which the patient provoked. If, for example, it is helplessness that is disowned, staff are apt to experience their own helplessness, in response to which the patient may exhibit further anxiety and passivity.

The patient's defensive operations create the conditions for conflict among staff. Projected and split off good and bad affects and images can produce a subtle, elusive, and generally unconscious process among staff members. Because different staff may be viewed differently by the patient and come to feel differently about the patient, the potential for intrastaff strife is considerable. The same potential exists between the patient's therapist and the ward staff.

Furthermore, staff members are subject to personal and internal responses to the rage and helplessness that borderline patients evoke. Highly capable therapists have reported the guilt, intense personal doubt, fears of criticism, and masochistic submission they and others have experienced in therapeutic work with borderline patients (4, 131, 132).

A unit's supervisory group must encourage staff to understand and recognize the internal experiences and the group processes that borderline defenses generate in clinicians. Unit supervisors must agree to examine staff feelings and then consistently weave them into the supervision. Staff meetings and case conferences must take care not to ignore the day-to-day emotional life of the unit (133, 134). Able unit leadership, in which staff members can feel contained, as they are expected to contain themselves and the patients, is essential for the successful hospital treatment of borderline patients. The clinical leaders must also have and articulate an appreciation of what can and cannot be done in the care of these patients.

Respect for the integrity of the clinician and the patient is crucial if we are to master the demands of working with borderline patients. As T.F. Main wrote (135):

Sincerity by all about what can and what cannot be given *with good will* [italics ours] offers a basis for management that, however, leaves un-touched the basic psychological problems, which need careful understanding, but it is the only way in which these patients can be provided with a reliable modicum of the kind of love they need, and without which their lives are worthless. More cannot be given or forced from others without disaster for all. . . .

It is important for such patients that those who are involved in their treatment and management be *sincere* with each other, in disagreement as well as agreement. . . .

Believing that sincerity in management is a *sine qua non* for the treatment of the patients I have described, I offer . . . one piece of advice. If at any time you are impelled to instruct others to be less hostile and more loving than they can truly be—*don't!*

Evaluation and Treatment of the Family

The family evaluation of borderline patients should include, whenever possible, the patients' parents, significant family members, and people with whom the patients currently live. As discussed earlier, the families of borderline patients may show marked psychopathology in their individual members or in the family's functioning as a group. The evaluator will want to assess the family and its members as well as try to understand the role that patients play in the unconscious life of their parents and in the current psychic equilibrium of the family.

In addition to examining the family members, the clinician must carefully examine the patient's immediate living environment. Frequently, these patients have been living with friends, intimates, or in some informal or professionally managed living situation. The patient's interpersonal environment must be assessed for the presence of toxic relationships and the absence of adequate structure and support.

The family evaluation is an opportunity to establish an alliance with individual members of the family and the family as a whole. The working alliance with the borderline patient is tenuous at best (91). This alliance may be strengthened by an effective working alliance with the family. Furthermore, when the family is negatively disposed to the hospital and its treatment staff, the working alliance with the individual borderline patient is seriously jeopardized.

Clinical opinion varies on how and when to provide family therapy for the families of borderline patients (44–47, 71). Though there seems to be uniformity about involving families in treatment, particularly when the patient is an adolescent or living with the family, disagreement centers on when to begin therapy and whether the family should be seen separately from or together with the individual patient.

An answer to these questions may emerge from the family assessment. Families of borderline individuals seem to divide into two types. In the first type (described by Gunderson (42)), there is a tight parental bond with exclusion and even neglect of the child. Family treatment is contraindicated from the outset with this family structure. Instead, the patient and parents are seen separately. This appears to limit unconscious parental anxiety about the child's intruding upon their dyadic relationship. Separating the child and family treatments also diminishes excessive angry projections.

In the second family type (described by Zinner and Shapiro (45, 46)) the family and borderline child are deeply enmeshed. In this type, the child and parents are overly involved with each other and show mutual and marked dependent trends. In this family, separation is a fundamental fear. The appropriate treatment for these enmeshed families is to meet with the parents and child together. Structuring therapy in this manner minimizes fears of premature separation and allows the family, as a group, to begin to disengage and begin a process of progressive autonomy.

Though the design for treatment may differ, both family treatments aim to help all the family members begin to work through the separation-individuation issues that were inadequately mastered. In addition, the therapist works to minimize the family's use of projective identification and splitting and to help them begin to understand that autonomy is different from hateful abandonment. Finally, the therapist can serve as a model of firmness, boundary maintenance, consistency, and concern.

Contact with Other Professional Agencies

Frequently, borderline patients have established contact with several human service agencies. Diffuse, split, and disorganized caregiving, perhaps not unlike the care they received from their families, adds to the patients' difficulties. When multiple agencies have been involved in the care of a borderline patient, it is advisable for the clinician to arrange a meeting of the different caregivers. Wishnie (72) has suggested that the purposes of this meeting include clarifying roles, disengaging unnecessary helpers, and promoting patient autonomy.

MEDICOLEGAL CONSIDERATIONS

The hospital treatment of borderline patients does not occur without regular consideration of the staff's professional responsibilities and their risks of liability. The borderline patient's use of projection and the disavowal of personal responsibility that accompanies this defense, as well as the impulsive and self-destructive behaviors that typify this syndrome, are the principle factors in creating medicolegal problems for these patients.

Borderline patients are especially difficult to approach medicolegally because their dynamic interactions with hospital staff, and with the legal system, are not often clearly recognized as pathological, as is the case with schizophrenic and depressed patients (136–138). Patient's feelings of entitlement can result in the conviction that the hospital is offering less than optimal care or even negligence. Splitting may result in certain staff becoming devalued and depicted as agents of professional malfeasance. Finally, transferences of psychotic proportions can cast physician and, in particular, nurses as the source of all the patient's difficulties.

Borderline dynamics of entitlement, splitting, and psychotic transference in themselves would not necessarily present medicolegal difficulties were it not for the essential treatment intervention of setting limits on the impulsive self-destructive behavior that these patients present when in their most desperate and regressed states. The importance of limits has been addressed clinically. From a medicolegal perspective, however, limits may be seen as punitive, arbitrary, or a deprivation of right to treatment. Furthermore, when patients respond to limits with suicidal threats or behavior, the hospital and its staff may appear to be responsible for inducing problems rather than seeking to remedy them. Discharge from a hospital as a form of limit setting is most problematic medicolegally when the patient continues to be at risk for suicide.

Furthermore, therapists may be particularly subject to violations of appropriate interpersonal boundaries with the borderline patient (119). Most egregious of these violations is that of sexual misconduct. Because this patient population frequently seeks care in an eroticized manner (through early conditioning or through the repetition compulsion seen in victims of abuse) therapist overinvolvement often occurs in a sexualized manner. Clinicians must be alert to the early signs of boundary blurring by the patient and to reciprocal boundary problems on the clinician's part. Any sexual contact by a therapist is unethical and inexcusable. Therapists should seek immediate

consultation and supervision whenever they recognize any sign of misconduct developing.

In all medicolegal dilemmas, sexual and otherwise, the solution lies in a well-considered treatment plan that is clinically, not legally, based (139, 140). Careful *documentation* of the patient's pathology and the thinking by which decisions for limits (including curtailing privileges, transfer, or discharge) were developed is critical: in the mind of the court, if it is not documented it did not occur. Finally, *consultation* (evidence that the professional staff were concerned enough to review the case with peers or supervisors) should be sought and documented for complicated or worrisome patients.

CONTROVERSIES IN THE TREATMENT OF THE HOSPITAL BORDERLINE PATIENT

Controversy about diagnosis and treatment is perhaps most apparent in the care of the borderline patient than it is with any other group of patients. Diagnostic confusion is common. Multiple schools of thought about treatment exist. Finally, countertransference reactions add to the clinician's dilemma.

1. Diagnostic Dilemmas. It is only in the past decade that valid and reliable instruments were developed for the diagnosis of borderline personality disorder. To complicate diagnostic confusion, borderline patients have very high rates of co-morbid disorders, especially substance abuse and affective disorder. Co-morbid disorders (because of their impulsive, self-destructive, and addictive behaviors) can be confused with borderline psychopathology; furthermore, both substance abuse and mood disorders can induce personality regressions that may mimic Axis II borderline pathology.

Treatment staff commonly disagree in

diagnosing borderline disorder. It is important to keep in mind that not all impulsive and difficult patients are borderline. Staff must be well-trained to recognize mood, addictive, and other psychotic disorders and understand their relationship to personality functioning. Frequently, discovery of a proper treatment of the former will result in personality recompensation.

2. Treatment Dilemmas.

a. The Use of the Hospital in Treating the Borderline Patient: The range of opinion on the use of hospital treatment for these patients is remarkable. Some advocate long-term care, some short-term care, some believe the hospital should not even be used (if at all possible).

"When is hospitalization necessary?" is the question that can lead the way out of this conundrum. Safety, diagnostic clarity, and therapeutic interventions that can be addressed only in a 24-hour setting are the general criteria for admission. This position is clinically based and serves us in negotiating admission with patients, their families, and those who pay for and manage insurance benefits.

b. Length of Stay: Our mandate as clinicians is to advocate hospital stays based on clinical rather than economic factors (141). Our view is that the patient should spend as few days as necessary in a hospital; "as few days as necessary" may be merely a few days for one patient, a few weeks for another, a few months for yet another, and even a year or two for certain other patients.

Hospital care has its potential benefits and risks. Patients can be brought back from suicidal precipices; treatments can be initiated, renewed, and revised; families can be engaged; and essential environment resources (such as structured programs, residences, and rehabilitation) can be mobilized. Hospitals can also foster atrophy of ego and will, and

pathological behaviors can spread contagiously through a patient milieu. Risk must be weighed against benefit and informed judgments of the likelihood of a favorable outcome developed. So is it with any medical treatment.

We believe that intermediate (greater than 60 days) and long-term (greater than six months) inpatient stays should be attempted only when lesser efforts have failed. Patient, family, and clinical staff must also see clinical evidence that treatment offers the promise of benefit, particularly when long-term, high-resource care is prescribed.

c. The Nature of the Inpatient Milieu: Inpatient settings have developed various reputations, some earned, some fanciful. Some of these settings are characterized as heavily limit setting, "touchy-feely," "holding," structured, or emotionally evocative, etc. Debates continue about what environment the patient, especially the borderline patient, requires.

To our knowledge, no evidence suggests that any treatment striving for regression is useful for acutely decompensated hospitalized patients. During this phase, they do not have adequate ego functioning to tolerate affective stimulations or evocative inquiry. In fact, these methods can further disorganize the patient. Acutely disturbed patients require predictability, role clarity, and hierarchy for their recompensation. They also need an emotionally supportive, or "holding," unit for *how it can facilitate treatment, not as an end in itself.* The "holding" properties of the unit enable patients to do the work of hospitalization, which, as this chapter notes throughout, focuses principally on assessment, consultation, and initiation of treatment.

d. The Capacity to Use the Hospital: There are patients who are not yet ready to use the care offered or who must sabotage any effort others make for their care. There are times, as well, when the borderline patient's behavior evokes our hopelessness about the benefits of care and our aversion and animosity. At such times, we risk deeming them inappropriate for or unable to use the hospital.

Careful clinical assessment and formulation of each patient's dynamics can help answer this clinical dilemma. History and predictions of outcome can aid in our evaluation. Researchers are beginning to offer tools that may add to our acumen in the years ahead (142, 143).

3. Research Dilemmas. Borderline psychopathology offers researchers abundant lines of inquiry. Clinicians need research that correlates psychotherapeutic and psychopharmacologic treatments with specific patients at specific times in the course of their disorders.

Perhaps the area of research most pressing to the hospital practitioner is measuring treatment outcome. More than ever we need to know what will work in order to inform our clinical interventions, meet standards of quality assurance, and justify our actions to insurance carriers and managed-care organizations. Short-term outcome measures could include reducing targeted symptoms and developing a working alliance. Units that specialize in longer-term care will need to develop criteria for admission and instruments to measure effectiveness of care.

COURSE AND PROGNOSIS

For the modal borderline patient hospitalized for the first time in late adolescence or early adulthood, the first 10 years are typically a time of instability (116, 127, 144). Major impairments in ego functioning (as measured by object relations and work performance) are characteristic. In follow-ups during the initial 2–5 years of illness, this patient population is functionally indistinguishable from schizophrenic patients. However, as these patients enter their 30s, their clinical picture typically stabilizes.

Follow-up of borderline patients after 10 years of clinical disorder reveals that approximately two-thirds will improve, especially in occupational functioning. For some, this improvement may come as they forego efforts at intimacy. A core vulnerability to regression persists, even in those who appear improved, particularly in response to losses, disappointments, and rejections.

Poor outcome has been correlated with alcohol and drug abuse, co-morbid affective disorder, antisocial behavior, incestuous or violent victimization, and aggressiveness. Good outcome is associated with high intelligence, attractiveness and likableness, artistic talent, and self-discipline.

Hospital use and repeated efforts at psychotherapy are important to successful long-term outcome (95, 145). In fact, many patients with successful outcomes appear to require repetitious, brief therapeutic efforts before they can settle into an effective, enduring treatment.

REFERENCES

1. American Psychiatric Association: *Diagnostic and Statistical Manual of Mental Disorders,* ed. 3, (DSM-IIIR), Washington, D.C., American Psychiatric Association, 1987.

2. Kernberg OF: Borderline personality organization. J Am Psychoanal Assoc, *15*:641–682, 1967.

3. Schmideberg M: The borderline patient, in Arieti S (ed): *American Handbook of Psychiatry,* vol. 1, pp. 398–416, New York, Basic Books, 1959.

4. Kernberg OF: *Borderline Conditions and Pathological Narcissism,* esp. pp. 111–152, New York, Jason Aronson, 1975.

5. Gunderson JG, Kolb JE: Discriminating features of borderline patients. Am J Psychiatry, *135*:792–796, 1978.

6. Stern A: Psychoanalytic investigation of therapy in the borderline neuroses. Psychoanal Q, *17*:467–489, 1938.

7. Glover E: A psychoanalytic approach to the classification of mental disorders. J Mental Science, *78*:819–842, 1932.

8. Rickman J: *The Development of the Psychoanalytical Theory of the Psychoses, 1893–1926,* London, Bailliere, Tindall, Cox, 1928.

9. Akiskal HS, Rosenthal TL, et al.: Characterological depressions: Clinical and sleep EEG findings separating "sub-affective dysthymias" from "character spectrum disorders." Arch Gen Psychiatry, *37*:777–783, 1980.

10. Stone MH: Contemporary shift of the borderline concept from a subschizophrenic disorder to a subaffective disorder. Psychiatr Clin North Am, *2*:577–594, 1979.

11. McGlashan TH: The Borderline Syndrome: II. Is it a variant of schizophrenia or affective disorder? Arch Gen Psychiatry, *40*:1319–1323, 1983.

12. Perry CJ: Depression in borderline personality disorder. Am J Psychiatry, *142*:15–21, 1985.

13. McNamara E, Reynolds CF, et al.: EEG sleep evaluation of depression in borderline patients. Am J Psychiatry, *141*:182–186, 1984.

14. Gunderson JG, Elliot GR: The interface between borderline personality disorder and affective disorder. Am J Psychiatry, *142*:277–288, 1985.

15. Soloff PH, Millward JW: Psychiatric disorders in the families of borderline patients. Arch Gen Psychiatry, *40*:37–44, 1983.

16. Davis GC, Akiskal HS: Descriptive, biological, and theoretical aspects of borderline personality disorder. Hosp Community Psychiatry, *37*:685–692, 1986.

17. Rifkin A, et al.: Lithium carbonate in emotionally unstable character. Arch Gen Psychiatry, *27*:519–523, 1972.

18. Lahmeyer HW, Reynolds CF, Kupfer DJ, et al.: Biological markers in borderline personality disorder: A review. J Clin Psychiatry, *50*:217–225, 1989.

19. Andrulonis PA, Glueck BC, et al.: Borderline personality subcategories. J Nerv Ment Dis, *170*:670–679, 1982.

20. Andrulonis PA, Donnelly J, et al.: Preliminary data on ethosuximide and the episodic dyscontrol syndrome. Am J Psychiatry, *137*:1455–1456, 1981.

21. Andrulonis PA, Glueck BC, et al.: Organic brain dysfunctions and the borderline syndrome. Psychiatr Clin North Am, *4*:47–66, 1981.

22. Meissner WW: *The Borderline Spectrum,* esp. pp. 301–331. New York, Jason Aronson, 1984.

23. Van der Kolk BA: Psychological Trauma, American Psychiatric Press, Washington, D.C., 1987.

24. Kardiner A: *The Traumatic Neuroses of War,* New York, P. Hueber, 1941.

25. Herman JL: Traumatic antecedents of borderline personality disorder, in Van der Kolk BA (ed): *Psychological Trauma,* pp. 111–126, Washington, D.C., 1987.

26. Herman JL: *Father-Daughter Incest,* Cambridge, Harvard University Press, 1981.

27. Masson JM: The Assault on Truth: Freud's Suppression of the Seduction Theory. New York, Farrar, Straus & Giroux, 1984.

28. Herman JL, Perry JC, Van der Kolk BA: Childhood trauma in the borderline personality disorder. Am J Psychiatry, *146*:490–495, 1989.

29. Bryer JB, Nelson BA, Miller JB, Krol PA: Childhood sexual and physical abuse as factors in adult psychiatric illness. Am J Psychiatry, *144*:1426–1430, 1987.

30. Stone MH: Borderline syndromes: A consideration of subtypes and directions for research. Psychiatr Clin North Am, *4*:3–13, 1981.

31. Gelinas DJ: The persisting negative effects of incest. Psychiatry, *46*:312–332, 1983.

32. Mahler MS: *On Human Symbiosis and the Vicissitudes of Individuation,* New York, International Universities Press, 1968.

33. Winnicott DW: The theory of the parent-infant relationship. Int J Psychoanal, *41*:585–595, 1960.

34. Winnicott DW: Ego distortion in terms of the true and false self, in *The Maturational Process and the Facilitating Environment,* New York, International Universities Press, 1965.

35. Winnicott DW: The use of an object. Int J Psychoanal, *41*:585–594, 1969.

36. Adler G: *Borderline Psychopathology and Its Treatment*, New York, Jason Aronson, 1985.

37. Modell AH: "The holding environment" and the therapeutic action of psychoanalysis. J Am Psychoanal Assoc, 24:285–307, 1976.

38. Kernberg OF: *Object Relations Theory and Clinical Psychoanalysis*, New York, Jason Aronson, 1976.

39. Soloff P, Millward J: Developmental histories of borderline patients. Compr Psychiatry, 24:574–588, 1983.

40. Gunderson JG, Zanarini MC: Current overview of the borderline diagnosis. J Clin Psychiatry, 48:5–11, 1987.

41. Morris H, Gunderson JG, Zanarini MC: Transitional object use and borderline psychopathology. Am J Psychiatry, 143:1534–1538, 1986.

42. Gunderson JG, et al.: The families of borderlines: A comparative study. Arch Gen Psychiatry, 37:27–33, 1980.

43. Walsh F: Family study: 1976: 14 new borderline cases, in Grinker RR, Werble B (eds): *The Borderline Patient*, pp. 158–177, New York, Jason Aronson, 1977.

44. Shapiro ER, Shapiro RL, et al.: The borderline ego and the working alliance: Indications for family and individual treatment in adolescence. Int J Psychoanal, 58:77–87, 1977.

45. Zinner J, Shapiro ER: Splitting in families of borderline adolescents, in Mack JE (ed): *Borderline States in Psychiatry*, New York, Grune & Stratton, 1975.

46. Shapiro ER, et al.: The influence of family experience on borderline personality development. Int Rev Psychoanal, 2:399–411, 1975.

47. Masterson JF: *Treatment of the Borderline Adolescent: A Developmental Approach*, New York, John Wiley & Sons, 1972.

48. Masterson JF: *Psychotherapy of the Borderline Adult: A Developmental Approach*, New York, Brunner/Mazel, 1976.

49. Gunderson JG, Singer MT: Defining borderline patients: An overview. Am J Psychiatry, 132:1–10, 1975.

50. Perry JC, Klerman GL: Clinical features of the borderline personality disorder. Am J Psychiatry, 137:165–173, 1980.

51. Gunderson JG, Siever LJ, et al.: The search for a schizotype: Crossing the border again. Arch Gen Psychiatry, 40:15–22, 1983.

52. McGlashan TH: The borderline syndrome: Testing three diagnostic systems. Arch Gen Psychiatry, 40:1311–1318, 1983.

53. Zilboorg G: The problem of ambulatory schizophrenias. Am J Psychiatry, 113:519–525, 1956.

54. Shapiro D: *Neurotic Styles*, New York, Basic Books, 1965.

55. Spitzer RL, Endicott J, et al.: Crossing the border into borderline personality and borderline schizophrenia. Arch Gen Psychiatry, 36:17–24, 1979.

56. Mirin SM: Substance Abuse and Psychopathology, Washington, D.C., American Psychiatric Press, 1984.

57. Nace EP: Personality disorder in the alcoholic patient. Psych Annals, 19:256–260, 1989.

58. Bean-Bayog M: Psychopathology produced by alcoholism, in Meyer RE (ed): *Psychopathology and Addictive Disorders*, pp. 334–345, New York, Guilford Press, 1986.

59. Dulit RA, Fyre MR, Haas GL, et al.: Substance Use in Borderline Personality Disorder, Presentation APA Annual Meeting, San Francisco, 1989.

60. Adler G: The borderline-narcissistic personality disorder continuum. Am J Psychiatry, 138:46–50, 1981.

61. Kohut H, Wolf HS: The disorders of the self and their treatment: An outline. Int J Psychoanal, 59:413–425, 1978.

62. Kohut H: *The Restoration of the Self,* New York, International Universities Press, 1977.

63. Vaillant GE: *The Natural History of Alcoholism,* Cambridge, Harvard University Press, 1983.

64. Sederer LI: Multiproblem patients: Psychiatric disorder and substance abuse, in Milkman HB, Sederer LI: *Treatment Choices in Alcohol and Drug Abuse*, pp. 163–181, Lexington, Mass., Lexington Press, 1990.

65. Kernberg O: A psychoanalytic classification of character pathology. J Am Psychoanal Assoc, 18:800–822, 1970.

66. Kernberg O: Technical consider-

ations in the treatment of borderline personality organization. J Am Psychoanal Assoc, 24:795–829, 1976.

67. Perry S, Cooper AM, Michels R: The psychodynamic formulation: Its purpose, structure, and clinical application. Am J Psychiatry, 144:543–550, 1987.

68. Melchiode GA: The psychodynamic formulation: How and why. Gen Hosp Psychiatry, 10:41–45, 1988.

69. Meissner WW: Internalization and object relations. J Am Psychoanal Assoc, 27:345–360, 1979.

70. Gunderson JG: Borderline personality disorder, in Kaplan HJ, Sadock BJ (eds): Comprehensive Textbook of Psychiatry, pp. 1387–1395, Baltimore, Williams & Wilkins, 1989.

71. Friedman HJ: Some problems of inpatient management with borderline patients. Am J Psychiatry, 126:299–304, 1969.

72. Wishnie HA: Inpatient therapy with borderline patients, in Mack JE (ed): Borderline States in Psychiatry, pp. 41–62, New York, Grune & Stratton, 1975.

73. Sadavoy J, et al.: Negative responses of the borderline to inpatient treatment. Am J Psychother, 33:404–417, 1979.

74. Cowdry RW: Psychopharmacology of borderline personality disorder: A review. J Clin Psychiatry, 48:15–22, 1987 (supplement).

75. Koenigsberg HW, Kaplan RD, Gilmore MM, et al.: The relationship between syndrome and personality disorder in DSM-III. Am J Psychiatry, 142:207–212, 1985.

76. Faltus FJ: The positive effect of alprazolam in the treatment of three patients with borderline personality disorder. Am J Psychiatry, 141:802–803, 1984.

77. Cowdry RW, Gardner DL: Pharmacotherapy of borderline personality disorder. Arch Gen Psychiatry, 45:111–118, 1988.

78. Gardner DW, Cowdry RW: Alprazolam-induced dyscontrol in borderline personality disorder. Am J Psychiatry, 142:98–100, 1985.

79. Soloff PH, George A, Nathan S, et al.: Progress in pharmacotherapy of borderline disorders: A double blind study of amitriptyline, haloperidol and placebo. Arch Gen Psychiatry, 43:691–697, 1986.

80. Teicher MH, Glod CA, Cole JO: Emergence of intense violent suicidal ideation in patients treated with fluoxetine. Am J Psychiatry, 147:207–210, 1990.

81. Liebowitz MR, Klein DF: Hysteroid dysphoria. Psychiatr Clin North Am, 2:555–575, 1979.

82. Gardner DW, Cowdry RW: Development of melancholia during carbamazepine treatment in borderline personality disorder. J Clin Psychopharmacol, 6:236–239, 1986.

83. Brinkley JR, et al.: Low-dose neuroleptic regimens in the treatment of borderline patients. Arch Gen Psychiatry, 36:319–326, 1979.

84. Frances A, Soloff PH: Treating the borderline patient with low-dose neuroleptics. Hosp Community Psychiatry, 39:246–248, 1988.

85. Teicher MR, Glod CA, Aaronson ST, et al.: An open assessment of the safety and efficacy of thioridazine in the treatment of patients with borderline personality disorder. Psychopharmacol Bull, In press.

86. Gunderson JG: Pharmacotherapy for patients with borderline personality disorder. Arch Gen Psychiatry, 43:698–700, 1986.

87. Kernberg OF: Severe Personality Disorders: Psychotherapeutic Strategies, New Haven, Yale University Press, 1984.

88. Margo GM, Manring JM: The current literature on inpatient psychotherapy. Hosp Community Psychiatry, 40:909–915, 1989.

89. Liebenluft TE, Goldberg RL: Guidelines for short-term inpatient psychotherapy. Hosp Community Psychiatry, 38:38–43, 1987.

90. Rogoff J: Individual psychotherapy, in Sederer LI (ed): Inpatient Psychiatry: Diagnosis and Treatment, ed. 2, pp. 240–262, Baltimore, Williams & Wilkins, 1986.

91. Adler G: The myth of the alliance with borderline patients. Am J Psychiatry, 136:642–645, 1979.

92. Sederer LI, Thorbeck J: First do no harm: Short-term inpatient psychotherapy of the borderline patient. Hosp Community Psychiatry, 37:692–697, 1986.

93. Zetzel ER: A developmental approach to the borderline patient. Am J Psychiatry, 127:867–871, 1971.

94. Friedman HJ: Psychotherapy of borderline patients: The influence of theory on technique. Am J Psychiatry, 132:1048–1052, 1975.

95. Waldinger RJ, Gunderson JG: *Effective Psychotherapy with Borderline Patients: Case Studies,* New York, Macmillan, 1987.

96. Pine F: *Developmental Theory and Clinical Process,* New Haven, Yale University Press, 1985.

97. Ogden TH: On projective identification. Int J Psychoanal, *60*:357–373, 1979.

98. Bion WR: *Experiences in Groups,* London, Tavistock Publications, 1961.

99. Havens L: Explorations in the uses of language in psychotherapy: Counterprojective statements. Contemp Psychoanal, *16*:53–67, 1980.

100. Buie DH, Adler G: The uses of confrontation with borderline patients. Int J Psychoanal Psychother *1*(3):90–108, 1972.

101. Adler G, Buie DH: The misuses of confrontation with borderline patients. Int J Psychoanal Psychother *1*(3):110–120, 1972.

102. Adler G: Helplessness in the helpers. Br J Med Psychol, *45*:315–326, 1972.

103. Valenstein AF: On attachment to painful feelings and the negative therapeutic reaction. Psychoanal Study Child, *28*:365–392, 1973.

104. Guntrip H: *Schizoid Phenomena, Object Relations and The Self,* New York, International Universities Press, esp. pp. 310–365, 1969.

105. Herzog JM: *A Neonatal Intensive Care Syndrome: A Pain Complex Involving Neuroplasticity and Psychic Trauma,* pp. 291–300, New York, Basic Books, 1981.

106. Bernstein SB: Psychotherapy consultation in an inpatient setting. Hosp Community Psychiatry, *31*:829–834, 1980.

107. Jacobs DH, Rogoff J, Donnelly K, et al.: The neglected alliance: The inpatient unit as a consultant to referring therapists. Hosp Community Psychiatry, *5*:377–381, 1982.

108. Stiver IP: Developing dimensions of regression: Introducing a consultant in the treatment of borderline patients. McLean Hosp Journal, *13*:89–107, 1988.

109. Rogers CR: The necessary and sufficient conditions of therapeutic personality change. J Consult Psychol, *21*:95–103, 1957.

110. Truax CB, Carkhuff RR: *Toward Effective Counselling and Psychotherapy: Training and Practice,* Chicago, Aldine Publishing Co., 1962.

111. Book HE: Empathy: Misconceptions and misuses in psychotherapy. Am J Psychiatry, *145*:420–424, 1988.

112. Abroms GM: Setting limits. Arch Gen Psychiatry, *19*:113–119, 1968.

113. MacDonald DM: Acting out. Arch Gen Psychiatry, *13*:439–443, 1965.

114. Henisz JE: *Psychotherapeutic Management on the Short Term Unit,* pp. 122–130, Springfield, Ill., Charles C. Thomas, 1981.

115. Pirdis MJ, Soverow GJ, et al.: Day hospital treatment of borderline patients: A clinical perspective. Am J Psychiatry, *135*:594–596, 1978.

116. McGlashan TH: The Chestnut Lodge follow-up study, III: Long-term outcome of borderline personalities. Arch Gen Psychiatry, *43*:20–30, 1986.

117. Stone MH, Hurt S, Stone DK: The natural history of borderline patients, I: Global outcome. Psychiatr Clin North Am, *10*:185–206, 1987.

118. Paris J, Brown R, Nowliss D: Long-term follow-up of borderline patients in a general hospital. Compr Psychiatry, *28*:530–535, 1987.

119. Fyer MR, Frances AJ, et al.: Suicide attempts in patients with borderline personality disorder. Am J Psychiatry, *145*:737–739, 1988.

120. Kullgren G, Renberg E, Jacobson L: An empirical study of borderline personality disorder and psychiatric suicides. J Nerv Ment Dis, *174*:328–331, 1986.

121. Kullgren G: Factions associated with completed suicide in borderline personality disorder. J Nerv Ment Dis, *176*:40–44, 1988.

122. Meissner WW: *Treatment of Patients in the Borderline Spectrum,* Northvale, N.J., Jason Aronson, 1988.

123. Maltsberger JT: *Suicide Risk,* New York, New York University Press, 1986.

124. Havens LL: Anatomy of a suicide. N Engl J Med, *272*:401–406, 1964.

125. Maltsberger JT, Lovett CG: Suicide in borderline personality disorders, in Silverman D (ed): *A Handbook of Borderline Disorders,* New York, International Universities Press, 1991.

126. Gunderson JG: *Borderline Personality*

Disorder, Washington, D.C., American Psychiatric Press, 1984.

127. Gardner DL, Cowdry RW: Suicidal and parasuicidal behavior in borderline personality disorder. Psychiatr Clin North Am, *8:*389–403, 1985.

128. Pollack IW, Battle WC: Studies of the special patient: The sentence. Arch Gen Psychiatry, *9:*56–62, 1963.

129. Groves JE: Taking care of the hateful patient. N Engl J Med, *298:*883–887, 1978.

130. Gabbard GO: Splitting in hospital treatment. Am J Psychiatry, *146:*444–451, 1989.

131. Maltsberger JT, Buie DH: Countertransference hate in the treatment of suicidal patients. Arch Gen Psychiatry, *30:*625–633, 1974.

132. Winnicott DW: Hate in the countertransference. Int J Psychoanal, *30:*69–74, 1949.

133. Sederer LI: Morale therapy and the problem of morale. Am J Psychiatry, *134:*267–272, 1977.

134. Weisman A: Morale and the human condition. Unpublished manuscript. Presented at Hunter College, New York, March 28, 1977.

135. Main TF: The ailment. Br J Med Psychol, *30:*144–145, 1957.

136. Gutheil TG: Medicolegal pitfalls in the treatment of borderline patients. Am J Psychiatry, *142:*9–14, 1985.

137. Gutheil TG, Appelbaum PS: *Clinical Handbook of Psychiatry and the Law,* New York, McGraw Hill, 1982.

138. Gutheil TG: Borderline personality disorder, boundary violations and patient-therapist sex: Medicolegal pitfalls. Am J Psychiatry, *146:*597–602, 1989.

139. Gutheil TG, Magraw R: Ambivalence, alliance and advocacy: Misunderstood dualities in psychiatry and law. Bull Am Acad Psychiatry Law, *12:*51–58, 1984.

140. Gutheil TG: *Malpractice liability in suicide: Legal aspects of psychiatric practice. 1:*1–4, 1984.

141. Sederer LI, St Clair RL: Managed health care and the Massachusetts experience. Am J Psychiatry, *146:*1142–1148, 1989.

142. Alexander LB, Luborsky L: The Penn helping alliance scales, in Greenberg LS, Pinsof WM (eds): *The Psychotherapeutic Process: A Research Handbook,* pp. 325–366, New York, Guilford Press, 1986.

143. Suh CS, Strupp HH, O'Malley SS: The Vanderbilt process measures: The psychotherapy process scale and the negative indicating scale, in Greenberg LS, Pinsof WM (eds): *The Psychotherapeutic Process: A Research Handbook,* pp. 285–313, New York, Guilford Press, 1986.

144. Stone MH, Hurt SW, Stone DK: The PI 500: Long-term follow-up of borderline inpatients meeting DSM-III criteria, I: Global outcome. J Pers Disorders, *1:*291–298, 1988.

145. Stone MH: Psychotherapy of borderline patients in light of long-term follow-up. Bull Menninger Clin, *51:*231–247, 1987.

5

Anorexia Nervosa and Bulimia Nervosa

Margaret S. McKenna, MD

DEFINITION

Considerable controversy exists over what contitutes an eating disorder. At this time within our culture, eating behavior and body image concerns are areas of special vulnerability, especially for women. Most women, if questioned about weight and shape, will report dissatisfaction, and often that report will reflect highly personalized views of their own bodies, if not outright distortion. Is this pathology? If so, it is so widespread that it offers no meaningful way to discriminate distress from disorder.

The definition of eating disorders is further complicated by our incomplete knowledge of their origins. Are eating disorders distinct disorders or points on a continuum? Do they describe unique pathologic states, are they variants of affective disorder, or expressions of acculturation gone awry? They have proved resistant to unitary explanations, remaining much harder to classify than many other disorders.

Psychiatry faces the challenge of defining those entities which represent truly dysfunctional psychophysiologic states. Each of these must have a cluster of characteristic findings which distinguishes it in a reliable and consistent fashion. These findings must be primary, not secondary to another disorder.

The ease with which eating behavior is disrupted, and the many ways in which this can occur, make definition and classification very difficult. This is well-illustrated by considering two major syndromes, anorexia nervosa and bulimia nervosa. Primary anorexia nervosa (AN) was first described several centuries ago and its classic features have remained relatively unchanged. However, what was once a rare disorder has increased significantly in frequency over the last two decades. As this has occurred variations in the typical pattern have become more evident. One key variation is the presence or absence of bulimic behavior (1). When first described, bulimia was recognized only as a behavior sometimes present in anorexia nervosa. But in the late 1970s bulimia emerged as a syndrome distinct from anorexia nervosa. The next decade was spent refining the definition of bulimia, from what began as an over-inclusive syndrome reported in epidemic proportions to what is now a narrower, more discriminating definition with the name bulimia nervosa. We now distinguish restricting anorexics, bulimic anorexics, and bulimics*. This reflects continuing efforts towards more precise definition.

This chapter uses the definitions of anorexia nervosa and bulimia nervosa as they are presented in the Diagnostic and Statistical Manual of Mental Disorders, Third Edition, Revised (DSM-IIIR) (2). Further refinements of these definitions may appear in DSM-IV. The key features of anorexia nervosa are: (a) refusal to maintain body weight of at least 85% of normal expected weight; (b) intense fear of weight gain; (c) distorted body perception; and (d) amenorrhea. Denial of illness is another cardinal feature of anorexia nervosa, one notably absent in bulimia nervosa. Bulimia nervosa is defined as: (a) recurrent episodes of binge eating experienced as out of control; (b) regular purging, fasting, or excessive exercise to prevent weight gain; (c) at least two episodes of binging and purging per week for at least three months; and (d) persistent over-concern with weight and shape.

The presentation, understanding, and treatment of eating disorders is in continual flux. This chapter summarizes our current understanding and highlights controversy and areas of uncertainty. At points, anorexia nervosa and bulimia nervosa are discussed separately; at others, there is enough overlap that they are addressed together.

DIAGNOSIS

The first step in making a diagnosis is taking a history. The presenting complaint—the deviant eating behavior—and associated behavior and circumstances must be documented in detail. Then it must be placed in the context of a patient's psychological functioning, family environment, and sociocultural pressures. Specific guidelines for a comprehensive assessment are presented in the section on Evaluation. This section presents vignettes of the "classic" diagnostic picture.

Anorexia Nervosa

A young woman, most commonly in her early teens, is forced to come for treatment by distraught family members or school personnel. She sits looking stony-faced at the floor, either hostile or indifferent to well-intentioned inquiry which she experiences as controlling and invasive. At first glance it may be hard to assess her weight loss, since she is engulfed in layers of oversized, ill-fitting clothing. She denies her emaciation; her conviction that she is still fat and needs to lose more weight is unshakable.

If she shares anything, it may be anger at all those in her life who seem to think they have a right to interfere with her eating, who think they know better than she what she ought to weigh. For her, the triumph of restraint over her raging hunger (which she denies) is evidence of her specialness, evidence that she can, after all, control her destiny. She feels she has found the solution to all her problems. Why would she want help?

Family may report that she has been making elaborate meals for others that she barely touches. She subsists on high-protein and rabbit foods. Amazingly, she seems to have excessive energy, exercising compulsively, sleeping little, continuing her over-committed routine with her usual perfectionist's standards and compulsive conscientiousness. She has withdrawn from friends, all of whom are afraid that if they comment on her weight loss they will alienate her. Family alternate between trying to force her to eat, reasoning with her, and ignoring her behavior. They are angered and frightened by this tyrant who has always before been compliant and eager to please. What has happened to their lovely daughter?

Someone may have commented that she

---

*For the sake of brevity, those with anorexia nervosa will be called anorexics, and those with bulimia nervosa bulimics.

had gained weight. Or she may have experienced dismay as her body matured. She may have sustained an injury that forced her to curtail a sports activity, or had surgery—something that jeopardized too much her already fragile sense of ownership of her body. Something suggested to her that if she just lost weight everything would be okay. By the time she presents for medical attention, she may have lost so much weight that her judgment and concentration are impaired by the effects of starvation, so that one cannot distinguish psychological from physiological compromise.

Bulimia Nervosa

The bulimic patient comes on her own, feeling desperate, having realized that what once felt like a useful strategy for weight control has taken over her life. She has been bulimic for years, often having started either in high school or early in college. No one knows her secret. Initially, it felt like a choice, something that could be used as needed and stopped at any point. Now the cycle of binging and purging has a life of its own beyond control and beyond understanding. She feels like a victim, helpless to battle this compulsion, a blend of need and habit, that overtakes her.

Binging and purging go along with not eating. Rarely are there any normal meals; sometimes breakfast is okay. Thinking about food all day, she fights off the urge or plans when and how to succumb. She rigidly controls her intake, often delaying eating each day for as long as possible, afraid that any food ingested will lead to a binge. Bodily signals of hunger and satiety are ignored as unreliable until they can no longer be recognized. It's all or nothing; one bite of a brownie is the same as eating a panful; the day is ruined so eat and eat, for today will be the last time. Binging is ritual—the same foods, a certain sequence, standing up or setting an elaborate place, reading or watching TV. Binging is anaesthesia; everything else is blotted out. Binging is respite or structure or gratification. Purging is undoing or penance or punishment or putting things in order "like housecleaning." Vomiting, hard at first, becomes almost reflex. She may have discrete episodes separate from meals or she may vomit every time she eats.

Usually her normal weight and her secrecy will mask the terrible struggle that dominates her thoughts and makes her feel alone, unknown, and a fraud. She is often highly successful in academics, work, sports, and extracurricular activities and frequently has a social life filled with activity but devoid of satisfaction. She desperately wants help to rid herself of this behavior she now despises; she has little awareness of her deep ambivalence about letting it go.

Individual presentations of both anorexia and bulimia nervosa may vary from the above descriptions, but the phenomenology of each disorder is in many ways remarkably constant.

DIFFERENTIAL DIAGNOSIS

With respect to these psychosomatic illnesses, differential diagnosis must consider other medical conditions and other psychiatric disorders.

Medical Conditions

Weight loss is a major sign in a variety of illnesses. Conspicuously lacking, however, are the relentless pursuit of thinness, the distorted body percepts, and the pride in the weight loss which characterize the anorexic patient. Medically ill patients accurately perceive the degree of their weight loss, are worried about it, and seek treatment voluntarily. A careful history is thus the most useful discriminating diagnostic tool in instances where the physical picture may be compatible with either anorexia nervosa or another illness. These instances include:

1. Malignancies: Weight loss is a consistent feature, but it is due to true loss of appetite. CNS (central nervous system) tumors, especially of the hypothalamus or third ventricle, are the most important differential. A CT (computerized tomography) scan or MRI (magnetic resonance imaging) is indicated if the picture of anorexia nervosa is atypical, neurological

deficits are found, or there is evidence of neuroendocrine dysfunction other than amenorrhea.

2. Chronic infection, such as tuberculosis.
3. Gastrointestinal problems: malabsorption syndromes, inflammatory bowel disease, hepatitis.
4. Primary endocrine disturbances:
   a. *Anterior pituitary insufficiency,* like anorexia nervosa, presents with a slowed metabolism and amenorrhea, but these are the only significant shared characteristics.
   b. Significant weight loss occurs in *hyperthyroidism,* but the full clinical picture is of a hypermetabolic state. Thyroid function tests will immediately differentiate the two conditions. An anorexic, it should be noted, will exhibit a thyroid conservation response secondary to starvation, which accounts for her *hypothyroid-like* presentation (bradycardia, cold intolerance, constipation, dry skin, diminished reflexes). This is not, however, a true hypothyroid state. TSH (thyroid-stimulating hormone) is normal, T_4 (thyroxine) is low-normal, and total T_3 (L-triiodothyronine) is low. Thyroxine is never indicated in the treatment of anorexia nervosa.
   c. *Panhypopituitarism* (Simmond's disease) rarely presents with significant weight loss. In addition, there is a loss of secondary sex characteristics which does not occur in anorexia nervosa. Lab tests show low growth hormone—which is elevated in about half of anorexics—hypothyroidism, or other end organ hypofunction.
   d. *Diabetes mellitus* may be considered because in both conditions weight loss occurs along with polydipsia and polyuria. The differentiating factor is the diabetic's overwhelming thirst versus the anorexic's attempt to assuage hunger by drinking low-calorie fluids.
   e. Patients with *Addison's disease* may most closely resemble anorexics. Both have weight loss, reduced food intake, hypotension, and occasionally hypoglycemia. The distinction is between true loss of appetite and the anorexic's aversion to weight gain. In addition, Addisonian patients have little energy while anorexics have an excess. Any uncertainty can be dispelled with tests of adrenal-cortical function.

Bulimia nervosa does not present with significant weight loss, and associated physiologic findings are generally less prominent, with the exception of electrolyte abnormalities and at times dehydration. Malabsorption syndromes and inflammatory bowel disease, which might mimic the effects of induced vomiting or laxative abuse, need to be ruled out. There are also certain neurologic disorders, such as epileptic equivalent seizures, Klüver-Bucy-like syndromes, and Kleine-Levin syndrome, that present with aberrant eating behavior. As with anorexia nervosa, a careful history and physical, with appropriate laboratory testing, can separate these disorders from bulimia nervosa.

Psychiatric Disorders

Patients with eating disorders usually experience depressive symptoms and often report either obsessive-compulsive behavior or significant impulsivity. The clinician must determine whether the disordered eating behavior is primary or secondary to another diagnosis. Because of the ongoing debate in the literature about the relationship of eating disorders to major depression and personality disorders, a consistent diagnostic framework (DSM-IIIR) is essential. It is entirely possible that a patient with an eating disorder will meet criteria for more than one Axis I diagnosis and an Axis II diagnosis as well.

EPIDEMIOLOGY

Inconsistent sampling methods, varying definitions, and the fact that many affected individuals never come to medical attention have hampered identifying accurately the population affected and the population at risk for eating disorders. Certain findings, however, have emerged repeatedly.

In both anorexia and bulimia nervosa, single white females from middle and upper class backgrounds are most commonly affected, although recent reports suggest an increasing incidence in non-whites and less class distinction (3–8). The disorders begin in adolescence or early adult life; anorexia nervosa commonly occurs somewhat earlier, often around puberty, while bulimia nervosa affects greater numbers of college-age women. Ninety to 95% of those affected are women. Affected males present a clinical picture remarkably similar to that of affected females and show either a similar or marginally worse long-term outcome (10, 11). However, a somewhat greater percent of males were actually overweight beforehand (9). Bulimic anorexics comprise one-third–one-half of all anorexics but do not differ significantly in demographic characteristics from restricting anorexics (3, 12, 13). Of those patients presenting with bulimia nervosa, one-third have had a definite history of anorexia nervosa (14).

Despite the difficulty in documentation, it seems clear that the incidence of anorexia nervosa is increasing (5), a phenomenon that lends weight to the role of sociocultural factors in the etiology of the illness. Two studies have reported a doubling in incidence, one from .55 (1963–65) to 1.12 (1973–75) per 100,000 per year (inpatients only) (15) and the other from .37 (1960–69) to .64 (1970–76) per 100,000 per year (all new treatment contacts) (4). A recent Swedish study (16) including nonmedical caregivers found a one-year incidence of anorexia nervosa of 2.6 per 100,000 in a suburban catchment area. The highest incidence reported has been from the Northeast Scotland psychiatric case register: rates of 1.6 per 100,000 from 1966–69 (17) increased to 4.06 per 100,000 from 1978–82 (5).

The epidemiology of bulimia nervosa has been obscured by the early failure to discriminate between bulimic behaviors, which are very common, and bulimia nervosa, which is much less so (18). Stricter diagnostic criteria, specifically the requirement of frequency, chronicity, and the presence of purging behavior, have moderated early reports of an epidemic affecting vast numbers of college women. A recent study using DSM-IIIR criteria on a large multi-college sample found 1% of women and .2% of men met criteria for bulimia nervosa (19). Other prevalence studies using similar criteria have reported rates of from 1–4% (20). A longitudinal study of college freshmen (21) found an incidence of bulimia nervosa of 4.2 cases per 100 women per year; a stable prevalence rate of 2.9–3.3% reflects the clinical course of the disorder, which is one of exacerbation and remission.

THEORIES OF ETIOLOGY

Eating disorders have defied efforts to establish etiology. Despite its appeal, a unitary hypothesis seems untenable at present. The weight of opinion in the current literature favors conceptualizing anorexia and bulimia nervosa as syndromes in which multiple etiologic factors converge. Rather than outlining competing theories of causality, this section, then, will review those etiologic factors that contribute to the clinical presentation.

Biological

Substantial evidence of hypothalamic dysfunction exists in patients with eating disorders, reflected in multiple endocrine disturbances. Most salient of these are abnormalities of gonadotropin, growth hormone, and corticotropin-releasing hormone secretion. Studies of neurochemical abnormalities suggest that reduced norepinephrine activity and turnover are found consistently in anorexia nervosa; data on dopaminergic and serotonergic activity in these patients are inconclusive (22). However, no single biologic defect has proved specific to the disorder and most of the abnormalities now appear to be secondary to weight loss and nutritional compromise (23). Virtually all measurable neuroendocrine abnormalities can be reversed by restoring weight (22). However, this does not eliminate the possibility that starvation effects unmask an otherwise existing but compensated central disturbance (24). Amenorrhea, which precedes significant weight loss in half to two-thirds of anorexics, may continue even after adequate weight gain. This indication of persistent hypothalamic dysfunction, enduring changes in norepinephrine activity, and evidence that starvation effect does not sufficiently explain growth hormone findings in AN all support continued research into mechanisms that may interact synergistically with starvation to produce the observed biological defects (24, 25).

Endocrine and neurochemical abnormalities, including amenorrhea, lowered serotonergic activity, and impaired secretion of cholecystokinin in response to a meal (22), have been described in bulimia nervosa. However, adequate data does not exist from which to draw conclusions. Research on the possibility of increased hunger or decreased satiety and the ways in which the endogenous opioid system may mediate binge-eating may yield fruitful results (26, 27).

The repeated observation of depressive symptomatology and affective instability in patients with eating disorders has prompted much debate about whether eating disorders, especially bulimia, are variants of affective disorder (28–30). While there continue to be strong proponents of this argument the weight of evidence at present does not support this conclusion (31–34).

There is no debate about the presence of dysphoria, low self-esteem, and self-castigation in patients with eating disorders. These cardinal features also occur in major depression. Despite symptom overlap, however, there are differences between eating disorders and major depression in symptom phenomenology, course, family history, and biochemical abnormalities (32). At least some depressive symptoms in eating disorders are related to weight loss or fluctuations in nutritional status; inadequate or bizarre food intake can lead to CNS changes that mimic affective disorder (35–37). Depressive symptoms may also be intrinsic psychological aspects of the disorders, either characterologic features contributing to their development or reactive ones contributing to their perpetuation.

Regarding eating disorders and major depression as distinct entities does not minimize the important association between them. Increased incidence of major depression has been well-documented in patients with eating disorders and their first- and second-degree relatives (38–42). These disorders may coexist and influence each other's course and expression or may occur at separate points in a vulnerable patient's lifetime. Recognizing an increased susceptibility to major depression among patients with eating disorders underscores the need to consider the possibility of dual diagnosis in this population.

Genetic

Eating disorders cluster in families (43). An increased prevalence of anorexia nervosa exists in first-degree relatives (sisters more often than mothers) of between 5–10% (44–46). A study including bulimia nervosa (44) found that 5% of female first-degree relatives of a proband with an eating disorder had a history of anorexia or bulimia nervosa. However, nothing in these figures distinguishes genetic from environmental influence. Does the family culture or an inherited factor increase the risk of developing anorexia nervosa?

Twin studies help to discern more accurately the genetic contribution. Reviews of twins with anorexia nervosa (47, 48) have found that between 35–55% of the monozygotic (MZ) twin pairs were concordant for the illness. Two studies (49, 50) compared MZ and dizygotic (DZ) pairs and found a significantly greater concordance for the MZ than DZ twins. The numbers of twin pairs remain small and methodological problems are substantial, making interpretation difficult. However, the family and twin studies together support an inherited vulnerability to anorexia nervosa. The nature of this vulnerability has not been established nor has the relationship between inherited factors and cultural and nongenetic family factors. It is quite possible that a genetically determined biological vulnerability, perhaps at the hypothalamic level, is expressed only in the context of behavior (such as extreme dieting) shaped by sociocultural or familial forces.

Psychodynamic

The feeding experience is the first human transaction, one that relies for its success on the infant's signaling of hunger and the mother's capacity to respond empathically. It is also a paradigm of the sort of interactive experience between mother and child fundamental to healthy development.

The nature of the deficits which occur in patients with eating disorders points to a failure in this interactive process early in development. The development of a coherent sense of self, with clear boundaries, sustaining self-esteem, a sense of competence, and the capacity to regulate tension is compromised. A fragile adaptation occurs, in which self-esteem is replaced by a continual search for external approval in a compliant, perfectionistic, dependent manner. The child's self, including her bodily self, may be experienced as indistinct from or an extension of the mother (by both of them). At some point in adolescence, the pressure of physical maturation and the renewed need to separate and establish autonomy combine to topple the tenuous equilibrium.

The development of an eating disorder can be understood as an effort to cope with these pressures. These young women experience their bodies as self-objects, echoing the earliest origins of the self in the body-self. Their bodies become the measure of all value, the battleground for autonomy and control, the organizing principle of the self. The battle over the taking in of food, which by its nature is something "not me" that becomes "me," expresses powerfully the difficulty with boundaries around the self. For the anorexic, a sense of personal effectiveness is attained through her capacity to dominate her own body and deny her hunger. The bulimic, in her apparent loss of control over food, is expressing split-off and disowned parts of the self. Neither is conscious of the meaning of these primitive, ritualistic behaviors; these patients have a startling lack of ability to identify and articulate their emotions or bodily sensations.

Hilde Bruch first noted these defects in interoceptive awareness (51). Along with body image disturbances and an overwhelming sense of ineffectiveness, they are the defects she described as essential in primary anorexia nervosa. Bruch's formulations (52, 53) are the basis for the current understanding of pathogenesis summarized above. Additional work, especially by self-psychologists, has added new dimensions and provided a theoretical language for her conceptualization (54–58).

While the above models are consistent with the dynamic picture of anorexia and bulimia nervosa, they do involve reconstruction of developmental events. It is uncertain whether these are descriptions of the psychology of the adult illness or its childhood pathogenesis.

Familial/Sociocultural

Family systems theory shifts the focus from individual pathology, postulating that eating disorders are caused by disturbances in the family system as a whole. Minuchin and Selvini-Palazzoli have offered compelling observations on the nature of transactions in families with an anorexic member (59, 60). Minuchin described five characteristics of these families which in his view contribute to developing and perpetuating the child's eating disorder: enmeshment, overprotectiveness, rigidity, lack of conflict resolution, and involvement of the sick child in unresolved parental conflict. Selvini-Palazzoli emphasized poor generational boundaries and the presence of covert coalitions and conflicts beneath a facade of family unity; individual identity is sacrificed and the disharmony denied.

Relatively few data-based studies exist to complement these observational reports; there is evidence for excessive closeness to one or both parents in a percentage (but not a majority) of cases and for anorexia serving to maintain an equilibrium with the family (61–63). Humphrey (64) compared restricting anorexics, bulimic anorexics, normal-weight bulimics, and normal families and found the families of both bulimic subtypes to be similar to one another and distinct from restrictor families (families of restricting anorexics). Bulimic families were much more disengaged and chaotic, highly conflicted, unexpressive, and very achievement-oriented. Relationships were more hostile-dependent. These families were more affectively labile and neglectful, while restrictor families were phobic, constricted, and controlling.

However accurate these descriptions may be of families with members who have eating disorders, they do not establish causality. Dysfunctional family patterns may perpetuate rather than cause the illness; the illness may have changed the family; and the observed patterns may not be specific to eating disorders (3, 65).

The family may also contribute to the development of an eating disorder through its function of transmitting culture. Cultural expectations and pressures are communicated by peer groups, media, and school/work settings as well. Sociocultural factors, which affect all of us, are clearly not a sufficient etiologic explanation for the development of an eating disorder. However, their impact is substantial and may well be pivotal in symptom choice for vulnerable young women.

In industrialized nations, the climate in which girls are developing may be the primary factor in the increased incidence of both anorexia and bulimia nervosa. Although the past 20 years have seen a dramatic increase in opportunities for women, a parallel increase in pressure to succeed according to male models has developed. The super-thin aesthetic which accompanies this pressure can be understood as a metaphor which associates nurturing and dependency (traditional female qualities) with a generous female form, and autonomy, self-discipline, and competence (traditionally male) with a very thin body. Patients with eating disorders embrace this aesthetic with unquestioning absoluteness. Being thin becomes the overriding measure of self-worth. Rather than challenge the cost of becoming a "superwoman" or the limits of a self defined solely by appearance, they suffer with tremendous internal emptiness, endorsing deprivation and the denial of need.

BIOPSYCHOSOCIAL EVALUATION

Even those patients who are ultimately hospitalized will usually be evaluated initially as outpatients. This is preferable, since the power dynamics are more muted in an outpatient setting. The assessment must be considered the beginning of treatment and as such must be sensitively tuned to the themes of autonomy and control so salient to these patients.

The first contact with the patient must set the tone for those to follow. Approach information-gathering by combining a matter-of-fact style with an attitude of genuine respect and curiosity. A structured interview is more appropriate than a nondirective stance. An open-ended interview can make a bulimic patient feel helpless, inadequate, and overwhelmed by undefined expectations; an anorexic, already wary, will become more so as she feels manipulated by attempts to extract her private thoughts. A structured interview offers reassuring clarity and clear evidence that the interviewer is experienced and knowledgeable about eating disorders. Asking questions that resonate with an experience the patients thought was theirs alone, or could never be understood, establishes a basic credibility and the possibility of connection.

History Taking

The first task of the assessment is to elicit a detailed picture of the eating disorder itself. One cannot assume anything; despite some commonalities, each patient has her own story to tell. What follows is an outline of the areas that should be covered and key issues to explore within each area (66). For most anorexic patients, a corroborative history should be obtained from the family since the patient will distort, conceal, and minimize her behavior.

Growth/weight history. Trace height and weight lifelong (to help establish "nor- mal" weight). Is weight stable or fluctuating? If weight loss exists, how rapid was the loss, and what percentage of premorbid weight does the loss represent? Are changes associated with specific life events (separation, illness or injury, puberty/menarche)? Is the patient satisfied with her present weight? If not, why not? How often does she weigh herself?

Eating behavior. Ask for yesterday's intake and patient's reactions to it. How chaotic is her eating pattern? Does she eat regular meals? Snack? Wait for as long as she can each day before eating? Can she tell when she's hungry or full? Are there forbidden foods or unusual food preferences? Does she eat alone or with others? Does she keep a running calorie count all day? What would she consider a normal dinner?

Dieting behavior. Does the patient fast? If she diets, how often and in what ways? How did she decide she needed to diet? Does she face athletic or occupational pressures to lose weight? Is she "always" on a diet?

Binging. When and how did she start binging? How often does she binge, at present and at her most frequent? Has she had symptom-free periods? What triggers a binge—certain foods, social situations, feelings? Are binges planned? What constitutes a binge—how much food, what kinds? Are binges part of meals or separate events? What are the rituals around her binging? What are her feelings before and afterwards? How long does a binge last? What stops a binge?

Purging. If the patient purges, how often does she do so? What methods does she use—vomiting, laxatives, diuretics? Did purging begin simultaneously with binging or later? Does she purge only after binges or after meals as well? In her experience, what is more central—the binging or the purging?

Body image. Is there a specific area of the body where dissatisfaction is focused? Does the patient avoid activities where her body will be seen (sex, athletics, sunbathing) or dress to conceal her body? Do her perceptions of her body differ from the way others see her? Distinguish distortion from dissatisfaction.

Exercise. How often and for how long? What types? Any competitive sports? Is the patient's exercise routine new or longstanding? Does she use exercise to compensate for binging or to lose weight? If she can't exercise, what is her reaction?

Alcohol or drug use. Inquire about specifics of substance, frequency and duration of use, and the patient's perceptions about it.

Menstrual history. Age of menarche? Periods of amenorrhea? Regularity, before and after onset of eating disorder? PMS (premenstrual syndrome)?

Physical problems related to eating. Hyperactivity? Weakness/fatigue? Lightheadedness? Cavities? Swollen parotid glands? Cold intolerance? Edema? Diarrhea/constipation? Increased urination? Skin changes? Bloating? Stress fractures?

Medical history. Thyroid/endocrine disorders? GI (gastrointestinal) problems? Previous eating disorder? Psychiatric illness? Medications?

Life adjustment. To what extent do eating problems interfere with school/work? Daily activities? Personal relationships? Family interactions? Feelings about herself? What are her strengths?

Course of illness. Is this an acute episode or a chronic problem?

Prior treatment. What help has she had and for how long? What was helpful, what wasn't? Has the patient tried to change her behavior on her own; if so, how? Who knows about her eating problems? Would she be willing to tell anyone else? What external supports are available to her?

Physical Examination

Because the behavior of patients with eating disorders has such direct physical consequences (67, 68) a full physical examination must be part of any evaluation. These patients should be managed in conjunction with a pediatrician or internist.

The signs and symptoms of anorexia nervosa are obvious. The physical exam must establish the degree of physical compromise. Height and weight, body temperature, pulse and blood pressure (lying and standing), and electrolyte measurements provide the most crucial information. Significantly compromised anorexics will present with a heart rate below 60, systolic blood pressure below 80, and temperature below 97°. Muscle-wasting, edema, yellowish skin with fine downy hair on face and arms, dehydration, and impaired peripheral circulation are common. Cardiac and GI systems should be carefully evaluated.

Laboratory evaluations are often remarkable for their lack of findings; mild, nonspecific changes are common even in the face of severe weight loss. Screening should include: CBC (complete blood count) with differential, urinalysis, BUN (blood urea nitrogen)/ creatinine, glucose, thyroid function tests, electrolytes, EKG (electrocardiogram). Other studies which may be indicated include liver enzymes, muscle enzymes, amylase, cholesterol, calcium, and magnesium. A spot urine sample can be helpful in detecting surreptitious use of diuretics or laxatives; a toxic screen may be important if substance abuse is suspected (69).

The patient with bulimia nervosa is usually of normal weight and presents with few physical findings. Volume depletion, dental caries and erosion of dental enamel, parotid gland enlargement, and electrolyte abnormalities are cardinal signs. Bulimics are most jeopardized by potassium depletion and the resulting risk of cardiac arrhythmias. If there is any suspicion of ipecac abuse, cardiomyopathy must also be considered. Screening tests are the same as for anorexics.

Psychodynamic Evaluation

Once the specifics of the patient's eating behavior are clear, the search begins for the context and meaning of the behavior. Careful psychological assessment is required to establish, for a given individual, the adaptive function of the behavior and the underlying conflicts contributing to its origin. No single formulation will fit all patients with eating disorders.

A dynamic understanding of the patient is usually incomplete early in treatment. The patient may be unable or unwilling to describe much about her psyche. Keeping in mind the need to be open to revision as treatment proceeds, the interviewer should explore the following areas:

Developmental history. Much of this may have to be obtained from parents, but compare patient's with parents' recollections. Important are: pregnancy and birth history, early attachment, developmental milestones (precocity or delay), degree of compliance, self-assertion, negativity, areas of competence, response to loss and separation, socialization, experience of puberty.

Experience of self. Does she have a distinct sense of self? Is there a private truth and a public persona (and is she aware of this?) Is there an internal gauge of self-esteem or is it totally dependent on external recognition and performance? What degree of self-hatred does she feel? How does she perceive her "body self"? What is her experience of being female? In her view, what is the purpose and meaning of her eating behavior? How does she view sexual maturity and being "grown up" in general? Look for pseudomaturity.

Defenses. What is the extent of denial? Defense configuration tends to fall in either a paranoid-obsessive mode (hypervigilance, projection, intellectualization, distancing) or a hysterical-impulsive mode (splitting, dissociation, flight/merger).

Affective experience. How aware is she of her affective state? (Distinguish lack of awareness from vigilance.) Intense or muted? How labile is she? Does she recognize feelings only in retrospect? Can she communicate them to others? What does she do with anger (usually suppressed or turned on herself?) Evaluate depressive symptoms and their relation to eating.

Quality of object relations. How clear are her boundaries? How isolated is she? What kinds of relationships has she formed, with adults, with peers? Any sexual involvements? Empathic capacity? How does she deal with interpersonal conflict (usually avoidance)? How does she perceive her relationship with each parent and siblings and her role in the family?

Cognitive style. Consider that starvation can compromise cognition; impaired cognition must be corrected before a meaningful evaluation is possible. How concrete is the patient's thinking? To what extent is her mental life dominated by thoughts about food, eating, weight and shape, or by a need to be "in control"? How rigid are her thought patterns? What kind of cognitive distortions are present? (Common are black and white thinking ["If I can't win the race I may as well not run"]; self-referential thinking ["Everyone is looking"]; catastrophizing; overgeneralization; magical thinking.) What is her capacity for self-observation? Does she have concerns that she can identify and share?

Co-morbidity. Identify co-existing Axis I and Axis II psychopathology. The patient may meet criteria for an affective disorder, substance abuse, obsessive-compulsive disorder, or a personality disorder in addition to the eating disorder diagnosis. This will have important treatment implications.

The psychological evaluation may be usefully supplemented with psychological testing, especially in the extended evaluation possible in an inpatient setting. Frequently used measures include: Eating Disorders Inventory (70); Symptom Checklist-90 (71); Beck Depression Inventory (72); Social Adjustment Scale (73); MMPI (Minnesota Multiphase personality inventory test).

Family Assessment

Whether or not a family is directly interviewed or included in treatment will vary with circumstances. The age of the patient, living arrangements, amount of contact among family members, and willingness to participate are all influential factors. Whether or not direct involvement occurs, information must be gathered about family history, patterns of interaction, and the emotional climate within the family.

Family history should ascertain the presence of medical and psychiatric illness, especially eating disorders (including obesity), substance abuse, and affective illness. Evidence of physical or sexual abuse should be noted. The inquiry should also address family attitudes and expectations about food, exercise, and appearance.

Looking at the family system can help to determine whether the patient's illness serves an adaptive function within her family, which, unless addressed, could serve to reinforce and perpetuate her behavior. Understanding structural and communication patterns may also have direct implications for intervention. Dimensions for assessment include:

1. Cohesiveness—boundaries, enmeshment/ distance, overprotectiveness
2. Roles
3. Parental relationship
4. Rigidity versus chaos
5. Patterns of communication—how stereotyped, covert versus direct, level of affective expression

6. Expectations and reinforcements
7. Ways of dealing with conflict
8. Impact of illness—on individuals and family as a whole; extent of family focus on eating disorder; attempts to intervene

Motivation for Treatment

No treatment recommendations can be formulated without considering the patient's motivation for change (66). The anorexic patient does not want to change. At the outset she will always resist treatment; working with her fierce need to remain in control will be a part of every intervention. Degree of emaciation, chronicity of illness, and response to previous treatment may help predict her capacity to engage. See if she can acknowledge distress about related areas, such as impaired concentration, isolation from peers, insomnia, depression, or irritability; if so, she has more reason to agree to treatment (74).

In some ways it is harder to assess a bulimic patient's motivation for change. While her stated wish is to change her behavior, she is highly ambivalent about doing so. It is worth asking, straightforwardly, what the patient expects from treatment. This yields information about how she views the problem, whether she has any understanding of the function it serves for her psychologically, and how ready she is to look at this and collaborate in efforts to change.

Many bulimics will have multiple "false starts" before they can successfully enter treatment. Key to assessing readiness are: degree to which symptoms are ego-syntonic, expectations for magical cure, and the patient's perception of the role of her behavior in weight maintenance. Some bulimics exhibit little distress, describing their behavior in a detached, matter-of-fact way; in this case there is not yet a task around which to ally. Others, who have become distressed, seek treatment urgently. However, many of these are seeking rescue, not treatment. They perceive themselves as helpless victims and expect the clinician to rid them of the problem. Bulimics at this stage cannot tolerate the idea that change will take time, be difficult, and require their active struggle. The clinician who assumes the full burden of responsibility will encounter a patient holding tightly to what he or she is trying to take away. Finally, it is useful to inquire whether or not the patient would be willing to gain five pounds in the process of treatment. Those who "would rather die" are probably poor candidates for treatment.

HOSPITAL TREATMENT

Decision to Hospitalize

Hospitalization is not automatically recommended for patients with eating disorders. The decision, an individual one, depends on clinical and strategic factors. A large proportion of anorexics are hospitalized; most bulimics are not. Indications for hospitalization (for both groups) include: a degree of physical compromise requiring medical intervention; symptoms so overwhelming they interfere with the patient's ability to function; concurrent major depression, severe character pathology, or active substance abuse; suicidality; the need for a medication trial in an unreliable patient; failure of previous outpatient treatment; the need for a more extended and comprehensive evaluation than is feasible as an outpatient; the need to put together a treatment team; the need to engage a recalcitrant family. Every effort should be made to arrange hospitalization on a voluntary basis. The hope for a therapeutic alliance is markedly compromised by involuntary commitment; such a stance should be taken only in life-threatening situations.

Hospitalization is rarely a definitive treatment for an eating disorder (75). It is one phase in a long-term treatment effort. As such, the hospital must be used in a way that maximizes the unique opportunities it provides. Foremost among these are increased containment, increased intensity, and improved integration of treatment modalities.

Changing Eating Behavior

The single most important feature of the hospital setting is the capacity to supervise and/or control a patient's eating behavior. In general the hospitalized patient needs external control of her eating, either because she has compromised her physical condition or because overwhelming symptoms have disrupted her ability to function.

Nutritional rehabilitation is the first priority in treating an anorexic patient (76). Until they are reversed, the cognitive, behavioral, and affective consequences of starvation (77) preclude meaningful change via other treatment modalities.

Several published protocols may serve as models for program design (77–81). Although substantial variations exist in the specifics of individual programs, most are based in an operant conditioning model with a balance of positive and negative reinforcers (82). A target weight is set and along with it the expectation of a specified amount and rate of weight gain (usually around 0.1 kg/day). The patient's weight and vital signs are obtained every morning after voiding, in the same attire. A body search for concealed objects may be necessary. (There are differing opinions about sharing weight with the patient; on the one hand sharing the information includes her, on the other it may increase her anxiety to hear concrete evidence of weight gain.) Initially, appropriate meals are planned by a dietitian without input from the patient, who is expected to eat under supervision and within a specified time frame all the food placed in front of her. If the patient cannot cooperate, a liquid supplement such as Sustacal is prescribed at regular intervals. In some cases the supplement is part of the refeeding protocol itself. Low vital signs or inadequate weight gain require activity restriction (bed rest at its most controlled) and loss of privileges. As weight gain progresses, the patient is given increasing responsibility step-by-step for making her own food choices. Some programs allow more patient control over intake from the outset and introduce restrictions or supplements only if weight gain is inadequate or vital signs low. Although some element of coercion is unavoidable during this phase, it can be minimized by framing it as an opportunity to relearn normal eating behavior and a necessary step on the way to regaining true control over food; control must include the choice to eat as well as to refrain from eating.

More than any specific provision, what is crucial to the success of the protocol is that it be relatively standard for all patients and that the staff who carry it out support it, understand it, and apply it consistently. Managing the anorexic patient requires enormous staff cohesion; any opportunity to split staff or negotiate details will be manipulated to the fullest. With an experienced, cohesive staff, however, most patients comply voluntarily with the refeeding protocol. Measures such as nasogastric tube feedings or hyperalimentation should be used only in life-threatening situations; they represent to the patient a total loss of control and a hostile, intrusive assault.

Bulimic patients also require a structured protocol to interrupt the cycle of binging and purging and relearn reasonable eating habits. Hospitalization imposes abstinence from binging and purging; despite initial anxiety, most bulimics experience relief in the presence of this external control. Using a therapeutic contract agreed upon by the patient makes her an ally in changing her eating patterns.

"The best defense against binging is to eat" (83). Patients should be expected to eat, under supervision, three meals and one or two snacks a day; food may be initially pre-selected but ultimately the patient makes her own choices. Exposure to "forbidden foods" is part of meal planning. Eating in the new setting provided by the hospital also interrupts the eating rituals that have developed. Patients must sit in an open area for a period following meals, without access to bathrooms. Initially all bathroom use is supervised to prevent purging. Although patients are not exposed to binging, they are sufficiently frightened of eating normal-sized meals that this approach operates as a modified exposure/response-prevention model.

Greater autonomy in food choice, greater freedom of movement off the unit, and unsupervised bathroom use all reinforce changing behavior patterns. The relief the patient feels when the anticipated "huge" weight gain does not occur is also reinforcing. Although some initial weight gain may occur, it is transient; many patients actually lose weight when they stop binging and purging.

Pharmacologic Interventions

A medication trial can be conducted in a safer, more reliable, and more aggressive fashion in an inpatient setting. Although a variety of agents have been studied in anorexic patients, there is no convincing evidence that medication has a significant role in treatment. Existing studies suggest that several psychotropic medications (tricyclic antidepressants, cyproheptadine, and lithium) may increase weight gain in the short term in conjunction with other treatments (84–86). Nothing indicates any effect on underlying psychopathology and long-term effects are unknown (87).

In contrast, the results of pharmacologic treatment of bulimia nervosa have been highly promising. Eleven of 13 placebo-controlled studies (88, 89) have found antidepressant medications effective in reducing the frequency of and, in some cases, eliminating binge eating and vomiting. This effectiveness is *not* related to the presence of major depression (90, 91).

Several important issues, however, remain unresolved. Because bulimic patients are especially sensitive to the side effects of tricyclics and MAO inhibitors, a significant proportion of those treated discontinue the drug (92, 93). In addition, only short-term efficacy has been demonstrated. The longest follow-up study (two years) (92) found that many patients had required a switch of medications because they had relapsed on the original drug. Also, it is not known whether improvement will be sustained when medication is discontinued after a reasonable treatment course (6–12 months) (94). Last, and most important, is the absence of information concerning which bulimic subtypes are likely to respond to medication (95). Until this knowledge is available, treatment decisions must be made pragmatically.

In general, patients compromised enough to seek hospitalization should be given a trial on medication. More specific indications for a medication trial are: failure to respond to other treatments; severe symptomatology; prominent affective symptoms such as anxiety or dysphoria; and patient request. Patient preference must always be considered; many bulimics refuse to relinquish control to a foreign agent, others are fearful of a "different addiction," and others welcome a biological explanation and the possibility of external relief from their symptoms.

Treatment should be initiated with fluoxetine or trazodone because of the lower incidence of side effects. If these are unsuitable, desipramine or nortriptyline are good choices. Although response often takes place within several weeks (96), a full course of treatment (6–10 weeks) should be undertaken, using blood levels where avail- able. MAO inhibitors must be used with great caution because of the need for careful dietary compliance; they are ideally initiated during hospitalization.

Researchers are also investigating the effectiveness of narcotic antagonists (which in animals attenuate hyperphagia) and fenfluramine (which enhances satiety) in bulimic patients (97, 98).

Milieu Treatment

The inpatient setting is uniquely suited to provide an intensive, integrated treatment. The patient is placed in an empathic, containing environment, apart from the disordered relationships, rituals, and cues that have helped perpetuate her illness. A multifaceted treatment is initiated. The members of the treatment team are in regular communication in order to treat the patient with consistency, according to a coherent model; each component of the model is valued explicitly.

The milieu most powerfully conveys the overall treatment philosophy. Despite the time and energy it entails, changing eating behavior must be subsumed under the goals of helping the patient with an eating disorder attain a genuine and autonomous sense of self, separate herself appropriately from her family, and come to understand the meaning her eating behavior has had for her (99). Until the patient recognizes that she has needs and feelings and conflicts that have been obscured by her preoccupation with food, any change in eating behavior or weight will be imposed and rapid relapse will follow discharge. This recognition comes slowly. Given current insurance limitations, real change is seldom consolidated before discharge. Under these conditions, assembling a treatment team, interrupting eating patterns, and establishing enough of an alliance to permit continued outpatient treatment are substantial accomplishments. Repeated briefer hospitalizations at crisis points in treatment may be necessary.

Milieu treatment makes extensive use of groups. These include groups specifically related to the eating disorder (psychoeducational, cognitive-behavioral, body image) and those addressing related areas such as assertiveness training, social skills training, relaxation techniques, and family relations. Group treatment, whatever its focus, offers several advantages: (*a*) an end to secrecy and isolation by sharing with peers; (*b*) reality-testing of distorted beliefs and self-percepts, which carries credibility because the feedback comes from other women with eating disorders; (*c*) an interpersonal context in which these women can begin to identify and communicate affect and where the links between eating behavior and relationships may become clear through the evolving relationships among group members (100).

Certain patients, however, cannot use a group. In general, groups are used less frequently with anorexics because of their denial, competitiveness around weight/eating, rigidity, and interpersonal isolation. Severe emaciation and impenetrable denial are contraindications for group treatment (101). Bulimics whose severe character pathology, suicidal ideation, or questionable motivation would make them unsuitable for an outpatient group can usually be adequately contained in an inpatient group.

Overall, groups are probably of maximal benefit when they are one part of a comprehensive treatment. It should be noted, however, that numerous short-term outpatient groups for bulimics have reported substantial declines in binge/purge episodes, though durability of response is not known (102). In addition, a recent carefully controlled study comparing a very intensive group treatment with placebo, imipramine, and group plus imipramine (103) reported impressive results with the group

treatment alone, superior to either imipramine alone or group plus imipramine.

Individual Psychotherapy

The barriers to psychotherapy with an anorexic patient are formidable yet the need for psychological growth is urgent. In her desperate struggle for control and individuality, the patient identifies her emaciated body as evidence of her success. She is withdrawn and isolated and not aware of the psychological meaning of her behavior. Any attempts to challenge her position are met with obstinate resistance (either directly or masked by superficial compliance). Thus the first priorities of psychotherapy are making emotional contact and then moving from antagonist to ally.

The therapist must first communicate interest in the patient as a person not just a skinny body. It will be hard to persuade the patient of one's genuine interest in understanding her experience and to divert her attention from total preoccupation with food and weight. This requires an active, empathic stance and an alert receptiveness to any communication she initiates. Early dialogue will inevitably focus on the patient's hospital experience. Respecting her perspective, exploring day-to-day occurrences, searching for aspects of her life experience that she feels comfortable discussing all contribute to slowly building an alliance and helping her find her own voice.

The therapist walks a difficult tightrope with respect to weight gain. He or she must respect the patient's need for control and anger at intrusion while simultaneously supporting the necessary nutritional rehabilitation. The therapist cannot stand apart; this risks splitting the treatment team and implicitly condones the patient's self-starvation. Meaningful change must include both weight gain and psychological growth. It is naive to believe that once underlying unconscious conflicts are resolved, weight gain will follow (104). These processes are intertwined and the therapist needs to be involved in both of them.

The tasks of therapy will change as the battle over food changes. If an alliance can be forged, the therapy will gradually move away from the defensive maneuvers around food and weight towards the underlying deficits in self-esteem, autonomy, and individuation. The therapist will try to help the patient discover and voice her feelings of helplessness, anger, and loneliness; will respond empathically; and will provide a trustworthy relationship. Changes in these areas require long-term treatment by an experienced therapist. The fact that long-term treatment may not be feasible has of course spurred interest in briefer treatment modalities; however, to expect rapid change in an anorexic patient is unrealistic.

For most bulimics, individual therapy has an important place in treatment. Behavioral change is important and the most easily measurable index of change. Meaningful, long-term improvement must also include greater self-acceptance, access to and tolerance of the affects that have been buried or acted out in binging and purging, and alternate ways of tension regulation. As with anorexics, the challenge of individual work with bulimics is to balance the focus between symptoms and psyche.

The technical aspects of therapy will be tailored according to individual need. Impulsive patients will require considerable containment; obsessional, perfectionistic ones will require a constant redirecting of attention to their inner experience. The therapist needs to be comfortable with pragmatic, symptom-focused strategies and also with utilizing the transference and other aspects of the therapeutic relationship (37).

Although formal cognitive-behavioral treatment (CBT) is used with anorexic pa-tients (105), it has been used and studied far more extensively with bulimic patients. Detailed descriptions are available for CBT programs tailored specifically for bulimic patients (106). The programs' effectiveness have been demonstrated in a number of studies (107–109).

Goals of CBT are to challenge the bulimic's distorted and irrational ways of thinking about food and about herself; identify triggers that initiate and maintain the binge-purge cycle; and devise specific ways to interrupt that cycle. Tools include self-monitoring via a food diary (intake, situations, thoughts and feelings); incremental goal setting (breaking the behavior down into small enough pieces to experiment with); meal planning; training in problem solving (anticipating a potential problem, generating several possible solutions and choosing one); developing alternatives to binging (e.g., contacting another person, decreasing food availability, exercising, sleeping); cognitive restructuring (identifying, examining, and challenging a dysfunctional thought or belief); and education about the disorder. The techniques can be implemented in either a group or individual treatment.

While cognitive-behavioral approaches clearly have an important place in the treatment of bulimia nervosa, they are probably most effective with highly motivated patients free of serious concurrent psychopathology. CBT requires active collaboration and substantial readiness to change.

Family Therapy

Family therapy is essential to the treatment of every anorexic patient living at home. The family has organized itself around the anorexic patient in ways that are either ineffective in helping her or actually perpetuate her difficulties. A negative cycle of guilt and recrimination becomes established. Hospitalization is helpful in several ways. First, it interrupts the family dynamic by removing the anorexic member. In some families this brings relief and a chance to regroup and they welcome assistance in becoming more effective. Second, the need for hospitalization forcefully underlines the seriousness of the situation. This message, along with clear expectations for family participation, can help to engage those families whose defensiveness or denial have hampered treatment.

Programs vary considerably in their expectations for family involvement and in their approach to family treatment. Some enforce a period of noninvolvement to provoke the dynamic instability that will occur in the family in the absence of the anorexic member (110). Others involve the family as full members of the treatment team, thereby diminishing the risk of reinforcing the parents' sense of helplessness and of parenting responsibilities getting delegated to the hospital (111). Most programs do involve the family from the outset, though without incorporating the family as fully as this model does in treatment decisions. Sadly, there are cases in which family pathology is so severe and intransigent that the anorexic patient has to be separated from her family (112).

When attempting to engage a family in treatment, it is crucial to avoid blame, to support each member's self-esteem, and to focus on problems that they consider directly relevant. The family needs help to communicate openly and directly, to strengthen the parental alliance, and to permit each family member to become more autonomous. Because the family has developed an equilibrium around its anorexic member, attempts to help the anorexic individuate without parallel assistance for the family who need to let her do so will trigger powerful attempts (in both patient and family) to preserve that equilibrium.

The best known models for treating anorexic families are the structural model of Minuchin (59) and the systemic model of Selvini-Palazzoli (60). They are both active, directive models that aim to change family structure and interactions. The structural therapist first joins with, then attacks, family subsystems. Reframing and enactment (e.g., a family lunch) are also used. The systemic therapist uses a circular questioning method both to gather and transmit information; then he or she prescribes an intervention, frequently paradoxical or ritualistic, designed to facilitate change without the direct pressure which so often elicits massive resistance (113, 114). Specific training in these techniques is needed to treat the anorexic family.

Family therapy is used less often with bulimic patients, in large measure because most bulimics no longer live at home. However, when feasible, it can be a powerful adjunct to individual therapy. Ongoing family therapy is indicated when a bulimic lives at home or remains highly dependent upon her family or when a parent or spouse is either chronically undermining or a potential ally. Many bulimics have tried to hide their behavior from their families and some families have ignored or minimized the evidence. In these cases, especially, bringing the secret struggle out into the open where it can be dealt with directly is a crucial step.

There has been only one controlled study of family therapy in anorexia and bulimia nervosa. Treating 80 patients with either family therapy or individual supportive therapy, Russell (115) found after one year that family therapy was more effective than individual therapy in anorexic patients whose illness was not chronic and who had become ill before they were 19. A more tentative finding was that individual supportive therapy was more effective than family therapy for anorexic patients with an older age of onset. There was no significant difference between the two treatments for the patients with bulimia nervosa or for young, chronic anorexics.

CONTROVERSIES AND SPECIAL PROBLEMS

The history of eating disorders research and treatment is a history of controversy. The controversies involve both how to conceptualize the disorders and how to treat them. The lack of definitive data in both these areas has further fueled the debates.

The current working acceptance of a multifactorial etiology of these disorders has helped bring disparate perspectives together. It has not, however, diminished the need to clarify the exact nature of the contribution of each factor. Just what is the relationship between eating disorders and affective disorder? How exactly do neurotransmitters, hormones, and the endogenous opioid system shape eating behavior? Are sociocultural factors enough to explain the overwhelming preponderance of women affected? To what extent are these disorders an illness of the family system rather than of an individual? Are there parallels with models of addiction? How does a coexisting personality disorder affect the development or expression of an eating disorder? Are bulimia nervosa and anorexia nervosa each a distinct disorder or are they points on a continuum?

The model of multifactorial etiology has led to the development of the multifaceted treatment approach described in this chapter. Yet the treatment team faces many unresolved dilemmas and the challenge of integrating sometimes incompatible goals. When should patients with eating disorders be hospitalized? How should the team respond to treatment refusal? What is the best way to balance behavioral, dynamic, and systemic approaches; or do these approaches undermine one another? What is the role of medication? How can the struggle for control be optimally managed? How is a target weight selected? What are sensible criteria for discharge? What are the best ways of involving the family? Does the chronically ill patient require a different treatment?

Each treatment center deals with these questions in the design of its program. Additionally, clinicians in these programs must grapple, individually and as members of a team, with the special problems posed by these patients. Splitting of staff, covert competition among patients, manipulative and deceitful behavior, failed alliances with treaters, impenetrable preoccupation with food, and ferocious struggle for control all require that staff maintain high levels of sophistication and communication in order to preserve a therapeutic stance.

What remains too often unaddressed is how hard it is to treat these patients. Certain predictable countertransference reactions occur which, if not recognized, can significantly undermine treatment efforts. Female therapists, vulnerable to the same cultural pressures as their patients, may find the patient's conflicts resonating with their own. They must be prepared to find their body a subject for discussion in the treatment, either as an object of envy, competition, or, if overweight, anxiety and devaluation. Male therapists may have difficulty empathizing with the patient's experience of her body and also may hesitate to discuss specifics for fear of being intrusive. They may especially be vulnerable to rescue fantasies or the wish to reason the patient out of her dysfunctional behavior. They may also be dismissed by the patient who assumes that hers is a problem no man could ever understand. Common in the experience of all treaters are: succumbing to a preoccupation with food that parallels the patient's; experiencing patient deceit as malicious; exhaustion; and, most important, rage in response to a pervasive sense of helplessness in dealing with these patients—rage at their resistance, rage at their lack of improvement, rage at their inaccessibility. The team approach offers the chance to anticipate and address these reactions and share the challenge, one usually too great for any therapist to carry alone.

COURSE AND PROGNOSIS

Differences in methodology and study design make it very difficult to compare results of outcome studies for anorexia nervosa. Although certain observations are warranted, no definitive statistics are available.

Meaningful assessment of outcome requires follow-up of at least four years; the success of initial treatment in accomplishing weight gain is quite satisfactory but does not predict longer-term results (116). At follow-up a majority of patients have improved their weight status; however, between a quarter and a third exhibit a chronic, intractable course. Mortality in more than half of available studies is 4% or less but may increase with long-term follow-up (117–118). Those who have successfully gained weight are often still preoccupied with food and weight and commonly report depressed and anxious feelings (119). In overall functioning, anorexics have much greater success in employment than in interpersonal relationships (120).

Thus an anorexic patient may have a single episode from which she recovers without sequelae, she may improve but not fully recover, or she may develop a chronic, refractory illness. What determines outcome? More severe illness, as indicated by longer duration, extreme weight loss, and failure to respond to treatment, carries a worse prognosis. Disturbed family relationships and concomitant personality disorders

have also frequently been associated with poor outcome (116). Answers to the questions whether younger patients have a better outcome than older and whether bulimic anorexics have a worse prognosis than restrictors are controversial (121).

One interesting study (122) approached the question of recovery from the perspective of the patient. Establishing an empathic relationship with either a therapist or someone in her everyday life was cited as the single most important element in recovery. Overall, however, not a single study exists that documents a clear relationship between treatment and outcome (123). It is not known whether treatment alters prognosis. In this context of uncertainty, most treatment decisions must be made pragmatically. However, the need for early, comprehensive intervention is indisputable.

In contrast to anorexia nervosa, the course of bulimia nervosa is episodic, with remissions and relapses. Follow-up over time is necessary to differentiate a symptom-free period from recovery. Existing studies indicate that bulimia nervosa is not a benign, time-limited condition; at least one-third of patients will still be affected several years after initial presentation (117).

At present there is not enough data to compare the relative effects of different treatments on long-term outcome. Treatment does, however, have a positive impact on outcome. A decrease in binge/purge episodes has been documented in response to a variety of interventions (124, 125). These results will become more meaningful when outcome criteria are widened to include psychological as well as behavioral change and when longer-term follow-up gauges the extent to which improvements are sustained over time.

Prognostic factors are beginning to be identified. Those bulimics with the most severe eating pathology at baseline appear to have the poorest outcome (124, 126). In one study (127), pretreatment level of self-esteem was a consistent predictor of outcome. Interestingly, the degree of associated depression is not a factor affecting outcome (117, 124, 127). A history of prior anorexia nervosa, duration of illness, and age at onset have also not predicted outcome. These are counterintuitive findings and highlight how much we still have to learn.

Anorexia and bulimia nervosa pose a diagnostic and therapeutic challenge of impressive magnitude, a challenge both frustrating and compelling. As increasingly frequent disorders with considerable morbidity, they demand our skilled and thoughtful attention.

REFERENCES

1. Garfinkel PE, Moldofsky H, Garner DM: The heterogeneity of anorexia nervosa: bulimia as a distinct subgroup. Arch Gen Psychiatry, 37:1036–1040, 1980.

2. American Psychiatric Association: *Diagnostic and Statistical Manual of Mental Disorders*, ed. 3, (DSM-IIIR) Washington, D.C., American Psychiatric Association, 1987.

3. Garfinkel PE, Garner DM: *Anorexia Nervosa: A Multidimensional Perspective*, New York, Brunner/Mazel, 1982.

4. Jones DJ, Fox MM, Barbigan HM, Hutton HE: Epidemiology of anorexia nervosa in Monroe County, New York: 1960–1976. Psychosom Med, 42:551–558, 1980.

5. Szmukler, GI: The epidemiology of anorexia nervosa and bulimia. J Psychiatr Res, 19:143–153, 1985.

6. Pumeriega AJ, Edwards P, Mitchell CB: Anorexia nervosa in black adolescents. J Am Acad Child Adolesc Psychiatry, 23:111–114, 1984.

7. Lacy JH, Dolan BM: Bulimia in British black and Asian women, a catchment area study. Br J Psychiatry, 152:73–79, 1988.

8. Dolan BM, Evans C, Lacey JH: Family composition and social class in bulimia. J Nerv Ment Dis, 177:267–272, 1989.

9. Andersen AE: Anorexia nervosa and bulimia nervosa in males, in Garner DM, Garfinkel, PE (eds): *Diagnostic Issues in Anorexia and Bulimia Nervosa*, New York, Brunner/Mazel, 1988.

10. Burns T, Crisp AH: Factors affecting prognosis in male anorexics. J Psychiatr Res, 19:323–328, 1985.

11. Oyebode MB, Boodhoo JA, Schapira K: Anorexia in males: clinical features and outcome. Int J Eating Disorders, 7:121–124, 1988.

12. Crisp H: *Anorexia Nervosa: Let Me Be*, New York, Grune & Stratton, 1980.

13. Casper RC, Eckert ED, Halmi, KA, Goldberg SC, Davis JM: Bulimia: Its incidence and clinical importance in patients with anorexia nervosa. Arch Gen Psychiatry, 37:1030–1034, 1980.

14. Fairburn CG, Cooper PJ: The clinical features of bulima nervosa. Br J Psychiatry, 144:238–246, 1984.

15. Willi J, Grossman S: Epidemiology of anorexia nervosa in a defined region of Switzerland. Am J Psychiatry, 140:564–567, 1983.

16. Cullberg J, Engstrom-Lindberg M: Prevalence and incidence of eating disorders in a suburban area. Acta Psychiatr Scand, 78:314–319, 1988.

17. Kendel RE, Hall DJ, Haily A, Babigian HM: The epidemiology of anorexia nervosa. Psychol Med, 3:200–203, 1973.

18. Schotte DE, Stunkard AJ: Bulimia vs bulimic behaviors on a college campus. JAMA, 258:1213–1215, 1987.

19. Drewnowski A, Hopkins SA, Kessler RC: The prevalence of bulimia nervosa in the US college student population. Am J Public Health, 78:1322–1325, 1988.

20. Connors ME, Johnson CL: Epidemiology of bulimia and bulimic behaviors. Addict Behav, 12:165–179, 1987.

21. Drewnowski A, Yee DK, Krahn DD: Bulimia in college women: Incidence and recovery rates. Am J Psychiatry, 145:753–755, 1988.

22. Fava M, Copeland PM, Schweiger U, Herzog DB: Neurochemical abnormalities of anorexia nervosa and bulimia nervosa. Am J Psychiatry, 145:963–971, 1989.

23. Fichter MM, Doerr P, Pirke KM, et al: Behavior, attitude, nutrition, and endocrinology in anorexia nervosa. Acta Psychiatr Scand, 66:429–444, 1982.

24. Newman MM, Halmi KA: The en-

docrinology of anorexia nervosa and bulimia nervosa. Neurol Clin, 6(1):195–212, 1988.

25. Kaye WH, Jimerson DC, Lake CR, et al: Altered norepinephrine metabolism following long-term weight recovery in patients with anorexia nervosa. Psychiatry Res, 14:333–351, 1985.

26. Kaye WH, Gwirtsman H, George DT, et al: Altered feeding behavior in bulimia: Is it related to mood and serotonin? in Walsh BT (ed): *Eating Behavior in Eating Disorders,* Washington, D.C., American Psychiatric Press, 1988.

27. Marks-Kaufman R, Kanarek RB: The endogenous opioid peptides: relationship to food intake, obesity, and sweet tastes, in Walsh BT (ed): *Eating Behavior in Eating Disorders,* Washington D.C., American Psychiatric Press, 1988.

28. Swift WJ, Andrews D, Barklage NE: The relationship between affective disorder and eating disorders: A review of the literature. Am J Psychiatry, 143:290–299, 1986.

29. Halmi KA: Relationship of eating disorders to depression: Biological similarities and differences. In J of Eating Disorders, 4:667–680, 1985.

30. Hatsukami DK, Mitchell JE, Eckert ED: Eating disorders: A variant of mood disorders? Psychiatr Clin North Am, 7:349–365, 1984.

31. Pope HG, Hudson JI: Is bulimia nervosa a heterogeneous disorder? Lessons from the history of medicine. Int J Eating Disorders, 7(2):155–156, 1988.

32. Strober M, Katz JL: Depression in the eating disorders: A review and analysis of descriptive, family, and biological findings, in Garner DM, Garfinkel PE (eds): *Diagnostic Issues in Anorexia Nervosa and Bulimia Nervosa,* New York, Brunner/Mazel, 1988.

33. Altshuler KZ, Weiner MF: Anorexia nervosa and depression: A dissenting view. Am J Psychiatry, 142:328–332, 1985.

34. Levy AB, Dixon KN, Stern SS: How are depression and bulima related? Am J Psychiatry, 146:162–169, 1989.

35. Laessle R, Schweiger U, Pirke KM: Depression as a correlate of starvation in patients with eating disorders. Biol Psychiatry, 23:719–725, 1988.

36. Eckert ED, Goldberg SC, Halmi KA,

Casper RC, Davis JM: Depression in anorexia nervosa. Psychol Med, 12:115–122, 1982.

37. Johnson C, Connors ME: The Etiology and Treatment of Bulima Nervosa, New York, Basic Books, 1987.

38. Hudson JI, Pope HG, Jonas JM, Yurgelun-Todd D: Phenomenologic relationship of eating disorders to major affective disorder. Psychiatry Res, 9:345–354, 1983.

39. Herzog DB: Are anorexic and bulimic patients depressed? Am J Psychiatry, 141:1594–1597, 1984.

40. Winokur A, March S, Mendels J: Primary affective disorder in the relatives of patients with anorexia nervosa. Am J Psychiatry, 137:695–698, 1980.

41. Hudson JI, Pope HG, Jonas JM, Yurgelun-Todd D: Family history study of anorexia nervosa and bulimia. Br J Psychiatry, 142:133–138, 1983.

42. Biederman J, Rivinus T, Kemper K, Hamilton D, MacFadyen J, Harmatz J: Depressive disorders in relatives of anorexia nervosa patients with and without a current episode of nonbipolar major depression. Am J Psychiatry, 142:1495–1496, 1985.

43. Strober M, Salkin B, Burroughs J, Morrell W, Sadjak J: A family study of anorexia nervosa and depression. Presented at the annual meeting of the American Psychiatric Association, Washington D.C., May 10–16, 1986.

44. Strober M, Morrell W, Burroughs J, Salkin B, Jacobs C: A controlled family study of anorexia nervosa. J Psychiatr Res, 19:239–246, 1985.

45. Crisp AH, Hsu LFG, Harding B, Hartshorn J: Clinical features of anorexia nervosa: A study of a consecutive series of 102 female patients. J Psychosom Res, 24:179–191, 1980.

46. Theander S: Anorexia nervosa: A psychiatric investigation of 94 female patients. Acta Psychiatr Scand, Suppl 214, pp. 1–194, 1970.

47. Vandereycken W, Pierloot R: Anorexia nervosa in twins. Psychother Psychosom, 35:55–63, 1981.

48. Nowlin NS: Anorexia nervosa in twins: Case report and review. J Clin Psychiatry, 44:101–105, 1983.

49. Holland AJ, Hall A, Murray R, Russell GFM, Crisp AH: Anorexia nervosa: A study of 34 pairs of twins and one set of triplets. Br J Psychiatry, *145*:414–419, 1984.

50. Holland AJ, Sicotte N, Treasure J: Anorexia nervosa: Evidence for a genetic basis. J Psychosom Res, *32*(6):561–571, 1988.

51. Bruch H: Perceptual and conceptual disturbances in anorexia nervosa. Psychol Med, *24*:187–194, 1962.

52. Bruch H: *Eating disorders: Obesity, Anorexia Nervosa and the Person Within,* New York, Basic Books, 1973.

53. Bruch H: *The Golden Cage: the Enigma of Anorexia Nervosa,* Cambridge, Harvard University Press, 1978.

54. Goodsit A: Self-regulatory disturbances in eating disorders. Int J Eating Disorders, *2*:51–60, 1983.

55. Goodsit A: Self psychology and the treatment of anorexia nervosa, in Garner DM, Garfinkel PE (eds): *Handbook of Psychotherapy for Anorexia Nervosa and Bulimia,* New York, The Guilford Press, 1985.

56. Sugarman A, Kurash C: The body as a transitional object in bulimia. Int J Eating Disorders, *1*:57–67, 1982.

57. Kohut H: *The analysis of the self,* New York, International Universities Press, 1971.

58. Casper RC: The psychopathology of anorexia nervosa: The pathological psychodynamic processes, in Beumont PJV, Burrows GD, Casper RC (eds): *Handbook of Eating Disorders, Part 1: Anorexia and Bulimia Nervosa,* Amsterdam, Elsevier, 1987.

59. Minuchin S, Rosman BL, Baker L: *Psychosomatic Families: Anorexia Nervosa in Context,* Cambridge, Harvard University Press, 1978.

60. Selvini-Palazzoli M: *Self-Starvation. From Individual to Family Therapy in the Treatment of Anorexia Nervosa,* New York, Jason Aronson, 1978.

61. Kalucy RS, Crisp AH, Harding B: A study of 56 families with anorexia nervosa. Br J Med Psychol, *50*:381–395, 1977.

62. Morgan HG, Russell GFM: Value of family background and clinical features as predictors of long-term outcome in anorexia nervosa: Four year follow-up study of 41 patients. Psychol Med, *5*:355–372, 1975.

63. Crisp AH, Harding B, McGuiness B: Anorexia nervosa. Psychoneurotic characteristics of parents: Relationship to prognosis. J Psychosom Res, *18*:167–173, 1974.

64. Humphrey LL: Family-wide distress in bulimia, in Cannon D, Baker T (eds): *Addictive Disorders: Psychological Assessment and Treatment,* New York, Praeger, 1987.

65. Stern SL, Dixon KN, Jones D, Lake M, Nemzer E, Sansone R: Family environment in anorexia nervosa and bulimia. Int J Eating Disorders, *8*(1):25–31, 1989.

66. McKenna MS: Assessment of the eating disordered patient. Psych Annals, *19*(9):467–472, 1989.

67. Mitchell JE: Medical complications of anorexia nervosa and bulimia. Psychiatr Med, *1*:229–255, 1983.

68. Mitchell JE, Seim HC, Colon E, Pomeroy C: Medical complications and medical management of bulimia. Ann Intern Med, *107*:71–77, 1987.

69. Bulik CM: Drug and alcohol abuse by bulimic women and their families. Am J Psychiatry, *144*:1604–1606, 1987.

70. Garner DM, Olmsted MP, Polivy J: Development and validation of multidimensional eating disorder inventory for anorexia nervosa and bulimia. Int J Eating Disorders, *2*:15–34, 1983.

71. Derogatis LR, Cleary P: Confirmation of the dimensional structure of the SCL-90: A study in construct validation. J Clin Psychology, *33*:981–989, 1977.

72. Beck AT, Ward CH, Mendelson M, Mock J, Erbaugh J: An inventory for measuring depression. Arch Gen Psychiatry, *5*:561–571, 1961.

73. Weissman MM: The assessment of social adjustment. Arch Gen Psychiatry, *32*:357–364, 1975.

74. Halmi KA: Treatment of anorexia nervosa: A discussion. J Adolesc Health Care, *4*:47–50, 1983.

75. Russell, GFM: The present status of anorexia nervosa. Psychol Med, *7*:353–367, 1977.

76. Andersen AE, Morse C, Santmyer K: Inpatient treatment for anorexia nervosa, in Garner DM, Garfinkel PE (eds): *Handbook of Psycho-*

therapy for Anorexia Nervosa and Bulimia. New York, The Guilford Press, 1985.

77. Keys A, Brozek, J, Henschel A, Mickelson O, Taylor HL: *The Biology of Human Starvation,* Minneapolis, University of Minnesota Press, 1950.

78. Levendusky PG, Dooley CP: An inpatient model for the treatment of anorexia nervosa, in Emmet S (ed): *Theory and Treatment of Anorexia Nervosa and Bulimia,* New York, Brunner/Mazel, 1985.

79. Collins M, Hodas GR, Liebman R: Interdisciplinary model for the inpatient treatment of adolescents with anorexia nervosa. J Adolesc Health Care, 4:3–8, 1983.

80. Pierloot R, Vandereycken W: An inpatient treatment program for anorexia nervosa patients. Acta Psychiatr Scand, 66(1):1–8, 1982.

81. Russell GFM: General management of anorexia nervosa and difficulties in assessing the efficacy of treatment, in Vigersky RA (ed): *Anorexia Nervosa,* New York, Raven Press, 1977.

82. Bemis KM: The present status of operant conditioning for the treatment of anorexia nervosa. Behav Modif, 11(4):432–463, 1987.

83. Johnson C, Connors ME: *The Etiology and Treatment of Bulimia Nervosa: A Biopsychosocial Perspective,* p. 231, New York, Basic Books, 1987.

84. Mills IH: Amitryptiline therapy in anorexia nervosa. Lancet, 2:687, 1976.

85. Halmi KA, Eckert ED, Falk JR: Cyproheptadine for anorexia nervosa (letter). Lancet, 1:1357–1358, 1982.

86. Gross HA, Ebert MH, Faden VB, Goldberg SC, Nee LE, Kaye WH: A doubleblind controlled trial of lithium carbonate in primary anorexia nervosa. J Clin Psychopharmacol, 1:376–381, 1981.

87. Hsu, LKG: The treatment of anorexia nervosa. Am J Psychiatry, 143:573–581, 1986.

88. Hudson JI, Pope HG: Psychopharmacological treatment of bulimia, in Fichter MM (ed): *Bulimia Nervosa: Basic Research, Diagnosis, and Treatment,* New York, John Wiley & Sons, 1990.

89. Hudson JI, Pope HG, Keck PE, McElroy SL: Treatment of bulimia nervosa with trazodone: Short-term response and long-term follow-up. Clin Neuropharmacol, 12(suppl 1):S38–S47, 1989.

90. Hughes PL, Wells LA, Cunningham CJ, Ilstrup DM: Treating bulimia with desipramine: A placebo-controlled double-blind study. Arch Gen Psychiatry, 43:182–186, 1986.

91. Blouin J, Blouin A, Perez E, Barlow J: Bulimia: Independence of antibulimic and antidepressant properties of desipramine. Can J Psychiatry, 34:24–29, 1989.

92. Pope HG, Hudson JI, Jonas JM, Yurgelun-Todd D: Antidepressant treatment of bulimia: A two year follow-up study. J Clin Psychopharmacol, 5:320–327, 1985.

93. Walsh BT, Gladis M, Roose SP, Stewart JW, Stetner F, Glassman AH: Phenelzine vs placebo in 50 patients with bulimia. Arch Gen Psychiatry, 45:471–475, 1988.

94. Mitchell PB: The pharmacological management of bulimia nervosa: A critical review. Int J Eating Disorders, 7(1):29–41, 1988.

95. Walsh BT: Antidepressants and bulimia: Where are we? Int J Eating Disorders, 7(3):421–423, 1988.

96. Pope HG, Hudson JI: Pharmacologic treatment of bulimia nervosa: Research findings and practical suggestions. Psych Annals, 19(9):483–487, 1989.

97. Mitchell JE, Christenson G, Jennings J, et al: A placebo-controlled, doubleblind crossover of naltrexone hydrochloride in outpatients with normal weight bulimia. J Clin Psychopharmacol, 9(2):94–97, 1989.

98. Russell GFM, Checkley SA, Feldman J, Eisler I: A controlled trial of d-fenfluramine in bulimia nervosa. Clin Neuropharmacol, 11(suppl 1):S146–S159, 1988.

99. Andersen AE: Contrast and comparison of behavioral, cognitive-behavioral, and comprehensive treatment methods for anorexia nervosa and bulimia nervosa. Behav Modif 11(4):522–543, 1987.

100. Oesterheld JR, McKenna MS, Gould NB: Group psychotherapy of bulimia: A critical review. Int J Group Psychother, 37(2):163–184, 1987.

101. Hall A: Group psychotherapy for anorexia nervosa, in Garner DM, Garfinkel PE (eds): *Handbook of Psychotherapy for Anorexia Nervosa and Bulimia,* New York, The Guilford Press, 1985.

102. Pyle R, Mitchell JE: Psychotherapy of bulimia: The role of groups, in Kaye WH, Gwirts-

man HE (eds): *The Treatment of Normal Weight Bulimia,* Washington, D.C., American Psychiatric Press, 1985.

103. Mitchell JE, Pyle RL, Eckert ED, Hatsukami D, Pomeroy C, Zimmerman R: A comparison study of antidepressants and structured intensive group psychotherapy in the treatment of bulimia nervosa. Arch Gen Psychiatry, *47*:149–157, 1990.

104. Bruch H: Psychotherapy in anorexia nervosa and development obesity, in Goodstein RK (ed): *Eating and Weight Disorders,* New York, Springer Publishing Company, 1983.

105. Garner DM, Bemis KM: A cognitive-behavioral approach to anorexia nervosa. Cognitive Therapy and Research, *6*:123–150, 1982.

106. Fairburn CG: Cognitive-behavioral treatment for bulimia, in Garner DM, Gurfinkel PE (eds): *Handbook of Psychotherapy for Anorexia Nervosa and Bulimia,* New York, The Guilford Press, 1985.

107. Fairburn CG: The current status of the psychological treatments for bulimia nervosa. J Psychosom Res, *32*(6):635–645, 1988.

108. Fairburn CG, Kirk J, O'Connor M, Cooper PJ: A comparison of two psychological treatments for bulimia nervosa. Behav Res Ther, *24*:629–643, 1986.

109. Wilson GT, Rossiter E, Kleifield EI, Lindholm, L: Cognitive-behavioral treatment of bulimia nervosa: A controlled evaluation. Behav Res Ther, *24*:277–288, 1986.

110. Strober M, Yager J: A developmental perspective on the treatment of anorexia nervosa in adolescents, in Garner DM, Garfinkel PE (eds): *Handbook of Psychotherapy for Anorexia Nervosa and Bulimia,* New York, The Guilford Press, 1985.

111. Sargent J, Liebman R, Silver M: Family therapy for anorexia nervosa, in Garner DM, Garfinkel PE (eds): *Handbook of Psychotherapy for Anorexia Nervosa and Bulimia,* New York, The Guilford Press, 1985.

112. Harper G: Varieties of parenting failure in anorexia nervosa: Protection and parentectomy revisited. J Am Acad Child Adolesc Psychiatry, *22*:134–139, 1983.

113. Selvine-Palazzoli MS, Boscolo L, Cecchin GG, et al: Family rituals: A powerful tool in family therapy. Fam Process, *16*:445–453, 1977.

114. Selvini-Palazzoli MS, Boscolo L, Cecchin G, Prata G: Hypothesizing—circularity—neutrality: Three guidelines for the conductor of the session. Fam Process, *19*:3–12, 1980.

115. Russell GFM, Szmukler GI, Dare C, Eisler I: An evaluation of family therapy in anorexia nervosa and bulimia nervosa. Arch Gen Psychiatry, *44*:1047–1056, 1987.

116. Hsu LKG: Outcome and treatment effects, in Beumont PJV, Burrows GD, Casper RC (eds): *Handbook of Eating Disorders, Part 1: Anorexia and Bulimia Nervosa,* Amsterdam, Elsevier, 1987.

117. Herzog DB, Keller MB, Lavori PW: Outcome in anorexia nervosa and bulimia nervosa: A review of the literature. J Nerv Ment Dis, *176*(3):131–143, 1988.

118. Theander S: Research on outcome and prognosis of anorexia nervosa and some results from a Swedish long-term study. Int J Eating Disorders, *2*:167–174, 1983.

Theander S: Outcome and prognosis in anorexia nervosa and bulimia: Some results of previous investigations, compared with those of a Swedish long-term study. J Psychiatr Res, *19*:493–508, 1985.

119. Hsu LKG: Outcome of anorexia nervosa. Arch Gen Psychiatry, *37*:1041–1046, 1980.

120. Schwartz DM, Thompson MG: Do anorectics get well? Current research and future needs. Am J Psychiatry, *138*:319–323, 1981.

121. Swift WJ: The long-term outcome of early onset anorexia nervosa: A critical review. J Am Acad Child Psychiatry, *21*:38–46, 1982.

122. Beresin EV, Gordon C, Herzog DB: The process of recovering from anorexia nervosa, in Bemporad JR, Herzog DB (eds): *Psychoanalyis and Eating Disorders,* New York, The Guilford Press, 1989.

123. Steinhausen H-C, Glanville K: Follow-up studies of anorexia nervosa: A review of research findings. Psychol Med, *13*:239–249, 1983.

124. Mitchell JE, Pyle RL, Hatsukami D, Goff G, Glotter D, Harper J: A 2–5 year follow-up study of patients treated for bulimia. Int J Eating Disorders, *8*(2):157–165, 1988.

125. Garner DM: Psychotherapy outcome research with bulimia nervosa. Psychother Psychosom, *48*:129–140, 1987.

126. Keller MB, Herzog DB, Lavori PW, Ott IL, Bradburn IS, Mahoney EM: High rates of chronicity and rapidity of relapse in patients with bulimia nervosa and depression. (letter) Arch Gen Psychiatry, 46:480–481, 1989.

127. Fairburn CG, Kirk J, O'Connor M, Anastasiades P, Cooper PJ: Prognostic factors in bulimia nervosa. Br J Clin Psychol 26:223–224, 1987.

6

Psychoactive Substance-Use Disorders

Steven A. Adelman, MD
Roger D. Weiss, MD

DEFINITION

The term *psychoactive substance-use disorders* refers to abuse of or dependence upon psychoactive substances that belong to the following three categories: (*a*) legal, nonmedicinal substances (e.g., alcohol, caffeine, and nicotine); (*b*) controlled substances available by prescription only (e.g., dextroamphetamine, methadone, benzodiazepines, and barbiturates); and (*c*) illicit substances (e.g., heroin and LSD [lysergic acid diethylamide]). Cocaine and marijuana, infrequently prescribed by physicians for legitimate medical purposes, may fall into either the second or the third category.

Abuse of a psychoactive substance refers to a pattern of usage accompanied by adverse consequences attributable to the substance use. When a person experiences either a greater degree of substance-related dysfunction or more chronic problems attributable to drugs or alcohol, substance dependence is said to occur. Although signs of physiological dependence (tolerance and

withdrawal) may exist as part of this syndrome, they are neither necessary nor sufficient to make a diagnosis of substance dependence.

Psychoactive substance abuse and dependence exist at one end of a continuum that begins with one-time experimentation and casual infrequent use. Frequent psychoactive substance use, unaccompanied by clear-cut adverse consequences, is a pattern of usage that exists in the middle of this continuum. Abuse and/or dependence are clearly present when an individual persists in using the substance despite impaired functioning due to the substance. *Loss of control*, which refers to repeated, compulsive substance use, accompanied by a growing preoccupation with obtaining and using the substance, is a clear sign of significant psychoactive substance dependence.

DIAGNOSIS

The most important tool in diagnosing a psychoactive substance-use disorder in a psychiatric inpatient is obtaining a comprehensive substance-use clinical history. Patients may conceal their problems with drugs and alcohol by denial or because they fear the interpersonal, vocational, or legal consequences of disclosure. The admitting physician may ignore or avoid the issue of substance use because of naivete, therapeutic nihilism, fears of angering the patient, or a desire to abbreviate the admissions process. For all of these reasons, it is essential that all clinicians routinely incorporate a detailed substance-use history as an important component of every inpatient psychiatric evaluation.

The substance-use history includes questions regarding the patient's use of alcohol, stimulants, sedative-hypnotics, opioids, marijuana, and hallucinogens, along with inquiries regarding the use of caffeine and nicotine. In addition to ascertaining the time course and extent of psychoactive substance use, it is critical to focus the history on the adverse consequences brought on by the use of these substances. Delineating the extent of substance-induced dysfunction and impairment is critical in establishing the diagnosis of a substance-abuse disorder and in determining the optimal level of treatment intervention.

Self-report techniques are valuable in screening for substance abuse (1). The best known self-report instrument is the Michigan Alcoholism Screening Test (MAST) (2). Instruments like MAST help patients with strong denial to begin acknowledging the existence of an alcohol or drug problem. The acronym CAGE represents the following questions:

1. Have you ever felt the need to   Cut down on drinking?
2. Have you ever felt   Annoyed by criticism of your drinking?
3. Have you ever had   Guilty feelings about drinking?
4. Have you ever taken a morning   Eye-opener?

The authors of CAGE contend that affirmative answers to three of these four questions confirm the diagnosis of alcoholism, and two affirmative answers are suggestive (3).

When a patient is unable or unwilling to furnish sufficient information either to rule in or out a substance-abuse diagnosis, information of critical significance may be readily provided by the individual's friends or family. Important evidence confirming the diagnosis is often present in the physical, mental status, or laboratory examinations. For example, a perforated nasal septum signals cocaine abuse, sudden onset of agitation and paranoia may indicate use of phencyclidine (PCP), and modest elevations of the gamma glutamyltransferase indicate alcoholism. Toxic screens of urine and blood upon admission should be ordered whenever the admitting clinician has any reason to suspect the diagnosis of a psychoactive substance-use disorder.

One may establish the severity of psychoactive substance use disorders with the help of the Addiction Severity Index (ASI), a structured interview proven to be a reliable and valid tool in clinical research (4). The ASI comprises six subscales, each covering a different domaine of substance-induced dysfunction. The six domains include medical problems, legal problems, psychiatric symptoms, interpersonal problems, vocational problems, and substance-specific problems (such as blackouts from alcoholism or insomnia from stimulant abuse). By focusing the clinical history on specific information regarding substance-related dysfunction in these six domains, diagnosing substance abuse becomes a relatively straightforward matter. Individuals with problems in one or more of these six areas, are, by definition, suffering from a psychoactive substance-use disorder for which intervention is needed.

DIFFERENTIAL DIAGNOSIS

Psychoactive substance-use disorders are psychiatry's great masqueraders; they may produce virtually any symptom picture a psychiatrist is likely to encounter. Failure to elicit a careful substance-use history can thus lead to misdiagnoses. The psychiatric symptoms, mental status findings, and presumed mental disorders that may be accounted for by an underlying psychoactive substance-use disorder are listed in Tables 6.1 and 6.2.

Psychiatric diagnoses coexisting with psychoactive substance-use disorders. Certain specific psychiatric disorders are associated with high rates of substance abuse. Young adult chronic patients, most of whom suffer from schizophrenia, schizoaffective disorder, or severe mood disorders with psychotic features, manifest rates of substance abuse approaching 50% (5). Individuals who suffer from antisocial personality disorder and adults with a history of attention deficit hyperactivity disorder also manifest higher than expected rates of substance abuse (6, 7).

Patients suffering from opioid abuse and cocaine abuse demonstrate higher than expected rates of major depressive disorder (8, 9). In women, depression coexists with

Table 6.1. Psychiatric Symptoms and Findings Associated with Substance Abuse

Erratic Behavior
Inappropriate Affect
Depressed, Elevated, or Labile Moods
Anxiety
Sleep Disturbances
Appetite Disturbances
Delusional Thinking
Suicidal Ideation or Behavior
Impulsiveness
Impaired Cognition
Poor Judgment
Disorientation
Vocational Problems
Sexual Dysfunction
Interpersonal Problems
Low Self-Esteem

alcoholism to a greater extent than it does in men (10). Other conditions which coexist with alcoholism to an extent exceeding chance alone are panic disorder and borderline personality disorder (11, 12). The etiological significance of such co-morbidity is addressed below.

The possible existence of a number of psychoactive substance-induced organic mental disorders further complicates the differential diagnostic evaluation of the inpatient substance abuser. When individuals manifest any of the symptoms or mental status abnormalities listed in Table 6.1, the

Table 6.2. Psychiatric Disorders Which May Be Erroneously Diagnosed When Substance Abuse Is the Primary Problem

Adjustment Disorder
Antisocial Personality Disorder
Avoidant Personality Disorder
Bipolar Disorder
Borderline Personality Disorder
Cyclothymic Disorder
Delusional Disorder
Dysthymic Disorder
Generalized Anxiety Disorder
Histrionic Personality Disorder
Major Depression
Panic Disorder
Schizophrenia
Sexual Disorders
Sleep Disorders

clinician must consider the possibility of a substance-induced organic disorder. In addition to the well-known intoxication and withdrawal syndromes, the following syndromes should be considered. Alcoholism may cause withdrawal delirium, hallucinosis, amnestic disorder, or dementia. Stimulants may cause delirium or delusional disorder. Hallucinogens may cause a delusional disorder, mood disorder, posthallucinogen perception disorder (flashbacks). The organic mental disorders engendered by sedatives, hypnotic, and anxiolytics resemble those caused by alcohol; those caused by PCP are like those of the hallucinogens.

EPIDEMIOLOGY

Alcohol

The Epidemiological Catchment Area (ECA) study conducted in three urban sites (New Haven, St. Louis, and Baltimore) yielded interesting data indicating the lifetime and six-month prevalences of alcohol abuse and dependence in the general population (13, 14). Diagnosed according to the *Diagnostic and Statistical Manual of Mental Disorders* (DSM-III), the overall lifetime prevalence of alcohol abuse/dependence in these three sites was 13.6%. The six-month overall prevalence was 5%.

The prevalence of alcohol abuse/dependence is significantly higher in younger adults over the age of 24 (13); men demonstrated a 5½-fold greater lifetime prevalence than women (24.2% versus 4.4%) (13). No difference in the prevalence rates of alcoholism was found comparing blacks to nonblacks (13). Although no consistent findings emerged from the ECA study regarding the relationship of alcoholism to education, Blazer et al. (15) noted greater rates of alcoholism in individuals with low socioeconomic and educational status, especially among Catholics of French or Irish

extraction. Other data suggest a low prevalence of alcoholism among Jews and a higher than expected prevalence among Native Americans (16). A comparison of alcoholics in treatment programs with individuals in the general population indicates that 25% of the former group are married, compared with 65.7% of the general population (17).

Cocaine and Other Stimulants

In the early and mid-1980s, use and abuse of cocaine skyrocketed in the United States. In 1988, the National Institute of Drug Abuse estimated that about three million Americans were current users of cocaine (defined as use in the 30-day period preceding the survey) (18). Eight million Americans had used cocaine within the past year (18). Surveys conducted in the mid-1980s indicate that nearly one in six Americans has tried the drug; for individuals between the ages of 25–30, the proportion who have tried cocaine approaches 40% (19, 20). Approximately one of every five people who tries cocaine progresses to a pattern of regular use, with one out of every four regular users progressing to frank abuse or dependence (21). The users of free-base or "crack" cocaine probably have greatest likelihood of progressing to a pathological pattern of usage.

Once thought of as a stylish drug for the rich and famous, cocaine has clearly become an equal opportunity "destroyer." The development of an easily administered, initially affordable, potently reinforcing preparation of free-base has led to a sophisticated nationwide "marketing" program that has left no segment of society untouched by cocaine. The distributors of crack have been particularly adept at selling their product to poor, young people in the inner cities, who are perhaps the greatest victims of the cocaine epidemic.

The use and abuse of other psychostimulants (e.g., dextroamphetamine, methylphenidate) appears to have remained stable throughout the cocaine epidemic. Recent data from the ECA study indicate that approximately 6% of the general population use psychostimulants without appropriate medical supervision (22); approximately one in three of these users qualifies for a lifetime DSM-III diagnosis of abuse or dependence (23). Demographically, amphetamine abusers fall into two categories: those who begin abusing by purchasing illicit amphetamines on the street and those whose abuse stems from initially appropriate medical usage (usually for weight reduction). The former group tends to be young, poor, and male; the latter group older, middle-class, and female.

Opioids

Most individuals who become dependent on opioids abuse street drugs such as heroin; a minority develop their substance use disorder in a medical setting and abuse prescription drugs like mepiridine or codeine. Methadone, available by prescription for the treatment of opioid dependence, may be abused by either type of abuser. Due to the illegality and stigma associated with opioid use, accurate epidemiologic data are difficult to obtain. One study estimates that between 1–3% of adults under age 26 have used opioids at least once (24). Two percent of the sample in the ECA study were heroin users (13, 22); the lifetime prevalence rate of opioid abuse or dependence was approximately 0.7% (23).

Most street users are poor, young nonwhite males with a premorbid history of school problems and antisocial behavior (25). This description of the typical street abuser contrasts with the profile of opioid abusers who obtain drugs in the medical setting. The latter tend to be middle-class women who suffer from chronic pain (26). Medical personnel who have easy access to controlled substances represent an important subgroup of this latter category (27).

Other Psychoactive Substances of Abuse

Sedatives, Hypnotics, and Anxiolytics. Recent data derived from the ECA study indicate that 3.7% of the sample were defined as users of scheduled anxiolytics and 4.2% users of other CNS (central nervous system) depressant drugs (13, 22). The lifetime prevalence of CNS depressant abuse or dependence in the general population is reported to be 1.1% (23). These medications are among the most commonly prescribed prescription drugs. They are routinely prescribed to individuals suffering from major mental disorders to improve sleep, reduce anxiety, and to combat akathisia, the common motor restlessness side effect of neuroleptics. Schuckit (28) reports that nearly one-third of individuals with a history of a major mental disorder report feeling psychologically dependent on these medications; between 5–10% develop a pattern of frank abuse.

Cannabis. The ECA study demonstrated that 16.7% of the sample used marijuana (13, 22); one-third of this group used the drug daily, and one in five met DSM-III criteria for a diagnosis of abuse or dependence (23). In 1988, the National Institute of Drug Abuse estimated that 12 million Americans had used marijuana in the preceding 30 days and 21 million had used the drug in the past year (18). Marijuana has commonly been thought of as a drug abused by teenagers and young adults. However, members of the 60s "baby boom" generation particularly liked cannabis. As a result, marijuana abuse has followed many members of this generation into midlife, raising the apparent age of abuse (29).

Hallucinogens. The use and abuse of hallucinogens peaked in the late 1960s.

Current evidence indicates that 3.6% of adults use hallucinogens (22). It is estimated that one in ten users has a history of daily use; because of the extreme alterations in mental status engendered by these drugs, virtually all daily users qualify for a diagnosis of abuse or dependence (22). Hallucinogen use is relatively common in teenagers and young adults. In 1982, the lifetime prevalence of hallucinogen use for individuals age 18–25 was 25% (28). In 1985, approximately 7% of high school students admitted to hallucinogen use. Other than the controlled use of peyote in the religious rituals of some Native Americans, no other cultural subgroup demonstrates a predilection for using hallucinogens.

Phencyclidine. Phencyclidine (PCP or "angel dust") is rarely the sole drug of abuse. In particular, users of PCP tend to abuse alcohol and marijuana (23). The typical PCP user is a young adult male (28). It is estimated that 10% of the adult population has used PCP at one time or another (30).

Inhalants. A variety of glues, aerosols, solvents, and other volatile compounds are abused, predominantly by older children and adolescents. Estimates suggest that 10% of children age 12–17 have abused inhalants at least once (31); boys and adolescents living in an urban setting show the highest prevalence (28, 31). Two other populations that appear to be particularly at risk are Native Americans and Spanish Americans (32). The typical inhalant abuser is poor and male, between 13 and 15 (31). Most inhalants are abused in group settings and other substances are often used concurrently. Poor school performance and antisocial behavior are commonly associated with inhalant abuse (33). One particular drug in this class, amyl nitrite, is thought to be commonly abused by homosexual males (31).

Anabolic Steroids. Anabolic steroids are widely used and abused by ahtletes at-tempting to increase the bulk and strength of their muscles. Although these compounds are not technically defined as psychoactive substances, they often cause disorders in mood and thought process when administered repeatedly in high doses. In one study of 41 bodybuilders and athletes, 22% demonstrated a clear mood disorder and 12% manifested psychotic symptoms (34). A study of anabolic steroid use among male high school seniors indicates a prevalence rate of 6.6% (35).

Polysubstance Abuse. For most psychoactive substance abusers, the use and abuse of more than a single psychoactive substance is probably the rule rather than the exception. In a sample of 171 individuals in an *alcohol* treatment program, Schuckit (28) found that 76% had used marijuana, 28% had used cocaine, and 17% had used hallucinogens. Hawkins et al. (36) found that 79% of soldiers treated for alcoholism reported using other substances; nearly half reported a pattern of heavy drug use. Individuals in methadone maintenance programs, PCP abusers, and patients suffering from psychiatric disorders may be at particular risk for developing polysubstance abuse (28). Clinicians working with substance abusers have noted that polysubstance abuse appears to be increasingly prevalent. As a result, treatment programs, which traditionally have treated one substance at a time, are under increasing pressure to remedy the growing problem of polysubstance abuse.

THEORIES OF ETIOLOGY

Psychoactive substance use disorders are a complex set of heterogeneous disorders that cannot be explained by a simple unitary etiological theory. A unique combination of biogenetic, psychological, familial, social, and cultural factors contributes to each case of substance abuse. Research on the etiology of substance abuse has focused on alcoholism because of its legality and high prevalence. The less prevalent and illicit forms of substance abuse are less amenable to standard research methodology. Therefore, the following discussion of theories of etiology centers on alcoholism. Many of the concepts and conclusions regarding the etiology of alcoholism have been applied to other psychoactive substance-use disorders. Future research may determine which particularly etiologic factors are common to all forms of substance abuse and which are unique to specific disorders.

Biogenetic Hypotheses

A large body of evidence indicates that vulnerability to alcoholism is an inherited trait. An individual with an alcoholic first-degree relative has a 3–4-fold greater risk of becoming alcoholic than someone with a negative family history, even if the individual at risk is adopted at birth by nonalcoholic parents (37). Studies of alcoholism in Scandinavia indicate two distinct inherited types: a mild form of alcoholism, occurring equally in men and women, and a severe form found mostly in men and often associated with criminality (38, 39). Finding a high rate of alcoholism in the parents of opioid abusers, Kaufman (40) has suggested that future family studies of drug abuse will indicate heritable patterns of biological vulnerability similar to those found in alcoholism.

The observation that vulnerability to developing alcoholism is a heritable trait has led researchers to explore possible biological mechanisms that might account for an individual's being at risk. A number of researchers have studied high-risk males, i.e., the nonalcoholic sons of alcoholic fathers. For the most part, these studies have shown that sons of alcoholic fathers demonstrate less extreme responses to a fixed dose of alcohol than do controls (41). The diminished response to alcohol in high-risk males was measured by subjective response (such as dizziness and perceived intoxication); cognitive and neuropsychological impairment; ataxia; electrophysiological changes (measured by EEG [electroencephalogram] and evoked potentials); and neuroendocrine response (e.g., cortisol levels and thyroid stimulating hormone response to thyroid releasing hormone infusion) (41). This globally attenuated responsiveness to alcohol in individuals with positive family history suggests that the ability to tolerate alcohol without significant neurophysiological disruption may increase the likelihood of developing alcoholism. In other words, people who are more adversely affected by alcohol at the outset are less likely to continue drinking heavily.

Theories regarding vulnerability to cocaine abuse are far more speculative than those attempting to explain alcoholism. A number of researchers posit that cocaine dependence may be promoted by the extreme dysphoria experienced by some users when the drug effect wears off (42). Thus, researchers hypothesize, individuals biologically prone to withdrawal dysphoria may repeatedly administer the drug and rapidly develop dependence in an effort to avoid the dysphoric withdrawal experience (43). In some cases, a history of preexisting mood disorder may increase an individual's propensity to experience particularly dysphoric withdrawal from cocaine.

Many of the commonly abused substances have potent effects on well-known neurotransmitter systems. These complex effects underly the pleasurable feelings that many substance abusers constantly seek to reproduce. For instance, the stimulants are believed to augment levels of dopamine and norepinephrine (21). Benzodiazepines attach to endogenous receptors and interact with the gamma-aminobutyric acid (GABA) system, while opioid drugs bind with endogenous opioid receptors (44, 45). Indeed, some research suggests that alcohol, too, may augment brain levels of endorphin-like compounds (46). Clearly, expanding our understanding of psychoactive substances activity at the molecular level is an important, ongoing effort which should add greater weight to the biogenetic theories of substance abuse and dependence.

Psychological Hypotheses

Although theoretically attractive, the concept of the so-called "addictive personality" has never been substantiated by rigorous research (47). The work of Vaillant (48) suggests that personality disturbance in substance abusers may be a consequence of the addiction, not a cause. As in the case of alcoholism, certain personality traits are in part determined by genetic factors (49). Thus, heredity may be the underlying factor that accounts for the apparent association between personality and substance abuse. Researchers have yet to prove that specific constellations of psychological factors predict the development of psychoactive substance-use disorders.

Khantzian (50) proposes that self-medication is an important etiological mechanism of addictive disorders. According to this hypothesis, individuals who abuse drugs do so to relieve intolerable affective states. Specifically, Khantzian suggests that opioid addicts are drawn to the anti-aggressive effects of the opioids, and that individuals abuse stimulants to negate inner feelings of depression, emptiness, and boredom (50). Although the self-medication hypothesis is consistent with clinical experience in treating certain patients with psychoactive substance-use disorders, little empirical evidence exists either to confirm or refute this hypothesis.

The tension-reduction hypothesis posits that alcoholics drink to reduce tension and avoid other feelings of dysphoria, including those that may accompany the al-cohol withdrawal syndrome. When studying active alcoholics, however, researchers have failed to substantiate the tension-reduction hypothesis (47).

The psychological factors relevant to establishing substance dependence may be distinctly different from those that perpetuate the dependence. For instance, the potent, positive reinforcement of the cocaine high may be more influential in developing cocaine dependence than the addicted individual's desire to avoid the dysphoria associated with withdrawal. Unfortunately, it is nearly impossible to perform research on individuals who are in the process of becoming drug dependent. Thus, it may be difficult to elucidate the psychological and behavioral factors that account for the initiation of psychoactive substance abuse and dependence.

Family and Social Hypotheses

Dysfunction is common in the families of addicted individuals (51). However, as with maladaptive personality traits, family dysfunction may be the consequence rather than the cause of substance abuse. Disturbed interactional patterns in the family of a substance abuser may impede the recovery progress and serve to perpetuate the dependence. For this reason sophisticated treatment programs evaluate and address family dysfunction in an effort to maximize the chances for recovery (52) (see "Hospital Treatment" below).

Adoption studies of alcoholism in Scandinavia indicate that low occupational status of adoptive parents is associated with alcoholism developing in their children, independent of genetic factors (38, 39). Zinberg (53) has written extensively on the importance of social controls in determining the extent of substance use in specific social subgroups. For instance, alcoholism is less common in groups who frown upon drunkeness (as opposed to drinking), who tend to use alcohol in relogous ceremonies, and for whom the normative drinking experience involves members of both sexes drinking together. Zinberg's work indicates that in addition to the biogenetic and behavioral factors discussed above, a variety of social, cultural, ethnic, and religious elements help determine whether or not a given individual develops a pathological pattern of drinking or drug use.

BIOPSYCHOSOCIAL EVALUATION

Biomedical Evaluation

As noted above, the psychoactive substance-use disorders are among the most prevalent mental disorders found in the general population (13, 14). In psychiatric patients, the prevalence of concurrent substance abuse is reported to be as high as 66% (54). For this reason, testing for substance abuse/dependence should be seriously considered whenever any patient is hospitalized on an inpatient psychiatric unit, regardless of the presenting complaints or diagnoses. The admission medical history, physical examination, and laboratory evaluation are invaluable tools for detecting and documenting psychoactive substance-use disorders and their complications.

Table 6.3 enumerates many of the physical complaints, findings, and medical diagnoses that suggest a coexisting psychoactive substance-use disorder. Even when patients deny a problem with drugs or alcohol, a careful history and physical examination may suggest a drug- or alcohol-induced medical problem. The reader is referred to basic textbooks of medicine for a more detailed review of the physical complications of substance abuse.

Laboratory evaluation. Most medical problems engendered by substance abuse will be apparent from the patient's history or physical examination. Compre-

hensive laboratory screening, including complete blood count, electrolytes, routine blood chemistries, chest x-ray, EKG (electrocardiogram), and urinalysis should be ordered when clinically indicated. Specialized studies (e.g., pulmonary function tests, EMGs [electromyograms], EEGs [electroencephalograms], etc.) should be ordered when clinically warranted.

Physiological dependence. Determining whether or not the new psychiatric inpatient is physiologically dependent on one or more psychoactive substances is one of the admitting psychiatrist's most crucial tasks. The hallmarks of physiological dependence are *tolerance* and *withdrawal*. *Tolerance,* which can be determined by history, is an indivdual's progressive need for greater and greater amounts of the substance in order to achieve the desired effects on the central nervous system. *Withdrawal* is a substance-specific physical syndrome that occurs when dependent individuals discontinue or drastically reduce their intake of a substance known to produce a withdrawal syndrome. Severe withdrawal syndromes are subjectively very unpleasant at best and may be life-threatening under certain circumstances. When the medical evaluation indicates the presence of physical dependence, detoxification (see below) is required to keep the patient safe and comfortable. The major withdrawal syndromes are listed below in Table 6.4.

Psychological Evaluation

PSYCHIATRIC

As described above, psychoactive substance-use disorders commonly coexist with other mental disorders (5–12). Consequently, inpatient evaluation should attempt to detect possible concomitant disorders, including but not limited to mood disorders, anxiety disorders, psychotic disorders, attention deficit hyperactivity disor-

Table 6.3. Medical Complaints, Findings, and Diagnoses Sometimes Associated with Substance Abuse (28, 55)

Abdominal Pain (A)
Abscesses (IV)
Acid/Base Imbalances (A)
Amenorrhea (All)
Anemia (A, IV)
Anorexia (All)
Arrhythmia (All)
Burns (All)
Bruising (A)
Bruxism (S)
Cerebellar Degeneration (A)
Cirrhosis (A, IV)
Cold Injury (All)
Constipation (O)
Diaphoresis (A, D, O, P)
Drowning (All)
Electrolyte Imbalances (A, IV)
Emboli (IV)
Endocarditis (IV)
Esophagitis (A)
Facial Edema (A)
Fetal Alcohol Syndrome (A)
Fetal/Neonatal Distress (All)
Gastritis (A)
Gastrointestinal Bleeding (A, IV)
Hepatitis (A, O, IV)
Hepatomegaly (A, O, IV)
HIV Infection (IV)
Hypertension (A, S)
Hypotension (O)
Infections (IV)
Infertility (All)
Insomnia (A, D, O, S)
Jaundice (All)
Lacrimation (O)
Lymphadenopathy (IV)
Miosis (O)
Muscle Wasting (A, IV, N)
Mydriasis (O, S)
Nasal Problems (C)
Neuropathy (A, N, O)
Nystagmus (A, D, P)
Pancreatitis (A)
Pharyngitis (M)
Pneumonia (A, C, O)
Pulmonary Dysfunction (C, O, M)

Renal Disease (IV, N)
Respiratory Depression (A, D, O)
Rhinorrhea (S, I)
Scleral Injection (M)
Seizures (A, O, S)
Sepsis (IV)
Sexual Dysfunction (All)
Sinusitis (M)
Skin Lesions (C, IV)
Somnolence (All)
Spider Angiomas (A, IV)
Splenomegaly (A, IV)
Tachycardia (A, M, S)
Tachypnea (S)
Tattoos (All)
Testicular Atrophy (A)
Tetanus (IV)
Thrombophlebitis (IV)
Tobacco Stained Fingers (All)
Traumatic Injuries (All)
Tremulousness (All)
Vitamin Deficiencies (All)
Weakness (All)
Weight Loss (All)
Wernicke's Syndrome (A)

KEY
A = Alcohol
All = All Abused Substances
C = Cocaine
D = CNS Depressants
IV = All intravenously administered substances
M = Marijuana
N = Inhalants
O = Opioids
P = Phencyclidine
S = Stimulants (including cocaine)

Table 6.4.   Clinical Features of Psychoactive Substance Withdrawal Syndromes (23)

(Note: Withdrawal syndromes vary in duration and intensity and may consist of any or all of the following signs and symptoms.)

Uncomplicated Alcohol Withdrawal
- a.   Coarse tremor, particularly in the upper extremities
- b.   Gastrointestinal distress
- c.   Feeling weak or ill
- d.   Elevated vital signs
- e.   Depressed, irritable, or anxious mood
- f.   Transient perceptual disturbances
- g.   Headache
- h.   Inability to sleep
- i.   Hyperreflexia
- j.   Generalized seizures

CNS Depressant Withdrawal

At least three of the following must be present:
- a.   Gastrointestinal distress
- b.   Feeling weak or ill
- c.   Elevated vital signs
- d.   Irritable or anxious mood
- e.   Postural hypotension
- f.   Coarse tremor
- g.   Generalized seizures
- h.   Marked inability to sleep

Withdrawal Delirium (Alcohol and CNS Depressants)

Frank delirium in conjunction with elevated vital signs.

Stimulant Withdrawal (including Cocaine)

Dysphoric mood and at least one of the following lasting at least 24 hours after last substance use:
- a.   Sleep disturbance
- b.   Fatigue
- c.   Agitation
- d.   Drug craving

Opioid Withdrawal

At least three of the following must be present:
- a.   Drug craving
- b.   Gastrointestinal distress
- c.   Myalgias
- d.   Lacrimation
- e.   Rhinorrhea
- f.   Dilated pupils
- g.   Yawning
- h.   Elevated temperature
- i.   Sleep disturbance
- j.   Piloerection
- k.   Sweating

der, and personality disorders. When an individual suffers from a "dual diagnosis," an integrated treatment approach that takes into account both disorders may be most effective (56). Several authors (57–59) have shown that identifying and treating a concomitant psychiatric disorder improves the treatment outcome of psychoactive substance-use disorders.

PSYCHODYNAMIC

Performing an accurate psychodynamic assessment and formulation in the clinical context of acute inpatient treatment of an active substance-use disorder is extremely difficult. Distinguishing longstanding characterological abnormalities from the consequences of substance abuse is a formidable clinical task. Vaillant (48) posits that even antisocial personality disorder may occur secondary to substance abuse, rather than as the primary psychological disturbance. Thus, in performing a psychodynamic evaluation of the newly abstinent patient, the clinician should carefully review historical data about the patient's psychological status before the onset of significant substance abuse.

This premorbid history, which may be obtained with the assistance of family members, should focus on the patient's level of ego functioning, the maturity of his or her defenses, the capacity to form significant relationships with others, and the depth and breadth of the patient's affective experiences. As the period of abstinence grows longer, observational data about the patient's functioning in the inpatient unit will grow in significance and may be used to refine psychodynamic hypotheses based on the history. These hypotheses are useful in shaping an individualized treatment program for each patient (see below).

BEHAVIORAL

Marlatt (60) stresses the importance of performing a behavioral evaluation determining the circumstances and behaviors that may lead to recurrent substance abuse in abstinent individuals. Because of the episodic nature of most psychoactive substance-use disorders, many hospitalized patients will be able to discuss previous periods of abstinence and the factors that led to relapse. Environmental cues, intolerable affective states, and interpersonal conflicts are among the most significant determinants of relapse (60). A careful behavioral analysis of the patient's "relapse history" provides data essential in formulating a treatment plan (see below).

NEUROPSYCHOLOGICAL

Chronic alcoholism commonly causes profound neuropsychological disturbances of cognitive, perceptual, and perceptual-motor functions (61). Chronic abuse of other substances may also lead to an impaired central nervous system, although much less information is available to document the extent and nature of these other substance-induced organic brain syndromes (28). Another cause of substance-related neuropsychological dysfunction is HIV (human immunodeficiency virus) infection, which may lead to tumors, CNS infections, and a nonfocal AIDS (acquired immune deficiency syndrome) encephalopathy (62).

Whenever the history, physical examination, or mental status examination suggest the possibility of neuropsychological dysfunction, the inpatient evaluation should include a battery of neuropsychological tests. Ideally, testing should take place as late in the hospitalization as possible, when the acute substance-related organic mental changes have diminished. Testing may include the Wechsler Adult Intelligence Scale (WAIS), the Wechsler Memory Scale (WMS), and the Halstead-Reitan Neuropsychological Test Battery (63). In alcoholics, the presence of ongoing neuropsychological dysfunction three weeks after admission is a significant predictor of poor long-term treatment outcome (64).

Sociocultural Evaluation

It is important for clinicians to assess the extent to which individuals' substance abuse adheres to the norms of their sociocultural milieu. For members of sociocultural groups that sanction heavy psychoactive substance use, overcoming denial of the severity and significance of pathological substance use is a common obstacle to initiating effective treatment. On the other hand, the knowledge and experience of recovering substance abusers from that group may encourage individuals with significant substance-related problems to get help. Once such an individual breaks through the barriers of sanctioned denial, he or she may benefit from the available subgroup of people engaged in the recovery process.

For people who belong to sociocultural groups that do not sanction heavy substance use, an atmosphere of "it can't happen to us" may prevail. In such a setting, individuals with a psychoactive substance-use disorder may easily be overlooked or made to feel their problem should be kept secret. The recovery process, less well known to members of such groups, may not be supported as readily as by groups more familiar with the problem. A patient's sense of shame about deviating from group norms and expectations is an additional barrier to treatment which should be assessed.

A patient's potential to make use of self-help groups such as Alcoholics Anonymous, Narcotics Anonymous, and other 12-Step programs is an important part of evaluation and treatment. If a patient is comfortable with groups of people and made good use of "social" therapies in the past, conventional group-oriented treatment may likely succeed. On the other hand, individuals who are schizoid, avoidant, or phobic may require an individualized treatment program that takes into account their particular difficulties with the social group approach.

HOSPITAL TREATMENT

Pharmacologic Therapies

DETOXIFICATION

When the initial evaluation of the patient indicates physiologic dependence on one or more psychoactive substances, the necessary first step of the treatment process is detoxification. In most cases, detoxification involves prescribing decreasing amounts of a relatively long-acting substance possessing pharmacologic properties similar to those of the abused substance(s). A newer detoxofication strategy which has come into vogue during the last 10 years in-

volves using noradrenergic or dopaminergic agonists such as clonidine and bromocriptine. Possessing minimal abuse liability themselves, these agonists are pharmacologically distinct from the substances of abuse they replace during detoxification.

Alcohol. Conventional alcohol detoxification involves using intermediate to long half-life benzodiazepines such as lorazepam or chlordiazepoxide (66). A typical regimen might involve prescribing 25–100 mg of chlordiazepoxide as often as every four hours in an attempt to normalize the patient's elevated vital signs. Once autonomic stability is achieved (usually within 24–48 hours), the dose of chlordiazepoxide may be reduced by about 25% per day. The usual time course for alcohol detoxification is 2–5 days. For alcoholics with hepatic dysfunction, oxazepam is the detoxification agent of choice. Intramuscular thiamine (100 mg) should be administered during the first three days of treatment, and multivitamins, folic acid, and thiamine should be given orally throughout the hospitalization. Patients manifesting the extreme autonomic instability and clouding of consciousness indicating alcohol withdrawal delirium are in a state of medical emergency. The acute care of such patients, which involves aggressive monitoring, fluid replacement, and intravenous benzodiazepines, is best conducted on an acute-care medical unit (65).

CNS depressants. It is important to recognize physiological dependence upon central nervous system depressants; failure to do so could lead to a life-threatening withdrawal seziure. Barbiturates are generally used for detoxification from CNS depressants (66). Typically, the dependent patient is given test doses of 200 mg of pentobarbital every two hours until somnolence is achieved. The amount of pentobarbital required to achieve somnolence is the 24-hour barbiturate requirement for the first two days of detoxification. The dosage of pentobarbital, which has an intermediate half-life, may be converted to an equivalent dosage of the longer acting phenobarbital (100 mg of pentobarbital is equivalent to 32 mg of phenobarbital). In either case, the barbiturates are administered four times daily; after the second day the daily dosage is reduced by about 10%.

Opioids. Detoxification from opioids may be accomplished with oral methadone or clonidine. With the former method, a 20-mg dose of methadone is administered; if the signs of opioid withdrawal are not diminished, an additional 5–20 mg may be required. One should be careful to base the administration of methadone on objective physical signs (such as dilated pupils and goose-flesh) and not merely on the addict's subjective symptoms. Once the withdrawal signs are suppressed, the methadone dosage is divided into a b.i.d. (twice a day) schedule and reduced by 10–20% daily. Opioid detoxification with methadone may last anywhere between five days and two weeks (28). Clonidine, which down-regulates the central sympathetic activity responsible for some aspects of the withdrawal syndrome, is an alternative to methadone detoxification. Clonidine is typically prescribed at a dose of 0.3–1.0 mg a day, for 7–10 days, and then tapered over a three- to four-day period (67).

Stimulants. There is no clinical consensus regarding the use of pharmacotherapy in treating the stimulant withdrawal syndrome. Although some clinicians prescribe tapering doses of amphetamine to patients dependent on oral stimulants, most clinicians avoid using medication for such patients. Studies indicate that the following pharmacologic agents may ameliorate the symptoms of anhedonia and dysphoria associated with withdrawal from cocaine: desipramine, imipramine, bromocriptine, and amantadine (68–71). At this time, however, none of the pharmacological strategies for diminishing symptoms of the cocaine withdrawal syndrome has entered standard clinical practice.

PHARMACOTHERAPY BEYOND DETOXIFICATION

Using psychotropic medications is generally discouraged during the immediate postdetoxification period. In the majority of substance abusers, most acute psychiatric symptoms diminish rapidly once abstinence is established. Beyond acute detoxification, there is virtually no place for benzodiazepines in this patient population. For patients who genuinely suffer from a concomitant major mental disorder, appropriate use of neuroleptic and/or thymoleptic medications is indicated once the patient is stabilized after detoxification. Investigations of various psychotropic agents (e.g., lithium carbonate) as a primary treatment for alcoholism have had disappointing results (72).

Disulfiram is sometimes a useful adjunct in treating alcoholism (73, 74). Disulfiram may be started while the individual is an inpatient in anticipation of discharge and to help prevent "slips" in the difficult readjustment period immediately following hospitalization. Naltrexone is a pure narcotic antagonist that binds with endogenous opioid receptors to block the effects of exogenous opioid drugs. Naltrexone following detoxification from methadone improves treatment outcome (75). Although outpatient compliance with naltrexone is often quite poor, opioid addicts with high social stability and a history of long drug-free intervals derive the greatest benefit from this compound (76, 77).

Milieu Management

On general psychiatric inpatient units, patients suffering from psychoactive substance-use disorders are sometimes regarded with mistrust and suspicion by unsophisticated staff members. They may view substance abusers as not truly mentally ill and manipulative, exploiting staff and patients. Attitudes like these may be in part responsible for the separate evolution of one treatment system for substance abusers and a parallel system for patients who suffer from other mental disorders.

Because of a great deal of overlap between these two supposedly separate populations (5–12), it is becoming increasingly evident that every psychiatric inpatient unit needs to develop expertise in treating substance abuse. Treatment methodologies known to be effective for substance abusers should be woven into the fabric of every inpatient psychiatric milieu. Empirical research indicates that the following milieu characteristics are associated with positive outcomes in treating alcoholism and drug abuse:

1. A strong group orientation in the milieu is more beneficial to patients than an intensive individualized treatment approach, even when programs offering the latter approach have a more favorable staff–patient ratio than programs with group-oriented milieu (78).
2. Patients treated by counselors with good interpersonal skills demonstrate a much better treatment outcome than patients treated by counselors with poor interpersonal skills (79). It is important to train and supervise unit staff in ways that build and maintain strong interpersonal skills.
3. Inpatient alcoholism treatment milieus that employ psychoeducational techniques and meetings have demonstrated more favorable treatment outcomes than milieus that do not offer these therapeutic modalities (80).
4. A variety of specific group therapeutic approaches are effective in treating alcoholism: focus groups which address issues of assertiveness and self-control,

client-centered groups, social skills groups, and desensitization/relaxation groups (81–84).
5. Milieu philosophies that encourage patient involvement in treatment (such as patients authoring treatment contracts) appear superior to approaches that stress staff directives (85).

In summary, research indicates that the inpatient milieu most favorable for treating substance abuse is one which utilizes AA, psychoeducational techniques, and a strong group orientation. The ideal milieu staff comprises highly trained and invested professionals who believe in empowering patients to assume some responsibility for their own treatment.

Individual Psychotherapy

As the recovering substance abuser's central nervous system readjusts to life without mind-altering substances, the patient's need for and ability to make use of one-to-one therapy grows. During the hospital phase of recovery, the appropriate psychotherapeutic approach consists of pragmatic, supportive, structured, cognitive, behavioral, and skill-based interventions. Focusing on the here-and-now, rather than the past, is essential. Techniques promoting uncovering, regression, and emotional catharsis should be avoided during the initial phases of recovery.

Early in recovery, one task of the individual therapist is to help stabilize the patient's confused emotions, out-of-control behaviors, and dysfunctional relationships at home and at work. An active, practical, problem-solving therapeutic approach helps achieve this goal. The therapist may also help the patient develop a set of individualized cognitive and behavioral strategies aimed toward preventing relapse (60). Last, the therapist should assist the patient in devising and adhering to a detailed aftercare plan that will insure continuity of the treatment after discharge (85).

Family Work

As noted above (37–40), psychoactive substance-use disorders often have genetic and familial bases. One important function of inpatient treatment is to educate patients and their families about the familial nature of these disorders. Such family education sometimes reduces the burdens of guilt and recrimination present in a family traumatized by the escalating substance abuse of one individual. Knowledge about the familial risk factor provides families with a rationale for early identification and aggressive treatment of substance abuse in relatives of the identified patient.

Significant family dysfunction usually accompanies clinically significant substance abuse resulting in hospitalization (51). Consequently, family evaluation is an essential part of treatment. Many such families will benefit from short-term, focused family therapy, either as a single family alone or in multiple family groups (52).

In the best of circumstances, a patient's employer may be conceptualized as a kind of "work family." Substance abuse may be as damaging and destructive to relationships in the workplace as it is at home. Involving employers in the treatment process has a beneficial effect on treatment outcome (86, 87). With the consent and participation of the patient, careful evaluation of the employment situation—paying special attention to the postdischarge reentry process—appears to be a valuable component of inpatient substance-abuse treatment (87).

CONTROVERSIES IN THE HOSPITAL TREATMENT OF PSYCHOACTIVE SUBSTANCE-USE DISORDERS

The nature of treating these disorders in the hospital may vary depending on the type of inpatient unit. Treatment may occur in a free-standing substance-abuse treatment unit, a specialized unit located in a general hospital, or a unit in a psychiatric hospital. Treatment in a psychiatric hospital may take place in a general unit serving all diagnostic groups, a specialized substance-abuse unit, or in a unit that focuses on dually diagnosed patients. Across this varied spectrum of treatment settings, two controversies prevail.

CONTROVERSY #1:

Is Inpatient Rehabilitation Necessary?

One review of 26 controlled studies comparing residential with nonresidential alcoholism treatment indicated that, overall, the two groups of patients fared equally well (88). A recent study in Rhode Island comparing extended inpatient alcoholism treatment with partial inpatient treatment also demonstrated similar outcomes for the two groups (89). These studies are frequently cited as evidence that inpatient treatment of substance abuse may be unnecessary and fiscally irresponsible.

Methodologically sound treatment comparison studies are merely prospective and randomize subjects to the different treatment groups under comparison. Such studies often contain exclusion criteria eliminating the most unstable patients (those for whom outpatient treatment is not a safe option) from the comparison (89). Because of the skewed subject pools which include only patients not demonstrating severe psychiatric symptomatology, these treatment comparison studies merely indicate that nonhospital treatment is as effective as hospital treatment for *certain* patients.

Despite their claim of equivalence in inpatient and outpatient treatment approaches, Miller and Hester (90) also concluded that hospital treatment was differentially beneficial for the most deteriorated patients with unstable social support systems. Recent studies by McLellan et al. have focussed on the value of matching treatment to the specific patient exhibiting a particular degree of psychiatric and substance-related dysfunction (90, 91). This work indicates that patients manifesting an intermediate degree of psychiatric dysfunction benefit preferentially from inpatient rehabilitation (91).

Future studies will better define the subpopulations of substance-dependent patients for whom hospitalization is clearly essential. At this time, hospitalization should be considered the treatment of choice for the following groups of patients: individuals with concomitant medical or psychiatric disorders that preclude safe outpatient treatment; individuals whose deficient family and social support systems would clearly disrupt any outpatient treatment effort; and individuals who have failed to respond favorably to bona fide outpatient treatment efforts (92, 93).

CONTROVERSY #2:

Should Cigarette Smoking Be Banned from Inpatient Units?

In recent years nicotine dependence has been recognized as a significant form of chemical dependency against which many alcohol and drug treatment techniques have been used. Multimodal rehabilitation programs may include support groups, individual counseling, relaxation exercises, and pharmacotherapy to lessen withdrawal symptoms. In a burgeoning therapeutic environment that views smoking as a bona fide addictive disorder, nonsmoking Alcoholics Anonymous groups have proliferated; inpatient treatment programs have begun to reckon with the issue of controlling or banning smoking during hospitalization of substance-dependent patients.

In one study, smoking was effectively banned on a 12-bed psychiatric crisis unit in Oregon (94) with no discernible effects on patterns of medication usage, need for seclusion or restraint, or discharges against medical advice. In this study, nicotine gum was prescribed and used freely. The unit staff enthusiastically endorsed the smoking ban and noted a decrease in staff time devoted to cigarette issues. A similar ban on a general hospital psychiatric unit was equally well received (95). A more moderate approach used in one inpatient alcohol treatment program restricted smoking to designated rooms (96); Patient or staff smokers lodged few complaints.

Lavin (97) has suggested that imposing smoking bans on unwilling psychiatric patients is normally indefensible. Although there is no consensus as to the most appropriate approach to smoking on inpatient units, current trends indicate that in the future this issue will be addressed in greater depth by many inpatient chemical-dependence treatment facilities. Some units may offer smoking cessation as a feature of an ambitious treatment program that addresses all of a patient's addictive behaviors.

COURSE AND PROGNOSIS

Variability typifies the course and prognosis of psychoactive substance-use disorders. When a patient's substance-abuse problem is sufficiently severe to warrant a diagnosis of dependence, the disorder is frequently chronic and has a significant chance of relapse. The favorability of the prognosis is inversely proportional to the chronicity of the disorder and the degree of substance-related psychopathology (90, 91). For this reason, it is clinically most rewarding to maintain a low threshold of identification and intervention in relatively early and mild cases of substance abuse.

DuPont (98) has described the development of a drug dependence syndrome with the following four stages: (a) experimentation and first-time use; (b) occasional use; (c) regular use; and (d) dependence. In this schema, the current diagnosis of abuse represents a dysfunctional pattern of *regular use*. Empirical research using the Addiction

Severity Index (1) has negated the overly pessimistic notion that psychoactive substance-use disorders have a progressively downward course (99). The degree and extent of the different types of substance-related problems wax and wane, especially early in the course of the disorders.

Once an individual demonstrates significant substance-related dysfunction in several different areas (i.e. medical, legal, interpersonal, vocational, psychiatric, and substance-specific, the long-term prognosis clearly worsens (4). Certain manifestations of a progressive problem unequivocally indicate the need for aggressive and immediate intervention. For alcoholism, such indicators include serious medical problems, loss of a job or spouse due to drinking, suicidal or homicidal behavior, and frequent blackouts or severe withdrawal symptoms. These complications most commonly develop in individuals who begin to abuse alcohol early in life and who possess a strong family history of alcoholism (100).

When a substance abuser shifts from a "medical" source of CNS depressants or opioids to an illicit source, this is a clear-cut indication of worsening prognosis. For users of illicit drugs other such indicators include: changing to intravenous administration, onset of criminal activity to subsidize drug purchases, and switching to a more potent and dangerous form of the substance (e.g., from intranasal cocaine use to smoking free-base).

Patients who suffer from psychoactive substance-use disorders in conjunction with other mental disorders (so-called *dually diagnosed* patients) have a less favorable course and prognosis than patients who suffer from a single disorder. Dually diagnosed patients manifest higher rates of hospitalization, violence, suicidal behavior, and poor medication compliance compared to patients with a single diagnosis (4, 101). Poor control of their psychiatric symptoms may also exacerbate the concomitant psychoactive substance-use disorder (102). Although the response of dually diagnosed patients to traditional substance-abuse treatment has also been unsatisfactory (103), newer forms of treatment specifically designed for this patient population have been encouraging.

Clinicians skilled at identifying pathological psychoactive substance use are in an excellent position to make effective treatment interventions that may shorten the course and dramatically improve the prognosis of patients with substance abuse. Although the psychoactive substance-use disorders are associated with a great deal of medical, psychiatric, and societal morbidity, these disorders are among the most preventable and treatable conditions that physicians are called upon to address. The impressive gains made by successfully treated substance-dependent individuals are extremely gratifying to patient, family, and physician alike.

REFERENCES

1. Rouse BA, Kozel NJ, Richards LG (eds): Self-report methods of estimating drug use: Meeting current challenges to validity. NIDA Res Monog #57, NIDA, Rockville, Md., 1985.

2. Selzer ML: The Michigan alcoholism screening test (MAST): The quest for a new diagnostic instrument. Am J Psychiatry, 3:176–181, 1971.

3. Ewing J, Mayfield D: CAGE. Am J Psychiatry, 131:1121–1122, 1974.

4. McLellan AT, Luborsky L, Woody GE, O'Brien CP: The addiction severity index. J Nerv Ment Dis, 168:26–33, 1980.

5. Safer D: Substance abuse by young adult chronic patients. Hosp Community Psychiatry, 38:511–514, 1987.

6. Lewis CE: Alcoholism, antisocial personality, narcotic addiction: An integrative approach. Psychiatr Dev, 3:223–235, 1984.

7. Gittelman R, Manuzza S, Shenker R, Bonagura N: Hyperactive boys almost grown up.

I. Psychiatric status. Arch Gen Psychiatry, 42:937–947, 1985.

8. Rounsaville BJ, Kosten TR, Weissman MM, Kleber H: Prognostic significance of psychopathology in treated opiate addicts. Arch Gen Psychiatry, 43:739–745, 1986.

9. Weiss RD, Mirin SM, Michael JL, Sollogub AC: Psychopathology in chronic cocaine abusers. Am J Drug Alcohol Abuse, 12:17–29, 1986.

10. Schuckit MA, Winokur G: A short-term follow-up of female alcoholics. Dis Nerv Syst, 33:672–678, 1972.

11. Quitkin FM, Rubkin JG: Hidden psychiatric diagnoses in the alcoholic, in Solomon J (ed): Alcoholism and Clinical Psychiatry, pp. 129–140, New York, Plenum, 1982.

12. Loranzer AW, Tulis EH: Family history of alcoholism in borderline personality disorder. Arch Gen Psychiatry, 42:153–157, 1985.

13. Robins LN, Helzer JE, Weissman MM, et al.: Lifetime prevalence of specific psychiatric disorders in three communities. Arch Gen Psychiatry, 41:949–958, 1984.

14. Myers JK, Weissman MM, Tischler GL, et al.: Six-month prevalence of psychiatric disorders in three communities. Arch Gen Psychiatry, 41:959–967, 1984.

15. Blazer D, Crowell BA, George LK: Alcohol abuse and dependence in the rural south. Arch Gen Psychiatry, 44:736–740, 1987.

16. Schaefer JM: Firewater myths revisited. J Stud Alcohol, 42:99–117, 1981.

17. Saxe L, Denise D, Esty K: The effectiveness and cost of alcoholism treatment: A public policy perspective, in Mendelson JH, Mello NK (eds): The Diagnosis and Treatment of Alcoholism, pp. 485–539, New York, McGraw Hill, 1985.

18. National Clearinghouse of Drug Abuse Information: National Household Survey on Drug Abuse, National Institute of Drug Abuse, Rockville, Md., 1988.

19. Abelson HI, Miller JD: A decade of trends in cocaine use in the household population. NIDA Res Monogr, 61:35–49, 985.

20. Gawin FH: Cocaine: Psychiatric update. Presented at the 139th Meeting of the American Psychiatric Association, Washington, D.C., May 11–16, 1986.

21. Gawin FH, Ellinwood EH: Cocaine and other stimulants. N Engl J Med, 318:1173–1182, 1988.

22. Anthony JC, Trinkoff AM: United States epidemiologic data on drug use and abuse, in Fischman MW, Mello NK (eds): NIDA Res Monogr, 92:241–266, 1989.

23. American Psychiatric Association: Diagnostic and Statistical Manual of Mental Disorders, ed. 3, (DSM-III R), Washington, DC, American Psychiatric Association, 1987.

24. Kandel DB, Logan JA: Patterns of drug use from adolescence to young adulthood: Periods of risk for initiation, continued use, and discontinuation. Am J Public Health, 74:660–666, 1984.

25. Halikas JA, Darvish HS, Rimmer JD: The black addict. 1. Methodology, chronology of addiction, and overview of the population. Am J Drug Alcohol Abuse, 3:529–543, 1976.

26. Lass H: Most chronic pain patients misuse drugs, study shows. Hospital Tribune World Services, 6:2, 1976.

27. McAuliffe WE, Rohman M, Santangelo S, et al.: Psychoactive drug use among practicing physicians and medical students. N Engl J Med, 315:805–810, 1986.

28. Schuckit MA: Drug and Alcohol Abuse: A Clinical Guide to Diagnosis and Treatment, ed. 3, New York, Plenum, 1989.

29. Lex BW, Griffin ML, Mello NK, Mendelson JH: Concordant alcohol and marihuana abuse in women. Alcohol, 3:193–200, 1986.

30. McCarron MM, Schulze BW, Thompson GA, et al.: Acute phencyclidine intoxication: Clinical patterns, complications, and treatment. Ann Emerg Med, 10:290–297, 1981.

31. Frances RJ, Franklin JE: A Concise Guide to Treatment of Alcoholism and Addiction, Washington, D.C., American Psychiatric Association, 1989.

32. Beavais F, Oetting ER, Edwards RW: Trends in the use of inhalants among American Indian adolescents. White Cloud Journal, 3:3–11, 1985.

33. Reed BJ, May PA: Inhalant abuse and juvenile delinquency: A controlled study in Albuquerque, New Mexico, Int J Addict 19:789–803, 1984.

34. Pope HG, Katz DL: Affective and psychotic symptoms associated with anabolic steroid use. Am J Psychiatry, 145:487–490, 1988.

35. Buckley WE, Yesalis CE 3rd, Friedl KE, Anderson WA, Streit AL, Wright JE: Estimated prevalence of anabolic steroid use among male high school seniors. JAMA, 260:3441–3445, 1988.

36. Hawkins MR, Kruzich DJ, Smith JD: Prevalence of polydrug use among alcoholic soldiers. Am J Drug Alcohol Abuse, 11:27–35, 1985.

37. Goodwin DW: Alcoholism and genetics. Arch Gen Psychiatry, 42:171–174, 1985.

38. Bohman M, Sigvardsson S, Cloninger RC: Maternal inheritance of alcohol abuse. Arch Gen Psychiatry, 38:965–969, 1981.

39. Cloninger CR, Bohman M, Sigvardsson S: Inheritance of alcohol abuse. Arch Gen Psychiatry, 38:861–868, 1981.

40. Kaufman E: The applications of biological vulnerability research to drug abuse prevention, in Pickens RW, Svikis DS (eds): NIDA Res Monogr, 89:174–180, 1988.

41. Monteiro MG, Schuckit MA: Populations at high alcoholism risk: Recent findings. J Clin Psychiatry, 49:(Suppl 9):3–7, 1988.

42. Resnick RB, Kestenbaum RS, Schwartz LK: Acute systemic effects of cocaine in man: A controlled study by intranasal and intravenous routes. Science, 195:696–698, 1977.

43. Weiss RD, Mirin SM: Cocaine, Washington, DC, American Psychiatric Association, 1987.

44. Tallman JF, Paul SM, Skolnick P, Gallagher DW: Receptors for the age of anxiety: Pharmacology of the benzodiazepines. Science, 207:274–281, 1980.

45. Bloom F, Segal D, Ling N, Guilleman R: Endorphins: Profound behavioral effects in rats suggest new etiological factors in mental illness. Science, 194:630–632, 1976.

46. Sjoquist B: Brain salsolinol levels in alcoholism. Lancet, 1:675–676, 1982.

47. Mello NK: The role of aversive consequences in the control of alcohol and drug self-administration, in Meyer RE (ed): Evaluation of the Alcoholic: Implications for research, theory, and treatment, NIAAA Res Monogr, 5:207–228, 1981.

48. Vaillant GE: Natural history of alcoholism, V. Is alcoholism the cart or the horse to sociopathy. Br J Addict, 78:317–326, 1983.

49. Butcher JN: Personality factors in drug addiction, in Pickens RW, Svikis DS (eds): NIDA Res Monogr, Biological Vulnerability to Drug Abuse 89:87–92, 1988.

50. Khantzian EJ: The self-medication hypothesis of addictive disorders: Focus on heroin and cocaine dependence. Am J Psychiatry, 131:1259–1264, 1985.

51. Moos RH, Moos BS: The process of recovery from alcoholism, III. Comparing functioning in families of alcoholics and matched control families. J Stud Alcohol, 45:111–118, 1984.

52. Kauffman E, Kaufmann P: Multiple family therapy: A new direction in the treatment of drug abusers. Am J Drug Alcohol Abuse, 4:467–478, 1977.

53. Zinberg NE: Social interactions, drug use, and drug research, in Lowinson JH, Ruiz PR (eds): Substance Abuse: Clinical Problems and Perspectives, Williams & Wilkins, Baltimore, 1981.

54. Caton CL, Gralnick A, Bender S, Simon R: Young chronic patients and substance abuse. Hosp Community Psychiatry, 40:1037–1040, 1989.

55. Hofmann FG: A Handbook on Drug and Alcohol Abuse: The Biomedical Aspects, New York, Oxford University Press, 1983.

56. Minkoff K: An integrated treatment model for dual diagnosis of psychosis and addiction. Hos Community Psychiatry, 40:1031–1036, 1989.

57. Gawin FH, Kleber HD: Cocaine abuse treatment: An open pilot trial with lithium and desipramine. Arch Gen Psychiatry, 41:903–909, 1984.

58. Giannini AJ, Malone DA, Loiselle RH, Giannini MC, Price WA: Treatment of depression in chronic cocaine and phencyclidine abusers. J Clin Pharmacol, 26:211–214, 1986.

59. Weiss RD, Pope HG, Mirin SM: Treatment of chronic cocaine abuse and attention deficit disorder, residual type, with magnesium pemoline. Drug Alcohol Depend, 15:69–72, 1985.

60. Marlatt, GA, Gordon JR: Determinants of relapse: Implications for the maintenance of behavior change, in Davidson PO, Davidson SM (eds): Behavioral Medicine: Changing Health Lifestyles, pp. 410–452, New York, Brunner/Mazel, 1980.

61. Parsons OA, Butters N, Nathan PE (eds): Neuropsychology of Alcoholism: Implications

for Diagnosis and Treatment, New York, Guilford, 1987.

62. Faultisch, ME: Psychiatric aspects of AIDS. Am J Psychiatry, 144:551–556, 1987.

63. Wilkinson DA: CT scan and neuropsychological assessments of alcoholism, in Parsons OA, Butters N, Nathan PE (eds): *Neuropsychology of Alcoholism: Implications for Diagnosis and Treatment,* pp. 76–102, New York, Guilford, 1987.

64. Sussman S, Rychtarik RG, Mueser K, Glynn S, Prue DM. Ecological relevance of memory tests and the prediction of relapse in alcoholics. J Stud Alcohol, 47:305–310, 1986.

65. Thompson WL: Management of alcohol withdrawal syndromes. Arch Intern Med, 138:278–283, 1978.

66. Ashton, H: Benzodiazepine withdrawal: Outcome in 50 patients. Br J Psychiatry, 82:665–671, 1987.

67. Charney DS, Sternberg DE, Kleber HD, Heninger GR, Redmond E: The clinical use of clonidine in abrupt withdrawal from methadone. Arch Gen Psychiatry, 38:1273–1277, 1981.

68. Gawin F, Leber H: Cocaine abuse treatment: Open pilot trial with desipramine and lithium carbonate. Arch Gen Psychiatry, 41:903–909, 1984.

69. Rosecan J: The treatmentof cocaine abuse with imipramine, L-tyrosine, and L-tryptophan. Presented at the Seventh World Congress of Psychiatry, Vienna, Austria, July 14–19, 1983.

70. Dackis CA, Gold MS, Sweeney DR, Byron JP Jr, Climko R: Single-dose bromocriptine reverses cocaine craving. Psychiatry Res, 20:261–264, 1987.

71. Tennants FS Jr, Sagherian AA: Double-blind comparison of amantadine and bromocriptine for ambulatory withdrawal from cocaine dependence. Arch Intern Med, 147:109–112, 1987.

72. Dorus W, Ostrow DG, Anton R, et al.: Lithium treatment of depressed and nondepressed alcoholics. Jama, 262:1646–1652, 1989.

73. Fuller RK, Williford WD: Life-table analysis of abstinence in a study evaluating the efficacy of disulfiram. Alcoholism, 4:298–301, 1980.

74. Fuller RK, Branchey L, Brightwell DR, et al.: Disulfiram treatment of alcoholism. JAMA, 256:1449–1455, 1986.

75. Rawson RA, Washton AM, Resnick RB, Tennant FS: Clonidine hydrochloride detoxification from methadone treatment: The value of naltrexone aftercare, in Harris LS (ed): Problems of Drug Dependence, NIDA Res Monogr, 34:101–108, 1980.

76. Greenstein RA, Arndt IC, McLellan AT, O'Brien CP, Evans B: Naltrexone: A clinical perspective. J Clin Psychiatry, 45:9 (Sec 2) 25–28, 1984.

77. Greenstein RA, Resnick RB, Resnick E: Methadone and naltrexone in the treatment of heroin dependence. Psychiatr Clin North Am, 7:671–679, 1984.

78. Stinson DS, Smith WG, Amidjaya I, Kaplan JM: Systems of care and treatment outcomes for alcoholic patients. Arch Gen Psychiatry, 36:535–539, 1979.

79. Valle SK: Interpersonal functioning of alcoholism counselors and treatment outcome. J Stud Alcohol, 42:783–790, 1981.

80. Finney JW, Moos RH, Chan DA: Length of stay and program component effects in the treatment of alcoholism. J Stud Alcohol, 36:88–108, 1975.

81. Brandsma JM, Pattison EM: The outcome of group psychotherapy with alcoholics: An empirical review. Am J Drug Alcohol Abuse, 11:151–162, 1985.

82. Ends EJ, Page CW: Group psychotherapy and concomitant psychological change. Psychological Monographs, No. 480, 1959.

83. Eriksen L, Bjornstad S, Gotestam KG: Social skills training in groups for alcoholics: One year treatment outcome for groups and individuals. Addict Behav, 11:309–329, 1986.

84. Olson RP, Ganley R, Devine VT, Dorsey GC: Long-term effects on behavioral insight-oriented therapy with inpatient alcoholics. J Consult Clin Psychol, 49:866–877, 1981.

85. Vannicelli M: Treatment contracts in an inpatient alcoholism treatment setting. J Stud Alcohol, 40:457–471, 1979.

86. Jaffe JH: Evaluating drug abuse treatment. NIDA Res Monogr, 51:13–28, 1984.

87. Moberg DP, Krause WK, Klein PE: Posttreatment drinking behavior among inpatients from an industrial alcoholism program. Int J Addict, 17:549–567, 1982.

88. Miller WR, Hester RK: Inpatient alcoholism treatment: Who benefits? Am Psychol, 41:794–805, 1986.

89. McCrady B, Longabaugh R, Fink E, Stout R, Beattie M, Ruggieri-Authelet, A: Cost effectiveness of alcoholism treatment in partial hospital versus inpatient settings after brief inpatient treatment: 12-month outcome. J Consult Clin Psychol, 54:708–713, 1986.

90. McLellan AT, Luborsky L, O'Brien CP: Alcohol and drug abuse treatment in three different populations: Is there improvement and is it predictable. Am J Drug Alcohol Abuse, 12:101–120, 1986.

91. McLellan AT, Luborsky L, Woody GE, O'Brien CP, Druley KA: Predicting response to alcohol and drug abuse treatments: Role of psychiatric severity. Arch Gen Psychiatry, 40:620–625, 1983.

92. Greater Cleveland Hospital Association, Cleveland admissions discharge transfer criteria: Model for chemical dependency treatment programs, Cleveland, Ohio, 1987.

93. Mee-Lee D: An instrument for treatment progress and matching: The recovery attitude and treatment evaluator (RAATE). J Subst Abuse Treat 5:183–186, 1988.

94. Resnick M, Bosworth EE: A smoke-free psychiatric unit. Hosp Community Psychiatry, 40:525–527, 1989.

95. Smith WR, Grant BL: Effect of a smoking ban on a general hospital psychiatric service. Hosp Community Psychiatry, 40:497–502, 1989.

96. Dawley HH, Williams JL, Guidry LS, Dawley LT: Smoking control in a psychiatric setting. Hosp Community Psychiatry, 40:1299–1301, 1989.

97. Lavin M: Let the patient smoke (letter). Hosp Community Psychiatry, 40:1301–1302, 1989.

98. DuPont RL Jr; Getting Tough on Gateway Drugs; A Guide for the Family, Washington, D.C., American Psychiatric Press, 1984.

99. McLellan AT, Luborsky L, Woody GE, O'Brien CP, Kron R: Are the "addiction-related" problems of substance abusers really related? J Nerv Ment Dis, 169:232–239, 1981.

100. Goodwin DW: Alcoholism and genetics. Arch Gen Psychiatry, 38:965–969, 1981.

101. Drake RE, Osher FC, Wallach MA: Alcohol use and abuse in schizophrenia: A prospective community study. J Nerv Ment Dis 177:408–414, 1989.

102. Osher FC, Kofoed LL: Treatment of patients with psychiatric and psychoactive substance-abuse disorders. Hosp Community Psychiatry, 40:1025–1030, 1989.

103. LaPorte DJ, McLellan AT, O'Brien CP, Marshall JR: Treatment response in psychiatrically impaired drug abusers. Compr Psychiatry, 22:411–419, 1981.

7

HIV Infection

Marshall Forstein, MD
Jay Baer, MD

DEFINITION

Human immunodeficiency virus (HIV), a retrovirus previously called lymphadenopathy virus (LAV) and human T-cell lymphotropic virus type III (HTLV-3), causes a spectrum of illnesses. Acquired immunodeficiency syndrome (AIDS) is the term now used to represent the most advanced consequence of HIV infection. With AIDS the immune system has usually irrevocably collapsed and the individual rendered vulnerable to a host of opportunistic infections, neoplasms, and neurological damage.

In 1987 the Centers for Disease Control (CDC) classified the spectrum of illnesses caused by HIV (1). The four groups include:

1. Acute infection: often silent, sometimes manifested by a flu-like syndrome;
2. Asymptomatic infection: occurring during a period which may be relatively short or as long as 10 years or more (2) with or without laboratory indications of immunological changes;
3. Persistent generalized lymphadenopathy: laboratory indications of abnormal cellular immunity may be present;
4. Other disease: divided into five subgroups which include the opportunistic infections, neoplasms, and neurological disease.

Table 7.1 summarizes the spectrum of diseases caused by HIV infection. The term HIV disease refers to any part of the spectrum of illnesses caused by HIV, including AIDS; AIDS indicates neuropsychiatric impairment, opportunistic infections, or neoplasms.

While the CDC classification system acknowledges neurological disease, it fails to describe adequately the range of psychiatric disorders seen in patients with HIV infection. To discuss assessing and treating these psychiatric disorders first requires understanding the natural history of HIV infection.

DIAGNOSIS OF HIV INFECTION

Before the recognition of HIV as the etiologic agent, diagnosing AIDS was based

Table 7.1.   Modified CDC Classification of HIV Infection[a]

Group I: Initial Infection
  Patients are designated as symptomatic seroconversion or asymptomatic seroconversion.
  Symptomatic infections may include mononucleosis-like syndrome, aseptic meningitis, rash, musculoskeletal
    complaints, hematological abnormalities, other clinical and laboratory findings.
  Asymptomatic infection may occur with or without hematological abnormalities.
Group II: Chronic asymptomatic infection
  Patients are designated as having a normal laboratory evaluation, specified laboratory abnormalities, or
    laboratory evaluation pending or incomplete.
  Laboratory abnormalities include: anemia, leukopenia, lymphopenia, decreased T-helper lymphocyte count,
    thrombocytopenia, hypergammaglobulinemia, cutaneous anergy.
Group III: Persistent generalized lymphadenopathy
  Patients are designated on the basis of laboratory evaluations in same manner as in Group II.
Group IV: Other diseases[b]
Subgroup IV-A: Constitutional disease
  Patients are designated as having fever > 1 month, involuntary weight loss > 10% of baseline body weight,
    diarrhea > 1 month, or any combination of these.
Subgroup IV-B: Neurological disease
  Category 1: CNS disorders: dementia, acute atypical meningitis (occurring after initial infections), myelopathy.
  Category 2: Peripheral nervous system disorders: painful sensory neuropathy, inflammatory demyelinating
    polyneuropathy
Subgroup IV-C: Secondary infectious disease
  Category 1: Patients are designated as having ≥ 1: *Pneumocystis carinii* pneumonia, chronic cryptosporidiosis,
    toxoplasmosis, extraintestinal strongyloidiasis, isosporiasis, candidiasis, (esophageal, bronchial, pulmonary),
    cryptococcosis, disseminated histoplasmosis, mycobacterial infection with *Mycobacterium avium* complex or
    Mycobacterium kansasii, disseminated cytomegalovirus infection, chronic mucocutaneous or disseminated
    herpes simplex virus infection, progressive multifocal leukoencephalopathy.
  Category 2: Patients are designated as having ≥ 1: Kaposi's sarcoma, non-Hodgkins's lymphoma (small,
    noncleaved lymphoma or immunoblastic sarcoma), primary lymphoma of the brains.
Subgroup IV-E: Other conditions
  Clinical findings or diseases not classifiable above may be attributed to HIV infection or may indicate a defect in
    cell-mediated immunity. Patients are designated on the basis of the types of clinical findings or diseases
    diagnosed, e.g., chronic lymphoid interstitial pneumonitis.

[a]CDC = Centers for Disease Control; HIV = human immunodeficiency virus
[b]Medical evaluation must exclude the presence of other intercurrent illness that could explain the symptoms.

upon case definition. An individual with no other reason for cellular immunodeficiency must have exhibited symptoms of at least one infection or malignancy from a specific list. Since the development of HIV antibody tests in 1985 and the more recent development of viral antigen tests and culture, laboratory diagnosis of asymptomatic infection has been possible.

Asymptomatic HIV infection is diagnosed most often using an enzyme-linked immunosorbent assay (ELISA) screening test to detect antibodies to HIV and a corroborating Western Blot (WB) or radioimmunoprecipitation assay (RIA) to confirm that the ELISA has detected specific HIV antibodies. Although it is still possible to

have a false positive test, technological refinements and standardized laboratory procedures have greatly minimized this happening (3). Advances in detecting several viral antigens, antibodies, and genomes will continue to modify laboratory diagnosis of HIV infection. As of this printing, the present state of available technology for widespread clinical diagnosis of HIV infection remains ELISA and a corroborative test (WB or RIA). However, confounding the clinical picture is the fact that rare individuals have had positive blood cultures for HIV without generating detectable antibodies (4).

Although rare, diagnosing HIV infection in the asymptomatic person may therefore go unnoticed even with appropriate testing. Furthermore, if testing is done in the window between when actual infection occurs and detectable antibodies form, the inaccurate data may be used to rule out HIV infection when it is actually present but undetected. Finally, laboratory diagnosis of HIV infection does not provide the necessary information to determine if particular symptoms are being caused by active HIV directly, by a secondary consequence of immunological compromise, or by a non-HIV-related medical or psychiatric disorder. Thus, even with laboratory evidence of HIV infection, additional laboratory, radiologic, and medical workup is necessary to determine the immediate etiology of presenting somatic or neuropsychiatric syndromes.

Virology of HIV

As a retrovirus, HIV comprises an RNA (ribonucleic acid) genome and multipartite protein envelope (5). Upon entering the bloodstream, the virus attaches to and is absorbed by T lymphocytes. Once infection is established, the viral genome is integrated into the host cell's genome via the enzyme reverse transcriptase. The virus may rest in the host cells for many years before entering a phase of active replication. During the period of accelerated growth, viral particles are mass-produced and the host cells are sacrificed. This process leads to a depletion of T lymphocytes and a failure of cellular mediated immune response. HIV is also capable of entering and damaging other cells of the immunological system (e.g., macrophages) and of the central and peripheral nervous systems.

Epidemiology of HIV Infection

TRANSMISSION

Initially, the transmission of HIV was poorly understood, contributing to a mass fear of contagion and fanning underlying social prejudices against those affected. HIV is now known to be passed during sexual intercourse (heterosexual and homosexual); from mother to fetus (intrauterine) or child (breast feeding); and in any activity in which infected blood can enter the bloodstream of another person (e.g., i.v. drug users sharing syringes, needlestick injuries to health-care workers, infusion of contaminated blood products that escape screening procedures).

The first cases of AIDS were reported in 1981 (6) when a peculiar form of immune deficiency was noted in young homosexual men. By late 1982, nationwide surveillance had begun, documenting what was to unravel as a worldwide public-health crisis which continues today.

While the majority of cases in the United States and Western Europe continue to appear in men of homosexual or bisexual orientation, the demographics of the epidemic are changing. In the 1990s an increasing percentage of cases in the United States will be reported in people who share needles or are the sexual partners of those who do. While gay and bisexual men continue to account for a substantial proportion of new cases, people of color are proportionately over-represented among newly diagnosed cases of AIDS. Males continue to outnumber females by almost 10 to one. In western Africa, where HIV clearly has been transmitted heterosexually, epidemiology has shown equal distribution of AIDS between males and females.

There is a relatively long period between initial HIV infection and the development of clinical illness. Although the actual reservoir of people infected with HIV is not completely known, it is clearly much greater than the overt number of AIDS cases reported in any given year. As of this printing, trends indicate a decreasing rate of new AIDS cases within certain segments of the gay male population and an increasing rate within the heterosexual population—largely, among i.v. drug users and their sexual partners (7). In particular, black and hispanic women of childbearing age are comprising a greater percentage of people infected, giving birth to an increasing number of HIV-infected children (8, 9).

Of increasing concern is evidence that sexually active adolescents are at risk for HIV infection, although the clinical manifestations are most often not seen for up to 10 years. This data becomes particularly important in the differential diagnosis of young adults presenting with psychiatric disturbance. We will say more about this later.

While sufficient research data is lacking, clinical evidence indicates that the prevalence of HIV infection is increasing in populations placed at risk for infection by their psychiatric disorders: persons with substance-abuse disorders, impulse control disorders, personality disorders with accompanying sexual behaviors that potentiate HIV transmission. Shelters for homeless people report increasing numbers of HIV-infected clients.

HIV AND NEUROLOGICAL COMPROMISE

Neurological symptoms have been documented in approximately 40% of people with AIDS. In 10% of all patients diagnosed with AIDS, neuropsychiatric symptoms may be the first clinical indication of disease (10).

Disorders of consciousness or cognition are evident in 68% of neurologically symptomatic patients. Headaches (55%), focal weakness (18%), incoordination (18%), and seizures (17%) are frequently found. In patients whose diagnosis of AIDS presented first with neurological symptoms, HIV encephalopathy accounted for approximately 16% and CNS (central nervous system) opportunistic viral infections for 11%. Patients with different underlying CNS op-

portunistic infections have varying frequencies of specific symptoms (11).

Dementia

HIV dementia complex (also known as subacute encephalopathy and AIDS dementia complex [ADC]) was first described by Navia and Price in 1986 (12). In 1987 the CDC added this syndrome to its list of AIDS-defining illnesses (1). While ADC may not be clinically apparent in all patients with AIDS, up to 90% of autopsies of deceased AIDS patients will show characteristic pathological changes in the brain (11). Patients who survive longest, especially without aggressive antiviral treatment, have the highest likelihood of developing HIV dementia complex.

Although it is now clear that HIV may enter the brain and cause dementia, much remains to be elucidated about the pathophysiology of this process. Controversy exists about when in the course of HIV infection cognitive compromise begins; several large studies of asymptomatic HIV-infected individuals reveal them to be indistinguishable on neuropsychological testing from noninfected controls (13, 14) while smaller studies reveal neuropsychological deficits in their "asymptomatic" populations (15).

However, consensus indicates that the more advanced the HIV-related illness is in an individual, the more likely significant neuropsychological compromise exists, frequently severe enough to warrant a diagnosis of dementia.

HIV dementia complex may have one or more cognitive, behavioral, motor, or affective abnormalities. Early on, patients commonly complain of forgetfulness, loss of concentration, and slowness of thought. Loss of balance, leg weakness, or psychomotor slowing may be present. Behavioral symptoms such as social withdrawal, apathy, personality changes, and depression are common and may be the only symptoms in the early phase. More rarely, organic psychosis may develop as a prominent early manifestation of HIV CNS infection.

The course of HIV encephalopathy is typically progressive, although newer anti-HIV and antiopportunistic infection therapies may have considerable impact on survival and CNS function. The course of dementia may accelerate, fluctuate, or have sudden onset in the context of acute systemic illness. Thus, an acute delirium, superimposed on a dementing process, may leave the patient more cognitively impaired than before even when the delirium clears.

As dementia progresses, cognitive function deteriorates and motor and behavioral abnormalities progress. Psychomotor slowing is frequently observed in the late stage of dementia. Weakness, tremor, incontinence, ataxia, hypertonia, frontal release signs, myoclonus, and seizures are end stage signs and symptoms. Psychiatric disturbances include depression and organic psychosis. The most severe cases include akinetic mutism, global cognitive impairment, and paraparesis.

Pathology of Subacute Encephalopathy

The histopathologic features of HIV infection in subacute encephalitis is that of a diffuse viral CNS infection. Areas most affected are the white matter and basal ganglia. The severity of dementia generally correlates well with the severity of histopathologic lesions of subacute encephalitis (16). Clinically, however, the severity of dementia does not always correlate well with the severity of disease documented by CNS visualizing techniques such as CT (computerized tomography) or MRI (magnetic resonance imaging).

Other Central Nervous System Pathology

In addition to primary infection by HIV, other opportunistic viral, fungal, bacterial, protozoal infections and neoplasms can cause CNS dysfunction. These insults can occur within the CNS itself or may occur systemically with CNS consequences.

The most common intracranial problems include: toxoplasmosis, cryptococcosis, and lymphoma. Herpes and cytomegalovirus (CMV) are also CNS pathogens seen in HIV infection. Common systemic illnesses that may compromise the CNS include Pneumocystis pneumonia (e.g., leading to hypoxemia), Kaposi's sarcoma, atypical Mycobacterium infection, wasting syndrome, chronic enteritis (leading to malabsorption), and Candida.

Iatrogenic Causes of CNS Dysfunction in HIV Infection

As newer antiviral agents, antimicrobials, chemotherapies for neoplasms, and immune modulators are used in the treatment of HIV, the CNS becomes more exposed to the effects of such interventions. Since effective medications must penetrate the blood-brain barrier, they can produce centrally induced adverse effects such as psychiatric symptoms and signs. Frequently seen psychiatric side effects of commonly used medications are listed in Table 7.2. While certain side effects are clearly attributable to specific medications, discerning what neuropsychiatric symptom results from medication rather than from the condition for which the medication is prescribed is often difficult.

In addition, a brain made vulnerable by HIV infection is more prone to the side effects of psychopharmacological agents used to treat psychiatric disturbance. For example, high-potency neuroleptics have a

Table 7.2.   Neuropsychiatric Effects of Commonly Prescribed Medications

Drug	Target Illness	Symptoms Affecting Mental State
Amphotericin B	Cryptococcosis Candidiasis Histoplasmosis	Fever, nausea, renal failure with secondary depression, delirium
Alpha-interferon	Kaposi's sarcoma	Depression, weakness, agitation
Acyclovir	Herpes	Headache, gastrointestinal distress, vertigo, malaise
Dideoxyinosine (DDI)	HIV	Peripheral neuropathy, agitation
Pentamidine	Pneumocystis carinii Pneumonia	Nausea, hypoglycemia, hypotension
Zidovudine (AZT)	HIV	Headache, restlessness, agitation, insomnia, mania

great likelihood of causing movement disorders, particularly in individuals with severe basal ganglia impairment by HIV. Pharmacological treatment is addressed in more detail later in this chapter.

HIV and Functional Psychiatric Disturbance

The presence of HIV infection has irrevocably changed the differential diagnosis of neuropsychiatric illness. Because of the following reasons HIV infection must be considered in the differential diagnosis of any psychiatrically symptomatic person with risk factors for transmitting HIV: a long, possibly asymptomatic, incubation period; the vulnerability to infection associated with sexual and drug using behaviors; and the neurotropic nature of the virus. However, the statistical chance of any single person having organic CNS illness due to HIV in the absence of other systemic findings is the exception rather than the rule.

At the same time as it yields the devastating immunological and neurological problems described above, infection with HIV also leads to severe psychological and social stress (17). Many communicable and terminal illnesses such as syphilis and cancer have for centuries been sources of social ostracism (18). AIDS is unique in its combining several sources of stigma in one disease. It was poorly understood (particularly in the early 1980s); it is associated with already stigmatized groups, such as homosexual men and intravenous drug users; it is disproportionately associated with oppressed racial and ethnic groups; it is sexually transmissable; and it is perceived as being uniformly lethal. The huge amount of stigma associated with an AIDS diagnosis may well exacerbate, if not cause, functional psychiatric disturbance and impede patients from pursuing support, including medical and mental health care.

Although it is difficult to estimate the frequency and severity of functional psychiatric disorders in individuals infected with HIV, a modicum of psychiatric literature and a wealth of clinical experience indicate such problems are far from rare. Numerous cases of depression, mania, anxiety, and psychosis are reported (19–25). Marzuk and associates (26) clearly showed that a diagnosis of AIDS should be considered a risk factor for suicide. A significant percentage of documented AIDS cases in the U.S. occurs in patients with past or current psychoactive substance-abuse disorders. Finally, people with preexisting major mental disorders have developed HIV disease and consequently have to struggle with psychiatric illness complicated by medical illness (19). Table 7.3 lists the spectrum of psychi-

Table 7.3.   Common Psychiatric Disorders in HIV-Infected People

I. Functional disorders
  A. Mood disorders
    1. Major depression
    2. Dysthymia
  B. Adjustment disorders
    1. With disturbance of emotions and/or conduct
  C. Anxiety Disorders
    1. Generalized anxiety disorder
    2. Panic disorder
    3. Posttraumatic stress disorder
  D. Psychoactive substance-use disorders
  E. Brief reactive psychosis
  F. Uncomplicated/complicated bereavement
  G. Preexisting major mental illness (e.g., schizophrenia)
II. Organic mental disorders
  A. Dementia
    1. Secondary to AIDS dementia complex (primary HIV infection)
    2. Secondary to other opportunistic infections or neoplasms
  B. Delirium
    1. Transient
    2. Chronic
  C. Psychoactive substance-induced organic mental disorder
  D. Organic affective disorder
  E. Organic anxiety disorder
  F. Organic delusional disorder
  G. Organic hallucinosis
  H. Organic personality disorder

atric disorders found in people with HIV disease. Clinicians must be alert to the likelihood of patients having more than one disorder at any given time or over the course of the illness.

BIOPSYCHOSOCIAL EVALUATION OF PERSONS INFECTED WITH HIV

Biological Evaluation

HISTORY OF MAJOR MENTAL ILLNESS

The clinician must inquire about a history of major psychiatric disturbance. A preexisting psychiatric disorder in a patient who becomes infected by HIV is likely to be active throughout the course of HIV-related illness.

HIV AS A PART OF THE DIFFERENTIAL DIAGNOSIS

The HIV serological status of a patient admitted to a psychiatric unit is generally not known. Now that HIV infection has been added to the differential diagnosis for altered mental state, the admitting clinician must consider HIV disease as a possible cause of psychiatric disturbance. The presence of HIV risk behaviors will help determine whether to approach the patient with a request for HIV antibody testing. Evidence of dementia mandates a full dementia workup which may include HIV serology. In many states, the decision to test a patient for HIV requires written informed consent, a process sometimes not possible with an acutely disturbed psychiatric patient. Furthermore, even when informed consent is possible, providers must evaluate the psychological capacity of the individual to handle not only the knowledge of long-term HIV infection but the initial effect of the tests results as well. Much of the psychiatric morbidity associated with HIV testing occurs over time as the irrevocable information is incorporated into how the individual copes with his uncertain and frightening future. A positive HIV test calls for a complete organic workup. A negative test does not necessarily rule out HIV as a factor in the presenting illness.

If a patient gives a history of infection or HIV is discovered during the course of assessment, several evaluations are necessary:

Overall assessment of extent of HIV-related illness. Consultation from an AIDS-knowledgeable internist or infectious disease specialist should be requested, unless the current medical status is available from the patients' primary care physician. History, physical exam, and laboratory studies will be needed to determine the extent of the damage to the immune system and identify HIV-related disorders. If present, the latter may well require treatment concurrent with treatment of the acute psychiatric disturbance.

Central nervous system evaluation. Patients infected with HIV are susceptible to numerous CNS insults which may be responsible for or contribute to the psychiatric disturbance that led to hospitalization. Although most of these will make themselves apparent in ways beyond behavioral disturbances (e.g., a man with Toxoplasma gondii abscesses in his brain is likely to develop headaches and/or neurological abnormalities), the psychiatric disorder may be the only presenting problem. Hence, a thorough neurological exam is required. Additional evaluation, such as CT scan or MRI of the brain, is often required to rule out treatable complications of HIV infection. As CNS neoplasms or infections can cause increased intracranial pressure, a brain imaging procedure is usually required before lumbar puncture is performed.

Psychodynamic Evaluation

A diagnosis of an HIV-related condition presents an individual with numerous psychological stresses. Although these may recur and overlap throughout the illness, many issues occur at characteristic times. The clinician must assess which issues are of paramount importance to the patient (see Table 7.4).

Even for well-adjusted individuals, diagnosis of an HIV-related condition incurs a massive assault on self-esteem. During an acute hospitalization, information about a positive diagnosis of HIV infection may be emotionally and/or cognitively unmanageable because of the acute psychiatric disturbance. Frequently, latent negative self-images are activated, such as those found in many forms of posttraumatic stress syndrome (27) (e.g., a homosexual man with

Table 7.4.[a] **Common Psychological Issues by Stages of HIV Infection**

I. New Diagnosis (of HIV infection; patient may or may not be symptomatic)
  A. Denial
  B. Massive self-esteem challenge
  C. Fears of rejection, often realistic and unrealistic
  D. Guilt and self-blame; illness as retribution
  E. Feelings of being contaminated and fears of contaminating others
  F. Affective numbing alternating with affective flooding
  G. Feeling overwhelmed, urgency re: many complex decisions
  H. Suicidal ideation: "When I become so sick, I won't want to live anymore," or "Maybe I should avoid all that pain."
II. Honeymoon
  A. Mood stabilization
  B. A balance of hope and denial: "Maybe there will be a cure," or "I'll be the one who beats this."
  C. Lifestyle changes
  D. Stress reduction
  E. Focus on "what really matters"
III. Midstage
  A. Loss of hope, emotional exhaustion
  B. Anticipatory grief: mourning the loss of important people, objects, the future
  C. Extent of treatment: living wills, durable power of attorney for medical care
  D. Unfinished business; putting one's affairs in order (practical and emotional)
  E. Fears of dying: suffering, being alone
IV. Terminal Care
  A. Minimization of pain and suffering
  B. Who will be there? Role of family, friends, providers
  C. Saying goodbyes
  D. Honoring patient's wishes
  E. Death
  F. Attention to those left behind in grief: family, friends, providers

[a]Adapted from Dilley JW, Shelp EE, Batke SL: Psychiatric and ethical issues in the care of patients with AIDS. Psychosomatics, *27*:562–566, 1986.

unresolved negative feelings about his sexuality may become enraged at himself for his sexual orientation).

Reviewing each patient's coping strengths and weaknesses and history of response to severe stress are as essential to the psychodynamic evaluation of an HIV patient for any patient admitted to inpatient service.

Sociocultural Evaluation

Careful review of each patient's support network is vital. Disruption of this network is a typical predisposing factor to psychiatric decompensation. People with HIV infection are multiplystigmatized because of risk factors and preexisting psychiatric illness when present. As a result, many are subject to discrimination in matters of housing, employment, and obtaining and maintaining insurance. The post hospital disposition of a psychiatrically ill patient with HIV infection is particularly problematic.

Because of prejudice patients with AIDS face the loss of emotional support, and because of illness they face the loss of self-esteem and perhaps the ability to function independently. Moreover, many people with AIDS have lost significant numbers of loved ones and peers to the disease they now suffer. For gay men in large cities, particularly, the phenomenon of compounded, unremitting grief has reached staggering proportions. Overwhelming grief may contribute to significant problems in patient's complying with medical treatments and may lead some individuals to withdraw emotionally from available social supports. Suicidal ideation is frequently present in people diagnosed with HIV seropositivity, AIDS, or dementia.

A review of income sources, living arrangements, source of medical and psychiatric care, additional services (e.g., delivery of meals to patients too fatigued to shop and cook for themselves), and optimal placement are routinely required. Often these life-sustaining basics have been disrupted, exacerbating the psychiatric disturbance. Patients often need visiting nurse and/or hospice care at advanced stages of illness.

Ethnic/Minority Issues

Individuals from minority groups contend with additional problems. These include barriers to medical and mental health care, poverty, and group-specific issues of denial and taboo surrounding AIDS. The meaning of the diagnosis of AIDS in each community must be understood in order to facilitate placement and mobilize necessary supports after hospitalization.

HOSPITAL TREATMENT

Psychopharmacology

Psychoactive drugs play a major role in the hospital treatment of psychiatric disturbances. Before discussing the pharmacological approach to several specific disorders, we offer some basic principles.

Generally, the tolerance and dosing of psychoactive agents in HIV patients not in an advanced state of physical or cognitive decline is similar to those of the non-HIV-infected population. However, patients with more advanced disease are particularly sensitive to drug side effects and frequently require lower dosages.

In people with AIDS a change in mental state can evolve quickly. For example, a patient may be cognitively intact one day, then develop sepsis or meningitis and become delirious the next. Thus, frequent monitoring of mental status and medication is important as the need for and tolerance of drugs change.

Most patients with symptomatic HIV infection will be receiving one or more "nonpsychiatric" medications for their condition. The introduction of new psychiatric or other medications may create a competition for protein binding sites and cause a significant (and unanticipated) increase in serum levels of either the newly introduced agent or the medications already on board.

DEPRESSION

Depression, frequently accompanied by suicidal ideation or action, is a frequent cause for psychiatric hospitalization. The symptoms of major depression—such as loss of energy or appetite, depressed mood, and cognitive complaints (e.g., poor concentration)—may be difficult to distinguish from dementia, another mood disturbance such as adjustment disorder with depressed mood, or the consequences of an acute medical condition.

All acute medical problems should be treated; unessential medications should be stopped, if possible, in order to assess the role they play in the depression. Diagnostically, it may be difficult to ascertain the nature of the depression; however, if functional impairment continues, psychopharmacological and psychotherapeutic interventions should be considered.

Depression is particularly likely to develop along with changes in an individual's medical condition. Defenses, including denial, which have sustained hope for the future may break down as dynamic issues emerge. Coexisting organic affective disorder and a depressive reaction to illness may complicate diagnosing and treating depression.

Selection of agent. Clinical experience and case reports, rather than research studies, inform the following observations and suggestions. In patients without advanced HIV disease, tricyclic antidepressants remain an effective treatment. Generally, it is preferable to use agents that incur minimum sedation and autonomic system side effects. Desipramine and nortriptyline usually serve well, in standard dosage regimens. For patients whose depression has a major component of anxiety or agitation, a more sedating agent such as doxepin or trazodone may be indicated.

Patients with more advanced disease usually suffer from significant fatigue and are less tolerant of autonomic nervous system side effects. The monamine oxidase inhibitors (MAOIs) are difficult to use in patients with HIV because of the tendency to cause hypotension.

Fluoxetine (Prozac) is also used successfully in patients with major depression. Prozac's relatively benign side effects can make it preferable to tricyclics or MAOIs. Fluoxetine occasionally causes agitation, described as hypomania or "speeding." Patients report feeling as if they have had too much caffeine. Sometimes this initial agitation abates after a few weeks, permitting fluoxetine's continued use. In patients in whom many pharmacologic agents may be used and changed frequently, fluoxetine has the disadvantages of a long half-life and a tendency to slow the metabolism of other medications. Bupropion (Wellbutrin) has not been well-studied in patients with HIV disease. Because of its increased risk of causing seizures, buproprion must be used cautiously in patients with clear evidence of brain disease. At least one anecdotal report (from Frank Fernandez, M.D., Baylor University, College of Medicine) suggests that bupropion may be as useful as psychostimulants and can be as safe, with proper attention to incremental changes and intervals between doses. Although AIDS patients exhibit an increased incidence of seizures, buproprion may be considered for those without evidence of seizures.

Psychostimulants are found to produce mood and neuropsychological test performance improvement in patients with symptomatic HIV disease involving an element of cognitive impairment (28, 29). Methylphenidate (Ritalin) may be given in divided morning doses, beginning with 5 mg per day, advancing to a maximum of 60 mg or more per day. Increases should be made every third day until a positive response occurs or side effects (anxiety, tachycardia, hypertension) limit the process. Patients may be maintained on psychostimulants over a period of several months. Although dextro-amphetamine has also been used with similar success, it may cause movement disorders in the HIV-infected person.

Physicians may worry about prescribing stimulants to people with a history of substance abuse, and pharmacists may be reluctant to fill such prescriptions without first confirming their validity with the physician. Experience has shown that even in an individual with a prior history of drug abuse, psychostimulants can be effective and appropriately managed, although not without some difficulty in patients with significant character pathology. Patients who respond well feel such improvement that they are reluctant to abuse the medications for fear of losing the benefits. Close monitoring of drug use, frequent visits for prescriptions, and clear parameters for use help to prevent misuse of these effective agents.

Electroconvulsive therapy (ECT) has not been widely studied as a treatment in depressed patients who are HIV-infected. ECT may be useful in depressed HIV-infected patients who are asymptomatic. In patients with intracranial lesions or neurocognitive impairment, ECT may be contraindicated.

Auxiliary agents. Patients who experience anxiety as a major component of their depression may require concomitant administration of an antianxiety agent such as alprazolam (Xanax) or lorazepam (Ativan). Low doses of short-acting agents are preferable (e.g., oxazepam) for reducing the risk of additional cognitive impairment. In patients who have significant sleeping problems, triazolam (Halcion) may be useful.

Patients who have major depression along with psychotic features will require an antipsychotic agent and an antidepressant. High-potency agents in modest dosages, such as 5–10 mg of haloperidol (Haldol) per day, usually suffice in patients without significant cognitive impairment (see below).

MANIA

Patients wtih HIV infection may develop a variety of mania that requires pharmacological intervention. Mania may occur with or without cognitive impairment, as a form of bipolar disorder or a consequence of drug therapy. Several psychiatrists (19, 22) have reported a syndrome of mania occurring in the context of dementia, which all too often heralds the incipient demise of the patient. In some cases the syndrome of mania may be caused or exacerbated by zidovudine or gancyclovir therapy (see below). However, it is clear that mania develops as part of the HIV disease process itself; mania was described in numerous patients before the advent of antiviral treatments. HIV-related mania can be adequately managed with midpotency antipsychotic agents such as perphenazine (Trilafon) or thiothixene (Navane) in low to moderate dosages. High-potency neuroleptics are not generally recommended in patients with cognitive impairment because of the high frequency and severity of extrapyramidal side effects in this population (19). Lithium therapy has been variably effective; if effective, the most acute symptoms of the syndrome are usually brought under control within a few weeks. However, often the patient will remain somewhat grandiose and delusional, with periods of lucidity and less problematic behavior.

Although carbamazepine may be considered, it must be carefully monitored because bone marrow problems are often already present in patients with HIV disease, particularly those taking AZT (azidothymidine) or other chemotherapeutic agents.

ORGANIC ANXIETY DISORDER

Patients with advancing HIV dementia may develop an anxiety syndrome characterized by agitation and overstimulation. Symptoms tend to worsen over the course of the day. In some patients, low doses of midpotency neuroleptics (e.g., perphenazine—8 mg per day) are tolerated and work well. Sometimes low doses of benzodiazepine (e.g., alprazolam—0.125 mg b.i.d. [twice a day] or t.i.d. [3 times a day]) are more successful. No single pharmacological approach to this problem is always successful.

DEMENTIA

Evidence suggests that AZT may be useful in treating HIV dementia complex. Documented cognitive impairment is considered reason alone for beginning AZT to slow loss of function. In conjunction, psychostimulants maximize cognitive capacity, sometimes making a significant difference in the ability of individuals to live independently or with less supportive services. For patients dually diagnosed with depression and dementia, psychostimulants are preferable to other agents.

DELIRIUM

Delirium may occur in demented and nondemented patients, often with the onset of an acute medical problem. Implicated medictions should be stopped if possible. While the search for a potentially reversible cause proceeds, low doses of a midpotency antipsychotic agent are recommended if the patient's symptoms (e.g., agitation, hallucinations) threaten his safety. This is particulalry important in light of one study (26) which revealed a significant incidence of suicide in the delirious hospitalized patient with HIV. A combination of haloperidol and ativan (both i.v.) has been used clinically with good outcome in acutely delirious patients (personal communication, Frank Fernandez).

PSYCHOTIC DISORDERS

Recurrent and new "functional" disorders such as schizophrenia, bipolar disorder, and brief reactive psychosis appear in nondemented patients with HIV disease. The pharmacological management of these disorders does not significantly differ from that of non-HIV-infected individuals, ex-cept as changes in medical status warrant and with the specific considerations noted elsewhere.

ZIDOVUDINE

Although this section is organized by syndromes, a few words about zidovudine (AZT) are necessary. Although this drug has rarely been implicated in causing secondary mania, it much more commonly causes a syndrome of irritability, insomnia, and anxiety during the first 4–6 weeks of therapy. In the majority of patients this syndrome will not prevent further zidovudine use, although some patients require benzodiazepine therapy to minimize these side effects. Recent studies, supporting lower doses of zidovudine treatment, may significantly reduce the frequency and severity of this syndrome. Recent studies have been optimistic about the effect of zidovudine on stalling or partially reversing HIV dementia and other complications of HIV itself (30).

Many psychiatric inpatients will be taking zidovudine. This does not usually prevent the co-administration of psychoactive medications as long as appropriate attention is paid to the interaction of medications and the effects on hepatic and renal metabolism. Serum levels of medication should be used whenever possible to minimize toxicity.

MILIEU MANAGEMENT

The presence of HIV-infected patients in the inpatient psychiatric unit is a stress for both staff and patients. Several issues must be addressed in order to insure optimum care and manage staff anxiety appropriately.

Confidentiality

Staff must respect the confidentiality of patients with HIV infection. This diagnosis should never be revealed to a patient's peers without the patient's permission. In most cases, no clinical benefit derives from revealing the HIV infection of patients to their peers. However, in some instances it is important for infected patients to be able to talk openly of their illness. Some patients choose to reveal their HIV status and may attempt to find support from the milieu; staff should never pressure patients to do so. When patients do choose to be open about their infection, the staff must insure that the consequences of the revelation become a part of the milieu treatment. Open discussion can teach all patients important information about sexual behaviors and drugs that may put them at risk for HIV.

Documentation is one area of clinical practice where rules of confidentiality are frequently violated. Laws vary from state to state regarding whether and how a clinician may transmit information of a patient's antibody status to other clinicians (e.g., in preparing to discharge a patient from the unit to a halfway house it is often routine to copy and send hospital admission records). Clinically, it is always best to determine whether information regarding HIV infection is germane to clinical care and, if so, gain the patient's written permission before transmitting.

Infection Control

Though the risk of HIV transmission in a psychiatric inpatient unit is small, it is frequently of disproportionate concern to staff and/or patients. The great majority of hospitals in this country have adopted universal precautions requiring staff to handle all bodily secretions as if they might be infected, protecting patients and staff not only from HIV but other illness as well. Applied to all patients, these precautions minimize the time spent agonizing over the relative risk involved in each episode of handling or cleaning up body fluids.

HIV infection does not automatically preclude sharing of bedrooms on the inpa-

tient unit. Many hospitals have policies regarding room sharing in general and for HIV-infected patients in particular. From a clinical vantage point, patients should be given private rooms if they are active in coughing and tuberculosis has not been ruled out and if they are not able to comply with handling body fluids (i.e., are incontinent).

A few activities in which a small but significant risk of HIV transmission exists are:

1. Needlesticks: In the tumult of a difficult seclusion and restraint, staff risk needlestick injuries. Current data suggest that the risk of infection with HIV from a needlestick from a known infected patient is approximately ½ of 1% (0.5%) (31). Therefore, it behooves an inpatient staff to orchestrate their medication of agitated patients with extra care, regardless of patient HIV serological status. To the extent possible, staff should give involuntary injections and remove and dispose of needles in an unhurried, controlled manner. We recommend that extra personnel be employed to insure patient immobility; the medication nurse should be the only staff member in motion from the time the injection is given until the time the needle is safely discarded. Safe disposal requires having an impenetrable needle discard container in the seclusion room or using needles that automatically self-cover with safety sheaths after use.

2. Unprotected Sex: Most, if not all, inpatient units proscribe sex between patients. This does not altogether prevent sexual activity from occurring on or off the unit; such activity can probably never be fully prevented. While sexually aggressive patients are usually identified and subject to extra monitoring, other patients with varying impairment in judgment may consent or be pressured

into sexual relations. Staff should carry out active AIDS education efforts to help minimize these occurrences (See Controversies section).

AIDS Education

Preventing HIV transmission on the unit itself is just one reason for making AIDS education part of the milieu program. Regular education sessions should be offered on a group and individual basis to all patients and staff. Emphasis should be on mode of transmission and ways to prevent infection even in those sexually active (patients will resume prior level of sexual activity after hospitalization). Educational meetings need to be tailored to the cognitive abilities of the patients; meetings, generally more useful to patients who are at least partly stabilized, should be offered routinely whether or not known HIV-infected patients are present on the unit. Psychiatrically disturbed patients with impulse disorders and individuals without sufficient defenses to ward off unwarranted sexual advances, (particularly in shelters, residential housing programs, and shared living situations) are at risk for HIV after hospitalization. The inpatient setting provides an important opportunity to counsel and educate patients about ways to protect themselves from HIV.

Peer Reactions

Even with an active AIDS education program, patients are often misinformed and quite fearful of contracting HIV from infected peers and will require consistent reassurance that casual contact is not hazardous to their lives. Patients may incorporate elements of their environment into their psychopathology; the presence of individuals known to been infected with HIV is no exception. The behavior of agitated, paranoid patients is particularly likely to escalate after they perceive that an HIV-infected person is nearby. Sometimes even a patient's known or presumed homosexuality can precipitate paranoid ideation and/or delusional thinking about HIV in other patients. More positively, patients can derive satisfaction and increased self-esteem from helping care for their medically ill peers; such activity can become an ingredient in their recovery.

Staff Reactions

Staff must manage the milieu issues described above. In addition to needing education and support to manage competently, staff anxieties must be acknowledged and managed so that patient care does not suffer.

Staff members are frequently stressed by having to work with medical illness, sexuality, illicit drug use, and death. Some may actually seek psychiatry as a means to handle or avoid these stresses. We recommend a two-pronged approach for staff support. One element is didactic; namely training sessions about HIV. The other element is more affect-oriented; namely, support groups in which staff can voice their fears and other emotional reactions to working with HIV. Both types of sessions should be offered as ongoing rather than single efforts and treated as a requirement of the work.

In addition, individual supervision is also helpful. Staff members can use supervision to sort out the strong countertransference reactions that may arise when working with HIV-infected patients or those at risk for HIV.

PSYCHOTHERAPY

Since HIV-infected patients come to the inpatient service with a wide variety of psychiatric diagnoses, the psychotherapeutic approach must vary as well (32). Varying modalities of treatment may be useful for different patients or at different points in the course of HIV infection. While it is imperative that therapists work closely with other clinicians, particularly medical personnel, care must be taken to preserve the privacy of the therapist-patient relationship. HIV patients often have intensely private and difficult issues to address which they fear will become exposed to others on the inpatient service.

Depression

HIV patients with depression always have something significant to be depressed about: they have a terminal illness. Therefore, work on the inpatient unit with depressed patients cannot aim toward a goal of complete resolution of mood disturbance. Instead, a realistic goal is mood improvement and instilling some amount of hope or way to continue with life. The clinician frequently feels caught between the urge to help patients live their remaining lives to the fullest and the urge to help patients accept that they are dying. Therapists must be open to discussing both objectives thereby helping patients accurately assess the realities of their illness and maintain sufficient defenses to avoid immediate despair. Aggressively diagnosing the depression and treating it pharmacologically may significantly enhance psychotherapeutic efforts.

A significant component of depression for many patients is the activation of latent negative self-images. Psychotherapy can be very useful in elucidating the source of these images and scrutinizing them critically. A psychoeducation model may be useful, particularly in the areas of drug addiction and coming to terms with homosexual experience and identity formation.

Suicidal ideation is common in HIV-infected individuals and usually arises at many times throughout the course of illness. It is common for people to feel suicidal when they first learn of (and are overwhelmed by) their diagnosis or when an exacerbating illness or other acute life stress makes life seem unbearable. Sometimes suicidal thoughts and behavior are delayed until after an initial period of adequate coping when the realization that HIV is a life-long infection sets in. Some patients who are not seriously medically ill will contemplate suicide for some unspecified time in the future when they envision becoming incapacitated by the disease. It is always important to inquire about and explore the suicidal thoughts of depressed HIV patients. Many are relieved to be able to talk about this subject. What is deemed intolerable and necessitating suicide varies tremendously from person to person. Some patients' reason for wanting to kill themselves are relatively straightforward to address (e.g., fear of intolerable pain can be allayed by a collaborative discussion with patients and their primary physician), while others are difficult to "fix." Patients benefit from an empathic discussion of their predicament regardless of solutions. Furthermore, because suicidal ideation often expresses the fear of losing control over one's life, actively discussing the fear can provide a sense of control that feels missing.

Clinicians must help sort out the difference between a treatable depression (which may be organic or reactive) and an accurate appraisal of the terminal aspect of HIV disease. The meaning of suicidal ideation in someone recently diagnosed as infected though asymptomatic is significantly different from someone recognizing the inexorable decline of body and mind. In the latter instance suicide may be less the fear of living and more the appropriate acceptance of the final stages of life; a wish to hasten that demise as an act of control and not burden others or a fear of total dependency on others. In working with the patient, the therapist can help the patient maximize healthy defenses against the impending sense of loss of self and differentiate between treatable and untreatable conditions.

Treating depression and other mental disorders in this population requires some amount of help organizing out-of-hospital supports in addition to individual or group psychotherapy. Helping the patient to connect to a peer support group of people who are HIV positive (with or without illness) can provide an important support in the transition out of the hospital. In most urban areas, AIDS service organizations or state public health departments may be a useful source of information about support groups and services. Increasingly, such community organizations are developing in rural and suburban areas as well.

However, the issues arising in patients suffering from depression may persist throughout the course of illness. Many of these matters may be pertinent to patients suffering from other psychiatric disorders discussed below.

Dementia

Therapists must assess the cognitive capabilities of the dementia patient and tailor their communications accordingly. For example, a person with severe dementia will not be able to process long, complex communications that occur in the context of considerable extraneous stimuli. Therapists should be careful not to overly challenge or condescend. They must also remember that the patient's abilities vary in the short term (e.g., the patient may be more lucid in the mornings) and decline in the long term. Sometimes it is the physical presence of the helper that is more successful in calming a patient than anything spoken.

One of the most devastating problems to confront is the sadness and terror experienced by patients who become aware they are losing cognitive capacity. By exploring these concerns early on and working with the patient to develop stategies for compensating for cognitive impairment, the therapist can help patients feel as if they are maximizing control over their lives for as long as possible. The clinicians' calmness and directness can help build an alliance that allows the patient increasingly to accept the necessary dependency that occurs with deterioration. By making an explicit "living will" regarding the type and degree of intervention patients want, they can feel more in control of their own destiny.

Often the issue of physical comfort and pain control are of paramount importance to patients with dementia, especially for those who have witnessed the demise of someone close. Physicians can assure the patient that pain will be controlled as much as possible. Just as in managing non-HIV dementia, consistency in routines and caregivers should be maintained.

Delirium

The managing of delirium in the HIV-infected patient is not substantially different from treating other deliriums. Patient insight is subordinated to patient safety, especially until the process is accurately diagnosed and resolved. Delirious patients may act impulsively and can be self-destructive. A psychotherapeutic alliance which may have contained suicidal ideation in a competent person cannot contain a delirious patient. Rapid diagnosis and treatment of delirium may prevent irreversible damage in a patient undergoing an underlying dementing process.

Psychotherapy can also be useful to help patients cope with the emotional aftermath of a delirium which often is a frightening experience and a reminder that the patient has lost control. Engaging the patient in how to manage future complications fortifies a sense of control and acknowledges the patient's need to accept help from others at critical times.

Psychosis

Patients with all types of psychotic processes are liable to struggle with postpsychotic depression. This is certainly true of patients wtih AIDS who must face the ongoing challenges of their medical illness after recuperation from their psychosis. Whenever possible, helping patients to understand the cause of the psychosis and how it has been treated will facilitate working through the shame and fear of being out of control.

Family Work

DEFINITION OF FAMILY

To a significant extent, patients define their families. Many patients with AIDS live in nontraditional family units (i.e., other than two parents of different gender with children). Gay men and women may live with same-sex life partners (significant others) that warrant the same attention and respect afforded a heterosexual patient's spouse. In addition, many patients will have an extended nonbiological family of friends who may be intimately involved in their care. Of course, the patient's biological family is the other crucial component of the working definition of family that the staff must utilize. For gay people, however, biological family members who have been estranged from the patient for significant periods of time may attempt to enter the patient's life during a time of illness and attendant crisis. While it is always in the interest of the patient to reconcile if possible, the patient must retain control (to the extent possible) over involvement with others. The patient and significant other often fear that a biological family member will displace a same-sex significant other in controlling decisions about medical interventions or even the disposition of the body after death. Staff can help make the patient's wishes explicit. Durable powers of attorney can be established early on in illness to facilitate reconciliation with family while sustaining control by the patient and/or significant other over treatment decisions.

GOALS OF FAMILY WORK.

Several basic tasks take place during a psychiatric admission:

History-gathering. This is basic to family work for all psychiatric disturbances, including those that are HIV-related. History-gathering through family is especially helpful when working with patients who are grossly psychotic or demented and therefore compromised as historians. Sometimes, subtle signs of dementia such as memory impairment or change in personality are first noticed by significant others.

Support for the family. The patient's family is often in turmoil about the patient's psychiatric disorder and will benefit from staff explanation of the illness and its treatment. Also, family members benefit from an opportunity to ventilate some of the intense feelings they experience as they live with or take care of their loved one with AIDS. In some instances, families first learn of AIDS and a person's homsexuality and/or drug use during the acute crisis that leads to hospitalization. Sometimes families require referral for their own sources of mental health care. In areas where HIV is prevalent, self-help and therapist-led groups are increasingly being offered for the various caregivers of people with AIDS.

Psychiatric units that treat several patients with HIV disease simultaneously should consider offering these patients' families a support group. If this is not feasible, referral to a local support group, usually sponsored by an AIDS service organization, may be offered.

Disposition planning. The treatment team must plan an appropriate disposition for the patient. Of course, this cannot be done without collaboration from the patient's support system. Patients with advanced disease frequently exceed the ability of loved ones to provide necessary care. The staff's ability to organize in-home services will often determine whether the patient returns home or is discharged to institutional care.

CONTROVERSIES IN TREATMENT

From its beginning, HIV has created many controversies that continue to plague patients, clinicians, and institutions. Political, economic, legal, and ethical issues continue to change the nature of the epidemic and bear directly on clinical decisions.

HIV Antibody Testing

A great amount of debate in American medicine has focused on when, why, and on whom HIV antibody testing should be performed (33). In the period immediately following the discovery of HIV, critics of the antibody test pointed out its significant liability for false positive and false negative readings. Technological advances have reduced (but not eliminated) these problems. Some experts have advised widespread antibody testing, arguing from a public health perspective. Testing would measure actual numbers of Americans who are infected, may reduce the infection's spreading, allows for early treatment intervention (with such drugs as zidovudine and pentamidine in aerosol form), and may improve the prognosis of individual patients. Others, who have raised objections to widespread testing, focus on the discrimination that often results once an individual is known to be infected (e.g., losing insurance, job, home) and on the mental health complications of learning one has a potentially terminal illness.

Research studies examining the relationship between antibody testing and behavioral change have primarily looked at self-selected gay males and lack long-term follow-up. Little is clearly understood about the relationship between testing, chronic substance abuse, and behavioral change. Likewise, the impact of testing on people with inadequte access to medical and psy-

chological services is unknown. However, all studies suggest a complex relationship between behavior, knowledge, and psychosocial supports. Antibody testing alone, with or without knowledge of one's personal risk for HIV, does not necessarily lead to appropriate behavioral changes.

Until one or another of the above concerns are refuted, which is unlikely in the immediate future, debate will likely continue about policies of widespread HIV antibody testing. In the meantime, clinicians must judiciously assess when the use of the test is appropriate (i.e., used to benefit the care of the patient) in each clinical situation.

Confidentiality Versus Duty to Warn

Clinicians working with infected patients can feel trapped between apparently conflicting ethical standards (34, 35). When a patient infected with HIV is having unprotected sex with a known other person and will not inform that person, what should the therapist do? The rubric of therapist-patient confidentiality posits that informing the person at risk violates the patient's trust and privilege. Many states have laws expressly forbidding release of information regarding HIV infection without the informed written consent of the patient. On the other hand, society's expectation that mental health practitioners warn victims of harm, demonstrated in the Tarasoff case (see Chapter 15), urges clinicians to warn and protect the "victim." Lawsuits are pending in which clinicians failed to warn "victims" of HIV infection.

The problem of whether or not to warn will plague inpatient staffs discharging infected patients unwilling to reveal their infection to their sexual partners. Efforts to engage patients in examining their reluctance to reveal their medical condition to their partner can sometimes resolve this dilemma. At other times, these attempts do not succeed. The American Psychiatric Association and the American Medical Association suggest that in the latter situation a clinician may violate the patient's confidentiality in order to protect another person, specifically if the clinician believes that the other person has no reason to suspect that consenting sexual activity would be risky.

Clinicians and public health officials also debate the use of psychiatric facilities and involuntary hospitalization to contain HIV-infected individuals lacking any major psychiatric disorder who may participate in activities which could transmit HIV. The APA takes the position that psychiatrists should not use involuntary hospitalization for this purpose. While laws vary from state to state, most states have public health statutes that provide for containing individuals with infectious diseases who endanger public safety.

Suicide

Suicide, historically difficult to study, is particularly difficult to study regarding AIDS (36). Despite such problems, Marzuk and associates document a sixfold risk of suicide in patients with AIDS compared with the general population (26). The study implies that a higher incidence of delirium exists in patients with AIDS, leading to impulsive, violent forms of suicide. The enormous stigma associated with the disease, often making patients feel (sometimes realistically) as if they have lost everything or that they will shame their families, may contribute to suicide attempts.

The presence of a terminal illness on the inpatient psychiatric unit complicates the day-to-day management of suicidal patients and raises thorny philosophical issues. Our society generally prohibits acts of suicide but permits competent patients with life-threatening illness to refuse medical treatment that might prolong their lives. Staff members may find themselves in the confusing position of hospitalizing patients against their will because they want to kill themselves and then supporting their decision to refuse treatment for a worsening, but perhaps treatable, medical illness.

Great controversy exists over the concept of rational suicide. Some in our society believe that terminally ill individuals should have the right to terminate their lives when they have had enough of fighting their disease. "Rational suicide" is regarded as a different entity than suicidal action which occurs in the midst of emotional turmoil or organic delirium and is more impulsive than reasoned. Others maintain that no suicide is "rational." Because many psychiatric inpatients are likely to be viewed as in turmoil and having acted impulsively, clinicians will feel relatively confident in their prohibiting further self-destructive behavior. At times, however, less distraught, more reasoned suicidal patients will appear and, particularly if they have advanced disease, will challenge the staff's sense of right and wrong and the goals of caregiving. Many countertransferential issues emerge, including the difficulty in watching young people lose function and experience increasing pain and/or realistic hopelessness about the future. Staff may have conscious or unconscious wishes that the patient die. Staff must feel free to discuss these matters wtih supervisors, in staff meetings, and as a part of the unit's didactic program.

Dedicated Care Units

Many organizers of inpatient medical units that solely provide care to patients with HIV disease believe that these dedicated units deliver better care than the care received by patients dispersed throughout a hospital. Although analogous studies of psychiatric units exist, there have been several reports of inpatient staffs maturing with increased experience with HIV-infected patients (37–39).

Debate continues over whether or not care of HIV patients should be centralized within institutions. From the vantage point of quality of care, worries of increasing patient stigma by creating a "ghetto" appear outweighed by evidence that the staff grows in expertise and compassion and provides better care. From the vantage point of staff burnout, what is better over time is not clear. The size of the hospital, whether the psychiatric unit is freestanding or part of a general medical setting, and the volume of known HIV-infected patients will all be important in determining how care is best delivered.

Substance-Abuse Rehabilitation

In addition to basic detoxification and chemical dependency treatment, questions arise of how best to engage HIV-infected individuals in decreasing risk behaviors (i.e., needle sharing, sexual activity under the influence of substances or for money to buy drugs) and in rehabilitation. For many drug-dependent people, the challenge of living with AIDS is hardly a source of motivation to give up drugs. Furthermore, for those who want treatment and enter programs, patient management is often more complex than for the nonmedically ill client. Advancing physical disability interferes with the ability to participate fully in the treatment program. Treatment on demand for substance abuse is essential for treating individuals who may be able to respond to the crisis. Clearly, although the ability to provide chemical dependence treatment on demand has enormous political, economic, and social implications, it is necessary for preventing the increasing transmission of HIV. For opiate-dependent patients who experience an increase in emotion and/or physical pain, daily methadone needs may increase (40). Additionally, the degree to which having HIV stigmatizes the individual within the drug treatment program itself

varies according to staff and client experience and understanding of HIV infection.

Access to Care

Is mental health care a right or a privilege? Do practitioners have the right to refuse to see patients because of perceived personal risk or other objection to dealing with an HIV-infected client? In an era of fiscal problems, mental health care is often the first to be eliminated by insurance carriers and government-sponsored programs. How will the swelling numbers of HIV-infected people be cared for?

Link of Psychiatric Diagnosis to HIV Risk Behavior

The prospect of offering AIDS education and reducing risky behavior in the entire population of patients with major mental disorders seems daunting. A better understanding of the link between psychiatric illness and risk behaviors would help clinicians refine their approaches to risk reduction. Current and commonly held views assert that patients with bipolar disorders (mania), significant character pathology, and substance-abuse disorders are at particularly high risk of participating in HIV transmission. More passive, dysfunctional patients on psychiatric units may be at risk for unwanted sexual exposure. Although research has yet to confirm such suspicions, experience suggests that the incidence of HIV infection is increasing in the homeless (in whom major mental disorders are prevalent).

COURSE AND PROGNOSIS

While the long-term prognosis for people with advanced HIV disease (AIDS) generally continues to be poor, the natural history of the infection is variable and under the influence of earlier medical interventions. While no single agent is yet curative or able to prolong life indefinitely, hope exists for a regimen of chemotherapies (in sequence or combination) that will prolong the asymptomatic state of HIV infection indefinitely or at least significantly. However, this success may increase the number of people living longer with a potentially transmissable infection and require lifelong changes in behavior that puts others at risk. Mental health and medical interventions will be needed by more people for a longer time.

The prognosis for someone with HIV will change as newer therapies become available and stategies are developed for coping with a chronic illness. Current studies strongly suggest early diagnosis and treatment of the medical and psychological problems associated with HIV infection are helpful. Aggressively assessing and treating the systemic, neuropsychiatric, and psychosocial problems of those who are HIV infected or at risk is clearly beneficial. Unfortunately, acccess to adequate medical care and funds to pay for expensive antiviral therapy and prophylaxis for opportunistic infections are not uniformly available to patients with chronic mental illness.

Mental health providers can have a significant impact on the quality of life of patients and significant others. Inpatient psychiatric units will play an increasing role in diagnosing and treating acute neuropsychiatric disturbances in people infected with HIV. Helping patients and significant others early on with difficult management issues and the psychological stress of living with a chronic disease so stigmatized and economically draining is a crucial aspect of comprehensive care. Helping patients who seek early intervention emotionally to manage the difficult medical procedures and treatments for HIV is also essential. Finally, when all that is medically possible has been done, mental health providers must not underestimate the importance of standing by the patient and providing a constant presence at a time when all else may be withdrawn. The clinician helps some people to live with this disease, others to die with it, and those left to grieve.

REFERENCES

1. Centers for Disease Control: Revision of the CDC surveillance case definition for acquired immunodeficiency syndrome. MMWR, 36(1S):3S–15S, 1987.

2. Bacchetti P, Moss AR: Incubation period of AIDS in San Francisco. Nature, 338:251–253, 1989.

3. Burke DS, Brundage JF, Redfield RR, et al.: Measurement of the false positive rate in a screening program for human immunodeficiency virus infections. N Engl J Med, 319:961–964, 1988.

4. Imagawa DT, Lee MH, Wolinsky SM, et al.: Human immunodeficiency virus type I infection in homosexual men who remain seronegative for prolonged periods. N Engl J Med, 320:1458–1462, 1989.

5. Ho DD, Pomerantz RJ, Kaplan JC: Pathogenesis of infection with human immunodeficiency virus. N Engl J Med, 317:278–286, 1987.

6. Gottlieb GJ, Ragaz A, Vogel JA, et al.: A preliminary communication on extensively disseminated Kaposi's sarcoma in young homosexual men. Am J Dermatopathol, 3(2):111–114, 1981.

7. Leads from the MMWR: Quarterly report to the domestic policy council on the prevalence and rate of spread of HIV and AIDS—United States. JAMA, 260:1845–1851, 1988.

8. D'aquila RT, Peterson LR, Williams AB, Williams AE: Race/ethnicity as a risk factor for HIV–1 infection among Connecticut intravenous drug users. J Acquir Imume Defic Syndr, 2:503–513, 1989.

9. Gardner LI, Brundage JF, Burke DS, McNeil JG, Visintine R, Miller RN: Evidence for spread of the human immunodeficiency virus epidemic into low prevalence areas of the United States. J Acquir Immune Defic Syndr, 2:521–532, 1989.

10. Levy RM, Bredesen DE, Rosenblum ML: Neurological manifestations of the acquired immunodeficiency syndrome (AIDS): Experience

at UCSF and review of the literature. J Neurosurg, 62:475–495, 1985.

11. Levy RM, Bredesen DE: Central nervous system dysfunction in acquired immunodeficiency syndrome, in Rosenblum ML, Levy RM, Bredesen DE (eds): *AIDS and the Nervous System*, pp. 29–63, New York, Raven Press, 1988.

12. Navia BA, Jordan BD, Price RW: The AIDS dementia complex. I. Clinical features. Ann Neurol, 19:517–524, 1986.

13. McArthur JC, Cohen BA, Selnes OA: Low prevalence of neurological and neuropsychological abnormalities in healthy HIV–1 infected individuals: Results from the Multicenter AIDS Cohort Study. Ann Neurol, Vol. 26 no 5 November 1989.

14. Goethke KE, Mitchell JE, Marshall DW, et al.: Neuropsychological and neurological function of human immunodeficiency virus seropositive asymptomatic individuals. Arch Neurol, 46:129–133, 1989.

15. Grant I, Atkinson JH, Hesselink JR: Evidence for early central nervous system involvement in the acquired immunodeficiency syndrome (AIDS) and other human immunodeficiency virus (HIV) infections. Ann Intern Med, 107:828–836, 1987.

16. De LaMonte SM, Ho DD, Schooley RT, Hirsch MS, Richardson EP: Subacute encephalomyelitis of AIDS and its relation to HTLV-III infection. Neurology, 37:562–569, 1987.

17. Dilley JW: Treatment interventions and approaches to care of patients with acquired immune deficiency syndrome, in Nichols SE, Ostrow DG (eds): *Psychiatric Implications of Acquired Immune Deficiency Syndrome*, pp. 61–70, Washington, D.C., American Psychiatric Press, 1984.

18. Sontag S: *Illness as Metaphor*, pp. 49–56, New York, Vintage Books, 1977.

19. Baer JW: Study of 60 patients with AIDS or AIDS-related complex requiring psychiatric hospitalization. Am J Psychiatry, 146:1285–1288, 1989.

20. Perry S, Jacobsen P: Neuropsychiatric manifestations of AIDS-spectrum disorders. Hosp Community Psychiatry, 37:135–142, 1986.

21. Gable RH, Barnard N, Norko M, O'Connell RA: AIDS presenting as mania. Compr Psychiatry, 27:251–254, 1986.

22. Kermani EJ, Borod JC, Brown P, Tunnell G: New psychopathologic findings in AIDS: Case report. J Clin Psychiatry, 46:240–241, 1985.

23. Dilley JW, Ochitill HN, Perl M, Volberding PA: Findings in psychiatric consultations with acquired immune deficiency syndrome. Am J Psychiatry, 142:82–86, 1985.

24. Rundell JR, Wise MG, Ursano RJ: Three cases of AIDS-related psychiatric disorders. Am J Psychiatry, 143:777–778, 1986.

25. Nurnberg HG, Prudic J, Fiori M, Freedman EP: Psychopathology complicating acquired immune deficiency syndrome (AIDS). Am J Psychiatry, 141:95–96, 1985.

26. Marzuk PM, Tierney H, Tardiff K, et al.: Increased risk of suicide in persons with AIDS. JAMA, 259:1333–1337, 1988.

27. Horowitz MJ, Wilner N, Marmar C, Krupnick J: Pathological grief and the activation of latent self-images. Am J Psychiatry, 137:1157–1162, 1980.

28. Fernandez F, Adams F, Levy JK, Holmes VF, Neidhart M, Mansell PWA: Cognitive impairment due to AIDS-related complex and its response to psychostimulants. Psychosomatics, 29:38–46, 1988.

29. Holmes VF, Fernandez F, Levy JK: Psychostimulant response in AIDS-related complex (ARC) patients. J Clin Psychiatry, 50:5–8, 1989.

30. Schmitt FA, Bigley JW, McKinnis R, et al.: Neuropsychological outcome of zidovudine (AZT) treatment of patients with AIDS and AIDS-related complex. N Engl J Med, 319:1573–1578, 1988.

31. Marcus R and the CDC Cooperative Needlestick Surveillance Group: Surveillance of health care workers exposed to blood from patients with the human immunodeficiency virus. N Engl J Med, 319:1118–1123, 1988.

32. Dilley JW, Forstein M: Psychosocial aspects of the human immunodeficiency virus epidemic, in Tasman A, Goldfinger SM, Kaufman CA (eds): *Review of Psychiatry, 9*, Washington, D.C., American Psychiatric Press, 1990.

33. Weiss R, Thier SO: HIV testing is the answer—what's the question? N Engl J Med, 319:1010–1012, 1988.

34. Perry S: Warning third parties at risk of AIDS: APA's policy is a barrier to treatment. Hosp Community Psychiatry, 40:158–161, 1989.

35. Zonana H: Warning third parties at risk of AIDS: APA's policy is a reasonable approach. Hosp Community Psychiatry, *40*:162–164, 1989.

36. Engelman J, Hessol NA, Lifson AR, et al.: Suicide patterns and AIDS in San Francisco. Presentation at IVth International Conference on AIDS, Stockholm, Sweden, June 12–16, 1988.

37. Amchin J, Polan HJ: A longitudinal account of staff adaptation to AIDS patients on a psychiatric unit. Hosp Community Psychiatry, *37*:1235–1238, 1986.

38. Baer JW, Hall JM, Holm K, Lewitter-Koehler S: Challenges in developing an inpatient psychiatric program for patients with AIDS and ARC. Hosp Community Psychiatry, *38*:1299–1303, 1987.

39. Cournos F, Empfield M, Horwath E, Kramer M: The management of HIV infections in state psychiatric hospitals. Hosp Community Psychiatry, *40*:153–164, 1989.

40. Batki SL: Methadone treatment and HIV infection. Focus A Guide to AIDS Research, 4(3):1–2, 1989.

8

Organic Mental Disorders

Barry S. Fogel, MD

ORGANIC MENTAL DISORDERS IN INPATIENT PSYCHIATRY

In recent years, organic mental disorders have become more prevalent on inpatient psychiatric units, and the inpatient psychiatrist's role in diagnosing and treating organic disorders has become more prominent. Several factors have contributed:

1. Increased prevalence of age-associated neurologic diseases, such as Alzheimer's and Parkinson's, frequently associated with depression or psychosis (1, 2).
2. Increased prevalence of drug-induced mental disorders due to the proliferation of prescription drugs and the cocaine abuse epidemic.
3. Increased recognition of organic problems because of new diagnostic technologies.
4. Increased availability and awareness of effective therapies for organically-based psychopathology (e.g., effective treatment for poststroke depression) (3).
5. Longer survival in neoplastic and autoimmune diseases in which either the disease or the therapy may cause psychiatric complications.
6. Changes in the organization and financing of health care leading to more rapid

extrusion of behaviorally complex patients from general medical settings.
7. The AIDS (acquired immune deficiency syndrome) epidemic (4).

This chapter will focus on selected issues of particular pertinence to the practice of general inpatient psychiatry in diagnosing and managing organic mental syndromes. The reader is referred to comprehensive texts on organic psychiatry (5) and neuropsychiatry (6, 7) for further details and discussing of syndromes less frequently encountered in general inpatient psychiatry, e.g., isolated parietal lobe dysfunction. Issues addressed here include the definition and limits of the "organic" category, diagnosis and management of delirium and dementia in inpatient psychiatry, frontal lobe syndromes, psychiatric syndromes caused by complex partial seizures (temporal lobe epilepsy), and evaluation of the general psychiatric inpatient for causal or contributory organic disease.

Definition and Limits of the "Organic" Category

The category of organic mental syndromes and disorders comprises mental syndromes caused by brain dysfunction re-

212

sulting from primary neurologic disease, drugs, or systemic illness (8). The category includes syndromes involving a diffuse disturbance of cognitive function, such as delirium or dementia, and syndromes with little or no cognitive disturbance, such as the organic personality disorder associated with temporal lobe epilepsy. The boundary between organic and other mental disorders shifts over time, both within the field of psychiatry and for particular patients. Historically, mental disorders have been reclassified as organic when a specific underlying brain dysfunction was found, such as when syphilitic infection was found to cause general paresis of the insane. For an individual patient, a major depressive episode may eventually turn out to be an early symptom of a systemic or neurologic disease, such as pancreatic carcinoma or Alzheimer's disease, justifying its reclassification as an organic mood disorder (9).

Despite the instability of the diagnostic boundary between organic and other mental disorders, the category has proved useful over time to identify a class of disorders often requiring a distinctive approach to management. Syndromes such as delirium that suggest a specific organic cause require an aggressive search for a specific and, it is hoped, remediable etiology (10). In other cases, such as Parkinson's disease, although the neurologic cause of a psychiatric disorder is not reversible, the neurologic disease has implications for the prognosis of the associated psychopathologic symptoms and for the therapy of those symptoms. The burgeoning field of neuropsychiatry focuses attention on the frequent psychiatric complications of neurologic diseases; neuropsychiatric research has established that location and type of brain injury may strongly influence the prognosis and phenomenology of organically caused disturbances of mood, behavior, or thinking (6).

As the revised third edition of the *Diagnostic and Statistical Manual of Mental Dis-* *orders* (DSM-IIIR) itself cautions, the presence of an organic diagnosis does not imply that developmental, environmental, or intrapsychic factors are unimportant, nor does it imply that abnormal brain function does not underlie major psychiatric disorders such as depression or schizophrenia. As will be discussed below, identifying *contributory* organic factors in cases of major primary mental disorders is an important ingredient in successful treatment planning.

DELIRIUM AND DEMENTIA

Delirium and dementia, syndromes characterized by generalized cognitive impairment, are the classic organic mental syndromes widely recognized by physicians of all specialties as indicating the presence of a neurologic or systemic disease. In addition to cognitive impairment, cardinal features of delirium include:

1. Prominent disturbance in attention and concentration.
2. Disorganized thinking or incoherence.
3. Acute or subacute onset.
4. Fluctuation often within minutes or hours.
5. Associated features, which can be florid, and include:
   a. Altered consciousness
   b. Perceptual disturbances
   c. Altered sleep-wake cycles
   d. Increased or decreased psychomotor activity
   e. Disorientation to time, place, or situation.

By contrast, patients with dementia have impaired memory and other cognitive functions disproportionate to disturbances in attention and consciousness. Attention and consciousness usually are normal in patients with mild dementia. Although the onset of dementia is often subacute or insidious, it may on occasion be sudden if caused by a specific brain injury such as head trauma or stroke. If fluctuation occurs, it is not rapid and usually attributable to specific changes in physical health, environment, or mood state.

In their prototypic cases, delirium and dementia are readily distinguishable. However, distinction is difficult in two situations: one, when delirium is superimposed upon dementia; the other, when the etiology of the dementia includes specific brain injury that produces prominent disturbances of attention and orientation such as a right parietal lobe stroke.

Delirium and dementia, *syndrome* diagnoses, can be diagnosed even when a specific organic cause for the syndrome is not known. Diagnosing dementia or delirium as a syndrome requires a subsequent thorough search for the underlying etiology, paying particular attention to finding those etiologies that can be reversed or arrested. The next sections will address diagnostic problems of delirium and dementia particularly relevant to inpatient psychiatric practice.

Delirium

Diagnostic problems associated with delirium differ according to whether the delirium is mild or severe. In the case of mild delirium, the initial problem is deciding whether the patient's mental syndrome represents a delirium or is better explained by an alternate mental diagnosis such as a brief reactive psychosis or a hypomanic episode. In more severe cases of delirium, with striking and fluctuating alterations of orientation and consciousness, the *syndrome* diagnosis is rarely in doubt; however, *etiologic* diagnosis is urgent—severe delirium suggests potentially life-threatening medical illness (10, 11).

The *syndrome* differential diagnosis for mild delirium is set forth in Table 8.1. Brief reactive psychosis and atypical psychosis are in fact diagnoses of exclusion because they can be completely mimicked by delirium. Mood disorders, both depressive and

Table 8.1. Syndrome Differential Diagnosis of Mild Delirium

Brief reactive psychosis
Atypical psychosis
Mania or hypomania with cognitive impairment
Depression with cognitive impairment
Dissociative disorders
Other organic disorders:
— psychoactive substance intoxication
— psychoactive substance withdrawal
— psychoactive substance hallucinosis
— dementia

manic, can at times be accompanied by such significant cognitive impairment, sleep disturbance, or agitation that they mimic delirium. Dissociative disorders, particularly if marked by amnesia and bizarre behavior, may resemble delirium; a specific differential diagnosis is between psychogenic fugue and epileptic fugue states. Among other organic disorders, many of the psychoactive substance-induced organic mental syndromes are classified as deliria or not based on a judgment about the relative prominence of disturbed cognition as opposed to other psychological and behavioral symptoms.

While a conclusive syndrome diagnosis between mild delirium and alternative diagnoses is not always possible on a single cross-sectional evaluation, the diagnosis of delirium is suggested by cognitive impairment disproportionate to other psychopathology and rapid fluctuations (from hour to hour) in attention and orientation. The most useful laboratory test to support the syndrome diagnosis of a mild delirium is the electroencephalogram (EEG) (12, 13). Most delirious episodes are associated with a characteristic change in the EEG—a slowing of the dominant background rhythm (13). When a baseline EEG is available, slowing of the background can be demonstrated in most cases of delirium. However, in milder cases of delirium, slowing of the background may still leave the patient's background rhythm within normal limits, leading to a false negative assessment when no baseline EEG is available. Some causes of delirium produce not only background slowing, but also characteristic specific EEG findings, such as triphasic waves in hepatic encephalopathy and recurrent seizure discharges in nonconvulsive status epilepticus (14, 15).

When a mild delirium is suspected but the *syndrome* diagnosis is not clear, the following steps may be useful:

1. Obtaining an EEG and comparing it with baseline tracings, if they are available.
2. Structured assessment of orientation and cognition every shift for 24–48 hours, using an instrument such as the Mini-Mental State Examination (16).
3. A sleep chart.
4. Diagnostic assessment of *suspected* organic etiologies such as electrolyte disturbance or drug intoxication.

In cases of severe delirium, the dramatic alterations and fluctuations in attention, orientation, cognition, and psychomotor state leave few differential diagnostic possibilities except for very acute and severe psychiatric disorders such as catatonic excitement or acute mania with confusional features (delirious mania) (17). On occasion, severe agitated depression in a patient with an underlying dementia may mimic severe delirium. However, because of the association of severe delirium with medical conditions that are dangerous if untreated, a full etiologic workup for delirium is warranted even when the patient is thought to have a primary psychiatric illness.

THE ETIOLOGIC WORKUP FOR DELIRIUM

While it is generally recognized that delirium may be induced by virtually any significant medical illness (see Table 8.2), a

Table 8.2. Etiology of Delirium

INTOXICATIONS
a. *Medications*—Anticholinergics, tricyclic antidepressants, lithium, sedative-hypnotics, antihypertensive agents, antiarrhythmic drugs, digitalis, anticonvulsants, antiparkinsonian agents, steroids and anti-inflammatory drugs, analgesics (opiates and nonnarcotic), disulfiram, antibiotics, antineoplastic drugs, cimetidine
b. *Drugs of abuse*—phencyclidine and hallucinogenic agents
c. *Alcohol*
d. *Poisons*—heavy metals, organic solvents, methyl alcohol ethylene glycol, insecticides, carbon monoxide

WITHDRAWAL SYNDROMES
a. *Alcohol*
b. *Sedatives and hypnotics*

METABOLIC
a. *Hypoxia*
b. *Hypoglycemia*
c. *Acid-base imbalance*—acidosis, alkalosis
d. *Electrolyte imbalance*—elevated or decreased sodium, potassium, calcium, magnesium

e. *Water imbalance*—inappropriate antidiuretic hormone, water intoxication, dehydration
f. *Failure of vital organs*—liver, kidney, lung, pancreas
g. *Inborn errors of metabolism*—porphyria, Wilson's disease, carcinoid syndrome
h. *Remote effects of carcinoma*
i. *Vitamin deficiency*—thiamine (Wernicke's encephalopathy), nicotinic acid, folate, cyanocobalamin

ENDOCRINE
a. *Thyroid*—thyrotoxicosis, myxedema
b. *Parathyroid*—hypo- and hyperparathyroidism
c. *Adrenal*—Addison's disease, Cushing's syndrome
d. *Pancreas*—hyperinsulinism, diabetes
e. *Pituitary hypofunction*

CARDIOVASCULAR
a. *Congestive heart failure*
b. *Cardiac arrhythmia*
c. *Myocardial infarction*

NEUROLOGICAL
a. *Head trauma*
b. *Space-occupying lesions*—tumor, subdural hematoma, abscess, aneurysm

c. *Cerebrovascular disease*—thrombosis, embolism, arteritis, hemorrhage, hypertensive encephalopathy
d. *Degenerative disorders*—Alzheimer's disease, multiple sclerosis
e. *Epilepsy*
f. *Migraine*

INFECTION
a. *Intracranial*—encephalitis and meningitis (viral, bacterial, fungal, protozoal)
b. *Systemic*—pneumonia, septicemia, subacute bacterial endocarditis, influenza, typhoid, typhus, infectious mononucleosis, infectious hepatitis, acute rheumatic fever, malaria, mumps, diphtheria, etc.

HEMATOLOGICAL
a. *Pernicious anemia*
b. *Bleeding diatheses*
c. *Polycythemia*

HYPERSENSITIVITY
a. *Serum sickness*
b. *Food allergy*

PHYSICAL INJURY
a. *Heat*—hyperthermia, hypothermia
b. *Electricity*
c. *Burns*

Table 8.3. Common Medication-Induced Deliria

Type	Usual Provoking Agents	Typical Features	Special Diagnostic Points	Specific Treatment	Prevention
Anticholinergic	Tricyclic antidepressants Low-potency neuroleptics Anticholinergic antiparkinson drugs Anticholinergic antihistamines OTC cold remedies	Agitation Visual hallucinations Fever Peripheral signs and symptoms Tachycardia, dry mouth, constipation, urinary retention, dry skin, dilated pupils	Peripheral signs may be mild or absent in elderly patients Lack of sweating and of rigidity may help differentiate from NMS May be caused by polypharmacy with each drug at a nontoxic level	Check EKG Physostigmine (see text)	Bias toward less anticholinergic alternatives within drug classes, e.g., amantadine over benztropine; nortriptylene over amitriptylene Patient education on risks of OTC agents
Lithium	Lithium aggravated by: neuroleptics, anticonvulsants (carbamazepine, valproate, phenytoin) Anticholinergic agents Drugs raising lithium levels (e.g., diuretics, ACE inhibitors)	Tremor, often coarse Involuntary movements Rigidity (especially if given with neuroleptics)	EEG abnormalities may be striking and lack paroxysmal features Syndrome may overlap with NMS: assessment for rhabdomyolysis is necessary if rigidity is pronounced May occur with "therapeutic" lithium level in presence of other drugs in preexisting neuroleptic disease	Special care for hydration Intervention for NMS if needed Monitor kidney	Conservative lithium dosage Recheck lithium levels after adding new drugs

Syndrome	Drugs	Signs and symptoms	Evaluation	Treatment	Prevention
Impaired dopaminergic transmission	Neuroleptics Metaclopromide Aggravated by: lithium, carbamazepine Serotonergic agents*	Agitation or catatonia Rigidity, especially in the neck Unstable vital signs Diaphoresis	CPK and urine myoglobin to be checked to evaluate rhabdomyolysis Sweating distinguishes from anticholinergic toxicity EEG may be abnormal Hypokinesia and quiet confusion in milder cases	Monitor CPK and kidney function Dopamine agonists: bromocriptine amantadine (in milder cases) Dantrolene for severe muscle rigidity Benzodiazepines if a drug is needed for agitation	Conservative neuroleptic dosage Amantadine therapy of milder extrapyramidal side effects**
Sedative-hypnotic	Benzodiazepines (especially short-acting) Barbiturates Street drugs, e.g., "Quaaludes"	Toxicity: Dysarthria Nystagmus Drowsiness or disinhibition Withdrawal: agitation, tachycardia and hypertension Seizures Tremor or myoclonus	"Toxic" blood levels not needed, especially in elderly or brain-injured Detailed drug history, including collateral sources, may help Conventional benzodiazepines may not "cover" alprazolam withdrawal	Intoxication: assess respiratory status Withdrawal: replace drug to stop symptoms, then taper slowly	Careful admission drug history Avoid sedative-hypnotic in elderly and brain-injured patients
Serotonin excess	combination of: MAOI and tricyclic antidepressants fluoxetine tryptophan	Tremor Nystagmus Dysarthria Myoclonus Fever	Distinguished from NMS by lesser abnormality of vital signs and rigidity is rare Myoclonus, "chattering teeth" or other signs of neuromuscular irritability are common	Cyproheptadine* Propranolol* benzodiazepines if a drug needed for agitation Dantrolene if NMS-like syndrome develops	Slow dosage titration if serotonergic drugs must be combined Long withdrawal period between stopping fluoxetine and starting MAOI; consider a fluoxetine level before starting MAOI

*Indicates a less firmly established connection.
**Option suggested by anecdote but not well-established.

relatively small number of medical and neurological conditions account for the majority of cases of delirium found in inpatient psychiatric units. An effective workup for the etiology of delirium must be organized to quickly diagnose common and reversible conditions; more diagnostic tests should be added if the delirium persists. Structuring the workup is particularly relevant regarding timing tests such as brain imaging and lumbar puncture that may be expensive, inconvenient, or uncomfortable.

The most common etiology of delirium encountered on general psychiatric inpatient units is *medication.*

MEDICATION-INDUCED DELIRIUM

Medication or its withdrawal can induce delirium which may be caused by either psychotropic drugs or drugs prescribed for concurrent medical conditions. The most common psychotropic drug-induced delirious states are caused by *anticholinergic toxicity; lithium toxicity; impaired dopaminergic transmission,* usually from neuroleptics given alone or in combination with other drugs; *sedative-hypnotic agents;* and *serotonin excess.* Important features of these five drug-induced deliria are presented in Table 8.3. The text will add additional fine points concerning each of the five conditions. Regarding the treatment recommendations of the table, it is assumed that all patients will receive good general supportive care, including monitoring of vital signs, attention to hydration, protection from self-injury, and, most importantly, removal of the offending agent. Patients whose medical instability exceeds the capacities of the inpatient psychiatric unit would be transferred to a medical ward or intensive care unit. The table concentrates only on those measures relatively specific to the etiologic drug class.

1. Anticholinergic toxicity (18–24).

The general features of anticholinergic toxicity, familiar to most psychiatrists, are summarized in the table. The following points are of special interest:

a. Anticholinergic toxicity frequently results from the additive anticholinergic effects of several drugs. An assay of total cholinergic receptor blocking activity, unfortunately not yet generally available, has shown to correlate with the presence of postoperative delirium (24). Therefore, levels in "therapeutic range" for each of several anticholinergic drugs do not rule out this syndrome.

b. Anticholinergic delirium is often considered in patients taking neuroleptics and anticholinergic antiparkinson medication. In this situation the key differential diagnosis is between anticholinergic toxicity and neuroleptic malignant syndrome (NMS). Dry skin and absence of muscular rigidity favor anticholinergic toxicity; rigidity and diaphoresis favor NMS (25).

c. Physostigmine challenge may be both diagnostic and therapeutic in this condition. One to two mg i.v. may rapidly improve mental state and peripheral signs. However, the technique has fallen out of favor because of potential complications of heart block, respiratory arrest, seizures, bronchospasm, and g.i. side effects (18). Physostigmine challenge would now deserve consideration only if the anticholinergic delirium were itself life-threatening. In this situation, the challenge should be administered in an acute medical setting with continuous cardiac monitoring.

2. Lithium toxicity.

Because lithium has such a low therapeutic index and the early signs of lithium toxicity may be nonspecific, a lithium level is indicated any time a lithium-treated patient shows a change in mental status (26–29). Additional special considerations are as follows:

a. Lithium is implicated in many drug interactions, both pharmacokinetic and pharmacodynamic. The important kinetic interactions occur when drugs such as diuretics or ACE (angiotensin converting enzyme) inhibitors raise lithium levels to the toxic range (30). Significant dynamic interactions occur with neuroleptics, anticonvulsants, and anticholinergic agents. In the presence of these drugs, lithium toxicity may occur at "therapeutic" serum levels.

b. Lithium toxicity has prominent neuromuscular symptoms, including tremor, rigidity, and involuntary movements. The more severe forms may overlap with neuroleptic malignant syndrome. When they do, assessment for muscle breakdown (rhabdomyolysis) is necessary, checking blood CPK (creatine phosphokinase) and urine myoglobin levels. NMS-like symptoms occurring on lithium should be treated as if they were NMS; the risks of renal and systemic complications are comparable.

c. Host factors are relevant to lithium toxicity: brain damaged, mentally retarded, or elderly patients are more likely to show toxic symptoms at "therapeutic" blood levels.

3. Toxicity from impaired dopaminergic transmission.

While NMS is now well-known to virtually all psychiatrists, it is important to appreciate that a spectrum of neuroleptic-induced CNS toxicity exists, including milder forms with varying combinations of delirious symptoms and extrapyramidal motor involvement (25, 31, 32). For example, a quiet confusional state with akinesia and mild muscular rigidity can be encountered. The following points deserve emphasis:

a. Drugs such as lithium and carbamazepine that affect dopamine receptor sensitivity (33) or reduce dopamine levels (34) may aggravate toxicity from dopamine receptor blockade.

b. In evaluating milder cases, the best place to look for rigidity is in the neck. A rigid neck may often be encountered before the limbs are conspicuously rigid. Also, tremulous rigidity, or "cogwheeling," an inconstant feature of neuroleptic toxicity, should not be required to diagnose extrapyramidal side effects.

c. Because NMS is life-threatening and its specific treatment is relatively benign, there should be a bias in favor of treating presumptive cases.

d. When treating an agitated delirium possibly caused by impaired dopaminergic transmission, benzodiazepines are the drug of choice for managing agitation (35).

4. Toxicity of sedative-hypnotic agents.

Occasionally, although sedative-hypnotic agents produce delirium from intoxication, more often delirium results from withdrawal (36–48). Elderly patients or patients with preexisting CNS (central nervous system) disease are at higher risk. Specific points worthy of attention are as follows:

a. Short-acting hypnotic drugs such as triazolam may produce confusional or amnestic states, even from single doses in patients without preexisting organic impairment (49).

b. Abrupt discontinuation of sedative-hypnotics sometimes takes place inadvertently upon admission or transfer to a psychiatric inpatient unit. Patients may deny or minimize outside drug use, or data on previous drug use may not be transferred properly when a patient is moved from one unit to another.

c. Alprazolam or clonazepam withdrawal may not be completely covered by older benzodiazepines such as diazepam. A patient suspected of alprazolam or clonazepam withdrawal should be replaced with clonazepam. The longer duration of action of the latter drug makes it easier to taper (50, 51).

d. Patients with benzodiazepine toxicity

deserve clinical assessment of pulmonary function, with an arterial blood gas test if there is any clinical risk of CO_2 retention (52).

5. Delirium from serotonin excess.
With the increasing popularity of monoamine oxidase inhibitors (MAOIs) and serotonin reuptake blocking drugs such as fluoxetine (Prozac), clinicians on inpatient units have begun to encounter delirium caused by serotonin excess. Although symptoms may occur spontaneously, more often they occur when drugs that enhance serotonin transmission are combined, such as when an MAO inhibitor is added to fluoxetine, tricyclics and fluoxetine are taken together, or tryptophan is taken together with one of the serotonergic antidepressants (53, 54). The ensuing "serotonin syndrome" consists of altered mental state (delirium) accompanied by tremor, nystagmus, dysarthria, myoclonus, and fever. On occasion, rigidity resembling NMS may occur (55).

No established treatment exists other than discontinuing the offending medications. Anecdotally, we have learned that both cyproheptadine and propranolol have been used to mitigate symptoms. When symptoms overlap with NMS, treatment for NMS should be considered. Two additional points deserve mention:

a. If a patient with presumed serotonin excess requires treatment for agitation, a benzodiazepine rather than a neuroleptic should be used because of possible adverse interaction between neuroleptics and serotonergic agents.
b. Many severe cases have been related to starting MAOIs after recent discontinuation of fluoxetine. Cases might be prevented by checking that fluoxetine (and norfluoxetine) levels are zero (i.e., below the laboratory's threshold for detection) before starting an MAOI.

NONPSYCHOTROPIC MEDICATIONS

A wide range of nonpsychotropic medications may cause delirium. Elderly patients, patients with preexisting brain disease, and patients receiving multiple drugs are particularly susceptible. Common offending agents are listed in Table 8.4.

Adverse CNS reactions to nonpsychotropic drugs usually occur at one of two times—either when the drug is started or increased or when other aspects of the patient's pharmacotherapy are changed. The diagnosis is more difficult in the latter situation because it requires that the clinician consider the many pharmacokinetic and pharmacodynamic interactions among the drugs the patient is receiving.

A general approach to patients with suspected drug-induced delirium begins by organizing the recent drug history. For inpatients, this includes looking at the medication Kardex, not just the physician's orders, since transcription errors occasionally occur. It also involves reviewing the history of drugs taken during the previous week or two, paying special attention to changes in dosage or the starting and stopping of other medications. If the patient has recently been admitted from home, request that family members or friends bring in the contents of the medicine cabinet in order to assemble the most complete drug history possible. In-

Table 8.4. Common Nonpsychotropic Medications Causing Delirium

Prednisone and other corticosteroids (56–58)
Cimetidine and other H_2-blockers (59–61)
Antiarrhythmics: quinidine, procainamide, lidocaine and tocainide (blood levels helpful) (62, 63)
Digoxin (blood level helpful) (64–69)
Cancer chemotherapy and immunosuppressive drugs (70)
Nonsteroidal anti-inflammatory drugs (especially indomethacin) (62, 71)
Salicylates (blood level is diagnostic) (72)
Narcotics (especially pentazocine and meperidine) (73–77)
Antiparkinson drugs (78–81)

clude over-the-counter drugs, medications prescribed by other doctors, and any medications left from previous episodes of illness that the patient may have used for self-medication.

If the diagnosis is not obvious from the medication history, obtain blood levels of medications for all drugs the patient is taking for. which levels are meaningful. When levels are interpreted, it should be borne in mind that toxicity may occur at a "therapeutic" blood level. In addition to host factors and drug interactions, interpretation of blood levels should also consider protein binding, particularly for drugs that are highly protein-bound. For such drugs, therapeutic and toxic effects depend on the level of free drug, which can be increased either by other drugs that displace the first drug from plasma protein or by a decrease in plasma protein resulting from malnutrition, anorexia, or severe systemic illness. In general, patients with a low serum albumin are at increased risk for toxicity at apparently therapeutic blood levels. Although levels of free drug are sometimes available, they often are difficult to obtain, expensive, and subject to interpretive problems.

Once drug toxicity is diagnosed, make all reasonable efforts to eliminate the drug, reduce its dose, or substitute a less psychotoxic agent. For example, for patients receiving H2-blockers such as cimetidine, sucralfate usually can be substituted; sucralfate, an anti-ulcer drug that is not systemically absorbed, has therefore no CNS side effects.

METABOLIC DISORDERS

While a long list of metabolic disturbances can produce delirium, the ones most commonly encountered on inpatient psychiatric services are electrolyte disturbances—particularly hyponatremia and hypercalcemia—and dehydration. Table 8.5 summarizes metabolic disorders frequently causing delirium in inpatient psychiatric services.

The table emphasizes the etiologies of metabolic disturbances most relevant to the inpatient psychiatric population. Some additional points deserve mention.

1. Mild hyponatremia, in which the serum sodium is between 130–135, is unlikely to produce delirium. Delirium can more confidently be attributed to hyponatremia when sodium is below 125. Even then, however, a medical condition such as cancer may be causing the hyponatremia while independently contributing to the delirium by another mechanism. A full medical and neurologic workup is usually needed, except in those cases when hyponatremia is directly linked to a recently started medication (86).

2. For evaluating patients for dehydration-caused delirium, a careful set of orthostatic vital signs is as important as any blood test and has the advantage of immediate availability.

3. For evaluating patients for hypoglycemia, blood glucose must be obtained at the time of maximum behavioral disturbance; glucose levels may fluctuate significantly, particularly in brittle diabetics. Resolution of symptoms by administering i.v. glucose is diagnostic and therapeutic. If any doubt exists about the patient's overall nutritional status, parenteral thiamine should be given along with the glucose.

4. Thiamine deficiency may be encountered in alcoholic and malnourished populations, the latter including the homeless mentally ill and people with severe eating disorders. The symptoms are nonspecific and the classic triad of ataxia, ophthalmoplegia and confusion often is not present (87). When there is the slightest doubt, administer thiamine.

5. Although patients with acute renal failure rarely present to psychiatric services, aggravations of preexisting chronic renal insufficiency may be encountered, particularly when dehydration, intercurrent infection, or potentially nephrotoxic medications

Table 8.5.   Metabolic Disorders Commonly Causing Delirium on Inpatient Psychiatric Services

Disorder	Test	Frequent Etiologies
Hyponatremia (86)	Sodium	Medication, especially carbamazepine and diuretics SIADH (a) due to neoplasms Congestive heart failure
Dehydration (82)	Elevated BUN (b): creatinine ratio (also check orthostatic vital signs)	Stress Poor oral intake caused by depression or psychosis Increased fluid losses from diuretics, fever, or diarrhea Eating disorders: self-induced vomiting, fasting, or laxative abuse
Hypercalcemia (83)	Calcium Albumin Ionized calcium (if albumin is low and/or calcium is borderline high)	Hyperparathyroidism Malignancy
Hypoglycemia (84)	Blood sugar *during* time of abnormal behavior	Oral hypoglycemics or insulin in diabetes Factitious liver disease Alcoholism
Thiamine deficiency (87)	No standard blood test; neurological examination may show ataxia or nystagmus; memory loss may be prominent	Alcoholism Malnutrition
Aggravation of kidney failure (85)	BUN; creatinine	Dehydration Medications Intercurrent illness
Liver failure (88)	SGOT (c), SGPT (d) Ammonia CSF glutamine EEG: slowing or triphasic waves Asterixis or tremor on neurological examination	Alcoholism Infectious diseases Aggravation by g.i. bleeding or dehydration

a. Syndrome of inappropriate secretion of antidiuretic hormone
b. Blood urea nitrogen
c. Serum glutamic-oxaloacetic transaminase
d. Serum glutamic-pyruvic transaminase

are present. These phenomena deserve particularly close attention when the serum creatinine on admission is greater than 2, since this implies that creatinine *clearance* is already reduced by more than 75%.

6. Patients with chronic liver disease, such as from cirrhosis, may have hepatic encephalopathy despite normal levels of "liver enzymes." In these cases, a venous or arterial ammonia level, a CSF glutamine, or an EEG may be helpful. Asterixis, diagnostically helpful when present, is not a constant feature (88).

7. Alcoholics, patients on total parenteral nutrition (TPN), patients with profound malnutrition, or patients with certain chronic medical illness may be vulnerable to less common metabolic disturbances such as hypophosphatemia (89). In these patients, order additional metabolic tests in keeping with the patient's known medical history. Conditions such as hypophosphatemia, which appear on comprehensive lists of causes of delirium, are remote considerations in patients without specific risk factors.

Resolution of Metabolic Delirium

Delirium from toxic or metabolic problems may not resolve immediately once the toxic or metabolic problem is corrected. Particularly in patients who are aged or have prior neurologic impairment, resolution of symptoms may take several days beyond normalization of "the numbers" (90). Nonetheless, failure of delirium to resolve after several days should raise the suspicion of an error in etiologic diagnosis or the presence of a second diagnosis such as dementia or a primary psychiatric disorder.

DELIRIUM FROM SYSTEMIC DISEASE

Major physical disease of any kind, including such diverse entities as trauma, myocardial infarction, and pancreatitis, may produce delirium without measurable changes in the chemical constituents of the blood (91). The likelihood of delirium is increased if the patient is in pain, has a fever, is dehydrated, or if the condition affects cardiac output. Therefore, the new onset of a delirium warrants a complete physical reassessment of the patient. Naturally, attention should be directed to areas where the patient has a preexisting disease or vulnerability. For example, delirious patients with known lung disease require assessment of arterial blood gases. In structuring a delirium workup, the principle is to begin with a physical and neurological examination and general screening tests, adding those additional tests and investigations linked to the conditions for which the patient is at greatest individual risk (see Table 8.6).

DELIRIUM FROM NEUROLOGICAL DISEASE

Delirium, an acute disturbance of brain function, can be produced by a wide variety of neurologic diseases. Ultimately, deliria not explained by drugs, metabolic problems, or systemic disease indicate a full CNS workup, including brain imaging, EEG, and often a lumbar puncture. However, because most delirious states found in psychiatric inpatient settings are not caused by primary neurologic disease, an early, ag-

Table 8.6. Laboratory Screening of the Delirious Patient

Metabolic Assessment

General: Electrolytes, BUN, creatinine, glucose, calcium, albumin, phosphate, magnesium

Specific: Blood gases (if lung disease known or suspected), ammonia or CSF glutamine (if liver disease known or suspected), trace elements (if patient on TPN), B_{12} and folate (if malnutrition or malabsorption are suspected), porphyrins (in patients with family history of porphyria or atypical syndrome of psychosis, neuropathy, and seizures)

Infectious Disease Screening:

General: CBC and differential, urinalysis, ESR (erythrocyte sedimentation rate), serologic test for syphilis

Specific: Chest x-ray (if pulmonary symptoms or known lung disease), cultures of body fluids (blood, urine, sputum, etc.), serologies (HIV, Epstein-Barr, herpes), CSF examination (if meningeal signs present)

Toxic Assessment:

General: Blood levels of medications and drugs, when they are known to be meaningful

Specific: Urine screening for recent drug abuse

Neurologic Assessment:

General: EEG

Specific: Brain imaging (CT or MRI) (in patients with focal neurologic signs, headache, seizures, risk factors for CNS complications, or otherwise unexplained delirium)
CSF examination (in patients with fever, meningeal signs, headache, or with special vulnerability to CNS infection)

gressive, and expensive workup for CNS disorders is not always appropriate. Make a distinction between "high risk" patients who need an immediate full CNS workup and those for whom the workup is necessary only if the delirium fails to clear and other more common causes are ruled out.

Neurologic causes of delirium include epileptic seizures and postictal states, migraine, stroke, brain tumor, head trauma, hemorrhage, neoplasm, and CNS infection, particularly encephalitis and meningitis. Sexually transmitted diseases affecting the brain, including HIV (human immune deficiency virus) infection and syphilis, may also present with delirium.

Because focal lesions such as strokes and tumors usually cause overt neurologic signs, diagnosis is not difficult. However, there are certain locations where focal brain injury may produce a delirium with few other signs. These locations include the right parietal lobe and the base of the occipital lobes (posterior cerebral artery territory) (92–94). With strokes in these locations, although hemisensory loss or visual field defects are theoretically detectable, they may be difficult to find if the patient's delirium prevents full cooperation with sensory testing. Isolated frontal lobe and temporal lobe lesions also may produce cognitive and behavioral changes disproportionate to changes in motor and sensory function; however, lesions in these locations usually do not cause delirium unless accompanied by seizure activity (5).

Delirium from seizures may either be caused by continual seizure activity (nonconvulsive status epilepticus) or be postictal, following a seizure that frequently is unobserved. Complex partial seizures, as well as full-blown convulsions, may produce postictal delirium.

The Neurologic Workup

The search for primary CNS pathology causing delirium virtually always includes a brain image, such as a CT (computerized tomography) scan or MRI (magnetic resonance imaging), followed by a lumbar puncture if infection is suspected. The lumbar puncture would be indicated if the patient had a fever, headache, stiff neck, or a primary illness known frequently to give rise to meningeal complications. For example, patients with cancer, HIV infection, or a past organ transplant would receive lumbar punctures. Also seriously consider lumbar punctures when assessing patients *without* headache, fever, or meningeal signs who are receiving immunosuppressive drugs that might prevent an inflammatory response to CNS infection.

Lumbar puncture should be supplemented by serologic tests for relevant infections, such as HIV antibodies, a VDRL (Venereal Disease Research Laboratories), and Lyme disease titers where appropriate. Regarding the choice between CT and MRI, MRI is more sensitive to a wider variety of CNS lesions (95). However, the MRI procedure requires the patient to spend a relatively long period in the claustrophobic environment of the scanner. Many delirious patients are not able to tolerate the MRI scan; if patients are medically unstable, an additional drawback is the difficulty in providing emergency medical attention in the MRI suite. If there are unresolved diagnostic issues, however, the MRI can be expected to reveal positive diagnostic findings in many cases where the CT scan is negative.

Perform an EEG in all cases of delirium where either the syndrome diagnosis or the etiology is not readily evident on initial assessment (12). In addition to confirming the syndrome diagnosis by showing slowing of the background, the EEG is the best screen for conditions such as nonconvulsive status epilepticus that can be specifically treated with anticonvulsant drugs. In evaluating a delirium, special EEG lead placements are not necessary, nor are sleep records. However, an important technical point is noting the patient's level of arousal during the EEG recording. Normal patients may show some degree of EEG slowing during drowsiness (96), so that accurate interpretation of mild EEG abnormality requires knowledge of the patient's level of alertness during the recording. Many physicians find the EEG unhelpful because formal readings are frequently equivocal or nonspecific. For best results read the EEG *description* rather than the interpretation, looking for crucial features such as background slowing and the presence or absence of paroxysmal features suggesting seizure activity.

When and How to Seek Neurological Consultation

Ultimately, any unresolved and unexplained delirium warrants consultation by a neurologist. Consultation is most helpful when properly timed and the questions clearly defined. Seek early neurologic consultation in cases where primary neurologic disease is highly likely and beyond the range of problems with which the treating psychiatrist is comfortable. In other cases, neurologic consultation usually is best deferred until the syndrome diagnosis of delirium is established and the most common and obvious medical etiologies have been ruled out. At that point, ask the neurologist specific questions such as what is the relevance of a specific EEG abnormality or the appropriateness of a lumbar puncture, and what CSF examinations should be done. Neurologic consultations obtained before the psychiatrist's initial etiologic evaluation are often disappointing because they require the neurologist to devote time to "boiler plate" suggestions for the standard delirium workup rather than focusing on specific, often subtle, diagnostic issues.

Other Diagnostic Problems

A frequently occurring diagnostic problem for inpatient psychiatry is severe behavioral disturbance in the presence of a relatively mild cognitive disturbance. When this occurs, the patient may be suffering from a delirium superimposed on a preexisting primary mental illness or personality disorder. In the author's experience, delirium, similar to intoxications, may particularly aggravate impulsive behavior in borderline or antisocial personalities. However, the presence of co-morbid pathology should not discourage a thorough workup for the etiology of the delirium.

Delirium Following ECT

Another diagnostic issue concerns the development of delirium following ECT. While a brief period of delirium is universal following anesthesia and certainly following an electrically induced convulsion, the persistence of delirium for more than a few hours following ECT may be caused by an interaction with concurrent lithium therapy, excessive anticholinergic medications, a co-morbid medical or neurological problem, an excessive number or frequency of ECT treatments relative to the patient's age and neurologic status, or excessive seizure duration (97–99). All of these issues deserve attention before additional convulsive treatments are administered.

TREATING SYMPTOMS

Although the primary treatment of delirium consists of removing or reversing the etiology, symptomatic treatment is often needed for behavioral symptoms. Principles of the symptomatic treatment of delirium (100) are summarized in Table 8.7.

Psychotherapeutic or educational interventions are often needed with the patient, the family, and sometimes other patients on the unit because of the strange and frightening character of delirious symptoms. Common concerns include patients' and families' fears that delirium implies an irreversible dementia. Also, patients may fear taking appropriate psychotropic medications after witnessing a frightening drug-

Table 8.7. Symptomatic Treatment of Delirium (97)

Environmental
  Continual reorientations:
    Clocks, calendars, family pictures at bedside
    Nurses' reminders of time, place, and situation
  Optimal stimulation:
    Transfer overstimulated patients to private rooms; decrease visits by family and friends
    Put understimulated patients in semiprivate rooms; increase frequency of visits
  Protection from injury:
    Frequent observation
    Remove potentially dangerous objects from room
    Restraints for severe agitation
Pharmacologic
  Low-dose neuroleptics for psychotic symptoms
  Sedatives for insomnia if needed and tolerated
Psychotherapeutic
  Brief supportive visits by physician during episode
  Explanation and "debriefing" after resolution
  Education and reassurance of concerned family members
  Education of, discussion by, other patients on the unit

induced delirium in another patient on the ward.

Dementia

Dementia becomes an issue in inpatient psychiatry either because a patient admitted for a primary psychiatric problem turns out to have cognitive impairment from a dementing illness or a patient with a known dementing illness develops a psychiatric complication or symptom requiring inpatient care. In the first case, primary concerns are distinguishing the syndrome of dementia from other mental disorders and identifying the etiology of the dementia, if possible. In the second case, the syndrome of dementia and its etiology may already be established, and the problem is finding an appropriate therapy for the most disabling or troublesome symptoms.

In its more severe manifestations, the syndrome of dementia is unmistakable. The patient has an acquired impairment in memory and other cognitive functions which produces significant disability in social and instrumental functions. Often, other neurological impairments are associated. Diagnostic problems arise when the patient has cognitive impairment without major functional consequences, or both cognitive and functional impairment are mild and overlap with the phenomena of normal aging or impairment from primary psychiatric illness.

As with delirium, patients with dementia have both syndrome and etiologic diagnoses. Diagnostic confusion results because the most common *etiology* of dementia, Alzheimer's disease, is often thought of as a synonym for the *syndrome* of dementia; in fact, it is possible to have pathologic changes of Alzheimer's disease without a dementia syndrome, or a dementia syndrome without Alzheimer's disease as its cause. Furthermore, cognitive impairment is not synonymous with dementia. Community studies have shown that a significant degree of cognitive impairment, as assessed by the Mini-Mental State Examination or even by neuropsychological testing, is compatible with normal everyday function (16, 101). The diagnosis of dementia must be considered in any psychiatric inpatient with subacute or chronic cognitive impairment in association with other psychopathology. Since early dementia is frequently associated with mood disorder or personality change (102, 103), the apparent presence of a primary psychiatric diagnosis should not discourage a dementia workup.

ETIOLOGIES OF DEMENTIA (104, 105)

The most common dementing illnesses encountered in inpatient psychiatry are summarized in Table 8.8. Included are the usual clinical and distinctive neuropathologic features and some useful diagnostic points. As Table 8.8 shows, most patients with dementia suffer from degenerative diseases not reversible at present. The crucial part of etiologic diagnosis for dementia patients is identifying those dementing disorders that *may* be arrested or reversed by specific medical treatment. Making distinctions among various untreatable diseases, such as that between Alzheimer's and Pick's diseases, is a less urgent consideration, although it occasionally may be useful for prognostic purposes.

THE CONCEPT OF TREATABLE OR REVERSIBLE DEMENTIA

Most of the pathologic processes that cause dementia are not reversible; the major degenerative diseases cannot even be arrested by medical treatment. Unfortunately, these nonreversible dementing illnesses account for the majority of dementia patients.

The major treatable dementias include dementias of infectious origin (syphilis, chronic meningitis, and perhaps AIDS dementia); metabolic problems, particularly hypothyroidism and B_{12} deficiency; and hy-

Table 8.8. Common Etiologies of Dementia

Etiology	Usual Clinical Features	Distinctive Pathologic Features	Useful Diagnostic Points
Alzheimer's Disease (affects about 50% of all demented patients)	Insidious onset Cortical dysfunction: aphasia, apraxia Relative absence of motor, sensory, and reflex changes Depression or psychosis in ⅓–½ of patients	Senile plaques and neurofibrillary tangles Cell loss and tangles in subcortical nuclei	Diffuse, nonspecific EEG changes roughly correspond to level of impairment; discrepancies warrant reconsideration of diagnosis; "cortical atrophy" on CT is neither necessary nor sufficient for diagnosis, but is usually present in advanced cases; cortical dysfunction can be found on neuropsychological testing if not evident clinically
Vascular Dementia (affects about 20–30% of all demented patients)	Stepwise or stuttering course Risk factors for stroke (smoking, hypertension, diabetes, sleep apnea) History of stroke or TIA (not always present) Motor, sensory, or reflex changes common Depression in ⅓–½; psychosis less common than in Alzheimer's disease	Definite infarcts—either cortical or subcortical, or diffuse softening of subcortical white matter (Binswanger's Disease)	EEG usually abnormal in cases with multiple cortical infarcts, but may be normal in purely subcortical disease; MRI is more sensitive than CT to subcortical vascular lesions, but also *less specific*; vascular dementia should not be diagnosed by MRI *alone*
Basal Ganglia Disease (Parkinson's Disease; Huntington's Disease; progressive supranuclear palsy)	Insidious onset Extrapyramidal motor signs invariably present, though occasionally less prominent than the dementia; cortical dysfunction less common than slowed thought, impaired concentration, memory disturbance, reduced verbal fluency, and depression	Basal ganglia cell loss (details are disease-specific)	Cognitive impairment may covary with motor signs, especially in Parkinson's disease; CT and MRI show the specific finding of covariate atrophy in Huntington's disease; also, virtually all Huntington's cases are familial; progressive supranuclear palsy is distinguished from Parkinson's disease by a more erect posture and by impairment of voluntary lateral eye movements
Hydrocephalus	Insidious onset History of predisposing factor (CNS infection, hemorrhage, trauma, congenital abnormality) Gait abnormality Urinary incontinence "Frontal lobe" features of impaired memory, abstract reasoning, and judgment Aphasia or apraxia unusual	Enlarged ventricles Increased interstitial fluid in periventricular white matter	Gait may have a distinctive "magnetic" quality, or may be spastic or ataxic; MRI shows characteristic changes in periventricular white matter; lumbar puncture shows high or high-normal opening pressure with relatively little difference between opening and closing pressures; symptoms may improve transiently following large-volume lumbar puncture (30–50 cc CSF removed)
Frontal lobe degeneration (Pick's disease; pure frontal lobe degeneration)	Insidious onset Early changes in personality and behavior Aphasia and apraxia occur late, if at all Memory loss improves with cues	Atrophy, cell loss, and gliosis concentrated in frontal region (and anterior temporal for Pick's disease) "Pick cells" in Pick's disease	CT or MRI may show frontal predominance of atrophy; neuropsychological testing may show disproportionate frontal impairment

227

Table 8.8. Common Etiologies of Dementia—continued

Etiology	Usual Clinical Features	Distinctive Pathologic Features	Useful Diagnostic Points
Dementia associated with alcoholism (up to 10% of dementia patients in high-risk population)	History often vague History of head trauma or malnutrition Long-term, high-quantity alcohol use	Cortical scars from head trauma Wernicke-Korsakoff changes in diencephalon Atrophy and cell loss	Diagnosis by history and exclusion; other alcoholism complications usually present (neuropathy, liver disease); memory and judgment prominently impaired
Metabolic (e.g., hypothyroidism, B_{12} deficiency)	Onset often subacute Specific cortical dysfunction not prominent General slowing and inefficiency of cognition Associated physical symptoms and signs	Depends on disorder, e.g., subacute combined degeneration of spinal cord in B_{12} deficiency	These conditions may co-occur with other etiologies; laboratory evaluation essential with attention to false-negative tests; nonspecific EEG changes usually present
Infectious (includes HIV encephalopathy, chronic meningitis)	Varies with etiology, but intellectual impairment (slowing, inaccuracy, poor concentration) Usually precedes specific cortical signs Evidence of systemic disease usually present	Depends on disorder	Diagnostic tests to be selected by risk; e.g., HIV in drug abusers, fungal infection in transplant patients; MRI more sensitive than CT to early changes in white matter; carefully plan CSF analysis before LP (lumbar puncture) to assure adequate volume of fluid

drocephalic dementia. Cognitive impairment caused by space-occupying lesions such as tumors or subdural hematomas and cognitive impairment caused by depression, though not likely to be mistaken by a well-trained clinician for a primary degenerative dementia, also are specifically treatable. Cognitive impairment from chronic drug intoxication, while again unlikely precisely to mimic a degenerative dementing process, is also reversible by removing the offending agents. Many of the same drugs that can cause delirium can produce more chronic cognitive impairments that mimic or aggravate dementia.

Dementia caused by vascular disease can be slowed or arrested, but not reversed, by correcting risk factors such as hypertension, smoking, sleep apnea, hyperlipidemia, or a source of emboli. Also consider antiplatelet agents if a history of definite strokes or TIAs (transient ischemic attack) is present. If new vascular lesions are prevented, some recovery from the functional effects of previous lesions is possible. Patients with dementia associated with alcoholism may improve with total abstinence and good nutrition.

The condition of patients with primary degenerative or vascular dementia may be aggravated by one or more of the factors listed as causes of treatable dementia. For example, patients with Alzheimer's disease frequently will look worse when undergoing a concurrent depression or when mildly hypothyroid. Although in these cases it could not be said that the depression or hypothyroidism caused the dementia or that the dementia was completely reversible, treating those problems could improve the patient's cognitive and instrumental function and overall quality of life.

THE DEPRESSION-DEMENTIA RELATIONSHIP

Because depression causes cognitive impairment, geriatric psychiatrists are enthusiastic about treating depression in cognitively impaired patients. However, the concept of "pseudodementia", once very popular, is now passé. The majority of patients who present with dementia and depression do in fact have two diagnoses; while treatment of the depression will improve cognitive function, it is unlikely to completely reverse the dementia (106, 107). A typical scenario is that of a patient with early Alzheimer's disease, who has not yet reached the point of a dementia syndrome, suffering an intercurrent depression. The cognitive impairment associated with depression increases the severity of cognitive symptoms to the point of a syndrome diagnosis. Through treating the depression, cognitive impairment returns to the pre-depression baseline, which may be abnormal but not quite warranting a dementia diagnosis. Over the next few years, the dementia progresses and ultimately the patient is demented regardless of whether concurrent depression is present.

STRUCTURING THE DEMENTIA WORKUP

The basic dementia workup aims at ruling out the most common and treatable causes of dementia and identifying other factors that might aggravate the cognitive or behavioral impairment of dementing diseases not specifically treatable. The elements of the basic workup are outlined in Table 8.9. Patients with unusual features such as those shown in Table 8.10 may deserve a more extensive workup which usually should be planned in consultation with

Table 8.9. The Basic Dementia Workup

Physical and neurological examination
Neuropsychological *screening* (see text)
Brain image: noncontrast CT or MRI
Blood tests: automated chemistry profile
  TSH
  Vitamin B_{12} and folate levels
  Syphilis serology
  HIV serology (for patients at risk)
EEG (waking)

Table 8.10. Reasons to Pursue More Extensive Etiological Investigation of Dementia

Early age of onset
Family history of heritable neurologic disease
Associated neurological or metabolic abnormalities
Involuntary movements or myoclonus
Seizures
Cognitive deficits atypical for Alzheimer's disease
Rapidly progressive or fluctuating course

a neurologist. Patients with specific risk factors, for example, those at high risk for HIV infection, should have additional tests appropriate to their risk factors. Items often included in extended workups are listed in Table 8.11, with typical indications.

A number of special points deserve mention in conducting the dementia workup. These are listed according to the tests and investigations.

1. CT versus MRI. Either CT or MRI are satisfactory tests for demonstrating treatable structural etiologies of dementia, such as tumor, subdural hematoma, or hydrocephalus. The MRI is more sensitive than the CT for demonstrating demyelinating disease and small subcortical white matter lesions of vascular dementia (108). However, because the MRI may reveal subcortical white matter abnormalities in

Table 8.11. "Special" Dementia Workup: Options and Usual Indications

Neurological consultation (for unusual features or second opinion)
MRI (for suspected lesions equivocal or not detectable on CT)
Sleep EEG (for detection of epileptic foci)
Comprehensive neuropsychological testing (for quantitating deficit or assessing atypical cases)
Noninvasive vascular studies (for suspected vascular dementia)
Lumbar puncture and CSF examination (for suspected infection or meningeal neoplasm)
Isotope cisternography (for suspected hydrocephalus)
SPECT and PET (for research assessments)
Cerebral biopsy (for atypical cases in young patients)
Cerebral angiography (for suspected CNS vasculitis)

apparently normal elderly people and patients with Alzheimer's disease (109, 110), the risk of overdiagnosing vascular dementia exists if one is inexperienced with MRI interpretation. Patients who are agitated or poorly cooperative may have difficulty tolerating the MRI procedure, which involves keeping the head in a tightly enclosed scanner for more than half an hour.

2. B_{12} levels. For a variety of technical reasons, a low–normal B_{12} level is compatible with a clinical diagnosis of B_{12} deficiency. If a patient has a history of gastrectomy or malabsorption or exhibits other signs compatible with B_{12} deficiency such as macrocytosis or spasticity and sensory loss in the lower extremities, a Schilling test deserves consideration even when the B_{12} is low–normal (111, 112).

3. Thyroid function tests. The TSH (thyroid stimulating hormone) level is now the test of choice for detecting hypothyroidism in neuropsychiatric patients. Patients with normal T_4 levels and elevated TSH levels may show clinical improvement with thyroid replacement (113).

4. VDRL. Patients with incompletely treated syphilis may show a normal VDRL in the serum. If the patient has a history of sexually transmitted disease, perform a serum FTA-ABS even if the VDRL is normal. Lumbar puncture is indicated if either blood serology is positive (4).

5. Role of the EEG. The EEG is infrequently helpful in ruling out treatable dementias because it adds little incremental diagnostic power to brain images, blood tests, and the clinical examination. However, it may be useful in distinguishing among different degenerative dementias, diagnosing superimposed delirium, making a prognosis about the rate of decline, or reassessing diagnosis in a case not evolving as expected (114). The basic principle for primary degenerative dementia is that the EEG worsens roughly in proportion to the cognitive impairment (115). Thus, in a mildly demented individual a markedly slow EEG suggests a different diagnosis or a superimposed delirium; in a patient with severe impairment, a normal EEG suggests a process other than Alzheimer's disease (116). Although patients with poorly controlled partial epilepsy can, of course, be diagnosed by EEG, their symptomatology is rarely mistaken for degenerative dementia.

ROLE OF NEUROPSYCHOLOGICAL TESTING

Neuropsychological testing is widely practiced in neurological research settings to quantitate and define regional cerebral dysfunction (see Chapter 14). However, extensive formal neuropsychological batteries are of limited value in the diagnosis and treatment of dementia in general psychiatric practice. More helpful in most cases is an extended screening examination that identifies areas of cognitive strength and weakness and assesses whether the pattern of cognitive impairment is or is not typical of Alzheimer's disease. Further, such extended screening evaluations can indicate areas of preserved cognitive function that might be employed in developing a rehabilitative strategy. For example, a patient with relatively preserved nonverbal memory but significant verbal memory deficits might be trained to use images and visualization as aids for remembering. A variety of extended screens have been developed; two are the High Sensitivity Cognitive Screen of Faust and Fogel and the battery developed by the Consortium for Research on Alzheimer's disease (117, 118).

PSYCHIATRIC COMPLICATIONS OF DEMENTIA

The most frequently encountered psychiatric complications are depression, para-noid psychosis, and superimposed delirium (1, 119). The most frequently troublesome clinical problem is agitation which, without a psychiatric diagnosis, may be caused by any of the above-mentioned complications or may reflect an organic personality disorder (120). In general, because treatment of co-morbid psychopathology in Alzheimer's disease is far more gratifying than treatment of Alzheimer's disease itself, diagnosis of co-morbid psychopathology deserves the attention it gets on inpatient psychiatric units.

TREATMENT OF DEMENTIA (121, 122)

The first step in treating dementia is to identify all specifically reversible medical factors that may cause or aggravate the patient's cognitive impairment. Treating these disorders often is the province of internal medicine or neurology. Second, for patients with nonreversible vascular dementias, interventions may still be possible for reducing risk factors of further vascular damage; interventions include smoking cessation, control of hypertension, or use of antiplatelet agents. These interventions are generally designed in conjunction with a patient's internist or neurologist. Co-morbid psychopathology, particularly depression, paranoid psychosis, or episodic agitation, is treated. Several points are offered concerning the treatment of psychopathology associated with dementia:

1. Depression. Because dementia diminishes cognitive capacities, treating depression with primarily psychotherapeutic interventions usually produces disappointing results in demented patients with moderate or severe depression; however, suitably adapted supportive therapy can mitigate milder depressions and can be used as an adjunct in treating more severe cases (123–125). The mainstay for treating more severe depressions is pharmacologic therapy or ECT (electroconvulsive therapy). In choosing drugs, more anticholinergic agents should be avoided because of the increased susceptibility of demented patients to delirium. Initial dosage should be low and dosage increments small, in order to avoid drug-induced confusional or agitated states. MAO inhibitors deserve consideration; they have been found effective in depression accompanying dementia and may be better tolerated than tricyclics in some patients (126). ECT is not contraindicated because of premorbid cognitive impairment. However, careful documentation of the dementia workup and pre-ECT cognitive function is desirable.

2. Paranoid psychosis. Neuroleptics are effective for treating paranoid psychosis in demented people (127–129). However, because patients with dementia are significantly more sensitive to neuroleptic side effects than nondemented patients, dosages *must* be kept low. If high-potency neuroleptics are prescribed, dopamine agonist antiparkinson medication may be needed to avoid profound rigidity and akinesia. (Anticholinergic antiparkinson medications are poorly tolerated in most demented patients.) It is advisable to limit using neuroleptics to treating paranoid and psychotic thinking. They are not desirable for general sedation because their neurotoxicity in demented patients is substantial (130). If the patient has agitation that persists despite adequate treatment of psychosis with a low-dose neuroleptic, consider using an alternate agent such as a benzodiazepine or antidepressant as an adjunct for treating agitation or insomnia.

3. Agitation. Agitation in dementia may be caused by agitated depression, excessive anxiety, psychosis, or aggravation of premorbid personality problems (116). Treat agitated depression vigorously with specific antidepressant drugs or ECT. Treat psychosis with neuroleptics. Benzodiazepines or other adjuncts can be added if ag-

itation is insufficiently controlled by a modest dose of neuroleptic. Agitation from anxiety warrants a trial of buspirone (116, 131–139); benzodiazepines are less desirable as a first choice because they often aggravate cognitive impairment. However, long-time benzodiazepine-dependent patients may respond to benzodiazepines and to nothing else.

4. Premorbid personality disorders. For personality disorders with high trait anxiety, buspirone or perhaps a beta-blocker deserve a trial; for borderline and schizotypal character pathology, low-dose neuroleptics may be appropriate (140, 141). Pharmacologic therapy is combined with behavioral and psychotherapeutic interventions to provide consistent yet sympathetic limit setting and minimize splitting.

INTERVENTIONS WITH THE FAMILY

Patients with dementia frequently are referred to inpatient psychiatric units when their behavior exceeds the capacity of family caretakers or paid caretakers to manage. Effective intervention requires incorporating the relevant family caretakers or institutional caretakers into treatment planning (142–144). This includes focusing treatment on behavioral symptoms of greatest concern to caretakers, further education of the caretakers regarding the patient's diagnosis and its implications, and working out a satisfactory posthospital disposition. Inadequate involvement of the family or paid caretakers in the hospital phase is a common reason for failure of an otherwise reasonable postdischarge plan.

In addition, family caretakers frequently suffer from clinically significant depression or other maladaptive stress reactions (145–147). Treating these problems specifically often enables the family caretaker to make better decisions and care more effectively for the patient. Not only are education and support groups such as those sponsored by the Alzheimer's Disease and Related Disorders Association relevant, but many patients benefit from formal supportive therapy or even drug treatment if they are depressed with significant somatic and vegetative symptoms. Proper psychiatric assessment of family caretakers is an important addition to the dementia workup on the inpatient psychiatric service.

ORGANIC MENTAL DISORDERS WITHOUT GENERAL COGNITIVE IMPAIRMENT

Apart from substance-related organic mental disorders, other organic conditions commonly encountered in general inpatient psychiatry include the organic personality disorders associated with frontal lobe dysfunction and temporal lobe epilepsy, organic mood disorders mimicking depression or mania, and organic anxiety disorders. Although organic causes of delusions are encountered occasionally, most often delusions of organic cause arise either in connection with delirium or dementia or in relation to psychoactive substance use. The organic personality disorders will be discussed first, followed by guidelines for evaluating patients with mania, depression, anxiety, or psychosis, for underlying organic factors.

Frontal Lobe Syndromes

The frontal lobes of the brain are an anatomic structure that reaches a uniquely high level of development in primates. Their functions include:

a. Abstract reasoning
b. Judgment
c. Organizing and planning complex behavior
d. Maintaining or shifting mental set purposefully
e. Persisting in a task despite distracting stimuli (148).

It is evident from this list of functions that frontal lobe damage may profoundly affect personality and behavior, often in ways that overlap with disturbances attributed to primary psychiatric illness.

The frontal lobes may be specifically damaged by stroke or tumor but bear the brunt of the damage in a number of conditions that affect the brain more widely, including closed head injury, multiple sclerosis, degenerative dementias, and intoxications (149). Furthermore, frontal lobe dysfunction may be prominent in some cases of severe primary mental illness, particularly schizophrenia (150) and bipolar disorder. Often, more than one factor contributes to frontal lobe dysfunction, such as in the case of a patient with head injury, alcoholism, and an acute depression.

The effects of frontal lobe damage on planning, insight, judgment, impulse control, and abstract thinking often give a peculiarly "psychiatric" flavor to frontal lobe patients. The magnitude of frontal lobe dysfunction may correlate with how likely patients are to act out upon impulses; in one recent study the presence of frontal lobe injury helped explain which psychiatric inpatients engaged in assaultive behavior (151).

Identifying frontal lobe dysfunction can be helpful in identifying specific organic diagnoses and planning treatment. Both problem identification and choice of treatment are aided by organizing frontal lobe symptoms into groups according to the region of brain affected. Table 8.12 describes behavioral symptoms commonly encountered with damage to each of four anatomic subdivisions of the frontal lobes. Associated with each are some therapeutic approaches proved useful in management.

FRONTAL LOBES AND
NEUROPSYCHOLOGICAL TESTING

Unlike patients with delirium or dementia, patients with localized frontal lobe damage or dysfunction may show a completely normal performance on conventional cognitive screening tests such as the

Table 8.12. Syndromes and Management Options with Damage to Different Frontal Lobe Regions

Region of Damage	Associated Behavioral and Cognitive Impairments	Treatment Considerations
Superior Mesial	Apathy; "pseudodepression"; disturbance of initiation; bradykinesia; aspontaneity; decreased speech; performance deficits; superficial cognitive processing; go-no-go deficit; decreased attention	Dopamine agonists Therapy to increase stimulation and reactivity: physical, speech, occupational Cuing to action
Dorsal Lateral	Significant cognitive impairments that may include decreased intellect, poor memory, apraxia, aphasia, disturbed attention, hemispatial neglect, extinction, poor judgment, impulsivity, lack of planning, decreased empathy, cognitive and emotional rigidity, affective disturbances, irritability	Mood stabilizers Environmental structuring Concrete behavioral therapies Simplified consistent routines
Orbital	"Pseudopsychopathic": impulsiveness, poor planning. Disturbed motivation; poor follow-through. Emotional lability, lack of empathy, possibly with decreased autonomic responses. Primarily social deficits: may be entirely normal in IQ, memory, perception, praxis	Mood stabilizers Environmental structuring Behavioral therapies
Posterior Ventromedial	Prominent memory disturbance Confabulation; emotional lability	Cuing to improve memory Reality orientation Mood stabilizers

Reprinted with permission from Stoudemire A, Fogel B (eds.): *Medical Psychiatric Practice, Vol. 1,* Washington, D.C., American Psychiatric Press, 1991.

Mini-Mental Status Examination and frequently have a completely normal IQ as well (110). The dysfunction can only be established by special testing that focuses on specific frontal lobe functions. The ability of tests to detect frontal lobe damage depends on a suitable match of the test with the anatomic subdivision of the frontal lobes affected by the lesion. Table 8.13 summarizes the tests most helpful in diagnosing involvement of each of the major subdivisions of the frontal lobe.

ESTABLISHING THE PRESENCE OF FRONTAL LOBE DYSFUNCTION

The presence of frontal lobe damage or dysfunction is suggested by a clinical history and pattern of behavior showing typical features of impaired planning, judgment, persistence, insight, or impulse control; neuropsychological findings are confirmatory. The demonstration of physiologic or anatomic abnormality of the frontal lobes is readily accomplished for conditions such as stroke and tumor, but may be more difficult in cases caused by closed head injury or neurotoxic exposure. Among brain imaging methods, MRI is most sensitive to white matter lesions and may show lesions not evident on CT scan. In theory, computerized EEG procedures might be more sensitive to regional disturbances of electrical activity over the frontal lobes. However, the technical complexity of this procedure, its numerous artifacts, and controversy over proper interpretation limit its clinical use at this time (152, 12). Likewise, although SPECT (single photon emission tomography) and PET (position emission tomography) may be sensitive to frontal dysfunction, limits on their specificity and lack of standards for interpretation argue aginst their routine clinical use at this time. Diagnosis of behavioral disturbance from frontal lobe damage is most secure when the clinical history, imaging findings, and neuropsychologic test results all agree.

Table 8.13. Commonly Used Neuropsychological Tests for the Frontal Lobes

Test	Description	Time to Administer	Strengths and Weaknesses
Wisconsin Card Sort (Heaton, 1981)	Subject needs to abstract, maintain, and shift card sorting principles	15–30 minutes	Sensitive to frontal lobe dysfunction Yields multivariate measures Normative values available Failure not specific to frontal lobes
Verbal Associative Fluency (Benton, 1968)	Subject needs to generate words beginning with certain letter within limited response time	5 minutes	Sensitive to frontal lobe dysfunction Easy to administer and score Normative values available Failure not specific to frontal lobes
Verbal Concept Attainment (Bornstein & Leason, 1985)	Subject chooses one word on each line that has conceptual similarity to words on preceding and following lines	30-minute limit	Sensitive to left frontal lesions Normative values available No special equipment needed Failure not specific to frontal lobes
Stroop Test (Perret, 1974; Golden, 1978)	A conflicting stimuli task in which subjects must suppress the reading of color words to name the color in which the words are printed	5 minutes	Sensitive to left frontal lesions Easy to administer and score Normative values available
Category Test (Jarris & Barth, 1984; Crockett et al., 1986)	Requires subject to abstract similarities and differences (principles) among stimuli and to formulate hypotheses	45 minutes	Sensitive to damage to many areas of the brain Not especially sensitive to frontal lobe dysfunction except when impaired in isolation Requires special equipment

Reprinted with permission from Stoudemire A, Fogel B (eds.): *Medical Psychiatric Practice, Vol. 1*, Washington, D.C., American Psychiatric Press, 1991.

IMPLICATIONS FOR DRUG THERAPY (145)

Patients with frontal lobe damage are particularly sensitive to adverse behavioral effects—especially disinhibition and impaired judgment from sedative-hypnotics and *benzodiazepines.* Whenever possible, avoid these drugs and consider nonbenzodiazepine therapies such as buspirone or antidepressants for treating anxiety.

Neuroleptics, too, have a lower therapeutic index in patients with frontal lobe damage. The frontal lobes are richly supplied with dopaminergic neurons, and an adequate dopaminergic input appears essential for normal frontal lobe function. Ex-

cessive dopamine blockade with neuroleptics may aggravate the symptoms of anatomic frontal lobe dysfunction, including apathy, impersistence, and difficulty maintaining mental set. Thus, the use of neuroleptics in patients with frontal lobe damage should be restricted to the treatment of psychotic symptoms; neuroleptics should not be used for general sedative purposes.

Inversely, patients with apathy or impaired attention caused by frontal lobe lesions may benefit from dopamine agonists such as bromocriptine (153–156) or stimulants such as dextroamphetamine or methylphenidate. These drugs deserve consideration in treating apathetic or inattentive frontal lobe syndromes, particularly when there is no history of psychosis or drug abuse.

Emotional lability caused by frontal lobe damage may be aided by mood-stabilizing anticonvulsants such as *carbamazepine* (157). Also, the benefits of *beta-blockers* for impulsive or violent behavior (158) may extend to patients with disinhibited violent behavior caused by frontal lobe damage.

Because depression aggravates focal cognitive deficits and some cases of depression may specifically be associated with impaired frontal lobe blood flow (159, 160), carefully diagnose and vigorously treat depression in patients with frontal lobe damage. Give preference to less sedating antidepressants such as secondary tricyclics and the newer nontricyclic antidepressants. In diagnosing depression, bear in mind that patients with frontal lobe damage may show shallow affect that sometimes distracts the clinician from the correct diagnosis. For example, a patient may sincerely voice suicidal ideation and anhedonia, yet laugh and joke in the same interview. In the context of frontal lobe damage, do not take the discrepancy of affect and described mood as evidence the patient is not depressed.

IMPLICATIONS FOR PSYCHOSOCIAL AND BEHAVIORAL THERAPIES (145)

Patients with frontal lobe damage frequently respond well to a definite structure and clear expectations and have the most trouble in poorly organized and highly distracting situations. On the inpatient unit, a patient with frontal lobe damage should undergo an early, individualized occupational therapy assessment, and a structured daily routine should be established.

The value of insight-oriented psychotherapy in patients with frontal lobe damage depends on the location and extent of the lesion. Some patients with dorsal-lateral frontal lesions are capable of improving their behavior if they understand their sit-

uation sufficiently, even if they have cognitive difficulties in *independently* understanding their practical and emotional situation. These patients may benefit from a concrete form of supportive therapy. By contrast, although patients with orbital frontal lesions may be able to attain or express awareness and insight into emotional and practical realities they may be unable to conform their behavior to their awareness. For these patients, pharmacotherapy and structuring the environment are usually more effective than efforts to build insight.

Because patients with frontal lobe damage so often require environmental manipulation, coordinating inpatient staff efforts is crucial; successful follow-up depends on work with the family or other significant people in the patient's life, to continue consistent and effective environmental contingencies. Often, interventions with nursing staff and family members must begin with explaining the organic nature of the patient's problem and the limitations on understanding and self-control that are consequences of frontal lobe damage. This permits a move away from blaming the patient or making overly psychological explanations of the patient's behavior.

Specific, targeted behavior therapy interventions are of greatest use either to develop or to extinguish specific targeted behaviors, such as developing better grooming or extinguishing inappropriate sexual remarks. In both cases, consulting with an expert behavior therapist may help in designing a behavioral treatment paradigm. Both operant conditioning and cuing approaches have been beneficial in selected cases (161, 162).

Personality Disturbances Associated with Temporal Lobe Epilepsy (163, 164)

Temporal lobe epilepsy, more accurately called complex partial epilepsy, is one of the most common chronic neurologic disorders, probably affecting between 1–2% of the general population. Patients with temporal lobe epilepsy are vulnerable to a variety of psychiatric complications including depression, anxiety, and schizophreniform psychosis. They frequently present to psychiatric inpatient units because of mood disorders or psychotic conditions; a less common but still frequent presentation is with pseudoseizures often associated with genuine epileptic attacks.

Diagnosing and treating mood disorders and psychotic disorders in patients with complex partial seizures follow the same general principles as treating those disorders in nonepileptic patients; however, take particular care to carefully monitor antiepileptic drug therapy and take steps to minimize adverse drug interactions between psychotropic and antiepileptic drugs (165). Diagnostic and therapeutic difficulties in treating patients with psychiatric manifestations of temporal lobe epilepsy often relate to the effect this condition has on the patient's personality. The occurrence of characteristic personality traits and profiles in patients with complex partial seizures is useful to the clinician both for suggesting diagnoses in patients not known to be epileptic and helping patients and families understand behavioral traits that may seem otherwise incomprehensible given the patient's family and developmental history. Psychiatric features of complex partial epilepsy are summarized in Table 8.14.

Patients with temporal lobe epilepsy may develop progressive changes in personality and behavior during the course of their illness. This can create unusual dynamic conflicts if the behavior that develops is counter to the patient's ego ideal or superego prohibitions. For example, the epilepsy-induced development of unconventional sexual interests in a patient with conventional morality could induce severe anxiety and guilt. Similarly, the progressive development of epilepsy-induced hyposexuality in a patient within a marriage based

Table 8.14. Psychiatric Features of Complex Partial Epilepsy

Increased incidence of depression and anxiety
Schizophrenia psychosis with preserved affective
  warmth
"Temporal lobe" personality
  Hypergraphia
  Religious or philosophical preoccupations
  Altered or diminished sexuality
  "Viscosity" or "stickiness" in interpersonal relations
  Hyperseriousness or overconscientiousness
Episodic psychomotor and psychosensory symptoms
Increased impulsiveness and suicidal behavior when
  depressed

on an active sexual life could trigger marital conflict.

The personality disturbances of temporal lobe epilepsy occur within a social and developmental context; rarely can a patient's traits be attributed exclusively to neurologic illness. Nonetheless, convincing evidence, both anecdotal and systematic, supports genuine changes of personality, or accentuation of personality traits, directly linked to the presence of a temporal lobe seizure focus. Theoretical explanations are offered for these changes, the most appealing based on notions of "hyperconnection," or excessive facilitation of limbic synapses from the continual discharge of the temporal lobe seizure focus (166).

On the inpatient psychiatric unit, awareness of temporal lobe personality traits by nursing staff can be useful in properly understanding and interpreting patient's ward behavior. For example, an epileptic patient might occasionally show impulsive behavior violating ward rules. However, excessively firm limit setting might be totally unnecessary if the patient's spontaneous response to such impulsive acts is intense guilt and remorse. In that situation, excessively firm or confrontational limit setting by staff might activate a different dimension of the patient's personality— a hypersensitivity to unfairness or injury that might trigger further escalation of conflict. Awareness that for temporal lobe patients impulsive or hyperemotional behavior may occur in the context of intense conscientiousness and moralism is useful in formulating the patient's dynamics and planning an appropriate response.

Evaluating Patients with Mood Disorders, Anxiety, and Psychosis for Causal or Contributory Organic Factors (167)

For each of the major primary psychiatric disorders, textbooks of organic psychiatry offer exhaustive lists of medical and neurological conditions that can cause mental symptoms mimicking that disorder. Depending on the inclination of the psychiatrist, this can lead either to inefficient and expensive workups for organic factors, a nihilistic position advocating a standard workup for everyone, or only testing those patients with blatant physical symptoms.

Both the overinclusive and nihilistic approaches may derive from the same misconception: that a sharp distinction exists between functional and organic mental disorders. In fact, a mental syndrome usually reflects the convergence of many factors, including genetics, developmental history, environment, individual psychodynamics, and physical health (9). Overemphasizing the physical covariate leads to generating excessively long lists of "organic causes" of mental syndromes; physician disappointment in how patients respond to the correction of a single organic factor leads to disillusionment with organic workups. Although the case of the patient with a subdural hematoma presenting as a psychosis occurs, it is an exception; more typical is the patient with depression accompanied by hypothyroidism, the treatment of which is necessary but not sufficient for a full remission of depressive symptoms. Studies of physical illness in psychiatric patients (168, 169) suggest that illness prevalence is high, even in patients allegedly "screened" for

medical illness before psychiatric unit admission. However, in most cases the physical illness is an aggravating or concurrent factor rather than a sole cause of the psychiatric syndrome.

Particular mental symptoms in connection with particular physical symptoms from *syndromes* that suggest particular organic diagnoses. As suggested above, the chronic and treatment-refractory depression in a patient with peculiar dizzy spells and memory lapses, who was hypergraphic and hyperreligious, would suggest temporal lobe epilepsy even if the patient did not offer a history of convulsions or other unequivocal seizures. A general approach to evaluating the psychiatric inpatient for organic factors is now offered. Further discussion is available in several recent monographs on differential diagnosis (7, 163, 170).

THE GENERAL EVALUATION FOR ORGANIC FACTORS

The general evaluation begins with a medical history and physical examination conducted *by the psychiatrist*. This examination is conducted following the psychiatric history and mental status examination, and addresses special attention to areas in which the patient has complaints. In the neurological examination, special areas of attention are gait, coordination, muscle tone, evidence of peripheral neuropathy or lower extremity sensory loss, and asymmetries of limb size, strength, tone, or coordination. This neurologic examination is needed because screening examinations by internists, family practitioners, and physicians' assistants often performed on psychiatric inpatient units are usually insufficiently attentive to mild neurological signs of psychiatric importance, including dyskinesia, "soft" neurologic signs of congenital encephalopathy, mild parkinsonism, and peripheral neuropathy. The psychiatrist's physical examination should focus especially on signs of endocrine disease such as changes in hair pattern and skin pigmentation, orthostatic hypotension, and abnormalities of the thyroid. As with the neurologic examination, the psychiatrist's awareness of conditions of particular psychiatric interest may pick up new findings outside the trio of heart, lungs, and abdomen that frequently dominates nonspecialist screening physicals on psychiatric units. The author has seen "medically cleared" patients with such diverse endocrine problems as goiter, adrenal insufficiency, and hypothyroidism.

Following the physical examination, laboratory tests are ordered, consisting of a core of tests supplemented by tests specifically suggested by the patient's age, personal history, symptoms, and signs.

LABORATORY ASSESSMENT FOR ALL PSYCHIATRIC INPATIENTS

The general laboratory assessment for all psychiatric inpatients is presented in Table 8.15, subdivided into general assessment and additional tests warranted by the patient's age, area of residence, or findings on physical examination. These tests should often be supplemented by specialist consultation which often leads to additional testing. Following a discussion of specialist consultation and the use of toxic screens and drug levels, special considerations are presented for the evaluation of depression, mania, anxiety, and psychosis. For each, a comprehensive table featuring differential diagnostic possibilities is followed by a discussion of general issues the author has found helpful in constructing more focused and limited differential diagnoses.

THE ROLE OF SPECIALIST CONSULTATION

In the author's experience, consultation with subspecialty services generally has been more rewarding than diagnostic consultation with general internists or primary

Table 8.15. General Laboratory Assessment for Psychiatric Inpatients

CBC with differential and ESR
Automated blood chemistry panel including: electrolytes, BUN, creatinine, calcium, liver enzymes, and glucose
TSH level (and T_4 & RT_3 if TSH assay is not ultrasensitive)
Urinalysis
Syphilis serology
EEG

Additional Tests (as indicated)

EKG for patients over 40 or with a history of cardiac disease or major risk factors (e.g., juvenile diabetes)
Chest x-ray for patients with known lung disease, long-term smoking histories, or pulmonary complaints
HIV serology for patients with a history of drug abuse, transfusions, or high-risk sexual behavior
ANA (antinuclear antibodies) and rheumatoid factor for patients with joint pain or polysymptomatic histories suggesting rheumatic disease
CT or MRI for patients with headaches or unexplained abnormalities on neurologic examination or EEG
Lyme disease serology for patients with polysymptomatic disease, from areas where Lyme disease is endemic
Sleep apnea evaluation for patients with unexplained excessive daytime drowsiness or markedly noisy sleep
CSF examination for patients with new psychiatric symptoms occurring with headache, stiff neck, and fever

practitioners. When obtaining a subspecialist consultation, it is crucial to inform the subspecialist of those elements of the patient's history, physical examination, and psychiatric syndrome that raise specific diagnostic possibilities, for example, systemic lupus erythematosus (SLE) or primary neurologic disease. Consulting subspecialists can then focus their consultative examination on the question at hand. Subspecialists usually are impressed when a psychiatrist has personally performed a physical examination and directed attention to specific symptoms and findings. Obtaining subspecialist consultation before embarking upon exotic, expensive, or unusual laboratory investigations is usually wise.

TOXIC SCREENS AND DRUG LEVELS

As noted above and discussed in the section on delirium, medications and drugs are among the most common causes of organic mental disorders encountered among inpatients. Although laboratory confirmation of the presence of drugs or excessive drug levels can be extremely helpful in differential diagnosis, several technical issues must be considered for a drug test to be properly interpreted (171, 172).

1. For detecting prior ingestion of a drug or substance, urine testing is far more sensitive than blood testing. However, urine testing offers no quantitative information.

2. The likelihood of detecting a drug depends on the sensitivity of the assay. Gas chromatography/mass spectroscopy (GC/MS) and radioimmunoassay (RIA) technologies are more sensitive but far more expensive than the simple thin layer chromatography (TLC) technique more generally available in hospital laboratories.

3. Drug testing should not be used for forensic purposes unless extraordinary care is taken in obtaining the patient's consent and assuring that testing samples are under continuous supervision from the time they are collected until the time the analysis is reported.

4. Blood tests are appropriate for diagnosing a *current* intoxication or adverse drug reaction, but not generally for establishing past exposure to a drug.

5. Medications and drugs can cause organic mental syndromes at "therapeutic" or "nontoxic" blood levels. The reasons include individual pharmacodynamic vulnerabilities, variations in protein binding, and interactions with other medications. A common diagnostic error is to rule out a medication-induced organic mental disorder because of a "therapeutic" blood level of the drug.

Special Considerations for Specific Mental Syndromes

DEPRESSION (See Table 8.16)

In evaluating depression, substance abuse deserves especially close attention because of its high prevalence and the frequent association of alcohol and drug abuse with major depressive syndromes developing during abstinence. Apart from substance abuse, adverse drug reactions, endocrine disease, occult cancer, and primary neurologic disease are the crucial diagnostic considerations.

When a depression develops for the first time or recurs with greater severity in a patient over 50, occult cancer should be considered; perform a full workup if the depression is associated with significant weight loss and systemic symptoms. In less clear-cut cases, direct a limited evaluation for occult cancer to areas where the patient is at highest risk, such as the lungs in a smoker or the breasts in any woman over 40. Perform appropriate tests, such as chest x-ray, mammography, and bowel radiography. An important related concern is that depressed patients often neglect recommended screening procedures for cancer, such as rectal examination and sigmoidoscopy, mammography and pelvic examination in women, and testicular examination in men. Make special efforts to ascertain that such examinations are up to date.

Depression As an Adverse Drug Reaction (173)

Depression is frequently precipitated or aggravated by prescription drugs; more than 100 drugs have been implicated, generally by clinical reports rather than controlled studies. Although the literature is problematic because of varying definitions of depression, consensus nonetheless indicates that several major classes of drugs produce or aggravate depressive symptoms in at least a clinically significant minority of patients. These drugs include methyldopa (Aldomet), propranolol, reserpine, corticosteroids, L-dopa, oral contraceptives, cimetidine, and digoxin.

Depression and Endocrine Disease (174, 175)

The most secure associations of depression and endocrine disease are with hypothyroidism and with Cushing's syndrome (hypercortisolism). In evaluating hypothyroidism, the TSH level is the test of choice; elevations in TSH deserve treatment whether or not accompanied by a low T_4 level. Although controversy remains whether patients with a normal TSH but abnormal TRH-stimulation (thyrotropin-releasing hormone) test benefit from thyroid supplementation, consider it in an otherwise treatment-refractory depression (109). In patients suspected of adrenal disease, an overnight dexamethasone suppression test is the best initial screen. Patients who fail to suppress 8 A.M. cortisol following 1 mg of dexamethasone the night before warrant further endocrine evaluation to distinguish Cushing's syndrome from adrenal hyperactivity caused by primary depressive illness (176).

Depression and Neurological Disease

Since depression is frequently the presenting symptom of degenerative neurologic diseases, such as Parkinson's, Huntington's, or Alzheimer's, patients with depression in midlife or old age warrant an especially careful neurological examination; pay particular attention to cognitive status, muscle tone, and involuntary movements. If cognitive deficits are found, reexamine for cognitive deficits following optimal treatment of the depression. Persistent deficits should trigger ongoing neurologic follow-up. Because depression frequently accompanies *multiple sclerosis* (177–179), multiple neurologic complaints in a younger patient with depression indicate an evaluation for this disorder.

MANIA (180) (See Table 8.17)

By far, the most common organic causes of mania are drugs and medications, particularly antidepressants, stimulants, and corticosteroids (181). Mania has been reported as a complication of drugs as diverse as muscle relaxants and over-the-counter (OTC) decongestants. Endocrine

causes of mania include hyperthyroidism and, rarely, Cushing's disease, although the latter usually presents with depression (182). Among the most frequent neurological causes are right hemisphere lesions, head injury, and multiple sclerosis (176, 183).

Regarding the workup for the manic patient, thyroid function tests occasionally can be misleading because an isolated elevation of T_4 may occur in the acute stages of mania (109). However, persistent elevation of T_4 or T_3, or a *low* TSH on an ultrasensitive assay would not be expected from mania alone. Endocrine consultation should usually be requested if the manic patient's thyroid function tests are persistently abnormal.

A related endocrine issue is that lithium can induce or aggravate thyroid disease and also cause hyperparathyroidism (184, 185). Therefore, when a lithium-treated bipolar patient develops new changes in mental status, repeat thyroid function and calcium tests.

Brain imaging to pursue a neurologic cause of mania is indicated when the neurologic examination shows abnormal signs or manic symptoms are mixed with specific neurologic complaints. Another situation requiring brain imaging is manic symptoms occurring in a patient at unusual risk for cerebral emboli or infection, such as someone with valvular cardiac disease or receiving immunosuppressive therapy.

ANXIETY (186, 187) (See Table 8.18)

As with mania, medications and other psychoactive substances are the most frequent organic causes of anxiety. Frequent offenders include caffeine, alcohol, decongestants, and bronchodilators. Anxiety may occur at therapeutic doses of these medications; patients with a personal or family history of anxiety or panic are particularly vulnerable. Cigarette smoking or the withdrawal of cigarettes can cause or aggravate anxiety. When a smoker is admitted to a

Table 8.16. Diseases Associated with Depressive Syndrome

Drugs and Toxins	Endocrine	Malignancy
Antihypertensives	Hypothyroidism	Brain tumor
Reserpine	Cushing's syndrome	Carcinoma of pancreas
Clonidine	Hyperthyroidism	Lung carcinoma
Propranolol	Diabetes mellitus	Carcinomatosis
Methyldopa	Addison's disease	Lymphoma
Guanethidine	Hyperparathyroidism	Carcinoid syndrome
Phenothiazines	Hyperaldosteronism	
Corticosteroids	Acromegaly	
Digitalis		
Sulfonamides		
Ranitidine		
Antituberculous agents		
Antineoplastic agents		
Hydralazine		
Lidocaine		
Bromides		
Anticonvulsants		
Narcotics		
Narcotic antagonists		
Indomethacin		
Methysergide		
Estrogens		
Diphenoxylate		
Dopamine agonists		
Heavy metal intoxication		
Phenylpropanolamine		

Metabolic	Epilepsy	Neurodegenerative
Anemia	Partial complex	Parkinson's disease
Renal failure		Alzheimer's disease
B_{12} deficiency		Blindness
Folate deficiency		Deafness
Hepatic failure		Pick's disease
Amyloidosis		Huntington's disease
Gout		
Anoxia		

	Immunologic	Infection
	Systemic lupus erythematosus	Neurosyphilis
	Multiple sclerosis	Hepatitis
	Rheumatoid arthritis	Herpes simplex
	Migraine	AIDS
	Periarteritis nodosa	Epstein-Barr virus
	Sarcoidosis	Tuberculosis

	Immunologic	
	Giant-cell arteritis	
	Regional enteritis	
	Ulcerative colitis	

Atherosclerotic

Stroke

Reprinted with permission from Schiffer RB, Klein RF, Sider RC: *The Medical Evaluation of Psychiatric Patients,* New York, Plenum Medical, 1988.

Table 8.17.   Medical and Neurologic Syndromes Associated with Secondary Mania

Drugs and toxins	CNS trauma
Corticosteroids	Immunologic
Dopamine agonists	Systemic lupus erythematosus
Decongestants	Multiple sclerosis
Bronchodilators	Endocrine
Alpha-methyldopa	Hyperthyroidism
Amphetamines	Cushing's disease
Methylphenidate	Brain tumor
Cocaine	Multiple cell types and anatomy
Tricyclic antidepressants	Metabolic
L-tryptophan/monoamine oxidase inhibitor	Hemodialysis
Flutamide	Postoperative state
Trazadone	B_{12} deficiency
Cyclobenzaprine	Calcium infusion
Monoamine oxidase inhibitors	Hypoxia
Thyroid hormone	Infection
Procarbazine	Neurosyphilis
Bromide	Cryptococcosis
Phencyclidine	Influenza
Metoclopramide	Fever
Cyclosporine	St. Louis type A encephalitis
Procyclidine	AIDS
Digitalis	CNS degenerative disease
Reserpine withdrawal	Spinocerebellar atrophy
Antidepressant withdrawal	Epilepsy
Baclofen	Stroke
Niridazole	
Alprazolam	

Reprinted with permission from Schiffer RB, Klein RF, Sider RC: *The Medical Evaluation of Psychiatric Patients*, New York, Plenum Medical, 1988.

general hospital or psychiatric facility with a no-smoking or limited-smoking policy, anxiety caused by smoking cessation may result.

Other causes of anxiety include hyperthyroidism, hyperparathyroidism, and hypoglycemia. Hypoglycemia causes chronic anxiety or typical recurrent panic attacks very rarely. In one study, panic disorder patients could distinguish symptoms of insulin-induced hypoglycemia from their typical panic attacks (188). However, hypoglycemia may cause *acute* anxiety in conjunction with sweating, tachycardia, and hunger. Falls in blood sugar levels may also trigger panic attacks in patients with panic disorder, although this phenomenon has been difficult to reproduce experimentally (183).

Panic attacks may occasionally be the manifestation of partial seizures with ictal fear or, even more rarely, the consequence of paroxysmal endocrine disorders such as pheochromocytoma (189, 190). When panic patients are seen in the inpatient setting, the opportunity to directly measure vital signs and observe the patient can establish whether the panic symptoms are accompanied by neurological or autonomic symptoms suggesting one of these diagnoses. However, even when these symptoms are not present, panic attacks with significant hypertension warrant an assessment for pheochromocytoma. An EEG with sleep is recommended for any patient with panic attacks not readily responsive to conventional antipanic therapy (McNamara and Fogel, 1990).

PSYCHOTIC SYMPTOMS (191–194) (See Table 8.19)

Paranoid psychotic symptoms in the absence of the syndrome of delirium can be produced by drugs and also may be encountered in a number of neurologic and

Table 8.18. Medical and Neurologic Syndromes Associated with Anxiety

	Generalized	Episodic
Drug and toxin	Hypnotic/sedative withdrawal	Caffeinism
	Nicotine withdrawal	Methyl xanthine use/abuse
	Indomethacin	Adrenergic agonists
	Tricyclic antidepressant withdrawal	Dopamine agonists
	Cycloserine	Cocaine
	Antipsychotic withdrawal	Metrizamide
	Baclofen	Oxymetazoline
	Isocarboxazid	Phencyclidine
	Akathisia (antipsychotic-induced)	Organic solvent inhalation
	Lidocaine	
Endocrine	Hyperthyroidism	Pheochromocytoma
	Hypoparathyroidism	Hypoglycemia
	Cushing's syndrome	Hyperthyroidism
	Addison's disease	
Cardiovascular		Mitral valve prolapse
		Arrhythmia
		Angina pectoris
Pulmonary	Chronic obstructive pulmonary disease	Pulmonary embolus
Metabolic	Hypoxia	Porphyria
	Electrolyte disturbance	
	Hypocalcemia	
Epilepsy		Partial complex seizures

Reprinted with permission from Schiffer RB, Klein RF, Sider RC: *The Medical Evaluation of Psychiatric Patients*, New York, Plenum Medical, 1988.

endocrine diseases. Drugs particularly implicated in producing psychotic symptoms without delirium include cocaine, amphetamines and other stimulants, dopamine agonists such as Sinemet and bromocriptine, hallucinogens, and corticosteroids. Among the more common neurologic and endocrine disorders are temporal lobe epilepsy, hypothyroidism, and vitamin B_{12} deficiency. All of these conditions would be initially screened for by the recommended general test battery. However, because a single normal EEG does not rule out temporal lobe epilepsy, identify patients who are at higher risk for that disorder who should receive repeated EEGs and careful, repeated inquiry about paroxysmal psychomotor and psychosensory symptoms. An epileptic origin for psychotic symptoms is suggested by a relatively preserved personality with warm affect, personality characteristics associated with temporal lobe epilepsy, and prominent stereotyped psychomotor and psychosensory symptoms persisting throughout the various phases of the patient's illness (195).

Psychotic symptoms may accompany a wide range of CNS infections and neoplasms, usually in association with cognitive impairment. Exceptions are for tumors and infections localized to the frontal and temporal regions, such as temporal lobe brain abscess or herpes simplex encephalitis (188). Lesions in these areas, particularly if accompanied by seizure activity, can come close to mimicking schizophrenia. Diagnostic clues favoring a more aggressive neurologic workup include acute onset, fever, and disturbance of memory more severe than expected in a functional psychosis.

The combination of psychotic symptoms with specific, discrete somatic complaints is the key to diagnosing more unusual organic psychoses. For example, abdominal pain, seizures, and peripheral neuropathy together with psychotic symptoms suggest a diagnosis of porphyria (196); tests for this disorder are not warranted in the routine workup of acute psychosis. In addition to specific historical or physical evidence for unusual diagnoses, less common

Table 8.19. Medical-Neurologic Diseases Associated with Acute Paranoid States

Partial complex epilepsy	Drugs and toxins
Trauma	Cocaine
Tumor	Marijuana
Stroke	Bronchodilators
Degenerative diseases	Alcohol
Alzheimer's disease	Amphetamines
Parkinson's disease	Anticholinergics
Narcolepsy	L-dopa
Paraphrenia	Isoniazid
Huntington's disease	Benzodiazepines
	Ephedrine
	Bromocriptine
	Infection
	Metabolic (few)

Reprinted with permission from Schiffer RB, Klein RF, Sider RC: *The Medical Evaluation of Psychiatric Patients,* New York, Plenum Medical, 1988.

physical causes of psychosis that should warrant a workup are a poor response to neuroleptics or unusual features of the psychopathology, such as rapid fluctuations of mental status or disproportionate disturbance of cognition and memory.

CONCLUSION

The diagnosis of contributing organic factors in patients who apparently suffer from a psychiatric diagnosis is greatly aided by an open-ended and continual reconsideration of organic issues. Rather than focusing on a one-time "clearance" of the patient, a modest initial workup followed by a periodic reevaluation of treatment outcome and residual symptoms is less likely to leave diagnostic gaps. Selection of more expensive or less usual tests should be based on the specifics of the patient's mental syndrome, personal history, family history, and abnormal examination findings. Whenever possible, combining the mental and physical symptoms to form a specific syndrome suggesting an etiological diagnosis will lead to a higher proportion of positive test results. Although continual attention to organic factors is a necessary condition for the

best therapeutic result, it is rarely sufficient; patients referred for psychiatric inpatient treatment often have genetic, familial, or intrapsychic reasons for their mental disturbance in addition to the organic factors discovered by a careful evaluation.

REFERENCES

1. Wragg RE, Jeste DV: Overview of depression and psychosis in Alzheimer's disease. Am J Psychiatry, 146:577–587, 1989.

2. Mayeux R: Mental state, in Koller WC (ed): *Handbook of Parkinson's Disease,* New York, Marcel Dekker, 1987.

3. Lipsey JR, Robinson RG, Pearlson GD, et al.: Nortriptyline treatment of poststroke depression: A double-blind study. Lancet, Feb 11:297–300, 1984.

4. Summergrad P, Glassman RS: Human immunodeficiency virus and other infectious disorders, in Stoudemire A, Fogel BS (eds): *Medical Psychiatric Practice, Vol. 1,* Washington, D.C., American Psychiatric Press, 1991.

5. Lishman WA: *Organic Psychiatry,* Cambridge, Blackwell Scientific, 1987.

6. Hales RE, Yudofsky SC (eds): *Textbook of Neuropsychiatry,* Washington, D.C., American Psychiatric Press, 1987.

7. Cummings JL: Clinical Neuropsychiatry, Orlando, Grune & Stratton, 1985.

8. American Psychiatric Association: *Diagnostic and Statistical Manual of Mental Disorders,* ed. 3, (DSM-IIIR), pp. 97–164, Washington, D.C., American Psychiatric Association, 1987.

9. Fogel BS: Major depression versus organic mood disorder: A questionable distinction. J Clin Psychiatry, 51:53–56, 1990.

10. Lipowski ZJ: Diagnosis of delirium, in *Delirium: Acute Brain Failure in Man,* Springfield, Ill., Charles C. Thomas, 1980.

11. Beresin EV: Delirium in the elderly. J Geriatr Psychiatry Neurol, 1:127–143, 1988.

12. McNamara ME: Advances in EEG-based diagnostic technologies, in Stoudemire A, Fogel BS (eds): *Medical Psychiatric Practice, Vol. 1,* Washington, D.C., American Psychiatric Press, 1991.

13. Kiloh LG, McComas AJ, Osselton JW,

et al.: *Clinical Electroencephalography*, ed. 4, pp. 165–166, London, Butterworths, 1981.

14. Kiloh LG, McComas AJ, Osselton JW, et al.: *Clinical Electroencephalography*, ed. 4, pp. 79–180, London, Butterworths, 1981.

15. Kiloh LG, McComas AJ, Osselton JW, et al.: *Clinical Electroencephalography*, ed. 4, p. 122, London, Butterworths, 1981.

16. Folstein MF, Folstein SE, McHugh PR: Mini-Mental State. J Psychiatr Res, *12*:189–198, 1975.

17. Bond TC: Recognition of acute delirious mania. Arch Gen Psychiatry, *37*:553–554, 1980.

18. Granacher RP, Baldessarini RJ: Psysostigmine. Arch Gen Psychiatry, *32*:375–380, 1975.

19. Safer DJ, Allen RP: The central effects of scopolamine in man. Biol Psychiatry, *3*:347–355, 1971.

20. Greenblatt DJ, Shader RI: Anticholinergics. N Engl J Med, *288*:1215–1219, 1973.

21. Dysken MW, Merry W, Davis JM: Anticholinergic psychosis. Psychiatr Ann, *8(9)*:452–456, 1978.

22. Spiker DG, Weiss AN, Chang SS, et al.: Tricyclic antidepressant overdose: Clinical presentation and plasma levels. Clin Pharmacol Ther, *18*:539–546, 1975.

23. Davies RK, Tucker GJ, Harrow M, Detre TP: Confusional episodes and antidepressant medications. Am J Psychiatry, *128*:95–99, 1971.

24. Tune LE, Holland A, Folstein MF, et al.: Association of postoperative delirium with raised serum levels of anticholinergic drugs. Lancet, *Sep 26*:651–652, 1981.

25. Sewell DD, Jeste D: The neuroleptic malignant syndrome: Clinical presentation, pathophysiology, and treatment, in Stoudemire A, Fogel BS (eds): *Medical Psychiatric Practice, Vol. 1*, Washington, D.C., American Psychiatric Press, 1991.

26. Johnson GF: Lithium neurotoxicity. Aust N Z J Psychiatry, *10*:33–38, 1976.

27. Reisberg B, Gershon S: Side effects associated with lithium therapy. Arch Gen Psychiatry, *36*:879–887, 1979.

28. West AP, Meltzer HY: Paradoxical lithium neurotoxicity: A report of five cases and a hypothesis about risk for neurotoxicity. Am J Psychiatry, *136*:963–966, 1979.

29. Appelbaum PS, Shader RI, Funkenstein HH, et al.: Difficulties in the clinical diagnosis of lithium toxicity. Am J Psychiatry, *136*:1212–1213, 1979.

30. Dasgupta K, Jefferson JW: The use of lithium in the medically ill. Gen Hosp Psychiatry, *12*:83–97, 1990.

31. Addonizio G, Susman VL, Roth SD: Neuroleptic malignant syndrome: Review and analysis of 115 cases. Biol Psychiatry, *22*:1004–1020, 1987.

32. Shalev A, Munitz H: The neuroleptic malignant syndrome: Agent and host interaction. Acta Psychiatr Scand, *73*:337–347, 1986.

33. Jimerson DC: Role of dopamine mechanisms in the affective disorders, in Meltzer HY (ed): *Psychopharmacology: The Third Generation of Progress*, New York, Raven, 1987.

34. Post RM: Mechanisms of action of carbamazepine and related anticonvulsants in affective illness, in Meltzer HY (ed): *Psychopharmacology: The Third Generation of Progress*, New York, Raven, 1987.

35. Goldberg RJ, Dubin WR, Fogel BS: Behavioral emergencies: Assessment and psychopharmacologic management. Clin Neuropharmacol, *12*:233–248, 1989.

36. Lipowski ZJ: Delirium: Acute Brain Failure in Man, pp. 268–275, Springfield, Ill., Charles C. Thomas, 1980.

37. Wilker A: Diagnosis and treatment of drug dependence of the barbiturate type. Am J Psychiatry, *125*:758–765, 1968.

38. Essig CF: Addiction to nonbarbiturate sedative and tranquilizing drugs. Clin Pharmacol Ther, *5*:334–343, 1964.

39. Maletzky BM, Klotter J: Addiction to diazepam. Int J Addict, *11*:95–115, 1976.

40. DeBard ML: Diazepam withdrawal syndrome: A case with psychosis, seizure and coma. Am J Psychiatry, *136*:104–105, 1979.

41. Winokur A, Rickles K, Greenblatt DJ, et al.: Withdrawal reaction from long-term, low-dosage administration of diazepam. Arch Gen Psychiatry, *37*:101–105, 1980.

42. Stewart RB, Salem RB, Springer PK: A case report of lorazepam withdrawal. Am J Psychiatry, *137*:113–114, 1980.

43. Flemenbaum A, Gunby B: Ethchlorvynol (Placidyl) abuse and withdrawal. Dis Nerv Syst, 32:188–192, 1971.

44. Heston LL, Hastings D: Psychosis with withdrawal from ethchlorvynol. Am J Psychiatry, 137:249–150, 1980.

45. Haizlip TM, Ewing JA: Meprobamate habituation. N Engl J Med, 258:1181–1186, 1958.

46. Ewart RBL, Priest RG: Methaqualone addiction and delirium tremens. Br Med J, 3:92–93, 1967.

47. Essig CF: Newer sedative drugs that can cause states of intoxication and dependence of the barbiturate type. JAMA, 196:126–129, 1966.

48. Shader RI, Caine ED, Meyer RE: Treatment of dependence on barbiturates and sedative-hypnotics, in Shader RI (ed): *Manual of Psychiatric Therapeutics*, Boston, Little Brown & Co., 1975.

49. Patterson J: Triazolam syndrome in the elderly. South Med J, 30:1425–1426, 1987.

50. Albeck JH: Withdrawal and detoxification from benzodiazepine dependence: A potential role for clonazepam. J Clin Psychiatry, 48:43S–48S, 1987.

51. Herman JB, Rosenbaum JF, Brotman AW: The alprazolam to clonazepam switch for the treatment of panic disorder. J Clin Psychopharmacol, 7:175–178, 1987.

52. Stoudemire A, Fogel BS (eds): *Principles of Medical Psychiatry*, pp. 105–106, Orlando, Grune & Stratton, 1987.

53. Graham PM, Ilett KF: Danger of MAOI with therapy after fluoxetine withdrawal. Lancet, Nov 26:1255–1256, 1988.

54. Price LH, Charney DS, Heninger GR: Effects of tranylcypromine treatment on neuroendocrine, behavioral, and autonomic responses to tryptophan in depressed patients. Life Sci, 37:809–818, 1983.

55. Stoudemire A, Fogel BS, Gulley LR: Psychopharmacology in the medically ill: An update, in Stoudemire A, Fogel BS (eds): *Medical Psychiatric Practice, Vol. 1*, Washington, D.C., American Psychiatric Press, 1991.

56. Hall RCW, Popkin MK, Stickney SK, Gardner ER: Presentation of the steroid psychoses. J Nerv Ment Dis, 167:229–236, 1979.

57. The Boston Collaborative Drug Surveillance Program: Acute adverse reactions to prednisone in relation to dosage. Clin Pharmacol Ther, 13:694–698, 1972.

58. Ling MHM, Perry PJ, Tsuang MT: Side-effects of corticosteroid therapy: Psychiatric aspects. Arch Gen Psychiatry, 38:471–477, 1981.

59. McMillen MA, Ambis D, Siegel JH: Cimetidine and mental confusion, N Engl J Med, 298:283–285, 1978.

60. Barnhart CC, Bowden CL: Toxic psychosis with cimetidine. Am J Psychiatry, 136:725–726, 1979.

61. Strum WB: Cimetidine and ranitidine. JAMA, 251:2212, 1984.

62. Lipowski ZJ: *Delirium: Acute Brain Failure in Man*, Springfield, Ill., Charles C. Thomas, 1980.

63. Stoudemire A, Fogel BS (eds): *Principles of Medical Psychiatry*, p. 489, Orlando, Grune & Stratton, 1987.

64. Volpe BT, Soave R: Formed visual hallucinations and digitalis toxicity. Ann Intern Med, 91:865, 1979.

65. Reus VI: Behavioral side effects of medical drugs. Prim Care, 6:283–294, 1979.

66. Shear MK, Sacks M: Digitalis delirium: Psychiatric considerations. Int J Psychiatry Med, 135:371–381, 1978.

67. Shear MK, Sacks MH: Digitalis delirium: Report of two cases. Am J Psychiatry, 135:109–110, 1978.

68. Portnoi VA: Digitalis delirium in elderly patients. J Clin Pharmacol, 19:747–750, 1979.

69. Eisendrath SJ, Sweeney MA: Toxic neuropsychiatric effects of digoxin at therapeutic serum concentrations. Am J Psychiatry, 144:506–507, 1987.

70. Adams F: Neuropsychiatric evaluation and treatment of delirium in cancer patients, in Goldberg RJ (ed): *Psychiatric Aspects of Cancer*, Basel, Karger, 1988.

71. Cuthbert MF: Adverse reactions to nonsteroidal antirheumatic drugs. Curr Med Res Opin, 2:600–610, 1974.

72. Steele TE, Morton WA: Salicylate-induced delirium. Psychosomatics, 27:455–456, 1986.

73. Foley KM: The practical use of narcotic analgesics. Med Clin North Am, 66:1091–1104, 1982.

74. Foley KM: The treatment of cancer pain. N Engl J Med, 313:84–95, 1985.

75. Miller RR, Jick H: Clinical effects of meperidine in hospitalized medical patients. J Clin Pharmacol, 18:180–189, 1978.

76. Miller RR: Clinical effects of pentazocine in hospitalized medical patients. J Clin Pharmacol, 15:198–205, 1975.

77. Bernstein JG: Medical-psychiatric drug interactions, in Hackett TP, Cassem NH (eds): Massachusetts General Hospital Handbook of General Hospital Psychiatry, St. Louis, C. V. Mosby, 1978.

78. Sweet RD, McDowell FH, Fiegenson JS, et al.: Mental symptoms in Parkinson's disease during chronic treatment with levodopa. Neurology, 26:305–310, 1976.

79. Lin JT-Y, Ziegler DK: Psychiatric symptoms with initiation of carbidopa-levodopa treatment. Neurology, 26:699–700, 1976.

80. Hausner RS: Amantadine-associated recurrence of psychosis. Am J Psychiatry, 137:240–242, 1980.

81. Koller WC (ed): Handbook of Parkinson's Disease, New York, pp. 311–313; pp. 319–321; pp. 393–397; Marcel Dekker, 1987.

82. Epstein M: Disorders of sodium balance, in Stein JH (ed): Internal Medicine, ed. 3, Boston, Little Brown & Co., 1990.

83. Bilezikian JP: Hypercalcemia, in Stein JH (ed): Internal Medicine, ed. 3, Boston, Little Brown & Co., 1990.

84. Clutter WE, Cryer PE: Hypoglycemia, in Stein JH (ed): Internal Medicine, ed. 3, Boston, Little Brown & Co., 1990.

85. Luke RG, Strom TB: Chronic renal failure, in Stein JH (ed): Internal Medicine, ed. 3, Boston, Little Brown & Co., 1990.

86. Narins RG, Krishna GC: Disorders of water balance, in Stein JH (ed): Internal Medicine, ed. 3, Boston, Little Brown & Co., 1990.

87. Harper CG, Giles M, Finlay-Jones R: Clinical science in the Wernicke-Korsakoff complex role in a retrospective analysis of 131 cases diagnosed in necropsy. J Neurol Neurosurg Psychiatry, 49:341–345, 1986.

88. Schenker S, Hoyumpa AM, Jr: Principal complications of liver failure, in Stein JH (ed): Internal Medicine, ed. 3, Boston, Little Brown & Co., 1990.

89. Ziyadeh FN, Goldfarb S: Disorders of phosphate homeostatis, in Stein JH (ed): Internal Medicine, ed. 3, Boston, Little Brown & Co., 1990.

90. Lefkoff S, Evans D, Liptzin B, et al.: Delirium: The occurrence and persistence of symptoms among elderly hospitalized patients. Submitted to N Engl J Med, 1990.

91. Lipowski ZJ: Delirium: Acute Brain Failure in Man, pp. 110–111, Springfield, Ill., Charles C. Thomas, 1980.

92. Horenstein S, Chamberlin W, Conomy J: Infarction of the fusiform and calcarine regions: Agitated delirium and hemianopia. Trans Am Neurol Assoc, 92:85–89, 1967.

93. Medina JL, Rubino FA, Ross A: Agitated delirium caused by infarction of the hippocampal formation and fusiform and lingual gyri: A case report. Neurology, 24:1181–1183, 1974.

94. Mesulam M-M, Waxman SG, Geschwind N, et al.: Acute confusional states with right middle cerebral artery infarctions. J Neurol Neurosurg Psychiatry, 39:84–89, 1976.

95. Bradley WG, Bydder G: MRI Atlas of the Brain, London, Martin Dunitz, 1990.

96. Niedermeyer E, Da Silva FL: Electroencephalography: Basic Principles, Clinical Applications and Related Fields, pp. 96–97, Baltimore, Urban & Schwarzenberg, 1982.

97. Hoenig J, Chaulk R: Delirium associated with lithium and electroconvulsive therapy. Can Med Assoc J, 116:837–838, 1977.

98. Mande MR, Madsen J, Miller AL, Baldessarini RJ: Intoxication associated with lithium and ECT. Am J Psychiatry, 137:1107–1109, 1980.

99. Fogel BS: Electroconvulsive therapy in the elderly: A clinical research agenda. Int J Geriatric Psychiatry, 3:181–190, 1988.

100. Fogel BS: Delirium, in Conn's Current Therapy, Rakel RE (ed), Philadelphia, W. B. Saunders, 1990.

101. Evans DA, Funkenstein HH, Albert MS, et al.: Prevalence of Alzheimer's disease in a community population of older persons. JAMA, 262:2551–2556, 1989.

102. Merriam AE, Aronson MK, Gaston P, et al.: The psychiatric symptoms of Alzheimer's disease. J Am Geriat Soc, 36:7–12, 1988.

103. Petry S, Cummings JL, Hill MA, et al.: Personality alterations in dementia of the Alzheimer type: A three-year follow-up study. J Geriatr Psychiatry Neurol, 4:203–207, 1989.

104. Pearce JMS: *Dementia*, London, Blackwell Scientific, 1984.

105. Cummings JL, Benson DF: *Dementia: A Clinical Approach*, Woburn, Butterworth, 1983.

106. Stoudemire A, Hill C, Gulley LR, et al.: Neuropsychological and biomedical assessment of depression-dementia syndromes. J Neuropsychiatry Clin Neurosciences, *Fall*:347–361, 1989.

107. Reifler BV: Mixed cognitive-affective disturbances in the elderly: A new classification. J Clin Psychiatry, 47:354–356, 1986.

108. Baker HL, Berquist TH, Kispert DB: Magnetic resonance imaging in a routine clinical setting. Mayo Clin Proc, 60:75–90, 1985.

109. Kertesz A, Black SE, Tokar G, et al.: Periventricular and subcortical hyperintensities on magnetic resonance imaging. Arch Neurol, 45:404–408, 1988.

110. Bondareff W, Raval J, Woo B, et al.: Magnetic resonance imaging and the severity of dementia in older adults. Arch Gen Psychiatry, 48:47–51, 1990.

111. Eichner ER: Megaloblastic anemias, in Stein JH (ed): *Internal Medicine*, ed. 3, Boston, Little Brown & Co., 1990.

112. Herbert V, et al.: Is there a "gold standard" for human serum vitamin B_{12} assay? J Lab Clin Med, 104:829, 1984.

113. Hein MD, Jackson IVM: Review: Thyroid function in psychiatric illness. Gen Hosp Psychiatry, 12:1–13, 1990.

114. Fogel BS, Faust D: Neurologic assessment, neurodiagnostic tests, and neuropsychology in medical psychiatry, in Stoudemire A, Fogel BS (eds): *Principles of Medical Psychiatry*, Orlando, Grune & Stratton, 1987.

115. Coban LA, Danziger W, Storandt M: A longitudinal EEG study of mild senile dementia of the Alzheimer type: Changes at one year and at 2.5 years. Electroencephalogr Clin Neurophysiol, 61:101–112, 1985.

116. Meary D, Snowden JS, Bowen DM: Neuropsychological syndromes in presenile dementia due to cerebral atrophy. J Neurol Neurosurg Psychiatry, 49:163–174, 1986.

117. Faust D, Fogel BS: The development and initial validation of a sensitive bedside cognitive screening test. J Nerv Ment Dis, 177:25–31, 1989.

118. Morris JC, Heyman A, Mohs RC, et al.: The Consortium to Establish a Registry for Alzheimer's Disease (CERAD). Part I: Clinical and neuropsychological assessment of Alzheimer's disease. Neurology, 39:1159–1165, 1989.

119. Giombetti RJ, Miller BL: Recognition and management of superimposed medical conditions, in Cummings JL, Miller BL (eds): *Alzheimer's Disease: Treatment and Long-Term Management*, New York, Marcel Dekker, 1990.

120. Fogel BS: Treatment of agitation, in Light E, Lebowitz B (eds): *The Chronically Mentally Ill Elderly*, New York, Springer, 1989.

121. Slaby AE, Cullen LO: Dementia and Delirium, in Stoudemire A, Fogel BS (eds): *Principles of Medical Psychiatry*, Orlando, Grune & Stratton, 1987.

122. Cummings JL, Miller BL (eds): *Alzheimer's Disease: Treatment and Long-Term Management*, New York, Marcel Dekker, 1990.

123. Sadavoy J, Lazarus LW, Langsley PR: Psychotherapy with the elderly, in Sadavoy J, Lazarus L, Jarvik L (eds): *Comprehensive Review of Geriatric Psychiatry*, Washington, D.C., American Psychiatric Press, 1991.

124. Teri L, Gallagher D: Cognitive behavioral interventions for depressed patients with dementia of the Alzheimer's type, in Depression in Sunderland T (ed): *Alzheimer's Disease: Component or Consequence?* Orlando, Grune & Stratton, In press.

125. Teri L: Behavioral assessment and treatment of depression in older adults, in Wisocki P (ed): *Clinical Behavioral Therapy with Older Adults*, In press.

126. Jenike MA: *Geriatric Psychiatry and Psychopharmacology: A Clinical Approach*, pp. 178–181, Chicago, Year Book Medical, 1989.

127. Barnes R, Veith R, Okimoto J, et al.: Efficacy of antipsychotic medications in behaviorally disturbed dementia patients. Am J Psychiatry, 139:1170–1174, 1982.

128. Devanand DP, Sacheim HA, Mayeux R: Psychosis, behavioral disturbance, and the use of neuroleptics in dementia. Compr Psychiatry, 29:387–401, 1988.

129. Petrie WM, Ban TA, Berney S, et al.: Loxapine in psychogeriatrics: A placebo- and

standard-controlled clinical investigation. J Clin Psychopharmacol, 2:122–126, 1982.

130. Raskind MA, Risse SC: Antipsychotic drugs and the elderly. J Clin Psychiatry, 47(Suppl):17–22, 1986.

131. Cole JO: The drug treatment of anxiety and depression. Med Clin North Am, 72:815–822, 1988.

132. Colenda CC: Buspirone in treatment of agitated demented patient. Lancet, *May 21*:1169, 1988.

133. Levine AM: Buspirone and agitation in head injury. Brain Inj, 2:165–167, 1988.

134. Liegghio NE, Yerangani VK, et al.: Buspirone-induced jitteriness in patients with panic disorder and one patient with generalized anxiety disorder. J Clin Psychiatry, 49:165–166, 1988.

135. Ritchie DE, Bridenbaugh RH, et al.: Acute generalized myoclonus following buspirone administration. J Clin Psychiatry, 49:242–243, 1988.

136. Robinson D, Napoliello MJ, Shenk J: The safety and usefulness of buspirone as an anxiolytic drug in the elderly versus young patients. Clin Ther, 6:740–746, 1988.

137. Schweizer EE, Amsterdam J, Rickels K, et al.: Open trial of buspirone in the treatment of major depressive disorder. Psychopharmacol Bull, 22:183–185, 1986.

138. Strauss A: Oral dyskinesia associated with buspirone use in elderly woman. J Clin Psychiatry, 49:322–323, 1988.

139. Tiller JW, Dakis JA, Shaw JM: Short-term buspirone treatment in disinhibition with dementia. Lancet, *Aug 27*:510, 1988.

140. Soloff PH, George A, Nathan RS, et al.: Progress in pharmacotherapy of borderline disorders. Arch Gen Psychiatry, 43:691–697, 1986.

141. Gunderson JG: Pharmacotherapy for patients with borderline personality disorder. Arch Gen Psychiatry, 43:698–699, 1986.

142. Rabins PV: Family-directed therapy, in Cummings JL, Miller BL (eds): *Alzheimer's Disease: Treatment and Long-Term Management*, New York, Marcel Dekker, 1990.

143. Szwabo PA: The family as an integral part of the management of central nervous system disorders, in Strong R, Wood WG, Burke WJ (eds): *Central Nervous System Disorders of Aging*, New York, Raven Press, 1988.

144. Gwyther LPL: Clinician and family: A partnership for support, in Mace NL (ed): *Dementia Care*, Baltimore, Johns Hopkins University Press, 1990.

145. Cohen D, Eisdorfer C: Depression in family members caring for a relative with Alzheimer's disease. J Am Geriatr Soc, 36:885–889, 1988.

146. Haley WE, Levine EG, Brown SL, et al.: Psychological, social, and health consequences of caring for a relative with senile dementia. Am Geriatr Soc, 35:405–411, 1987.

147. George LK, Gwyther LP: Caregiver well-being: A multidimensional examination of family caregivers of demented adults. Gerontologist, 26:253–266, 1986.

148. Stuss DT, Benson DF: *The Frontal Lobes*, New York, Raven Press, 1986.

149. Fogel BS, Eslinger P: Diagnosis and management of patients with frontal lobe syndromes, in Stoudemire A, Fogel BS (eds): *Medical Psychiatric Practice, Vol. 1*, Washington, D.C., American Psychiatric Press, 1991.

150. Weinberger DR: Schizophrenia and the frontal lobe. Trends Neurosci, 11:367–370, 1988.

151. Heinrichs RW: Frontal cerebral lesions and violent incidents in chronic neuropsychiatric patients. Biol Psychiatry, 25:174–178, 1989.

152. Morihisa JM: Advances in neuroimaging technologies, in Stoudemire A, Fogel BS (eds): *Medical Psychiatric Practice, Vol. 1*, Washington, D.C., American Psychiatric Press, 1991.

153. Echiverri HC, Tatum WO, Merens TA, et al.: Akinetic mutism: Pharmacologic probe of the dopaminergic mesencephalofrontal activating system. Pediatr Neurol, 4:228–230, 1988.

154. Catsman-Berrevoets CE, von Harskamp F: Compulsive presleep behavior and apathy due to bilateral thalamic stroke: Response to bromocriptine. Neurology, 38:647–649, 1988.

155. Albert ML, Bachman D, Morgan A, et al.: Pharmacotherapy for aphasia. Neurology, 37:175, 1987.

156. Crimson ML, Childs A, Wilcox RE, et al.: The effect of bromocriptine on speech dysfunction in patients with diffuse brain injury

(brain stem). Clin Neuropharmacol, 11:462–466, 1988.

157. McAllister TW: Carbamazepine in mixed frontal lobe and psychiatric disorders. J Clin Psychiatry, 46:393–394, 1985.

158. Hales RE, Silver JM, Yudofsky SC: Beta-blocking agents and the treatment of aggression, in Cummings JL, Miller BL (eds): *Alzheimer's Disease: Treatment and Long-Term Management*, New York, Marcel Dekker, 1990.

159. Fogel BS, Sparadeo F: Focal cognitive deficits accentuated by depression: A case study. J Nerv Ment Dis, *173(2)*:120–124, 1985.

160. O'Connell, Van Heertum RL, Billick SB, et al.: Single photon emission computed tomography (SPECT) with ^{123}I[IMP] in the differential diagnosis of psychiatric disorders. J Neuropsychiatry Clin Neurosciences, *1*:145–153, 1989.

161. Sohlberg MM, Sprunk H, Metzelaar K: Efficacy of an external cuing system in an individual with severe frontal lobe damage. Cog Rehab, *6*:36–41, 1988.

162. Whaley AL, Stanford CB, Pollack IW: The effects of behavior modification vs. lithium therapy on frontal lobe syndrome. J Behav Ther Exp Psychiatry, *17*:111–115, 1986.

163. Benson DF, Blumer D: Amnesia: A clinical approach to memory, in Benson DF, Blumer D (eds): *Psychiatric Aspects of Neurologic Disease, Vol. II*, Orlando, Grune & Stratton, 1982.

164. Spiers PA, Schomer DL, Blume HW, et al.: Temporolimbic epilepsy and behavior, in Mesulam M-M (ed): *Principles of Behavioral Neurology*, Philadelphia, F. A. Davis, 1985.

165. Fogel BS: Combining anticonvulsants with conventional psychopharmacologic agents, in McElroy SL, Pope HG (eds): *Anticonvulsants in Psychiatry*, Clifton, N.J., Oxford Health Care, 1988.

166. Bear D: Temporal lobe epilepsy: A syndrome of sensory-limbic hyperconnection. Cortex, *15*:357–384, 1979.

167. Schiffer RB, Klein RF, Sider RC: *The Medical Evaluation of Psychiatric Patients*, New York, Plenum Medical, 1988.

168. Hall RC, Gardner ER, Stickney SK, et al.: Physical illness manifesting as psychiatric disease. Arch Gen Psychiatry, *37*:989–995, 1980.

169. Koranyi EK: Morbidity and rate of undiagnosed physical illness in a psychiatric clinic population. Arch Gen Psychiatry, *36*:414–419, 1979.

170. Roberts JKA: *Differential Diagnosis in Neuropsychiatry*, Chichester, John Wiley & Sons, 1984.

171. Swift RM, Griffiths W, Camara P: Special technical considerations laboratory testing for illicit drugs, in Stoudemire A, Fogel BS (eds): *Medical Psychiatric Practice*, Washington, D.C., American Psychiatric Press, 1991.

172. Miller NS, Gold MS, Belkin BM: Clinical laboratory testing in drug abuse and addiction. Annals Clin Psychiatry, *1*:227–236, 1989.

173. Pascualy M, Veith RC: Depression as an adverse drug reaction, in Robinson RG, Rabins PV (eds): *Aging and Clinical Practice: Depression and Coexisting Disease*, New York, Igaku-Shoin, 1989.

174. Gottlieb GL, Greenspan D: Depression and endocrine disorders, in Robinson RG, Rabins PV (eds): *Aging and Clinical Practice: Depression and Coexisting Disease*, New York, Igaku-Shoin, 1989.

175. O'Shanick GJ, Gardner DF, Kornstein SG: Endocrine disorders, in Stoudemire A, Fogel BS (eds): *Medical Psychiatric Practice*, Orlando, Grune & Stratton, 1987.

176. Biglieri EG, Kater CE: Disorders of the adrenal cortex, in Stein JH (ed): *Internal Medicine*, ed. 3, Boston, Little Brown & Co., 1990.

177. Rabins PV: Depression and multiple sclerosis, in Robinson RG, Rabins PV (eds): *Aging and Clinical Practice: Depression and Coexisting Disease*, New York, Igaku-Shoin, 1989.

178. Joffe RT, Lippert GP, Gray TA, et al.: Mood disorders and multiple sclerosis, in Jensen K, Knudsen L, Stenager E, et al. (eds): *Mental Disorders and Cognitive Deficits in Multiple Sclerosis*, London, John Libbey, 1989.

179. Minden SL, Orav J, Reich P: Characteristics and predictors of depression in multiple sclerosis, in Jensen K, Knudsen L, Stenager E, et al. (eds): *Mental Disorders and Cognitive Deficits in Multiple Sclerosis*, London, John Libbey, 1989.

180. Cummings JL: *Clinical Neuropsychiatry*, pp. 190–193, Orlando, Grune & Stratton, 1985.

181. Krauthammer C, Klerman GL: Sec-

ondary mania. Arch Gen Psychiatry, 35:1333–1339, 1978.

182. Hasket RF, Rose RM: Neuroendocrine disorders and psychopathology. Psychiatr Clin North Am, 4:239–252, 1981.

183. Schiffer RB, Wineman NM, Weitkamp LR: Association between bipolar affective disorder and multiple sclerosis. Am J Psychiatry, 143:94–95, 1986.

184. Brambilla F, Catalano M, Lucca A, et al.: Clonidine-induced growth hormone release, in Johnson FN (ed): Lithium and the Endocrine System, Basel, Karger, 1988.

185. Fitzpatrick LA, Spiegel AM: Parathyroid hormone secretion, in Johnson FN (ed): Lithium and the Endocrine System, Basel, Karger, 1988.

186. Goldberg RJ: Anxiety in the medically ill, in Stoudemire A, Fogel BS (eds): Principles of Medical Psychiatry, Orlando, Grune & Stratton, 1987.

187. Stein MG: Panic disorder and medical illness. Psychosomatics, 27:833–840, 1986.

188. Schweizer E, Winokur A, Rickels K: Insulin-induced hypoglycemia and panic attacks. Am J Psychiatry, 143:654–655, 1986.

189. McNamara ME, Fogel BS: Anticonvulsant-responsive panic attacks with temporal lobe EEG abnormalities. J Neuropsychiatry Clin Neurosciences, In press.

190. Starkman MN, Zelnik TC, Nesse RM, et al.: Anxiety in patients with pheochromocytomas. Arch Intern Med, 145:248–252, 1985.

191. Cummings JL: Organic psychosis. Psychosomatics, 29(Winter):16–26, 1988.

192. Cummings JL: Secondary psychoses, delusions, and schizophrenia, in Clinical Neuropsychiatry, Orlando, Grune & Stratton, 1985.

193. Roberts JKA: Disorders of perception, in Differential Diagnosis in Neuropsychiatry, Chichester, John Wiley & Sons, 1984.

194. Strub RL: Mental disorders in brain disease, in Frederiks JAM (ed): Handbook of Clinical Neurology, Vol. 46: Neurobehavioral Disorders, Amsterdam, Elsevier, 1985.

195. Toone BK, Garralda ME, Ron MA: The psychoses of epilepsy and the functional psychoses: A clinical and phenomenological comparison. Br J Psychiatry, 141:256, 1982.

196. Roberts JKA: Differential Diagnosis in Neuropsychiatry, p. 318, Chichester, John Wiley & Sons, 1984.

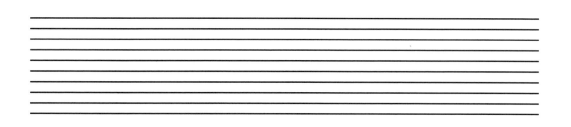

Section II

Specific Aspects of Inpatient Psychiatry

The Family

Ira D. Glick, MD
John F. Clarkin, PhD*

THE FAMILY MODEL OF INTERVENTION

The nature and quality of work with the family has varied enormously through-out the history of inpatient work. The regard and help given families has reflected prevailing theories of individual patient psychopathology as well as the capacity of hospitals to temporarily "adopt" patients from their families. Shorter lengths of stay (1) and a now-developed literature on *hospital* and *family* theory and practice, have combined to inform us of: (*a*) the limits of hospital practice; and (*b*) the importance of including and allying with families for the effective short *and* long-term posthospital care of the hospitalized psychiatric patient.

This chapter (adopted, in part, from Ira D. Glick and D. R. Kessler: *Marital and Family Therapy,* ed. 3, chap. 24, pp. 370–389, Boston, Allyn and Bacon, 1987) will focus on the new model (or orientation) of the evaluation and treatment of families on a short-term (weeks, not months or years)

psychiatric unit (2). The model is empirically rather than theoretically based (where data exist). General guidelines for inpatient family work will be provided, and specific approaches for specific diagnostic disorders elaborated. Table 9.1 contrasts the individually oriented model with the family-oriented model as they are utilized in a hospital setting (3).

Background

Although psychiatric residents, psychology interns, and social work students currently in training may not realize it, not that many years ago—the 70s— the family with a member in a psychiatric hospital was regarded at best as purveyors of hospital information to the social worker and as hospital bill payers. At worst, they were seen as malignant, pathogenic individuals who had played a major role in causing the patient's symptoms and who tended to make nuisances of themselves by interfering with the patient's treatment.

The staff acted *in loco parentis.* They often inappropriately blamed the family for the patient's symptoms. The family was fre-

*We are indebted to Alfred Lewis, M.D., for many helpful suggestions and comments and to Lee Combrick Graham for case examples.

255

Table 9.1. Family Therapy in Individually Oriented Hospitals and Family-Oriented Treatment in the Hospital: A Comparison

Issue	Individually Oriented Hospitals	Family-Oriented Hospitals
Locus of pathology	In the neurobiological system or psychodynamics of the individual	Dysfunctional individual behavior related to dysfunction in family interactions as well as individual neurobiological and psychodynamic factors—a biopsychosocial model
Locus of change and healing	In the biosystem or the intrapsychic system of the individual	In the individual within the family as a significant piece of the individual's ecology
Diagnosis	DSM-III-R, Axes I, II, III	DSM-III-R, Axes IV and V, and characterization of family interactions in relation to the symptoms or complaints
Role of the staff	To care for and provide therapy for the patient	To facilitate changes in the family through family interaction or planned interactions with patient
Visits	During visiting hours, informal	Visits are a part of the treatment. Those people who visit are a part of the treatment plan
Role of family therapy	A modality to work on those aspects of the patient's problem which seem to be related to family functioning	The orienting therapy of the overall treatment program
Discharge planning	Related to the condition of the individual and his/her ability to function outside the hospital	Related to the condition of the family and its ability to provide safety and continued growth for members

quently not allowed to visit during the early part of hospitalization. In turn, the psychiatric hospital was associated with much fear and stigma and, in many cases, families were only too happy to stay away. Before effective somatic treatments were available, hospital stays were much longer and already fragile family ties were broken. At the time of discharge, hospital staff members tended to want to remove the patient from the family setting, because they viewed the family as an adversary. Even more commonly, patients were sent back to adversarial families without having the adversarial problems addressed.

In other cultures, families are sometimes considered a vital part of the psychiatric hospitalization of any of their members (4). Because of a scarcity of trained professionals, families are needed in the hospital to care for the needs of the identified patient. They, in fact, often stay with the patient in or near the hospital. The assumption in other cultures is that the patient is an integral part of the family network, and it is unthinkable that the patient would return anywhere else but to the family (5).

Although during the last 20 years, family intervention has increased in inpatient settings (6), that move has not been without problems. In an article published in 1977, Anderson (7) outlined some of the difficulties, many of which still remain to some degree:

Regrettably, however, the family therapy literature is not particularly helpful to those working on inpatient units; such concepts as "defining the family as the patient" tend to alienate both the medical staff of an institution and the already overwhelmingly guilt-ridden families. The polarized approaches of family therapists, who generally operate on a "system" model, which overemphasizes interactional variables, and of psychiatrists, who generally operate on a "medical" model, which overemphasizes individual variables, disregard the complex and complementary interplay of biological, psychodynamic, and interactional factors. . . . A collaborative relationship between families and the hospital staff could be developed by the establishment of treatment contacts and by combining these two models, thus accepting the patient's illness as the focus *while* recognizing the importance of family variables.

This quote states extremely well the problem of integrating theories of etiology and pathogenesis. This problem is shared alike by patient, family, and hospital staff. Some advances have been made since 1977. For example, the research on expressed emotion (EE) in the family environments of schizophrenics has put biological and environmental influences into perspective, focusing treatment strategies (8, 9). In addition, research designs that include pharmacotherapy in various doses plus family intervention (10) recognize and provide data on the importance of therapeutically attacking biological and social fronts simultaneously.

The newest trend (a welcome one) is to involve the family almost as a "colleague" on the treatment team. More on this later. Accordingly, our prescription for hospital treatment of families has undergone major changes since the last edition. Important changes have occurred in hospital practice (most importantly, shorter length of hospital stays and patients mentally more ill and physically more disabled than before). Correspondingly, the families of these patients are different. Hospital staff has the impression that families are less functional now. Staff estimate that more than one-third of families of the seriously mentally ill now hospitalized have a psychotic member themselves.

Function of the Psychiatric Hospital Vis-À-Vis the Family

Brief psychiatric hospitalization, which is the norm in this country, provides a safe and controlled environment in which to treat acute symptoms of depression, mania, suicidal ideation, alcoholism, severe personality disorder, schizophrenia, and psychotic thought and behavior (2). In addition, the hospitalization serves major functions for the family of the patient. By hospitalization the identified patient is temporarily removed from the family environment when it seems no longer able to contain the patient. In acute family crises, hospitalization may be a means of decreasing behaviorial eruptions, offering substantial relief to a desperate family headed for serous deterioration. This enforced separation is undertaken with the goal of evaluating and changing the situation to improve the family's patterns of interaction (11).

Hospitalization can also dramatically symbolize the problems of patient and family, bringing the problems to a point that calls out for attention and resolution. As such, psychiatric hospitalization often disrupts a rigidly pathologic pattern of family interaction; while the family is thrown temporarily into turmoil, this very turmoil leaves family members open to change which is likely to be more substantial and happen more quickly than without hospitalization. Hospitalization permits observation, evaluation, and discussion of family interaction patterns around the patient and instills motivation for seeking marital and family treatment after the patient's return to a better functioning family setting. Hospitalization may also set the stage for overt (as opposed to previous covert) consideration of separation in deadlocked marital or parent-child interactions.

In our opinion the staff should consider at least four family-relevant functions when a patient with a serious mental illness is hospitalized (12):

1. Treat the patient.
2. Evaluate (and sometimes) treat the families. Identify families with special diffi-

culties who need immediate or intense support.

3. Develop an alliance with the families, which can later be shifted to the health care system.

4. Provide psychoeducation to the families (we regard therapy and consultation as distinct interventions.)

In performing the above functions, especially the second, it is important that the therapist identify *patterns* the family uses for coping with the patient's mental illness and intrafamilial differences in coping that cause family conflict (such as what happens when one parent sees the patient as "mad," and the other sees the patient as "bad"). In addition, the family response must be viewed in the context of the culture from which it derived. Finally, a good clinician needs to recognize that family coping patterns change over time.

Clinical Pearl: Families with a member who has a serious mental illness can cope successfully. It is fatuous for a clinician to presume that because a patient has a serious mental illness something *must* be wrong with the family. Family members of the National Alliance for the Mentally Ill do not accept the assertion of many family therapists that the whole family "is the patient"; Alliance family members prefer to serve as "members of the treatment team" (personal communication of D. Richardson).

Later in the chapter these tasks will be further elaborated upon as goals.

Family Influences on the Hospitalization Process and Their Function for the Family

While not trying to imply that the family interactions are a major, or sole, cause of serious individual symptoms, it seems clear that hospitalization of the family member can serve important functions for a disturbed family system.

1. The family is in a crisis, and the hospitalization can be an attempt to solve the crisis (13–15). For example, some dysfunctional couples have described both the outcome of a psychotic episode of one of them and the process of coping with it as a strongly positive experience for them (16).

2. The family extrudes the identified patient from the family in an often misguided attempt to solve a crisis.

The M family consisted of mother, boyfriend, and two teenage daughters. The eldest daughter had anorexia nervosa. The other sibling was functioning well in high school. The mother had longstanding chronic paranoid schizophrenia and was extremely dependent on her own mother. The mother had been divorced about 10 years previously and had finally found a boyfriend.

After the mother formed a relationship with her boyfriend and was seriously considering marriage, she began to argue with the elder daughter more frequently. The daughter began eating less and became paranoid. The mother then contacted a pediatrician, stating that the daughter was seriously ill and needed hospitalization. The mother confided to the family therapist she was unable to take care of the identified patient's demands because she was fearful of losing her boyfriend *since caring for her daughter would prevent her from spending time with her boyfriend.* The pediatrician hospitalized the daughter.

This case illustrates how one family member can extrude another member from the family in order to take care of her own needs. The mother was afraid of losing her boyfriend and therefore restructured the family by having the identified patient hospitalized.

3. The family uses the hospital to get treatment for a member other than the identified patient. The hospitalized member

is not necessarily the only "sick" one (or at times, not even the "sickest" one) in the family (17). A family approach allows for observing and evaluating all significant others, with appropriate treatment (including medication) for the family and for the non-patient individuals who may require it. Therapists concentrating on treating one individual may entirely overlook or not have access to even gross, florid psychological disturbance in a close relative. When therapists view their role as that of therapist to a family unit, this sort of blind spot is less likely to occur.

4. The family uses the hospital as a resource to regain a "lost" member. For example, a father who drinks and is never home is finally convinced to go into a hospital for treatment. Although the family's motivation is to have him back as a functioning father and spouse, the family may also need to keep him "sick" for its own needs and homeostasis.

5. The hospital is used as a neutral arena to change longstanding maladaptive patterns of family functioning. An example is the family with an alcoholic member. Hospitalization of the identified patient will sometimes allow an underlying family pattern to change. Of course, for this to happen, the hospital staff must plan the appropriate family interventions; simply separating the identified patient and the family is necessary but often not sufficient for change.

6. If the identified patient has a chronic progressive or deteriorating condition such as childhood or adult schizophrenia, for example, the family may use the hospital as a respite to relieve family burdens.

If these assumptions about the needs of the family in respect to the hospitalization are correct, it follows *that in such cases the treatment program is inadequate unless it includes the family.*

The Process of Family Treatment by the Hospital Team

The process of family intervention by the hospital team involves steps similar to those of outpatient family treatment: connecting with the family, assessment, defining the problem, setting goals, treatment, and referral for assistance following discharge. However, in the context of hospitalization what is different is the extent of pathology of one member, the seriousness of the event, and the crisis for the family, all of which require special mention and attention. It should be emphasized that a significant difference between inpatient and outpatient family treatment is the need in the former for more intensive psychoeducation about a specific illness and a specific treatment for that illness. Of course, treatment should be individualized and fit the needs of the particular family. Give particular attention to the needs of single-parent families and remarried families who have to cope with serious long-term mental illness. The Alliance for the Mentally Ill has found that approxiately 60% of its members are single parents. Most of these single parents express the opinion that the illness caused the marital breakup.

Although all the necessary research has not yet been done, preliminary work suggests that different interview techniques exist for different types of families. As a rule of thumb, psychoeducational techniques are indicated more for families in which one member has a schizophrenic or affective disorder, and psychodynamic and structural techniques are indicated more for patients with personality disorder.

ALLYING WITH THE FAMILY

Contact with the family should start very early, *preferably before hospitalization,* when the family is trying to arrange admission or certainly by the time of admission.

Discharge planning is a major concern from the beginning of therapy. Many hospital personnel have had the experience of beginning discharge planning late in the course of hospitalization, only to discover that the family, implicitly or explicitly, resists having the patient go home. It usually has to be pointed out to the family that hospital treatment of the identified patient involves (or requires) treatment of all family members. This also may be made a condition of admission. A family representative may be appointed as the central communicating link with the primary therapist in the hospital, outside of formal treatment sessions.

A more relevant question is whether to use a psychoeducational or a consultative approach and in which order? Grunebaum and Friedman (18) suggest that the first encounter should be psychoeducational rather than consultative. Therapists need the family "in order to learn about the history of the patient's illness and the family's story. They need us to teach them about what they are facing, often for the first time." Grunebaum and Friedman view "consultation" as a technique more appropriate later in treatment.

EVALUATING THE FAMILY

Evaluation of the family should involve the presence of the identified patient unless he or she is so psychotic this is impossible or too disturbing. The evaluation will follow the usual outline for hospital work—construction of a family genogram with particular emphasis on the immediate events, especially family interactions and changes, leading up to the hospitalization. The evaluation should be constructed in a way that provides information whether further family intervention is needed during hospitalization and, if so, what the potential focus of that intervention would be.

Most importantly, the family evaluation process requires the clinician to help move the family from a frightened defensive stance in which they presume they will draw blame to a position of collaborating with the treatment team. It also requires helping the family find the best possible coping mechanisms for handling the patient's symptoms. The coping mechanisms are often the best of difficult alternatives, i.e., even if the treatment team views the alternative as "not good," it may be the best one possible.

NEGOTIATING GOALS OF FAMILY INTERVENTION

Keeping in mind that hospitalization is brief, the therapist must quickly focus on the general goals of family intervention and goals most specific to the individual family at hand. Negotiating these goals with the family should be accomplished by the end of the evaluation session or in the next session. Negotiating must be done with confidence, delicacy, firmness, and empathy. Families, frequently upset about the condition of the patient, may see no need for the hospitalization; they may see no need for their participation in therapy because the patient is the only sick one, or they may be hostile to the hospital for not quickly "curing" their family member. In the worst case scenario the family consciously or unconsciously wants to extrude the patient. Usually this occurs because of the *burden* of dealing with the chronic illness. A treatment contract is needed at this point in the hospitalization process.

Education about the illness in order to reduce family guilt over creating the condition, information about the length of hospitalization, and expectation for change will reduce anxiety and allow realistic focus on the future. Realistic expectations for change may reduce unrealistic expectation of cure and subsequent disappointment and devaluing of the hospital and its staff. Education about needed family assistance will help in discharge, planning, and posthospital treatment compliance. Sessions can vary in length from 30 minutes to 1 hour and scheduled on a daily, biweekly, or weekly basis, depending upon need and/or anticipated discharge date.

We have found that psychoeducation rarely proceeds as smoothly as its description might imply. Frequently families resist participating in treatment, deny the patient's illness, or magnify its severity and intractability. Then the real complexities of family intervention appear or, perhaps better stated, the real challenge occurs. At this point, the family intervention switches from being primarily educational to interpretive and, at times, confrontational. The goal at this point is to overcome or circumvent family resistance to treatment.

Common Goals and Techniques of Inpatient Family Intervention

Six overriding goals dictate the focus of family intervention when one family member is an inpatient. These goals set the course of the work with each family so that the aim and thrust of intervention are clearly defined from the beginning of hospitalization. While our own inpatient family intervention research (19) has focused on two major diagnostic groups (schizophrenic spectrum patients and major affective disorders), these goals are not so much specific to diagnostic groups as they are specific to the serious problems, in general, presented to the family by a member in crisis hospitalized for major pathology.

Such a family, whatever the diagnosis, faces multiple *tasks:* (a) forming a conceptual understanding of the patient's illness; (b) deciding about the family's influence on the illness; (c) making some alliance with hospital treatment staff (in order to express and work through guilt, if a factor, or to undo guilt feelings from previous hospitalizations during which the staff *did* place blame); (d) beginning to conceptualize the possible future course of the illness and adjusting any previous images and expectations of the ill member; (e) deciding on what postdischarge treatment will be needed for the patient; and (f) making some decisions about what living arrangements will most benefit the discharged family member. These tasks are enormous, especially on first hospitalization. Without specific, organized attention from the therapeutic staff, these decisions are often faced without professional help despite the fact that the cost for the hospitalization is enormous.

The six goals of inpatient family intervention are designed to meet family needs in a systematic fasion. If these family needs are addressed, we hypothesize that the family can be a major asset in the patient's recovery. If these family needs are not met, in extreme cases the family may react with hostility and chaos and become an irritant to the patient, possibly leading to future exacerbation of symptoms rather than becoming an asset to the patient in the crucial posthospitalization phase. The six *family treatment goals,* with their corresponding treatment strategies and techniques, are as follows.

Goal 1: Accepting the Reality of the Illness and Understanding the Current Episode

While so obvious, this goal is the cornerstone of the other goals. Unless the family achieves some acceptance and understanding of the seriousness of the episode that caused hospitalization, their conception of the patient in terms of setting future goals and their acceptance of needed future treatment following hospitalization will be compromised.

Family therapists can choose from a number of techniques to accomplish this goal. They can actively engage the family and patient and form a working alliance. This is a "must"; all else is compromised without it. This can be accomplished by recognizing and expressing the burden of stress experienced by the whole family. Therapists can explore each family member's perception and understanding of the illness. While therapists may not agree with the family member's understanding of the illness, they can identify and empathize with the family's previous attempts to cope with the illness. In order to reduce inordinate feelings of responsibility for the illness, therapists can provide the family with facts about the illness, and (especially in the case of schizophrenia and major affective illness) articulate the biological, genetic causes. Once the family has some trust in the therapist and realizes that he or she is not attempting to blame the family for the current episode, the therapist can explore with the family the emergence and development of the current symptomatic episode in order to begin to identify external and internal family stresses.

The therapist can also educate the family about the course of the disorder, including early warning signs, progression, and future recurrences.

Goal 2: Identifying Stresses Precipitating the Current Episode

Once the family has even tentatively accepted the reality of the illness, the next step is to identify precipitating stressors of the present episode (while still fresh in the family's mind). The abstract notion that stress can influence a patient vulnerable to psychiatric illness becomes a concrete reality in the family's daily life. When this link between theory and reality is forged, progress will more likely occur.

Strategies and techniques for achieving this goal are mainly educative, cognitive, and problem solving. The therapist can encourage the family to think about recent stresses, in and outside the family, that may have contributed to the patient's regression. In addition, the therapist and family can rank the stresses in order to clarify their importance and thus assign priorities to necessary brief interventions. In the best of situations, the family comes to a consensus about the most important recent stresses and their role in the patient's illness.

Goal 3: Identifying Likely Future Stressors, Within and Outside the Family, That Will Impinge on the Identified Patient

Goals 1 and 2 are concerned in great detail with the immediate and remote past: recognizing the illness and stressors that might have contributed to the illness' eruption. Once these goals have been partly accomplished, there is a natural pull on the part of the family and therapist to consider the immediate future. In fact, in some cases the pull to focus on the future (e.g., discharge) comes too early in the hospitalization; this generally signals defensive denial that must be met with refocusing on goals 1 and 2 before proceeding to goals 3–6.

It is important to emphasize that family attitudes, not only toward the patient but also toward treatment, have an impact on outcome. For example, positive parental attitudes about hospital treatment correlate with patient improvement while resistance to treatment correlates with discharge against medical advice (20–22). In addition, Greenman et al. (23) have found that certain parental concerns *on admission* have an impact on patient behavior. Interestingly, they are gender-linked: specifically, mothers were concerned with limit setting, i.e., preventing impulsive and self-destructive behavior; fathers "had difficulty supporting treatment or setting limits about the need for treatment because they were afraid that taking such a position would anger the patient, leading to a loss of their relationship with the patient."

Goal 4: Elucidating Family Interaction Sequences That Stress the Identified Patient

Telling the family that they probably put stress on the patient is accepted intellectually and vaguely, at best. However, when in the immediacy of the moment the family is shown how their actions or behavior are disorganizing the patient (e.g., becoming paranoid, becoming disorganized, or smashing an object), learning can take place.

In the past decade an impressive body of evidence has suggested that families high in expressed emotion run an increased risk of relapse of the identified patient family member. Originally, although high EE was thought to be specific to schizophrenia, recent research demonstrates that the problem can be found in families with chronic affective disorder and other disorders (24). We speculate that increased EE is found in almost all chronic psychiatric illnesses. In any case, a number of techniques lower EE, and it has been found that lowering EE will result in better patient outcome.

While the goals (1–3) are approached by cognitive and educative strategies, the attempt to demonstrate how current family interaction stresses the patient more closely approximates systems or traditional family therapy. After pointing out when such an interaction occurs in the session (e.g., "Every time you criticize him, as you did just now, he puts his head down and murmurs something that sounds like nonsense under his breath"), a family's perception of being blamed, and responding with resistance and hostility, can be softened by doing one or all of several things. The therapist can educate the family members about the fact that current family interaction does *not* *cause* the disorder but is likely to *trigger* current symptoms. In addition, the therapist

can empathize with the family's frustration and anger toward the patient's behavior which leads them to criticize. We can then tell them that they need to find (with our help) better ways to try to influence the patient.

Goal 5: Planning Strategies for Managing and/or Minimizing Future Stresses

By the middle or toward the end of hospitalization family members sometimes believe that the past is over. However, the therapist must remind them that what happened in the past could happen in the future and planning is needed to ensure that history does not repeat itself.

The therapist can invite and initiate discussion of the possible return of symptoms and how the family can cope with them. Family members must discuss their expectations of the patient's future level of functioning; for some families expectations must be lowered realistically, for others hope will be stimulated. The therapist can also help families anticipate potential stresses related to the patient's reentering the community, including employment, education, social functioning, etc.

Goal 6: Accepting the Need for Continued Treatment Following Discharge from the Hospital

This goal, central to preventing relapse and rehospitalization, comes full circle with goal 1 (reducing denial of the illness). Families who have seen a patient go through numerous hospitalizations have no problem anticipating the future possibility of rehospitalization. However, these families may be so discouraged and burdened that they need support and encouragement. For families going through a first hospitalization there is more danger of denying future episodes, thus more chance of denying the need for aftercare.

The therapist can use a family technique of visualizing possible replays in the future of just what led to the present hospitalization. How would the patient tell the family or vice versa? What are the early signs that something is going wrong? Who would they contact? Additional education about typical courses of the condition may further emphasize the need for aftercare.

Not every family will need work on all goals. Some families will be so damaged and defective that only a few basic goals can be approached. However, in our experience most cases can fit into this general schema.

The ultimate goal of family intervention is to extend the therapeutic milieu of the hospital into the family setting after discharge. If the family can become more sophisticated in understanding precipitating stresses, dealing with high expressed emotion, and insuring that the patient continues therapy, the transition from the intensive treatment milieu of the hospital to a less intensive community treatment setting is greatly facilitated. This is especially important in an environment in which hospitals find it advisable to reduce hospitalization in order to limit regression and, especially, to reduce health care costs through early discharge.

Particular Decisions in Hospital Family Intervention

TIMING

Two issues of timing are important—when to make contact and when to start therapy. Contact with the family should start during the *decision-making process* leading to hospitalization (e.g., in the emergency room). Family therapists disagree about when during the psychotic process should family sessions begin with the patient present. Some believe that family therapy with the patient present should begin only when the active symptoms begin to diminish (25). Although this seems reasonable, in our experience this can be used to rationalize putting off family treatment; many patients, even in a psychotic state, become *more* coherent during well-planned and focused family sessions.

STAFFING

Who should do the family therapy? In our opinion, the primary hospital therapist is in the best position to conduct family therapy because he or she has the best overall grasp of the case. In our opinion, the advantages of one therapist doing both the individual and family therapy far outweigh the disadvantages. However, time constraints, lack of experience, or the need for supervision if the therapist is a trainee, may not always make this possible and alternative solutions may have to be devised. The solution usually involves having the unit social worker—trained in the modality and well-positioned—to deliver the family therapy.

Family therapy has been carried out by all members of the hospital treatment team. During visiting or other scheduled times, nurses can meet with the patient and family. Occupational and recreational therapists can suggest family interventions—activities which the family can do together—that can facilitate family change. They can prescribe activities such as preparing a meal together or going on a picnic. Professional staff of every discipline can have crucial roles in changing long-standing behavior patterns in the family system.

The hospital milieu is especially advantageous for observing and pointing out family interaction patterns. Accurate, on-the-spot observation of the family may reveal that patients have good reasons for their symptoms. For example, an adolescent's repeatedly recreating his family constellation on the psychiatric unit demonstrates to him that this is similar to the way he reacts to his mother.

How can the need for maximal communication among staff members reconcile with the need for confidentiality of patient and therapist? Communication among staff is crucial for effective treatment. The family should be told that the therapist will use all the material available from both the individual and family to help the family function better.

How about a cotherapist? Some therapists believe that family therapy in a hospital setting is the most difficult kind of psychotherapy. They recommend that every family therapist have a cotherapist to share the emotional strains of family therapy. Cotherapy in a hospital setting may be more practical than in a private office practice.

One member of the family should be designated as the *family representative*. One member of the ward staff can be assigned as liaison to the family and should be available to the family at mutually convenient times such as nights and weekends. These role assignments are crucial in situations in which there are "factions at war" within the family. Such collaboration, involving much work and family receptiveness, is often impractical.

FAMILY TECHNIQUES AND THEIR HOSPITAL UTILIZATION

A variety of family therapy techniques now available are virtually mandatory for use in the modern hospital. These include:

1. Individual family therapy
2. Multiple family-group therapy and conjoint couples group (26)
3. Family psychoeducational workshops (also known as family survival skills workshops or family support groups) (27)
4. Family psychodrama and family sculpture—nonverbal techniques often more helpful than cognitive techniques when treating a hospitalized (especially nonverbal) sample of patients.

Family treatment is rarely the primary therapy for hospitalized patients. For psychotic patients, family treatment is usually prescribed along with medication and other rehabilitative therapies. For nonpsychotic patients it is usually part of a treatment package consisting of individual therapy, rehabilitation therapy, and other interventions.

CASE EXAMPLE: A 17-year-old boy was admitted after having been extremely agitated and disoriented at home, refusing to eat or sleep. The working diagnosis was of a schizophrenic disorder. In the hospital he continued to be wary, eating only when his mother ate with him and avoiding participation in activities involving other patients. The staff had decided to administer neuroleptic medication. They sat down with the boy and his mother and explained their observations and concerns. They then described the drug and the effects they hoped it would have. They also discussed side effects and remedies for these and focused specifically on how the boy and his mother would be able to evaluate the effectiveness of the drug. Specifically, if the boy were to find out that he could think more clearly and understand what is going on around him, then the medicine would be working. He could also help the staff decide what will be the best dose.

The boy hesitated and his mother had some questions. However, finally she told the boy that she thought he should try it and he agreed. Two days later he said that he felt better and wanted to stop the medication. The staff told him that there had not really been enough time to evaluate it. They spoke again with him and his mother. Again she told the boy that she wanted him to take the medication. Again he agreed to do so. A week later he said he felt better but wondered if an increased dose would help him sleep better; in another conference with him and his mother a new dosage schedule was arranged.

The medication discussions provided the boy and his mother with a different kind of relationship. His mother had been consulted as a parent and her competence to evaluate and help her son was underscored. On the other hand, the boy had a new experience of negotiating with his mother. Decisions were not made for him; instead, he was included with his mother in an active decision-making process. As the hospitalization progressed he felt freer to question his mother and the staff, and the answers he received helped to clarify the confusion of his psychotic state. The neuroleptic and the contextual experiences described may have worked synergistically.

It is important to note that family intervention in a hospital setting is hard work. The resistant behavior emanating from the family is often intense, while the benefits are often not recognized until well after the patient is discharged. Family therapy also requires good communication, socialization, and control skills by the family therapist and is very time consuming, to boot.

The next question involves "choice" of family therapy model—psychoeducational versus psychodynamic versus structural approaches. Our position is that all three are useful in treating a hospitalized patient. However, because of the brief duration of most hospitalizations and the cognitive impairment of the identified patient, we principally recommend psychoeducational approaches, reserving psychodynamic and structural approaches for the latter stages of longer hospitalizations (three months or more) or for the posthospital phase.

A good description of the need for psychoeducation is found in the following communication from a parent of a patient with schizoaffective disorder.

When my daughter and son-in-law entered the clinic where their new-born son—diagnosed with spina bifida and hydrocephalus—would be cared for, the chief nurse said, in effect, "You will be with this child every hour of the day. We will teach you what to look for, and then you will be coming to us and telling us what is wrong with your baby." When my other daughter accompanied her son to the allergist about the boy's asthma, the doctor gave specific instructions about the dosage of medicine to fit the need, and the desired response. The doctor

told her when to go up and come down with the medication dosage and what to consider an emergency. As a pathologist who has worked closely with a son who has schizoaffective mental disorder, and as his psychiatrist, I believe it is important that the parent or family member be equally involved in the treatment of many mental disorders. The principle is that when a patient is treated by a physician, he and often his family member should be given esoteric medical education and training to enable them to better carry out the intentions of the treatment program.

By the nature of mental illness, the often complicated medicine administration program and treatment often needs to vary from day to day, week to week, or month to month. The person ill often cannot evaluate his own responses and needs the advice of those around him if he is not visited daily by his psychiatrist. The person ill may reach wrong conclusions about his treatment options; but with an educated close family member, the course is likely to be correct and likely keep the patient out of a more intense medical setting.

It is true that some people find it difficult to think in terms of symptoms and effects as far as illness and treatment are concerned. But if treatment is worth anything, it must produce a desired effect which can be recognized. Proper education of the patient and his family member requires their detailed knowledge of what is wrong, how it is to be corrected, and what response may be expected.

A Working Model of Inpatient Family Intervention

The GAP (Group for the Advancement of Psychiatry) Committee on the Family has succinctly summarized the new family model:

Hospitalization should be viewed in most cases as an event in the history of the family, an event that can be devastating or valuable depending upon the skills and orientation of the therapeutic team. Hospitalization viewed in this way becomes central in understanding the role of the patient in the family system and in supporting the family as well as the patient. The hospital becomes an important therapeutic adjunct not only for severely dysfunctional individuals and their families, but also for families stuck in modes of relating that appear to interfere with the development and movement of individual members. For these families, hospitalization aims to disrupt the family set; this disruption can be used to help the family system to change in more functional ways.

Family-oriented programs can be implemented within existing hospital resources, though there is a general trend toward adapting and revising hospital environments to include family members in patient care. (This trend is also noted in other specialties, such as "rooming in" in obstetric and pediatric units.) Effective programs involve the staff, from admission clerks on up, in building an alliance with the family. Stewart describes this as "the engagement of the family with the institution in a relationship that achieves mutual understanding and support and establishes clarity, acceptance, and commitment to mutually agreed upon goals for the treatment of the hospitalized patient" (28). This active reaching out is different from a commitment to change-oriented family treatment. Involvement of the family (as we are describing) makes possible the avoidance of staff overidentification with the patient against the family, as well as reducing the stigma of psychiatric hospitalization and increasing system-wide motivation for aftercare.

Many different types of staff/family interaction are possible and helpful. One may separate the tasks of alliance building, formal family therapy sessions geared to change, and staff and family interaction around medications, visits, and so forth, which can also have a therapeutic function (29).

An example of an innovative, well-functioning family-oriented approach in an inpatient setting can be found in Table 9.2.

Guidelines for Recommending Family Therapy in a Hospital Setting

The guidelines for recommending family therapy in a hospital setting are similar to those for outpatient settings. More-

over, if the family is present and available it is more effective to use family evaluation and often some form of family intervention than to withhold it (30).

A careful distinction has to be made between evaluation and family treatment, given the brief length of stay for most hospitals. As a rule of thumb, every family should be evaluated, then educated about family treatment. Whenever possible and when indicated, treatment should be started in the hospital, though most goals will be accomplished after discharge.

Prototypic situations that call for some form of family intervention during hospitalization include the following:

A suicidal and depressed adolescent living in the parental home is hospitalized following a car accident. There is some suspicion that the father is alcoholic and that the parents are not aware of the adolescent's depression nor of the adolescent's day-to-day functioning.

A 22-year-old male college student is hospitalized following an acute psychotic episode in the fall of his first year away from home. Family sessions are indicated with the parents to educate them about the unexpected illness, to help them and the patient evaluate their mutual expectations for his performance, and to encourage follow-up psychiatric care which the son has never before needed.

A 39-year-old divorced woman living with her two children, ages 11 and 13, is hospitalized following a paranoid psychotic break in which she stabbed herself in the abdomen in the presence of the children. Family sessions with the children are needed to assist the mother, now in a denial phase, to communicate with them about her illness episode and talk about the future. An urgent need also exists for the children to discuss their feelings about witnessing their mother stab herself.

A 23-year-old female who lives with her parents is hospitalized following an exacerbation of schizophrenic symptoms occasioned by her younger sisters leaving for college. The patient also had gone off her medication. The parents are suspected of high "expressed emotion" (they are critical of their daughter and one parent is

Table 9.2.   Inpatient Family Intervention (31)[a]

Definition: Inpatient family intervention (IFI) is work with patients and their families together in one or more family sessions. It aims at favorably affecting the *patient's* course of illness and course of treatment through increased understanding of the illness and decreased stress on the patient. It has been carried out by inpatient social workers, first-year psychiatry residents, or both together as co-therapists.

Description:

I.   *Assumptions*
1. IFI does *not* assume that the etiology of the major psychotic disorders lies in family functioning or communication.
2. It *does* assume that the *present-day* functioning of a family with which the patient is living or is in frequent contact can be a major source of stress or support.

II. *Aims*
1. IFI aims to help families to understand, live with, and deal with patients and their illness; to develop the most appropriate possible ways of addressing the problems the illness presents and its effects on the patient; to understand and support both the necessary hospital treatment and long-range treatment plans.
2. It aims to help patients understand family actions and reactions and to help patients develop the most appropriate possible intrafamily behavior, in order to decrease their vulnerability to family stress and decrease the likelihood that their behavior will provoke it.

III. *Strategy and Techniques*

A. *Evaluation*
1. Evaluation is accomplished in one or more initial family sessions, with the patient present when conditions permit. Information gained from other sources is also used.
2. The patient's illness and its potential course are evaluated.
3. The present effect and the possible future effect on the family are determined.
4. The family's effect on the patient is evaluated, with particular reference to the stress caused by expressed emotion and criticism.
5. Family structure and interaction and the present point in the family life cycle are evaluated in order to determine whether particular aspects of the patient's role in the family are contributing to exacerbate or maintain the illness or otherwise impair the patient.

B. *Techniques*
1. The family and patient are usually seen together.
2. Early in the hospitalization an attempt is made to form an alliance with the family that gives them a sense of support and understanding.
3. *Psychoeducation:* (a) The family is provided with information about the illness, its likely course, and its treatment; questions are answered. (b) The idea that stress from and in the family can exacerbate the illness is discussed. (c) The ways in which conflicts and stress arise within each family are discussed, and a problem-solving approach is taken in planning ways to decrease such stress in the future. (d) The ways in which the illness and the patient's impaired functioning have burdened the family are discussed and plans made to decrease such burden.
4. In some cases, the initial evaluation of subsequent sessions suggest that particular resistances due to aspects of family structure or family dynamics interfere with accomplishing (2) and (3) above. If it is judged necessary and possible, one or a series of family sessions may attempt to explore such resistances and make changes in family dynamics. Such attempts may use some traditional family therapy techniques. Such families may be encouraged to seek family therapy after the patient's discharge.

[a]The material in this table has been taken in part from a study, *Inpatient Family Intervention: A Controlled Study,* funded in part by an NIMH Grant (MH 34466), and was drafted by Drs. J. Spencer and I. Glick.

constantly with her). Family treatment is started during the hospitalization to increase the likelihood of efficacious after-care, including medication and family therapy.

Indications for family therapy come from the patient, the family, and the interaction between the family and the patient's illness. Patient-related criteria would include current living conditions (e.g., living with spouse or family of origin) and life-cycle issues (e.g., patient is a young adult trying to separate or an older adult living with and very dependent upon the family of origin). Family criteria include family conflict which appears to contribute to the patient's difficulties or significant psychiatric illness of one or more other family members. Criteria related to the interaction of family and the patient's illness are exemplified by deficit behavior around the illness (e.g., family denial of illness, family not supporting the vulnerable patient, family not supporting treatment for the patient's illness, and danger that the patient will harm a family member).

As to contraindications, it should be noted that even though family intervention may be indicated during hospitalization, many situations exist in which the intervention does not seem necessary nor the treatment of choice after discharge. When the patient is living alone but needs the family support during hospitalization, individual treatment will often be recommended upon discharge. When the individual patient is striving (with a good chance for success) for independence from parents, individual and family treatment may be best. The patient struggling to individuate may benefit from continued family treatment during which family resistance to individuation can be addressed. If the parents are severely in conflict (with this coming to the fore as the patient individuates) marital treatment may be recommended for them.

Results

Glick and associates have reported the only controlled study of family intervention in an inpatient setting. Inpatient family intervention (with a heavy family psychoeducational component) was compared to hospitalization without family intervention for patients with schizophrenic and affective disorders (31). The sample included 169 patients and their families for whom family intervention was indicated. The families were randomized into one of the two treatment conditions (mentioned above). Assessments were made at admission, discharge, and 6 and 18 months postadmission, using patient and family measures from the vantage points of patient, family, and independent assessors.

In terms of effectiveness, there was both good and bad news (31–34). Overall family intervention in the hospital setting was found to be effective; but *not* for everyone. And for some patients' and families it appeared not to add anything to standard hospital treatment.

Results for the full sample of 169 psychiatric patients suggest that adding family treatment to standard hospital treatment *was* effective, but not uniformly across all patient groups. At discharge, the positive effect of IFI (inpatient family intervention) was largely restricted to female patients with affective disorder and their families, although it was present to a lesser extent in good prehospital functioning schizophrenics and "others." At follow-up the statistical interactions indicated that this therapeutic effect was largely restricted to female patients with schizophrenia or major affective disorder. The effect of family treatment on male patients with these diagnoses was minimal or slightly negative. Also of note, the IFI effect on schizophrenia did not appear until the 18-month postadmission follow-up point and, in contrast to the discharge results, the effect was most striking in the poor prehospital functioning group. Similarly (in contrast to the discharge results) for patients with affective disorder, the follow-up results revealed positive findings favoring the inpatient family intervention, but only in the bipolar subgroup. Composite means showed that family treatment was somewhat better for the families of patients (primarily females) with the major psychoses, while families of patients with other diagnoses did better without family intervention.

It is important to emphasize that most

clinical research on hospital treatment(s) has (appropriately) focused on outcomes for patients. With the exception of the Glick et al. study referred to above, it is not known what the outcomes are for families. Although this issue has not been studied systematically, one hypothesis-generating, three-country study of family outcome after an episode of major affective disorder found that not only is the family less financially well off because of hospitalization costs, but usually functioning no better or even worse and, without psychoeducation, unprepared for the next episode (35).

Our clinical experience suggests that the specific interventions of psychoeducational groups can help the often demoralized family of the chronic patient to reestablish itself as a viable unit and lessen their burden of shame, guilt, despair, and isolation (36).

Treatment of Nonpsychotic Psychiatric Illnesses

Most of this chapter has focused on the hospital treatment of the family with a patient who has a major psychosis. Other situations require family intervention. The two most common are families with a member hospitalized with (a) severe personality disorder and/or (b) substance abuse. The most common personality disorders are schizotypal, obsessive compulsive, and borderline personality disorder.

SCHIZOTYPAL PERSONALITY DISORDER (SPD)

This disorder is thought to be a less severe version of schizophrenia. Although treatment principles are essentially the same, the lack of psychotic features makes it difficult for the family to accept the notion of underlying organic (rather than moral) failings. Accordingly, a great deal of time is spent in psychoeducation and laying the groundwork for posthospital family intervention.

OBSESSIVE COMPULSIVE DISORDER (OCD)

Recently, obsessive compulsive disorder was found to be caused by underlying selective basal ganglia dysfunction. Often (and erroneously) the family believes the symptoms, i.e., the obsessions and compulsions, can be voluntarily controlled. Controlled studies demonstrate the effectiveness of medication and behavioral therapy for managing the disorder. Family therapy, plays an important adjunctive role of decreasing patient anxiety, increasing coping skills, and improving family functioning by providing education and support.

BORDERLINE PERSONALITY DISORDER (BPD)

Research in the past decade suggests strong evidence of disturbed biological underpinnings in this clinical entity. Accordingly, as with other organic diseases, in the absence of adequate perceptual and cognitive equipment, it has been proposed that "oscillations of attachment" exist (37). These are thought to stem from trouble in regulating interpersonal distance. In addition, in many patients who are hospitalized, self-destructive behavior is a prominent symptom. Reducing this symptom is often a focus of treatment and, according to empirical studies, family help is necessary; family intervention is necessary in most cases of patients hospitalized with BPD (see also Chapter 4).

ADDICTIVE DISORDERS

These disorders have been extensively covered elsewhere in this text (see Chapter 6). The following facts are now well accepted (38):

1. The problems of alcohol and substance abuse affect and are affected by the patient's family situation.
2. Although the exact effectiveness of marital and family intervention is unknown,

most clinicians accept the notion that intervention is a necessary component for any patient hospitalized for an addictive disorder.

3. The objectives of family work are: changing the abuse patterns and related behaviors of the patient and the communication and interaction patterns of the family.

4. Of the few controlled studies done on alcohol or substance abuse, the family approach seems more effective than individual psychotherapy for both types of abuse.

5. An increased emphasis has been placed on recognizing family members as primary patients deserving treatment in their own right and not simply as adjuncts to treatment (because of the stresses of living in such a family). Therefore, for the long haul preventative family work seems indicated.

6. Family treatment techniques include not only psychoeducational but structural and psychodynamic techniques. Participation in spouse groups such as AL-ANON are mandatory for maintenance.

Other Types of Family Involvement as an Alternative to Psychiatric Hospitalization

At times of family crisis, psychiatric hospitalization of a family member is one solution. With the gradual shift of psychiatric services out of the hospital and into the community, other alternatives have emerged. In some cases, schizophrenic patients can be kept out of hospitals by sending the treatment team to see them in their homes (39, 40). Day hospitalization with a focus on family treatment is another alternative to psychiatric hospital admission (41). Day hospitals also have moved toward using family therapy as a primary method of treatment because their population is chronic and difficulties with family relationships are common.

CASE EXAMPLE: In the L family there were two brothers, A and M. Their father had died, and their mother was grieving. A lived by himself, managing marginally; M, the other son, came to a day hospital for managing his schizophrenia.

Treatment at the day hospital was oriented around helping M obtain volunteer work. Whenever the volunteer counselor and his therapist at the day hospital came close to finding a job replacement for him, they noticed that the patient's symptoms escalated, i.e., he would start screaming, become paranoid, and collapse on the street. Further investigation of these symptoms revealed that on the nights before the patient was to go to his appointments, his mother would, in painstaking detail, describe her anxiety about not knowing his whereabouts and how her heart would not pump as a result. She told him that although she would not want to stop him from work, she needed to know he was safe in the day hospital rather than at some volunteer job where she could not call him.

This case is typical for many chronic patients whose level of functioning is marginal. Any change in that level is often perceived as a threat by the family.

Often a change in the balance of family forces precipitates the request for hospitalization. Understanding the shift can thereby result in strategies to prevent extrusion of the identified patient. Although hospitalization may be avoided, continued family work is needed to change behavior patterns that exacerbate the identified patient's condition.

Reading for the Family

During the past decade, a number of excellent books have been written for families with mentally ill members. We recommended a partial list collected by the National Alliance for the Mentally Ill (NAMI):

DEPRESSION, AND MANIA

Depression and Its Treatment: Help for the Nation's No. 1 Mental Problem by John Greist and James Jefferson, New York, Warner Books, 1985.

Lithium and Manic Depression, Lithium Information Center, Madison, Wis., Univ. of Wis. (Center for Health Sciences), 1988.

Overcoming Depression by D. Papolos and Janice Papolos, New York, Harper & Row, 1987.

SCHIZOPHRENIA

Surviving Schizophrenia: A Family Manual, Revised Edition by E. Fuller Torrey, New York, Harper & Row, 1988.

Schizophrenia: Straight Talk for Families and Friends by Maryellen Walsh, New York, Warner Books, 1986.

CHILDREN AND ADOLESCENTS

Children and Adolescents with Mental Illness: A Parents Guide by Evelyn McElroy, Kensington, Md., Woodbine House, 1988.

Strategies: A Practical Guide for Dealing with Professionals and Human Service Systems by Craig U. Shields, Richmond Hill, Ontario, Human Services Press, 1987.

FAMILIES AND COPING STRATEGIES

The Caring Family: Living With Chronic Mental Illness by Kayla Bernheim, Richard Levine, and Caroline Beale, Chicago, Contemporary Books, 1982.

Families Helping Families: Living with Schizophrenia by Nona Dearth et al., New York, W.W. Norton, 1986.

Coping with Mental Illness in the Family: A Family Guide by Agnes B. Hatfield, Arlington, Va., NAMI, no date.

Hidden Victims by Julie Johnson, New York, Doubleday, 1988.

Finally, some hospitals have developed manuals for patients and family which describe management and treatment of mental illness; we heartily concur with this trend.

Controversies in Treatment

1. Is the family "in treatment," a part of treatment, or a member of the treatment team? Although this issue is complicated, our position is that good treatment involves all three. First, most families have at least some problems coping with the illness of the identified patient and some families have problems separate from the identified patient. Second, by virtue of the family's *presence* in this treatment (as compared to individual or drug treatment), they are a *de facto* part of the treatment. (Nevertheless, consent to treatment should be obtained.) Finally, Wynne et al., (42) advocate the position that given the long-term nature and seriousness of chronic mental illness and the family's experience with dealing with a particular member, the family has a certain expertise with its unique problems. This is called "complementary" expertise. The family's expertise and trust of the treatment team need to join in order to develop an effective treatment strategy for that particular patient.

From the family's point of view, initially at least, they feel most comfortable as "partners" with the treatment team. Later on, the family may feel "ready" to become part of treatment or enter into treatment themselves. Often this occurs *after* hospitalization when the patient has stabilized.

In short, the best treatment is one that subtly blends all three components into the best possible outcome for both patients and families.

2. Should the initial goals of family therapy be oriented around family change or family consultation? This controversy, a long-standing one, emanates from the traditional model which focused on the family as etiologic. The best way to engage family members is to make contact with them "where they are," provide psychoeducation, and respond to requests for information and support. From there the therapist can move on to whatever else the family desires. In a sense the initial consultation is a way to ally with the family.

3. From an etiological viewpoint, many family therapists believe that schizophrenia and other major functional psychoses are purely family-systems, psychological, and social problems. Are they? In part, this belief is based on the observation that without medication improvement or recovery from an illness means that the illness has no biological basis. Many diseases in medicine are caused by biological factors that have a history of exacerbations, remissions, and, in some cases, "spontaneous cures"; cancer is one of them. Our position agrees with Stein's (43) that these illnesses, "like virtually every disease, are influenced by biological, psychological, and social factors." Treating schizophrenia requires all of these interventions—biological, psychological, and social—and anything else that can benefit it.

4. Many families believe that major mental illnesses are solely "brain" illnesses. This belief creates a conceptual gap in the minds of families offered a psychosocial treatment such as family therapy. To them the question is why would a biochemical problem be treated with a psychosocial treatment? The answer, of course, is that for any family—regardless of its own internal pathology—living over a sustained period of time with a member who has cognitive and other brain function defects creates major problems in management for both the patient and the rest of the family. The bottom line for hospital therapists is that they must be sensitive to this particular "need" of the family and combine a family intervention with a somatic intervention.

Although both are useful, (from the families' point of view) the latter will "more correctly" treat the "brain" illness.

5. How much does family intervention add to medication in the treatment of most hospitalized patients. Most studies that have looked at this issue conclude that each modality is additive (44). Each treatment adds something to the equation—medication is effective for most of the positive (and possibly negative symptoms), while family intervention helps with the secondary interpersonal problems resulting from the deficit. Our position is that the two complement each other. A related issue is the trade-off between the risks versus the benefits of medication. Over the long run, most patients hospitalized for the major psychoses, obsessive-compulsive disorders, and even anxiety disorders discover that the symptoms of the illness are worse than the side effects of either medication or family therapy. However, this issue is really a matter of patient and family choice, i.e., some families prefer living with a problem rather than painful attempts at dealing with it; some patients prefer living with the disability from the illness than with the side effects of medication (most notably tardive dyskinesia, TD).

An interesting issue related to this question is whether family intervention can result in lowering the dose of medication needed and presumably reduce the risk of TD. The Treatment Strategies in Schizophrenia Collaborative Study is attempting to answer this question. A three by two design, the study involves the use of standard-dose versus low-dose neuroleptic versus an early onset strategy coupled with two kinds of family strategies (a weekly, applied, behaviorally oriented family treatment compared to a monthly supportive measure). The answers should be forthcoming in the near future. Early impressions indicate that the greater the family involvement in either the applied or supportive form of treatment, the fewer the patient's symptoms and the less need for medication.

Conversely, long-term drug maintenance often helps the patient participate more meaningfully in family therapy. Importantly, patients on lower doses of medication are found to be more socially responsive and involved in therapy.

6. Controversy exists about the objectives of family therapy in the hospital setting. We referred to this issue earlier in the chapter and return to it here to discuss an important nuance. Previously, for hospitalized patients, the notion (oversimplified here) was that family therapy would cut to the "core" of the family problem, and if the family caused the problem, therapy would "cure" the patient. Obviously, we no longer focus on "curing" the patient, but rather on reducing the risk of relapse and improving the quality of life for *both* patient and family. We strongly support this position and try to set up as our objective helping *both* patient and family achieve the maximum functional capacity they *each* can. As such, we walk a tightrope between pushing patient independence "too far versus too little," given the severity of illness. Likewise, we encourage families to pursue their lives as best they are able without a "total" all-compassing focus on the patient.

7. Family therapy in the hospital is criticized as lacking evidence of effectiveness. Therefore, the enormous resources in time, staff, and money should not be allocated to this modality. Although that accusation (up to recently) is mostly true, clinical experience and our recent study (referred to earlier in the chapter) suggest that the controversy about family therapy's effectiveness should be reformulated. The central question is *for whom* is inpatient intervention indicated? Our work suggests that intervention works best for females

with affective disorder (especially bipolar disorder) and females with chronic schizophrenia. The families of *all* patients with schizophrenia and bipolar disorder seem to benefit from family intervention. Consequently, our position is that until further studies are done family therapy should judiciously be prescribed based on the literature, the clinical experience of the staff, and an evaluation of each case on admission.

REFERENCES

1. Glick ID, Hargreaves WA: *Psychiatric Hospital Treatment for the 1980s: A Controlled Study of Short Versus Long Hospitalization.* Lexington, Mass., Lexington Press, 1979.

2. Glick ID, Klar HM, Braff DL: Guidelines for hospitalization of chronic psychiatric patient. Hosp Community Psychiatry, 35:934–936, 1984.

3. Group for the Advancement of Psychiatry: *The Family, the Patient, and the Psychiatric Hospital: Toward a New Model*, p. 24, New York, Brunner/Mazel, 1985.

4. Bell J, Bell E: Family participation in hospital care for children. Children, 17:154–157, 1970.

5. Bhatti RS, Janakiramaiah N, Channabassavanna SM: Family psychiatric ward treatment in India. Fam Process 19:193–200, 1980.

6. Harbin HT: Families and hospitals: Collusion or cooperation? Am J Psychiatry 135:1496–1499, 1978.

7. Anderson CM: Family intervention with severely disturbed inpatients. Arch Gen Psychiatry, 34:697–702, 1977.

8. Falloon IRH, Boyd J, McGill C, Strang JS, Moss HB: Family management training in the community care of schizophrenia, in Goldstein MJ (ed): *New Developments in Interventions with Families of Schizophrenics*, San Francisco, Jossey-Bass, 1981.

9. Falloon IRH: Communication and problem solving skills training with relapsing schizophrenics and their families, in Lansky MR (ed): *Family Therapy and Major Psychopathology*, New York, Grune & Stratton, 1981.

10. Goldstein MJ, Rodnick EH, Evans JR, May RA, Steinberg MR: Drug and family therapy

in the aftercare of acute schizophrenics. Arch Gen Psychiatry, 35:1169–1177, 1978.

11. Rabiner E, Malminski H, Gralnick A: Conjoint family therapy in the inpatient setting, in Gralnick A (ed): *The Psychiatric Hospital as a Therapeutic Instrument*, pp. 160–177, New York, Brunner/Mazel, 1969.

12. Kahn EM, White, EM: Adapting milieu approaches to acute inpatient care for schizophrenic patients. Hosp Community Psychiatry, 40:609–614, 1989.

13. Sampson H, Messinger, S, Towne RD: Family processes and becoming a mental patient. Am J Sociol, 68:88–96, 1962.

14. Sampson H, Messinger S, Towne RD: The mental hospital and family adaptations. Psychiatr Q, 36:704–719, 1962.

15. Langlsey D, Kaplan D: *The Treatment of Families in Crisis*, New York, Grune & Stratton, 1968.

16. Dupont R, Ryder R, Grunebaum H: Unexpected results of psychosis in marriage. Am J Psychiatry, 128:735–739, 1971.

17. Bursten B: Family dynamics, the sick role, and medical hospital admissions. Fam Process, 4:206–216, 1965.

18. Grunebaum H, Friedman H: Letter. Hosp Community Psychiatry, 4:20, 1989.

19. Glick ID, Clarkin JF, Spencer JH, Haas G, Lewis A, Peyser J, DeMane N, Good-Ellis M, Harris E, Lestelle V: Inpatient family intervention. A controlled evaluation of practice: Preliminary results of the six-months follow-up. Arch Gen Psychiatry, 42:882–886, 1985.

20. Goldstein E: The influence of parental attitudes on psychiatric treatment outcome. Social Casework, 60:350–359, 1979.

21. Daniels RS, Margolis PM, Carson RC: Hospital discharges against medical advice. Arch Gen Psychiatry, 8:120–130, 1963.

22. Akhtar S, Helfrich J, Mestayer RF: AMA discharge from a psychiatric inpatient unit. Int J Soc Psychiatry, 27:143–50, 1981.

23. Greenman DA, Gunderson JG, Canning D: Parents' attitudes and patients' behavior: A prospective study. Am J Psychiatry, 146:226–230, 1989.

24. Miklowitz DJ, Goldstein MJ, Nuechterlein KH, Snider KS, Mintz J: Family factors and the course of bipolar affective disorder. Arch Gen Psychiatry, 45:225–231, 1988.

25. Guttman H: A contraindication for family therapy: The prepsychotic or postpsychotic young adult and his parents. Arch Gen Psychiatry, 29:352–355, 1973.

26. Davenport YB: Treatment of the married bipolar patient in conjoint couples psychotherapy groups, in Lansky MR (ed): *Family Therapy and Major Psychopathology*, New York, Grune & Stratton, 1981.

27. Anderson CM, Hogarty GE, Reiss DJ: Family treatment of adult schizophrenic patients: A psychoeducational approach. Schizophr Bull, 6:490–505, 1980.

28. Stewart RP: Building an alliance between the families of patients and the hospital: Model and process. Natl Assoc Private Psychiatr Hosp J, 12:63–68, 1982.

29. Group for the Advancement of Psychiatry: *The Family, the Patient, and the Psychiatric Hospital: Toward a New Model*, pp. 27–29, New York, Brunner/Mazel, 1985.

30. Gould E, Glick ID: The effects of family presence and family therapy on outcome of hospitalized schizophrenic patients. Fam Process, 16:503–510, 1977.

31. Haas GL, Glick ID, Clarkin JF, et al.: A randomized clinical trial of inpatient family intervention, II. Results at discharge. Arch Gen Psychiatry, 45:217–225, 1988.

32. Spencer JH, Glick ID, Haas GL: A randomized clinical trial of inpatient family intervention, III. Overall effects at follow-up for the entire sample. Am J Psychiatry, 145:1115–1121, 1988.

33. Glick ID, Spencer JH, Clarkin JF, et al.: A randomized clinical trial of inpatient family intervention, IV. Follow-up results for subjects with schizophrenia. Schizophrenia Research, 3:187–200, 1990.

34. Clarkin JF, Glick ID, Haas GL, et al.: A randomized clinical trial of inpatient family intervention, V. Results for affective disorders. J Affective Disord, 18: 17–28, 1990.

35. Glick ID, Burti L, Suzuki K, Sacks M: Effectiveness in psychiatric Care: I. A cross-national study of the process of treatment and outcomes of major depressive disorder. J Nerv Ment Disease, In press.

36. McLean C, Grunebaum H: Parent's response to chronically psychotic children. Paper presented at the American Psychiatric

Association Annual Meeting, Toronto, 1982.

37. Melges F, Swartz MS: Oscillations of attachment in borderline personality disorder. Am J Psychiatry, 146:1115–1120, 1989.

38. U.S. Department of Health and Human Services: Sixth Special Report to the U.S. Congress on Alcohol and Health, DHHS Publication No. (ADM) 87-1519, p. 129, Washington, D.C., Superintendent of Documents, U.S. Government Printing Office, 1987.

39. Pasamanick B, Scarpitti, F, Dinitz S: Schizophrenics in the Community, New York, Appleton-Century-Crofts, 1967.

40. Davis A, Dinitz S, Pasamanick B: The prevention of hospitalization in schizophrenia: Five years after an experimental program. Am J Orthopsychiatry, 42:375–388, 1972.

41. Zwerling I, Mendelsohn M: Initial family reactions to day hospitalization. Fam Process, 4:50–63, 1965.

42. Wynne L, McDaniel SH, Weber TT: Professional politics and the concepts of family therapy, family consultation and systems consultation. Fam Process, 26:153–166, 1987.

43. Stein L: The effect of long-outcome studies on the therapy of schizophrenia critique. J Marital Family Therapy, 15:133–138, 1989.

44. Glick ID, Clarkin J, Haas G, Spencer J, Chen C: A randomized clinical trial of inpatient family intervention: VI. Mediating variables and outcome. Submitted for publication.

Dynamic Therapies on the Inpatient Unit

L. Mark Russakoff, MD
John M. Oldham, MD

Psychodynamics has long been applied to treating psychiatric inpatients. Harry Stack Sullivan (1) was one of the pioneers of applying Freudian theory and practice in the inpatient setting. He found that significant modifications of technique were necessary in such a setting; as a result, he formulated his own theory of therapy, the Interpersonal Theory. Frieda Fromm-Reichmann (2), a colleague of Sullivan's and also one of the pioneers in using psychodynamic theory in treating inpatients, described her approach in a now classic work. Other approaches were described by Brody and Redlich, who edited a collection of papers from a conference on the psychotherapeutic treatment of schizophrenia, and by Hill, who presented his integration of intensive psychotherapeutic treatment of schizophrenia (3, 4). Rosen's (5) approach of aggressive and unmodified interpretation of diagnosed conflicts, predicated upon a simple dynamic model, shocked many people (including his patients) and never found much support in practice. Burton's (6) collection of papers reflects the enthusiasm for intensive psychotherapy that many people shared. Searles (7) wrote extensively on the intensive treatment of schizophrenia and was widely acclaimed as a psychotherapist. Gunderson and Mosher (8) edited a collection of articles on the psychotherapy of schizophrenia during a period in which psychotherapy was under siege as a treatment for this condition. Pao (9) summarized the views of a number of clinicians and recommended a particular model for intensive inpatient treatment.

However, much of this work on the dynamic treatment of schizophrenic patients predated the availability of antipsychotic agents or occurred while debate about the effectivenss of antipsychotics was still raging. With the widespread use of antipsychotics and the concomitant pressure to decrease lengths of stay in the hospital, in some facilities dynamic treatment fell from preeminence to contempt. In the latter situation, the motto became "the right drug, in the right patient, at the right dose" as the only appropriate treatment. In these cases, psychotherapeutic intervention was limited to obtaining medication compliance; the meaning of events in the patient's life was considered to be either of little consequence or an aspect to be dealt with as an outpatient. The psychotherapy literature did not address the role that psychodynamics and psychodynamically oriented treatment could play with the short-term inpatient. Advocates of short-term hospitalization (promedication, antidynamics, medical model) polarized against advocates of long-term hospitalization (antimedication, proin-tensive psychotherapy, therapeutic community). Certainly principles generated from healthier patients were misapplied to situations of more severely ill patients; intensive treatment mindlessly applied can lead to adverse outcomes (10).

Our experience in running a short-term diagnosis and treatment unit led us to believe that the two poles—medication and the medical model, psychotherapy and the therapeutic community model—could blend, preserving the best features of both (11, 12). However, as we reviewed the literature, we found that little was written on the subject of dynamic treatment of short-term inpatients. Most texts of psychodynamics and psychotherapy focus on the problems and dynamics of outpatients. However, qualitative and quantitative differences exist between outpatients and inpatients in their symptomatology, dynamics, and levels of severity of psychopathology. The earlier cited psychotherapy literature dealt primarily with long-term inpatients.

Thus, we found ourselves without much guidance for developing a dynamic therapy model for brief inpatients. Many models of human behavior exist, some of which are dynamic models. Some of the suggested models are behavioral, psycho-dynamic, interpersonal, and biological. Psychoanalysts have developed several psy-chodynamic models. However, not all models comfortably fit all the varieties of behavior observed clinically in patient settings. Therefore, we recommend using a series of models, organized hierarchically, for understanding the behaviors of patients. We suggest an especially important place for the object relations (OR) model which has gained in popularity during the past 20 years but was not explicitly used in much of the earlier literature. Following Gedo and Goldberg (13), we would find the behavioral model most suitable for the most severely disturbed, disorganized individuals for whom verbal interventions have limited meaning.

The simple psychoanalytic structural model—id, ego, superego—fits best for the more adaptively functioning, mildly disturbed (the "neurotic"). In the simplified form of this model, an integrated and coherent sense of self is assumed. Conflict may be construed between various structures—id versus ego or wish versus defense. From the technical standpoint, the therapist operating from this model would focus on preconscious, disavowed wishes. Since we do not see this model as especially useful for dealing with inpatients, we will not elaborate on it here.

OBJECT RELATIONS MODEL

The model which we have found to be most frequently appropriate for understanding hospitalized patients is the OR model (14). This model proposes that individuals who do not have an integrated, coherent sense of self experience themselves instead in a fragmentary fashion. These fragments are referred to as "part-self representations." Individuals experience the fragmentary self as a complete representation of themselves, at least for the moment. For example, during a depression a person who typically vacillates between rage and severe dysphoria may feel totally inadequate, worthless, fearful, and incompetent. After being confronted by a therapy aide, the patient may switch into a state of rage, belittling, devaluing, and otherwise abusing the aide. Implicit during rage is the patient's belief that he or she is worthy and powerful. If explored in either state, patients are likely to spontaneously describe only one perspective of themselves, as if the other side did not exist.

The OR model further postulates that the part-self representations do not operate in a vacuum, but are linked to "part-object representations." The connecting links are conceptualized as affects. Pictorially, the model postulates "fundamental units" comprising a part-self representation, a part-object representation, and the affect which links them:

Part-self———Affect———Part-object
representation   representation

The part-object representations parallel the part-self representations in their structure and function. That is, the person will perceive only a fragmentary aspect of the other person—the object—and experience that aspect as the total person. For example, if individuals perceive themselves as being mistreated, they are likely to conceive of the other (the object) as cruel, dangerous, and hostile. Any other aspects of the other—caring, considerateness, etc.—are likely to be denied.

A corollary of the concept of the fundamental unit is that its ingredients may be accessed by any of three routes: activation of the part-self representation; activation of the part-object representation; and activation of the affective state. For example, if the fundamental unit were constituted as below

Helpless———Fearful———Cruel
(self)   (object)

and the individuals were placed in a situation in which they felt helpless, then they would likely experience other important people as cruel and be fearful of them. These experiences are likely to occur independently of the realistic factors, i.e., how cruel the important others are. This situation typically occurs when very successful and aggressive people are hospitalized with severe and potentially debilitating illnesses, e.g., acute and severe major depressive disorder. Patients may respond to their sense of helplessness and fearfulness by perceiving the nursing staff as cruel and uncaring. On medical services, the same dynamics may be implicated with executives hospitalized for acute myocardial infarctions. Such patients are often quite challenging for the staff.

Conflict in the OR model is modified from the simple, structural model. In the simple, structural model, conflict typically occurs between the various psychic structures: ego versus id, id versus superego, ego versus superego. Conflict is typically unconscious; the contents are repressed. In the OR model, conflict is between fundamental units. Rather than being repressed and unconscious, the conflicting units (labelled 1 and 2 below) are split off and denied. Pictorially, the image would be:

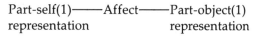

Part-self(1)———Affect———Part-object(1)
representation   representation

******* Splitting with denial *******

Part-self(2)———Affect———Part-object(2)
representation   representation

In part, the difference between splitting with denial versus repression is that in the former, the individual at times is very much aware of the attitudes, feelings, and thoughts that at another time are unavailable or denied. Denial occurs with elements of consciousness; repression deals with elements in the dynamic unconscious. The significance of this difference lies in how the processes are managed psychotherapeutically.

The difference between the simple structural psychoanalytic model and the OR model is clearest in the situation of the patient with paranoid rage. The example below illustrates the ramifications of the two approaches:

"Classically, in dynamic psychiatric interviewing, the formula has been to follow the *affect*. Thus the phrase "How did you feel about . . .?" has been the stock and trade of the dynamically oriented psychiatrist. As affect changes or intensifies, the therapist would pursue it, independent of the logical connectedness of the material. In fact, if the logical connections were tight, one would presume that these expressions of affect represented an avoidance of dealing with some issue.

Object relations theory would suggest that in more severely disturbed patients, the formula requires yet another modification; the therapist should follow the patient's explicit or implicit sense of self and others. That is, as mentioned in Chapter 3, the therapist should clarify the *part-self and part-object representations*. In our experience, this approach generally is experienced as being more empathic than the approach of following only the affect. In fact, when the "follow the affect" approach is joined with the classical Rogerian technique of reflecting the affect, the results can be disastrous. For example, a patient told his therapist that the hospital staff was treating him poorly, that his parents were the crazy ones, and that he himself had no problems at all. The therapist said to the patient, "You seem angry." The patient became enraged with the therapist, stating, "Of course I'm angry. You'd be too if you were in my situation. Don't you understand anything?" The therapist again, following the affect, and reflecting it back to the patient, noted that the patient was becoming even angrier. With that, the patient insisted on getting a new therapist and terminating the session. Shortly thereafter, the patient required placement in seclusion as he continued to escalate in his agitation.

A different therapist handled a similar circumstance using the principles espoused here. The patient complained to the therapist that the social worker was plotting with his family to put him away in a state hospital. The patient seemed threatening to the therapist, who sensed that the patient not only believed that such a plot was evolving, but that the therapist was a party to it, too. The therapist responded by noting that it seemed that the patient viewed himself as a helpless victim. The patient stated that that was right! He was powerless in the face of his parents and the social worker and was being treated unfairly by them. The therapist further noted that the patient seemed to feel that he could trust no one, that other people did not take his concerns seriously. The patient replied that he'd been burned too often. The therapist noted that the mistrust extended to the therapist himself, that it almost didn't pay for the therapist to answer the patient's questions since the patient had already decided what the answers were. The patient relaxed noticeably and said he wasn't sure, but was certainly afraid of what he'd overheard before. He said that in the emergency room where he had been taken by the police, he had overheard a discussion between the psychiatrist and his parents about the state hospital. The therapist remarked that it must clearly have been a frightening experience for the police to have taken him to the emergency room. To have heard that conversation could only have fueled his fears. However, the therapist informed him, when the decision was made to send him to this hospital, the plans for the state hospital had been shelved." (12, pp 62–64)

CENTRALITY OF NARCISSISTIC ISSUES

Many people treat good health as a "right" and are angry when they find themselves or others ill. Their anger can be understood as evidence of a wound to their self-esteem from being ill. When the illness is one which attacks the very sense of a person—his or her personality—the wound is only the greater. Thus, for many people, illness itself is a narcissistic mortification; being mentally ill means suffering the worst type of illness. The experience of hospitalization can often accentuate this sense of failure. We have observed that an inevitable loss of self-esteem results when a person is hospitalized for mental illness. Even the patients who seem to engineer their readmission have at the core a severe problem with self-esteem. As part of the reality of psychiatric hospitalization one is subject to many rules and regulations, including rules that severely curtail patients' liberties. In particular, for example, removal of items which might be used for self-injury emphasizes the fact that the staff, not the patient, "calls the shots." Additionally, hospitals are organized so that the work can be done with some degree of efficiency. Unfortunately, this leads to a certain amount of regimentation in the lives of the patients—medications are administered at times convenient for the staff. These actions can induce feelings of helplessness in the patients, feelings which often are intolerable. If the degree of helplessness is substantial and intolerable, patients may either respond to or defend against it by feeling despair or rage. The behavior of a patient who seemed to want to be hospitalized in order to obtain psychic relief and then turns on the staff can often be understood as reflecting this mechanism. The correlative of helplessness is powerlessness, also a feeling very poorly tolerated in individuals with low self-esteem. This feeling of powerlessness is typically converted into a sense of the powerfulness of others, i.e., the staff, who then should be able to grant all wishes. The failure of the staff to be able to demonstrate their powerfulness or their lack of willingness to perform some task may then provoke the patient's rage. Inseparable from the helplessness and powerlessness is the experience of dependency on others. Some people resist this feeling, creating the situation of hostile dependency. Others collapse into it, expecting to be passive during the treatment process.

COMMON DEFENSE MECHANISMS

Inpatients use the full range of defense mechanisms. However, some "primitive" defense mechanisms are more commonly used than others. *Projective identification* is a commonly used mechanism (15). Briefly, in this mechanism, patients unconsciously attribute to the object some consciously undesired or anxiety-provoking aspect of themselves, and then identify with that aspect of the object. Typically, patients will project onto the object (e.g., the therapist or other important staff member) aspects that are disavowed in themselves. However, patients will then react to the object as if the object is motivated by these disavowed feelings. To the extent that the patient is more likely to project onto an individual unacceptable feelings that are a closer fit to what the object actually feels, there is often a blurring in the object of just what is part of a dynamic process occurring between the patient and the object and what is realistic. Projective identification has the quality of controlling the object, in contrast to simple *projection* in which the affects are totally ridden from the patient and further contact with the object avoided.

Denial, a frequently used defense, forms the basis for many of the defenses in more primitively disturbed individuals. Denial usually refers to mental content that has at some time been conscious, as opposed to *repression* which may represent a method of not allowing unconscious material ever to reach consciousness. In denial, the person disclaims knowledge of something from reality or consciousness. When denial is of the obvious and impenetrable, it is referred to as having psychotic proportions.

Splitting is a process requiring the participation of denial. As was described above, in splitting the fragmentary knowledge of oneself and of the object are experienced as complete and the contradictory aspects are denied. Splitting is the defense mechanism often associated with "all or none" and "black or white" styles of thinking. Splitting is often used by patients with borderline personality disorder and patients with any of the psychoses.

TECHNICAL ASPECTS OF INDIVIDUAL PSYCHOTHERAPY

The immediate goal of dynamic therapy is to provide an *understanding* of behaviors. It is important to be clear that although we expect this understanding to be useful and helpful, we cannot be certain that this will be the case. Thus, we engage patients with the promise of improving their understanding of their behaviors, but without the promise that they will be helped. Their inclinations and desires will determine what they do with the understanding. We offer them the opportunity to gain this understanding with the expectation and hope that they will use it to help themselves; new understandings can provide new options for the person. Since some patients defy the staff to help them, the staff's sidestepping the issue of helping them—help experienced as occurring against their will—may paradoxically make helping them possible.

In the simple structural model, the goal of therapy can be construed as bringing into consciousness what is unconscious. This task can be enjoyable for both patient and therapist, generating the possibility of the "Ah, ha!" experience. However, in the OR model, since the conflict consists of elements that are held within consciousness, the task is not that of bringing material from unconsciousness to consciousness, rather one of *clarifying* the split off aspects of the self and others, *confronting* the split at times, and *interpreting* the defensive purpose of such a split. The most frequently used intervention is likely to be clarification. Occasionally it is necessary to confront split-off aspects. In brief inpatient stays, interpretation can also be used.

CONDUCT OF INDIVIDUAL PSYCHOTHERAPY

Structural Aspects

Frequency of psychotherapy sessions is likely to vary over the course of hospitalization. If the patient is admitted in an acutely psychotic state, initial sessions are likely to be brief and supportive. Although some patients can use these sessions for true psychotherapy, many patients cannot tolerate or constructively use the sessions until their reality testing has improved.

Duration of sessions is important. If the patient cannot use or tolerate longer sessions, daily, 5-minute sessions may suffice. Although one should not underestimate the significance of such sessions to patients, one must be modest and realistic about what will be accomplished psychotherapeutically. As the patient stabilizes, extending the length of sessions to 30 or 45 minutes two to three times a week seems to work best.

It is best if a *location* is chosen which meets the needs of the patient and staff for safety and confidentiality. If the patient is very labile, a quiet corner of the unit may suffice for brief sessions; other staff can be available if the patient begins to lose control. Some patients may need to be seen in the quiet room, with other staff at the doorway. For more extended sessions, a private office is necessary.

Content Aspects

Early sessions with the patient must focus on filling in pieces of history which have not been previously obtained. It is important to have a clear understanding of the *events that led to admission* and what these events meant to the patient. In the process of obtaining this information, the question must be asked if the patient can learn anything about his or her vulnerabilities and about signals that the situation was deteriorating. If the possibility exists of catching a relapse early, it is important to learn quickly just what occurred, before a process of sealing over begins. It is important to recognize that in some patients a sealing over of the story of their decompensation occurs, which may denote their defensive style. Later on, it may be countertherapeutic to push the patient into confronting these events and how they unfolded. Some patients will prefer to have a "laundry list" of signals, the source of which they prefer not to contemplate.

The *meaning of being hospitalized* is an issue that quickly comes to the fore in discussions. Here, the narcissistic mortification of being ill and hospitalized can be addressed. Some patients can deal with this issue only in the privacy of individual sessions. Others feel that "since it has never happened to you it's easy for you to say that (hospitalization is not the worst thing that can happen to you)," and see no point in talking to a therapist about the issue. For these patients, group psychotherapy can be most helpful; the negative feelings can be explored with others who reached a different conclusion and developed other methods to cope with their experience. The significance of hospitalization, of course, may differ along many parameters, including whether the patient is newly ill or chronic. For some chronic patients, hospitalization may mean relief or an opportunity to regress. For others, it is another "kick in the teeth." Pat formulations are not of use; the meaning for the specific patient needs to be understood.

GUIDELINES FOR THE CONDUCT OF INDIVIDUAL SESSIONS

The classic instruction in psychoanalysis is to "talk about whatever is on your mind." This instruction needs some adaptation in the therapy of inpatients. It certainly is important to know what is in the forefront of the patient's attention. Particularly in the hospital, where patients can easily misinterpret bureaucratic procedure for deliberate insult, the ability to clarify and allay anxieties can be most helpful. However, modifications will be needed because hospitalization will be brief; frequently inpatients need more structure to the therapy session to prevent anxiety-provoking psychotic regression. Thus, in individual and group psychotherapies the appropriate *focus of therapy* is on the following three issues:

1. Problems that brought the patient into the hospital;
2. Problems that emerge from being in the hospital; and
3. Problems that occur or are anticipated upon discharge.

A patient who chooses to talk about another area and seems to want to devote substantial time to the other area would be considered avoiding the therapeutic task, unless the relevance of the issue can be defined. Some patients believe that during their hospital therapy they should be getting to the bottom of their problems by attempting to understand all the details of their upbringing. Such patients would be told that although these are in fact issues the patient might want to delve into at a later date, for hospitalization, it is necessary to focus on the three issues listed above. Another way of thinking about whether or not an issue is an appropriate subject for discussion is to think about the relationship of the issue to *adaptation* for patients. How much is this issue linked to the failures of patients to adapt to their life situations? For example, the patient with an eating disorder who does not talk about her eating problem and failure to gain weight, but chooses to focus on what to do on a pass for which she is ineligible, would be questioned about her choice of subject. The initial questions would be clarifications. Were she not to address how her issue relates to her initial tasks, she would be confronted with her avoiding the issue of her eating habits and weight.

As stated above, the primary technical intervention is the use of clarification. But what should the therapist be on the lookout to clarify? As a derivative of the OR model, the focus of attention is on the part-self representations. That is, the therapist is constantly asking, "What does this say about the patient's view of him- or herself?" Very often, the question can be answered by asking the patient "And how did that affect your view of yourself?" If the part-self representation is totally unclear, one might ask "How did you feel about yourself then?" Sometimes the part-self representation must be inferred from the content of what is said or how it is said. It may be lightly camouflaged in the statements of the patient, and the clarification may resemble a Rogerian-type reflection of what the patient said: "So you felt pretty badly about yourself then." Although such an intervention may seem to be merely restating the obvious, not infrequently patients will vehemently disagree with the intervention and flip to the other side of the conflicted view of themselves, the other part-self representation. As therapists reflect back to patients through clarification the other side of the conflict, patients may be implicitly confronted with the contradictory views they hold of themselves. That may in and of itself lead to a somewhat more integrated self-view.

It is especially important to search out the part-self representations which contain significant elements of the "devalued self" and the "inflated other." The reason this particular constellation is important is that the part-self representations that represent the devalued self are likely to be linked to self-defeating and otherwise self-destructive attitudes. The "inflated other" is merely the flip side of the fundamental unit which is likely to contain the devalued self. The common "inflated other" is the idealized view of the therapist. In contrast to Kohut's description of healthier outpatients in psychoanalysis, we have found that patients who devalue themselves often idealize the therapist; when the patient must leave the therapist—a frequent occurrence at the time of discharge or staff rotation—the sense of the patient's personal inadequacy rises to the surface, complicating treatment on disposition planning.

GROUP PSYCHOTHERAPY

Group therapy can be a very useful means of intervention in hospitalized patients, either short-term or long-term (16). However, some inpatient programs eschew the use of groups, offering only individual and family psychosocial therapies. We see four specific advantages to the use of group therapy in brief hospitalizations.

1. Most patients admitted to the hospital have had recent problems in relating to others. The interpersonal-social focus of group therapy is a natural way to explore these issues and learn about ones's impact on others and how to modify it. Although group therapy is not the only means of addressing this issue, group therapy highlights it. Using a here-and-now focus permits the group to act as a social laboratory in which patients learn and try out new ways of interacting, with assistance available.

2. Research on group therapy has identified some factors specific to group therapy and experienced by patients as linked to success in therapy. These factors are universality and altruism. By universality, we mean the sense that you are not alone in having your troubles. Many patients feel extremely alienated from others;

hearing from others in an intimate setting that they are not so different can be helpful. The altruistic component—the opportunity to be helpful to others—is also highly rewarding. That this should be so is simply understood from the OR model: the person in the role of helper is positively construed.

3. Group therapy offers an opportunity for therapists to diagnose countertherapeutic forces that invariably emerge on units, i.e., perform a "milieu biopsy." This opportunity is shared with the community meeting (see below) but group therapy offers a closer view with greater opportunities for exploration. The group therapy can also be a site for intervention to correct countertherapeutic trends. Since the dynamics of small groups differ significantly from those of large groups, it may be easier to intervene even in processes that have taken hold of the community.

4. Some people act dramatically differently in individual contacts than they do in group situations. It is not infrequent for nurses to report markedly different patient behaviors from what an individual therapist sees in the office. Sometimes, the group offers the opportunity to diagnose special patterns which are only visible in the group setting. For some borderline patients, this may be extremely important.

Group psychotherapy is no less complicated than individual psychotherapy. Yalom's book (16) provides an interesting point of view specifically dealing with inpatients. For general introductory material on group psychotherapy, we refer the reader to Yalom and Weiner—both of whom focus on outpatient groups (17, 18).

Types of Groups

Many types of group therapy activities exist. Broadly speaking, one can classify the types of groups into three classes: task oriented, interpersonal, and expressive. Task-oriented groups typically have a concrete focus and are problem-solving in orientation. They tend to be easier to run and are suitable for patients with severe disturbance for whom cooperative effort may be a goal in itself. Dynamics tend to be ignored and the focus is on the individual's participation more than the group as a group. Group dynamics are typically experienced as an interference or annoyance. Interpersonal groups can be further divided into socialization, educative, and exploratory groups. Socialization groups, often useful for severe and chronically disturbed patients, are predicated upon the belief that any reasonable social interaction is beneficial in and of itself. Sometimes these groups are merged with medication groups, where the medications for the patients are reviewed and renewed. Other times, the group functions like a social club in which people share coffee and donuts. The educative model has been extensively described by Maxmen (19). These groups have a strong didactic component; the therapist uses the participants as case studies to teach the patients about their problems. Although Maxmen does not feel that dynamic group therapy is useful for brief inpatient work, we think that components of the educative model are quite useful and can be incorporated into a dynamic group therapy. Exploratory interpersonal groups leave the level of discourse and understanding at the level of the interpersonal and do not explore the intrapersonal (intrapsychic) dynamics. These groups operate on the model that what is important is interaction with others; the intrapsychic aspects are epiphenomena. These groups merge into the expressive category. Expressive groups typically require fairly high-functioning patients. In order for patients to be able to participate in such groups, they must be able to tolerate substantial increases in anxiety. The focus is on the irrational and transference issues are emphasized. The therapist tends to be rather passive; the time frame for the group is usually long-term. Group dynamics are explored along with individual dynamics. When such groups are used with severely disturbed patients, the groups are characterized by substantial regression and acting out. Of course, these behaviors would be interpreted in such a group.

Our position is that the nature of the patients on a modern inpatient unit will vary greatly from week to week. Therefore, the nature of the group is likely to change because the capacity of the group is directly linked to its membership. Thus, if many discharges have occurred and the patients who are then admitted are all severely ill and unable meaningfully to explore relationships or examine—even didactically—the events that have so recently troubled them, the new group is more likely to be task-focused (resolving conflicts over lights in bedrooms, sharing the stereo) or a socialization group. As these patients improve and less ill and more capable patients are admitted, the group may shift to a more interpersonal, educative, or expressive model. No matter how the group is conducted, we have found that grasping group dynamics is helpful in managing the patients and the milieu.

Small Group Dynamics

Many models of group dynamics have been proposed. Tuckman's (20) summary of the processes of forming, storming, norming, and performing is easy to remember and often useful in helping recognize the stages that groups go through. However, we have found that Bion's (21) model is most applicable and useful for understanding group processes on inpatient services. Since Bion's work is predicated upon an OR model, a convenient fit understandably exists between the group dynamic model and our model for individual dynamics. Bion looked at the group as a whole, as if it were an organism itself. He noted that although the group typically had a task, recurrent

forces distracted the membership from that task or consumed the group's attention. He referred to the group as acting as if it were making specific *basic assumptions* about its purpose and mode of conduct. Describing the groups relative to the basic assumptions they seemed to operate under, he characterized four group states: the *work group*, in which the group was performing its task, and three *basic assumption groups*, in which the group did not work at its assigned tasks. The three basic assumption groups were labelled basic assumption dependency, basic assumption fight or flight, and basic assumption pairing.

It is possible to compare the three basic assumption groups relative to the unstated aim of the group, qualities of leadership, and themes and issues for the group (see Table 10.1) (22). With respect to the *aims* of the group, the basic assumption dependency group acts as if the group will attain security through, and have its members protected by, one individual. In contrast, the basic assumption fight-flight group acts as if its goal is to preserve itself which can be done only through fighting or running away. In the basic assumption pairing group, the aim is to reproduce, to bring forth the savior.

Leadership varies with group state. In the basic assumption dependency group, the leader is portrayed and perceived as omnipotent and idealized. In contrast, the leader of the basic assumption fight or flight group acts paranoid, as if hostile forces are present without or, perhaps, within. The basic assumption pairing group has no leader; the leader is unborn.

The *themes and issues* for the groups vary, consistent with basic assumptions and leadership. In the basic assumption dependency group, the members are portrayed as inadequate and complexity is eschewed. The group may maintain the quality of a religious cult, with the leader of the group its head. In the basic assumption fight or flight

Table 10.1.   Basic Assumption Groups, Wilfred Bion (22)

	Aim of Group	Leader	Themes and Issues
Dependency	To attain security through and have its members protected by one individual	Omniscient, omnipotent, idealized	Members inadequate; complexity eschewed; quality of religious cult
Fight-Flight	To preserve itself, which can be done only by fighting or running away	Paranoid	Action is essential, individual is sacrificed to the group; anti-intellectual; feeling of rage, fear, anger common
Pairing	To reproduce, to bring forth the Messiah, the savior	No leader	Issue is sexual, no one is bored; hopeful; optimistic; unborn leader will save group from despair, etc.

group, action is deemed essential and the individual is sacrificed to the needs of the group. The group tends to be antiintellectual. Feelings of rage, intense fear, and anger are common. For the basic assumption pairing group, the issue is sensed to be sexual and no one is bored. The affective state tends to be hopeful and optimistic; the fantasy is that the pair within the group will create as yet an unborn leader who will save the group from despair.

In using Bion's model, we find it helpful to attempt to diagnose the state of the group at any point and supplement that assessment with assessments of the individuals' participation in the dynamics. It would not be enough to note that the group is functioning from a basic assumption dependency position; one would need to understand the way that relates to the specific dynamics of each member of the group. Does the depressed patient feel encouraged by participating in the group fantasy that the omnipotent leader brings hope, or is the patient's personal sense of failure and inadequacy highlighted by the group dynamics? In Tavistock training groups, the consultant to the group interprets the group process metaphorically. This type of intervention is not appropriate for inpatient group therapy. Once the therapist has assessed group dynamics and discerned the group's basic assumption state, the therapist must decide if it would be useful to the

group as a whole to clarify its dynamics. If the therapist senses that the group is not performing its task but is being diverted by one of the basic dynamic mechanisms, the therapist would clarify this process for group members. Since it can be quite difficult to differentiate group dynamics from other dynamic processes that can affect group members, the therapist may find the clarification to be incorrect or even mutating the group process. Statements such as "it seems that group members feel that the hospital can do it all for you" may focus the group members on their participation in their care, with the concomitant message that they play an important role in their own treatment, i.e., they are not helpless and inadequate.

Structural and Technical Parameters

The *site* of group therapy must be given due attention. Some sense of privacy is necessary for the conduct of the group; a busy corridor on the unit is unsatisfactory. The site must accommodate the number of patients and therapists. Because the group members are likely to be quite ill, the site should be fixed, providing a sense of reliability. The *duration* and *frequency* of sessions must balance the ability of the patients to tolerate group situations with the time required for an issue to be brought up, developed, and adequately discussed. Although some group therapists recommend group sessions of 1½ hours, we have found this duration too long for most acute inpatients. In our experience 45 minutes is the practical minimum length. As for frequency of sessions, others have recommended up to five meetings per week. We have found that two or three meetings a week are sufficient to accomplish our tasks.

The issue of *membership* is a difficult one. The two contrasting positions are either to include everyone who can participate—universal attendance—or screen for a selected membership. If universal attendance is chosen, one can use the group for the milieu biopsy. The group has the advantage of not being "sanitized" of the more difficult individuals; all the likely protagonists are present. To the extent that the sense of universality contributes to the group's effectiveness, nonexclusion is consistent with the fantasy. Likewise, to the extent that patients screened out of the group will feel rejected, the iatrogenic injury is avoided. The screening approach suggests that membership is a privilege; the universal approach suggests it is an obligation. Screened groups tend to be easier to conduct and generally will function at a higher level for longer periods of time because more difficult patients are typically screened out. Obviously, although screened groups cannot be used for an accurate biopsy of the milieu, important information can still be gained. However, the use of screening does create two classes of patients which can foster the use of projective mechanisms, an "us versus them" mentality.

Therapist factors must also be considered. In many training situations more than one therapist is used to accommodate training needs. We favor using two therapists not only for training needs, but for two additional reasons. First, since we have universal attendance at group therapy, the groups can often be difficult to manage. In this circumstance, having a cotherapist is often helpful. Second, patients will experience less disruption when one of the therapists is ill or on vacation. A frequently arising complication when more than one therapist is used is that the therapists typically will organize themselves hierarchically (or be structured that way by the group members) and will at least occasionally move in competing directions. Cotherapists need instruction and supervision in how to collaborate. When the therapists are not senior and experienced clinicians, it helps to have senior clinicians occasionally rotate through as therapists. Such a rotation offers the other staff members an opportunity to see how experienced therapists work and signals patients and staff that the modality is valued. The last common issue relating to the therapists is whether or not the therapists need to be hospital based. In our opinion at least one therapist—or, if only one therapist is used, that therapist—should be hospital based. We feel this way since the therapist needs a close working relationship with the staff and to have available all possible information, both formal and informal, in order to be effective.

Content of the therapy sessions should not be unstructured. Do not tell patients that the group is a place where they can talk about whatever is on their mind. The time constraints of brief hospitalization make it necessary to instruct group members that the group is a place to discuss problems that led to and develop during hospitalization and problems that develop or are anticipated upon leaving the hospital. It is not an accident that the "agenda" is the same for individual and group psychotherapies. Unless the issue can be related to the areas above, another issue would be seen as a resistance. Issues that relate to the distant past or far off into the future are typically efforts to avoid painful topics of the present. The focus is technically not a here-and-now approach, since topics from the weekend, night before, etc., might be discussed in the group.

Process and Procedural Aspects

In short-term units a rapid turnover in the groups is likely to occur. It is important for therapist and patients to know who is expected to be present. Thus, we recommend that *attendance* be noted at the beginning of each group. Although this procedure does not require a roll call, it should be acknowledged who was expected but has not attended. Sometimes, the absence of a group member—now in seclusion or transferred to a medical floor—may be of great significance but avoided. Absence of a cotherapist can be a highly significant event in some patients' lives.

New members of the group should be *introduced.* The new group member should be *oriented* to the group and specifically informed about the site, time, duration, frequency, and proper content. Ideally, one of the other group members performs the orientation. The patient is asked to introduce him- or herself to the group by means of a brief explanation of what led to hospital admission. At this point in group therapy, we feel that the educative model (Maxmen) can be fused with our approach to help patients learn about their illnesses and how the illnesses evolved. Although one should expect the patient's description to be only partially illuminating, patients should learn what they need to know in order to understand an illness episode.

Patients about to be *discharged* should expect to discuss their feelings about their hospitalization, feelings about leaving the hospital, and their discharge plans. Since separation experiences universally have substantial impact on people, this item is regularly placed on the agenda.

Any *critical incidents* from the unit since the last group, especially the prior 24

hours, should be placed on the agenda whether patients bring these issues up or not. Patients may not bring such an issue up because it is too frightening. If such an incident has taken place, therapists should start with a recitation of the facts as they are best known. The group can provide an excellent opportunity to explore and correct distortions regarding staff and hospital operations.

From the point of view of the group therapy process we think therapists should attempt to focus on the *group as a whole.* Direct your intervention to the group as a whole whenever possible. Some group therapists have recommended that only individually oriented interventions be used in inpatient groups. However, we view that as repetitive of the individual therapy experience. Group-centered interventions may be linked to individually directed interventions if it is felt to be appropriate and useful. Reflect all such interventions back to the group membership for comment or correction. No doubt it is a mistake only to use group-centered interventions; patients will feel ignored and dehumanized. However, group-centered interventions mobilize the special nature of groups and permit explorations not possible with individually directed interventions alone.

It might seem obvious, but an important and sometimes neglected factor is the responsibility of the therapist to *maintain order and decorum* during the session. Although frequently this task is not discussed in other literature on group therapy, it is especially important in situations with acutely disturbed inpatients and when group therapy attendance is universal. At times of great tension, the therapist may feel like a control rod in a nuclear reactor. Although a certain degree of permissiveness is allowed, such permissiveness cannot include threats or violent acts. The therapist must actively convey the culture and mores of the group since rapid turnover and severely ill members will less likely be able to sustain a pro-social point of view.

Groups that accept all acute inpatients will need direction from therapists to maintain *allegiance to reality.* By this we mean that acute inpatient groups can easily fall under the sway of a psychotic patient—or patients—and begin to accept and promote a severely distorted view of the world (or unit). We have found that three incidences often recur in which therapists fail to help the group to reality test. In the first instance, a new patient admitted to the unit tells about the sequence of events that led to his admission, and the story is delusional. Rather than confront the new patient with his distortions—directly or indirectly—group members may accept them and build upon them. It is the therapist's responsibility to maintain reality testing for the group and point out the unlikely aspects of the story. Therapists often feel controlled by the group as it embraces the psychotic beliefs; this instance is one of the occasions in which the presence and support of a co-therapist can be very helpful. In the second instance, a patient's speech is incoherent. If the therapist is silent, patients—already feeling inadequate—may feel that their inability to understand the patient is simply further evidence of their inadequacy. At these times, it may be liberating to the group members to hear from the therapist that the therapist is unable to understand the patient, that the patient seems to have serious problems conveying what she wants to say. The third instance parallels the second; a patient has behaved in a frightening way or some incident has occurred, terrifying the patients collectively. Under these circumstances, clarifying that the events are very frightening or terrifying can help the patients' reality testing by validating their experience. Clarification is necessary since patients may experience their fright as part of their illness, not as a realistic response to scary events. The failure to provide such clarification may lead to iatrogenic deterioration since the boundary between reality and fantasy is blurred.

The final technical issue we wish to comment upon is the issue of scope of the focus. Most dynamic therapy texts emphasize the continuity of experiences from early life to current behaviors and from session to session. Because of the regressive nature of illnesses that bring patients into the hospital, patients operate in a dedifferentiated fashion and are less available for genetic interpretations of the classic mode. Consistent with our emphasis on the here-and-now, we recommend that group therapists orient themselves and the group to a *single-session focus.* By this we mean that the therapist should ordinarily resist the temptation to refer to earlier group sessions in making interpretations. Not that such interpretations are necessarily problematic; simply, with the turnover that typically occurs on such acute units, such interventions often confuse patients as opposed to helping clarify processes. Stated another way, such interventions often seem to do more for the therapists than for the patients.

COMMUNITY MEETINGS

Following World War II a heightened interest in social factors emerged as well as an interest in how they related to mental illness. The experiences from wartime—at the front line and in understaffed hospitals—suggested that social forces were quite powerful in determining people's behaviors. Stanton and Schwartz (23) showed that social forces within the hospital could have profound detrimental effects on patients. They emphasized the importance of the hospital organization and clear communications. Studying a different hospital, Caudill (24) concluded that the traditional psychiatric hospital structure was dysfunctional and required a radical revision. Rubinstein and Lasswell (25) studied innovative changes at the same hospital which Caudill had studied. The therapeutic milieu was under intense scrutiny and hospital organizations were in flux. Denber (26) edited a series of papers from a research conference on therapeutic communities. Attempts were made to bridge the gap between psychosocial therapies and medication therapy, all of which were new. Others have attempted to synthesize the critical elements of therapeutic communities and understand their contribution to clinical care (27–29). One of the innovations from the therapeutic community movement that was almost universally adopted was the community meeting.

Community meetings are historically rooted in Maxwell Jones' therapeutic community (30). As adopted in the United States, these meetings of the staff and patients were very large groups which were simply structured—a leader, a set time and place, and a fixed duration. Little relationship existed between what Jones had described and how the model was implemented in the United States. Edelson (31, 32) struggled with the integration of individual, group, and social dynamics to arrive at a formulation to guide clinicians through the various psychosocial activities. His formulation of the community meeting was quite structured, with a severely limited focus. He sharply differentiated tasks—sociotherapeutic and psychotherapeutic—with the hope of rendering more comprehensible the complicated processes and reactions. Discussing the experience of participating in one of the simply structured meetings, Klein (33) likened the experience to attending a "tea party with the mad hatter." Likewise, Bernard (34) commented on the toxic effects of a community meeting with inadequate structure. With decreasing lengths of stay and increasingly acutely ill patients, community meetings have fallen from favor in many inpatient settings. Community meetings in some inpatients settings were the site of chaos. Interestingly, the

American version of Jones' community meeting was quite removed from Jones' original concept. In Jones' book, the community meeting is described as quite structured. When one recalls that the patients for whom this format was designed were psychologically healthier than those typically hospitalized in the United States, the dissatisfaction most people experienced with community meetings is not surprising. Rapoport (35) studied Jones' therapeutic community and characterized it by four principles: permissiveness, communalism, democracy, and reality confrontation. However, in contrast to the principles espoused, Rapoport reported that the primary function of the community meeting seemed to be to exercise social control. Patients regularly reported that they experienced the meeting as a courtroom. The staff's response—it is not a courtroom because no sentence is pronounced—was dismissed by the patients. The staff also saw the community meeting as an important channel of communication.

Of course, the patient population with whom Jones worked was distinctly different from the populations for which the therapeutic community principles were applied in the United States. In England, Jones had initially worked primarily with men in postwar circumstances suffering from character disorders. His length of stay by current standards was relatively long. Clearly these were not the usual circumstances that apply in acute hospital work. Later, Jones (36) recommended the use of multiple, task-oriented small groups for work with chronic schizophrenic patients.

Large Group Dynamics

In order to understand community meetings—purposes, complications, structure, and techniques—it is necessary to have a rudimentary understanding of large group dynamics (37). Most people have had personal experience with large groups and are familiar with many of the experiences that large groups induce. Probably the most common sources of such experiences are school situations. The large groups may take place during classes, lectures, or recreational times such as in a school yard. Probably the most common example of a classic large group process occurs in a large lecture hall. A professor is lecturing and you have a question about the material. Many people become very anxious about asking questions. Is it a good question? Can I formulate the question properly? Will I make a fool of myself? If you decide to ask the question, often you feel that the answer is not sufficient. Many times, you do not ask the question in class, but go up to the professor after the class and ask it. If the question was poorly formulated before, why is it any better formulated now? If the question was a bad one during the lecture, what in delaying it made it improve? The explanation for these phenomena lies in large group dynamics.

Large group dynamics lead to *common experiences.* In large groups, people often feel themselves to be lost or frightened. They feel out of touch with important aspects of themselves and others. Turquet (38) has referred to this as the sense of "losing one's wits." There is a fear of domination by the group and often a common rejection of direction by the group or leadership of the group. People feel immature, sometimes reacting to this feeling with a sense of competitiveness or helplessness. Similarly, one feels deskilled, disoriented as to one's proper role. One feels one's contribution— or in the above example from the classroom, one's question—has been either ignored and lost or unappreciated and incompletely responded to by the group or its leader.

The *defense mechanisms* commonly used in large groups are projective identification, splitting, denial, psychotic thinking, and primitive envy. It is clear that the defenses common to large groups are also defenses commonly seen in acute inpatients. However, it is critically important to understand that the defenses which are tapped in large groups are defenses which are used by normal people in large groups. The fact that normal people will be induced to use these primitive defenses suggests that the emotional pressure on the patients is likely to be irresistible. Already dedifferentiated, the experiences of the patients are all the more powerful.

Purposes of Community Meetings

Jones (30) stated that:

The most important thing is to arouse the patient's interest and if possible his active participation so that he changes from a passive or defeatist attitude and actually tests out the possibility of change in his real life problems. [page 56]

As we noted above, Rapoport (35) reported that the purpose of the community meeting seemed to him to be more of social control. Kisch et al. (39) described eight functions or purposes of community meetings: to identify the unit as a whole; to identify and raise issues that may be infringing on the rights of some or be detrimental to the morale and rapport between staff and patients and patients with one another; to reveal personality and social behavior problems of individuals that are invisible in the one-to-one setting of a therapy office; to confront inhibitions in speaking; to provide a safe forum to practice new behaviors; to provide an opportunity to discover the universal existential problems of emotional life; to deal with common issues such as stigma, insecurity in home visits, and dependency fears; and to evaluate and educate one another on the effective and ineffective aspects of the program. Working on an intermediate-term unit with a severely ill population, Gilman et al. (40) saw community meetings as useful for clarifying regressive countertherapeutic forces; clarifying overt, negative transference; confronting and occasionally interpreting countertherapeutic forces and negative transferences; assisting with reality testing; reducing the regressive pulls of the large group; correcting practical difficulties, i.e., problem solving; and transferring information.

In our experience on a short-term inpatient service, we emphasized the following purposes: enculturation, opportunity to participate in effective action, information transfer, clarifying roles and relationships, and reality testing. The community meeting provides an opportunity to describe for the entire community what the values of the unit are and to enact those values through various evaluations and decisions. This process is one of *enculturation.* Since the turnover of patients is great, there must be a continuous effort to maintain a specific perspective and to clarify what that perspective is for both patients and staff. The community meeting has the advantage of being public—no secrecy exists about the thinking that underlies a decision and just what the decision is. Decisions made in rounds—to which many staff members cannot attend and to which patients are not privy—are subject to significant distortions and misinterpretations.

The *opportunity to participate in effective action* is helpful for patients' self-esteem. It demonstrates the rationality of the system and the competency of all the participants. As noted above, it is linked to the enculturation phenomena, since some of the actions will implement the values of the unit. Such participation can also reduce stigma—from the staff and from other patients—as patients see that they can function effectively and in cooperation with nonpatients.

Information transfer serves several purposes. The primary antidote to various distortions is reality input; the community

meeting creates the opportunity to provide patients and staff with information to limit distortions. Providing maximal information to patients and staff in a single setting reduces some of the barriers to communication. Patients typically feel empowered by directly receiving information that affects them.

Clarifying roles and relationships becomes important with inpatients because the structure of the hospital milieu may be difficult to comprehend. Expectations about the nursing staff, psychiatrists, therapeutic activities personnel, and social workers may all lead to misunderstandings and animosity. The community meeting provides an opportunity for such expectations to be clarified and corrected. Additionally, the role of the patient in the milieu can be explored and understood. In particular, the urge to regress and be taken care of by the staff can be explored, confronted, and interpreted. For occasions when patients injure themselves while on the unit or on pass, the community meeting often provides an excellent forum for the community as a whole to learn about what had occurred, the response of the staff, and the rationale for their actions. For those patients who fantasize that by virtue of hospitalization, they have shed all responsibilities and that the staff in their omnipotence can do all, anger and resentment can be clarified and confronted.

Reality testing is the function of testing fantasies and beliefs against reality. The realistic limits of what can be accomplished in the hospital, what the staff can do, and what one can expect of friends and family are all topics that may emerge in community meetings. The imperfections of the staffs' performance may surface, and it is often helpful to acknowledge such imperfections and place them in the context of the patients' total treatment. Errors must be acknowledged and corrected when possible. Oftentimes, the thrust of the patients' complaints will be that there is no room for any error, an attitude not conducive to reasonable interpersonal relations.

Large Group Versus Small Group Dynamics

Large group dynamics contrast sharply with small group dynamics and lead to specific structural recommendations for community meetings (see Table 10.2). In small group settings, *feelings* of intimacy, support, and comfort are commonly experienced. In contrast, large groups are more conducive to feelings of alienation, anger, and anxiety. Rather than feeling a sense of support in a large group, people often feel on their own and unsupported by the group. Although *participation* in small groups may be difficult for some, that difficulty is often easily overcome through the support felt from the other members. In large groups, the participant often feels extreme anxiety, even on the border of terror. With the support of the small group, members may feel their *sense of themselves* enhanced or stabilized. In contrast, in the large group sense of self is lost, self-consciousness is heightened and painful, and identity is threatened.

Table 10.2.   Group Dynamics: Large Versus Small

Parameters	Small	Large
Affect	Intimacy, comfort, support	Alienation, anger, anxiety; unsupported
Participation	Natural and easy	Terrifying
Sense of Self	Enhanced or stabilized	Loss of sense of self, intense self-consciousness, identity is threatened

Table 10.3.   Parameters of Types of Community Meetings

Parameters	Highly Structured	Simply Structured
Primary Focus	Reality	Fantasy
Structural Level	Ego/Superego	Id
Purpose	Decisions	Understanding
Means	Information	Interpretation

Structural Parameters and Community Meetings

It is instructive to compare the simply structured community meetings popular from the 1950s–1970s with more highly structured meetings (see Table 10.3). During the 1950s, the primary focus of the community meeting was to elicit fantasies from the patients and interpret them. From a psychosexual structural viewpoint, the emphasis was on id functioning. The principal means of intervention was interpretation; the goal was greater understanding of the affective state of the community (construed of as solely constituting patients). With the more highly structured meetings we described (41), the primary focus is on reality. From the psychosexual structural viewpoint, emphasis is on the ego and superego functions. The community attempts to make decisions when appropriate. The primary means of intervention are providing information and clarification.

Leadership of the community meeting must be clearly defined. Any ambiguity will foster regression among both the patients and the staff, a primitization of defenses. The tasks of the leader are to make the situation safe for conducting meetings; initiate and maintain a therapeutic environment; maintain reality testing; and clarify issues as they arise. The *structural* elements necessary for conducting effective meetings are defined and capable leadership; defined time for beginning and ending the meeting; adequate duration of the meeting; appropriate and adequate seating; and internal organization of the meeting itself.

Technical Aspects—the Conduct of Community Meetings

We recommend that a number of things occur regularly during community meetings. *Attendance* at the community meeting is important both for patients and staff. All staff significantly involved with care of the patients should regularly attend. Staff should treat attending community meetings as equivalent in importance to attending individual sessions. If staff know that on a given day they will have to miss the meeting or be late, they must inform the leader of the meeting in advance, if possible. Given the rapid turnover on units, patient attendance must also be monitored. The absence of a patient—because of medical complications or a setback and placement in seclusion—needs to be addressed in the meeting and fully discussed if it is a concern to the community.

New members of the community must be *introduced*. It is simply rude to have a group meeting with participants who are not identified to other members. Additionally, it helps initiate new members into the process to be formally acknowledged. In the acute unit setting, we think it appropriate simply to introduce people by name without going into explanations of what led to their hospitalizations. Staff members should explain what their role will be vis-à-vis the patients.

An *agenda* is necessary; it should be created openly and minimally read out loud so all participants know what will be discussed. The failure to have an openly announced agenda can paralyze meetings; participants have no way to gauge their participation in discussions. Sometimes members will defer participation in a discussion to save time for another issue which then is not on the agenda. Agendas also make it possible for more disorganized patients to keep track of issues.

Information gathering is an important technique in conducting community meetings. One of the processes that impressed us when we observed the more classic, simply structured community meetings was how quickly leaders would intervene with interpretations without pursuing or clarifying the facts upon which the expressed attitudes were based. It is important in the information-gathering stages of each discussion to make sure that a common body of information exists upon which patients and staff can then proceed with their discussion.

Closure of discussions is also important. Large groups can be chaotic and disorganizing. Issues may not be resolved in a single discussion. Nevertheless, it is important for the leader of the community meeting to signal clearly to participants that discussion on a particular topic will cease and the community will now proceed to the next item on the agenda. Ideally, the closure will occur with some statement about the results of the discussion—that a conclusion had been reached, a conclusion cannot be reached but the topic will be resubmitted for discussion if interest persists, or that the community had made a particular decision.

Separation experiences have profound meanings for all people—staff and patients alike. Realizing how these experiences can be quite powerful and cut across all levels of personal functioning, we insist upon discussing impending staff vacations and patient discharges. We have seen how disorganized some patients become when a valued staff member is suddenly not present for prolonged periods of time. Our rule has been that planned staff absences of one week or longer should be announced in advance. When discussing such separations with patients who are particularly sensitive to such losses, the importance of team effort in treating the patient is often helpful. *Supportive beginning and ending* of the meeting is helpful in setting the tone of the unit. When possible, starting with an unprovocative item helps set a tone for the meeting. Similarly, ending with an upbeat item will also affect the way patients conduct themselves on the unit.

CONCLUSIONS

We have attempted to describe our point of view that a solid grounding in the principles of psychodynamics is extremely useful in understanding, planning, and implementing biopsychosocial therapy within a short-stay inpatient unit. We have found the framework of object relations theory particularly applicable to this work, and we have reviewed the fundamentals of this approach and its application in an inpatient setting. Against a backdrop of the essentials of medical evaluation and pharmacotherapy, individual and group psychotherapy must be understood by therapists on an inpatient unit and applied in appropriate ways. We have reviewed our approach to individual psychotherapy, group psychotherapy, and community meetings, along with references to individual, small-group, and large-group dynamics as they occur within the hospital milieu.

References

1. Sullivan HS: *Schizophrenia as a Human Process,* New York, Norton, 1962.
2. Fromm-Reichmann F: *Principles of Intensive Psychotherapy,* Chicago, University of Chicago Press, 1950.
3. Brody EB, Redlich FC (eds): *Psychotherapy with Schizophrenics,* New York, International Universities Press, 1952.
4. Hill LB: *Psychotherapeutic Intervention in Schizophrenia,* Chicago, University of Chicago Press, 1955.
5. Rosen J: *Direct Analysis: Selected Papers,* New York, Grune & Stratton, 1953.
6. Burton A (ed): *Psychotherapy of the Psychoses,* New York, Basic Books, 1961.
7. Searles H: *Collected Papers on Schizophrenia and Related Subjects,* New York, International Universities Press, 1965.
8. Gunderson JG, Mosher LR (eds): *Psychotherapy of Schizophrenia,* Northvale, N.J. Jason Aronson, 1975.
9. Pao P-N: *Schizophrenic Disorders: Theory and Treatment from a Psychodynamic Point of View,* New York, International Universities Press, 1979.
10. Drake RE, Sederer LI: The adverse effects of intensive treatment of chronic schizophrenia. Compr Psychiatry, 27:313–326, 1986.
11. Oldham JM, Russakoff LM: The medical-therapeutic community. J Psychiatr Treatment Eval, 4:347–353, 1982.
12. Oldham JM, Russakoff LMR: *Dynamic Therapy in Brief Hospitalization,* Northvale, N.J. Jason Aronson, 1987.
13. Gedo JE, Goldberg A: *Models of the Mind,* Chicago, University of Chicago Press, 1973.
14. Kernberg O: *Object Relations Theory and Clinical Psychoanalysis,* New York, Jason Aronson, 1976.
15. Ogden T: On projective identification. Int J Psychoanal, 60:357–373, 1979.
16. Yalom ID: *Inpatient Group Psychotherapy,* New York, Basic Books, 1983.
17. Yalom ID: *The Theory and Practice of Group Psychotherapy,* ed. 3, New York, Basic Books, 1985.
18. Weiner MF: *Technique of Group Psychotherapy,* Washington, D.C., American Psychiatric Press, 1984.
19. Maxmen JS: An educative model for inpatient group therapy. Int J Group Psychother, 28:321–338, 1978.
20. Tuckman BW: Developmental sequence in small groups. Psychol Bull, 63:384–399, 1965.
21. Bion W: *Experiences in Groups,* Basic Books, New York, 1959.
22. Rioch MJ: The work of Wilfred Bion on groups. Psychiatry, 33:56–66, 1970.

23. Stanton AH, Schwartz MS: *The Mental Hosptital: A Study of Institutional Participation in Psychiatric Illness and Treatment*, New York, Basic Books, 1954.

24. Caudill W: *The Psychiatric Hospital as a Small Society*, Cambridge, Harvard University Press, 1958.

25. Rubinstein R, Lasswell HD: *The Sharing of Power in a Psychiatric Hospital*, New Haven, Yale University Press, 1966.

26. Denber HCB (ed): *Research Conference on Therapeutic Community*, Springfield, Ill., Charles C. Thomas, 1960.

27. Almond R: *The Healing Community: Dynamics of the Therapeutic Milieu*, New York, Jason Aronson, 1974.

28. Cumming J, Cumming E: *Ego and Milieu: Theory and Practice of Environmental Therapy*, New York, Atherton Press, 1967.

29. Gunderson JG, Will OA Jr, Mosher LR (eds): *Principles and Practice of Milieu Therapy*, New York, Jason Aronson, 1983.

30. Jones M, Baker A, Freeman T, et al.: *The Therapeutic Community: A New Treatment Method in Psychiatry*, New York, Basic Books, 1953.

31. Edelson M: *Ego Psychology, Group Dynamics and the Therapeutic Community*, New York, Grune & Stratton, 1964.

32. Edelson M: *Psychotherapy and Sociotherapy*, Chicago, University of Chicago Press, 1970.

33. Klein RH: The patient-staff community meeting: A tea party with the mad hatter. Int J Group Psychother, *31*:205–222, 1981.

34. Bernard HS: Antitherapeutic dimensions of a community meeting in a therapeutic community. Psychiatr Q, *55*:227–234, 1983.

35. Rapoport RN: *Community as Doctor: New Perspectives on a Therapeutic Community*, Springfield, Ill., Tavistock Publications, Charles C. Thomas, 1960.

36. Jones M: *Beyond the Therapeutic Community: Social Learning and Social Psychiatry*, New Haven, Yale University Press, 1968.

37. Kreeger L (ed): *The Large Group: Dynamics and Therapy*, Itasca, Ill., Peacock, 1975.

38. Turquet P: Threats to Identity in the Large Group, in Kreeger L (ed): *The Large Group: Dynamics and Therapy*, Itasca, Ill., Peacock, 1975.

39. Kisch J, Kroll J, Gross R, et al.: Inpatient community meetings: Problems and purposes. Br J Med Psychol, *54*:35–40, 1981.

40. Gilman H, Russakoff LM, Kibel H: Bipartite model for community meetings: The separation of tasks. Int J Therapeutic Communities, *8*:131–140, 1987.

41. Russakoff LM, Oldham JM: The structure and technique of community meetings: The short-term unit. Psychiatry, *45*:38–44, 1982.

11

Occupational Therapy

Sharan L. Schwartzberg, EdD, OTR FAOTA
Janet Abeles Kahane, MEd, OTR

The clinical picture of a mental disorder is always associated with an impaired pattern of social or occupational functioning. Patients often present complaints about a loss of interest or pleasure in daily activities and difficulties in occupational performance. For the staff, these complaints and evidence of a diminished ability to function are in part the foundation of a diagnosis and treatment plan. At the same time, as a result of admission to a psychiatric inpatient unit, patients' usual routines of homemaking, self-care, work, and leisure activities are also disrupted.

This chapter will describe a therapy explicitly designed to focus on problems in occupational performance and daily living skills—namely, occupational therapy. First, occupational therapy is defined and then described within the framework of an historical overview and theoretical analysis of various conceptual models used in psychiatric inpatient settings. The assumptions of these psychiatric models and corresponding occupational therapy models are explained. Next, an occupational behavior approach to inpatient occupational therapy is proposed. Through a program example, the purpose,

methods, and value of such an occupational therapy program are detailed and illustrated. Finally, contemporary problems in occupational therapy are discussed, and some concluding remarks are made regarding the future of occupational therapy and inpatient psychiatry.

DEFINITION

Occupational therapy is the art and science of using purposeful activities to minimize pathology, teach performance component skills necessary for occupational performance and role adaptation, maintain or enhance function, and promote health (1–3). Thus purposeful activities are goal-oriented processes of doing, involving interaction with both the human and nonhuman environments (4). The performance component skills are the sensorimotor, cognitive, psychological, and social skills needed for occupational performance. Such performance involves life task activities of self-care, work, and play or leisure necessary for the satisfaction of personal needs and social roles (5). In particular, psychiatric occupational therapy in the acute inpatient setting focuses on functional evaluation, symptom reduction, supporting function or maintenance of abilities to relate to the human and nonhuman environments, mobilization for rapid return to the community, and discharge planning (2, 3).

HISTORICAL OVERVIEW

Although the former contemporary definition of occupational therapy helps to explain current practice, it is interesting to note that occupations or activities have been used as a form of treatment for the physically and mentally ill throughout recorded history (6). However, the value of activities therapy is not as well understood as the more widely accepted methods of verbal group therapy (7), individual psychotherapy, and psychopharmacologic treatment. Nevertheless, it was in the first decades of the 20th century that individuals wishing to reestablish mid-18th century moral treatment principles labeled these "second moral treatment" programs occupational therapy—an alternative for physicians who were dissatisfied with the prevailing medical model view of mental illness as an incurable disease of the brain (8). Over the years, various forces acted to change the face of occupational therapy. These changes have broadened the theoretical frames of reference in occupational therapy practice. Examining psychiatric models and their parallels in occupational therapy leads to examining the assumptions underlying various schools of thought.

Assumptions

Given the historically close alliance between occupational therapy and medicine, similarities in the conceptual models of these professions in the specialty area of mental health are no surprise. Close examination of these models can clarify the relationship between occupational therapy and inpatient psychiatry.

PSYCHIATRIC MODELS

Lazare (9) outlines four conceptual models of clinical psychiatry: medical, psychologic, behavioral, and social. As this discussion is concerned with modern day inpatient practice, we would add a fifth model—biopsychosocial. Using this configuration of clinical psychiatry, we can make several assumptions regarding occupational therapists' primary concern: occupational performance; that is, depending upon one's conceptual bias, the perceived relationship between mental illness and dysfunction in occupational performance varies (see Table 11.1).

As Lazare (9) points out, the ideology of the psychiatrist is one factor that implicitly determines which model is selected for patient evaluation and treatment. A similar case could be made in regard to the occupational therapist; however, an additional variable exists within the hierarchy of hospital practice. That is to say, it is more likely that occupational therapists are conceptually bound by their professional ideology *and* the orientation of the psychiatrist in charge of the inpatient unit. As a result, we see similarities in the clinical models of occupational therapists and psychiatrists.

OCCUPATIONAL THERAPY MODELS FOR PSYCHIATRIC INPATIENT SETTINGS

As was discussed earlier, a relationship exists between assumptions about mental illness and occupational performance dysfunction. A closer inspection of models in psychiatry and occupational therapy also reveals parallels (Table 11.2). Seven occupational therapy models for inpatient psychiatry are presented because they most broadly represent actual practice. Each will be briefly illustrated and explained. We wish to emphasize that our intent is not to compare the empirical validity of the models or imply that they are superior to other models. Our purpose is simply

Table 11.1.   Assumptions about Mental Illness and Occupational Performance

Psychiatric Model	Assumptions
Medical Model (9)	Mental illness is a physical disease caused by some defect in the nervous system or biochemical mechanism of genetically predisposed individuals. Disturbances in motor behavior are primary symptoms of neurophysiological defects, and disturbances in work, play, and self-care are secondary psychological symptoms (10, 11).
Psychologic Model (9)	Impaired development of early relationships and resultant unconscious conflicts confound the ability to care for self and derive gratification from or sublimate aggressive impulses in socially acceptable work and play activities (12–15).
Behavioral Model (9)	Abnormal work, play, or self-care behaviors are a result of inadequately learning performance components or cognitive, sensorimotor, psychological, and social skills necessary for occupational performance (16).
Social Model (9)	Disordered work and play environments foster mental illness and contribute to deteriorated habits of living—the absence of a pleasurable and balanced routine of work, play, rest, and sleep (17).
Biopsychosocial Model	Occupational performance problems are the sequelae of the dynamic interaction between biological, psychological, and social components of a mental disorder (18). Psychogenic and sociogenic factors involved in occupational performance, such as stress, loss, or sudden change in activity level or stimuli, can trigger and hence precipitate an episode of mental illness in genetically predisposed individuals (10).

to describe commonly reported theoretical models for short- and long-term inpatient settings and emphasize their suitability for short-term care.

1.   *Neurobehavioral model.*

CASE EXAMPLE: In the first occupational therapy session, Mr. T., age 43, with a diagnosis of schizophrenia, was unable to copy a simple mosaic title design or catch a large beach ball. He appeared to have a limited attention span (15 minutes) and an inability to think abstractly; was easily distracted; and demonstrated abnormal posture, poor balance, and a pattern of restricted movement. Furthermore, he did not interact with the therapist unless asked a specific question and his affect remained flat throughout the evaluation.

The occupational therapy inpatient treatment goals established were to begin a program to (a) increase range of motion, (b) increase spontaneous movement, and (c) improve posture. Treatment involved a daily 15–30 minute, developmentally sequenced program of sensory input through individual and group gross motor activities. The activities, structured by the therapist, involved repetitive pleasurable action, limited choice and distractions, and were physically demonstrated with repeated, simple verbal directions—continuously refocusing Mr. T.'s attention on the activity outcome. The activities were primarily games involving a beach ball, balloon, parachute, jump rope, and beanbag chair. After several weeks of treatment, Mr. T. appeared to be more active and socially responsive. He was referred to an occupational therapist in the day hospital for continued neurobehavioral treatment.

Table 11.2.   Occupational Therapy and Psychiatric Models

Psychiatry	Occupational Therapy
Medical Model (9)	Neurobehavioral Model Cognitive Disabilities Model (25)
Psychologic Model (9)	Psychodynamic Model
Behavioral Model (9)	Behavioral/Educational Model Developmental Model
Social Model (9)	Occupational Behavior Model
Biopsychosocial Model	Biopsychosocial Model

As demonstrated by the case example, this model concerns the relationship between biological functions and task performance (2). According to Clark (19), "the theoretical premise is that normalization of sensory and motor patterns, and their integration for interaction with the environment, will promote adaptive development of conceptualization, manipulative, and social skills." Function or dysfunction is viewed as the ability or inability to process information from the environment in order to act (19). Task performance evaluations are used to evaluate perceptual motor and sensory-integrative functions affected by the central nervous system (20). In treatment, developmentally sequenced sensorimotor activities are used to normalize the nervous system (19, 21–24). It is of interest to mention that Kaplan (20) observes "although some acutely ill inpatients demonstrate neurological deficits, short-term treatment is generally incompatible with neurologic reintegrative approaches."

2. Cognitive disabilities model.

CASE EXAMPLE: Ms. Smith is a 16-year-old high school student admitted to the inpatient unit after family and school complaints about her irrational talking, inability to concentrate on school work, and refusal to attend classes or come out of her room. She is reported by classmates and teachers as being strange, talking to herself, and socially isolated.

Using a series of structured activities Allen Cognitive Level Test [ACL] (25), the occupational therapist evaluates the patient to determine Ms. Smith's cognitive capacity to perform her school work, live at home and care for herself with family support, and interact independently with friends. In addition, the question of whether attending her mother's college alma mater is a realistic aim for the near future has to be answered.

3. Psychodynamic model.

CASE EXAMPLE: Seven patients are seated around a table about to share free associations to their freely created clay objects. The occupational therapist asks the patients to say whatever comes to their minds and to talk about what their clay object looks like and what it makes them think of or what it reminds them of.

The major theoretical premise of the psychodynamic model is that activities can provide insight and opportunities for needed expression and sublimation, thereby fostering personality change and symptom abatement (26–28). Measures of function and dysfunction are the ability or inability to seek and obtain gratification of needs and self-satisfaction (29). As the case example illustrates, projective activities are used for uncovering unconscious processes (26, 30). However, Kaplan (20) maintains that projective evaluation techniques are suitable for initially evaluating the longer-term psychiatric patient and do not appear suitable for a short-term evaluation concerning adjustment to community living. Treatment programs include short-term group and individual activities that provide an opportunity for aggressive impulses to be expressed appropriately and directly, engaging in conflict-free activity and testing living skills in an environment of thinking, feeling, and action (27, 31).

4. Behavioral/educational model.

CASE EXAMPLE: An occupational therapist is reviewing situations patients may encounter as they return to former jobs after hospitalization. Two patients have just volunteered to role play "the first day back on the job." One will be the recently discharged patient and the other the patient's job supervisor. All the patients have just seen a videotape depicting a former psychiatric patient successfully overcoming barriers toward her reemployment.

In this model the theoretical premise is that behavior is learned. In addition, more adaptive occupational behaviors can be taught and learned through here-and-now activities and the practice of isolated behavioral skills. Adaptive behavior requires the presence of knowledge, skills, and values needed for living in the community; maladaptive behavior presents the absence of such knowledge, skills, and values (32). Performance evaluations assess functional behavior in work, leisure, or self-care (20, 30, 32). Activities therapy treatment (32) focuses on increasing knowledge, skills, and values needed for future living. As the case example, demonstrates, the methods employed include learning through doing, the immediate here-and-now human and non-human environment, and the teaching-learning process (32). The short-term setting can provide an opportunity for learning behaviors necessary for immediately adjusting to community living; however, a short length of stay does not allow for much repetition or range in the learning process.

5. Developmental model.

CASE EXAMPLE: The occupational therapy department at "General Hospital" offers two levels of inpatient group treatment. The lower-level task groups are composed of patients who have difficulty concentrating and are unable to make decisions, share materials, and offer support to other group members. The occupational therapist selects and sets up activities, with simple, familiar procedures, which easily end successfully. The activities demand little concentration, can be completed in one session, and do not require group interaction. The therapist also attempts to fulfill members' emotional and social needs. The higher level task groups involve patients in cooperative activities. Members are expected to give and receive feedback, arrive at a consensus about the group project, and be able to share group leadership, membership, and task roles. The therapist serves as a role model, teacher, and activity resource consultant.

In the developmental model, it is assumed that performance component skills are multidimensional and learned in a stage-specific developmental progression that can be simulated through developmentally sequenced purposeful activities (33–

35). Function or dysfunction represents the presence or absence of age- or stage-appropriate adaptive skills or behaviors (29).

According to Kaplan (20), "in the short-term setting, the appreciation of developmental factors is critical in correctly understanding an individual's current situations. However, decisions need to be made about which abilities are most crucial to evaluate for a given individual because of time factors." Treatment programs simulate a developmental progression of purposeful activities in adaptive skill areas, and behavioral methods of teaching-learning are applied (34, 35). As the case example demonstrates, in acute care, such progressions are of value for activity analysis and adaptation. However, the major contribution of the developmental model appears in psychiatric rehabilitation programs where one is more likely to find a longer length of stay and larger homogeneous developmental subgroups of patients.

6. Occupational behavior model.

CASE EXAMPLE: Mrs. B., a 65-year-old mother of three independent children, was admitted to the hospital a month after her husband's death. She complained of loss of interest in her usual homemaking activities, had difficulty making simple decisions, was hardly eating or sleeping, felt isolated and depressed, and had suicidal thoughts. In an interview the occupational therapist learned that Mrs. B. had won several baking contests. She gently urged Mrs. B. to stop by the kitchen at 2 p.m. that afternoon. A group of patients were planning to bake pies and had expressed concerns about the best way to proceed.

Proponents of this model assume that life roles organize behavior and individuals are curious and intrinsically motivated to explore their environment. They also believe patients can learn necessary habits and skills through exploration and practice with occupational tools, behaviors, and environments (36–38).

Function consists of temporal (39) and occupational adaptation in performing life roles satisfying to self and others. Dysfunction constitutes unsatisfactory social roles, skill and habit deficits, and an imbalanced use of time—a daily life routine, disorganized or lacking in pleasure (17). Evaluation usually consists of history-taking regarding habit patterns; occupational role solidification and performance, past and present; and past, current, and future interests, values, and goals (20, 40–44). The history aims toward identifying target problems in the environment and in an individual's performance that contribute to role dysfunction. Treatment programs provide learning experiences that encourage temporal and occupational exploration and adaptation; they aim toward developing competency in work, play, and self-care activities by having individuals experience a balance of such activities in the hospital milieu (17, 37, 38, 45, 46).

The occupational behavior model is generally incompatible with a medical orientation and thus presents many communication problems for occupational therapists working in general hospital psychiatric inpatient units. However, it provides a means for beginning an analysis of the relationship between an individual's mental disorder and occupational performance deficits and, as the case example implies, acknowledges a patient's assets and the necessary ingredients of a hospital milieu that maintains and promotes health.

7. Biopsychosocial model. This model assumes individuals are dynamic and open biopsychosocial systems intrinsically motivated to "do" and have an effect on the environment. Also, the model believes that a health-satisfying environment of purposeful activities in conjunction with opportunities to learn adaptive skills for doing can help an individual "reconstitute" to an adaptive level of behavior (8, 16, 18, 47–51).

Function is viewed as the ability to adapt to the sequela of a mental disorder or one's biopsychosocial configuration—hence, to be able to participate in community life or environmental systems and achieve personal and social goals. Dysfunction is the inability to engage in satisfactory roles and occupational performance as a dynamic result of the interaction between biological, psychological, and socioenvironmental circumstances. Likewise, the physical disease process itself can be triggered by psychogenic and sociogenic factors related to occupational performance dysfunction.

In evaluations, therapists analyze the interactions between internal (biological-psychological) and external (social) mechanisms by assessing both the strengths and weaknesses in an individual's past and present occupational performance, life roles and skills, interests, goals, and available human and nonhuman resources. Usual evaluation methods include history-taking and observation of patient performance in occupational therapy and unstructured and semistructured unit activities (32, 42–44). Treatment methods include: using purposeful activities in individual treatment and in open and closed functional task groups (52, 53), the therapeutic relationship, activity analysis, and activity adaptation in the form of graded structured activities and graded structured relationships.

PROGRAM MODEL

The occupational therapy program represents a case example of occupational therapy in a free-standing psychiatric hospital. The program evolved from an occupational behavior model with a current emphasis on skills. It illustrates occupational therapy for adolescents and adults at a 62-bed private psychiatric teaching hospital located in Wellesley, Massachusetts (54). It does not describe a model for inpatient occupational therapy with children. The hospital is clinically organized into two separate but interrelated programs: the adolescent program and the adult services program. In addition to the two clinical inpatient programs, the hospital integrates with these services a women's program and a dual-diagnosis psychiatric/substance-abuse program. There are two inpatient adolescent units and two inpatient adult units. The bed capacity on each of the two adolescent units is 15, on the open adult unit it is 10, and on the locked adult unit 22. The two adolescent units are alike with respect to their patient populations and treatment philosophy. The adolescent programs, for patients between 12 and 18, combines a comprehensive therapeutic milieu with an active family systems treatment model. The two adult units, for patients age 18 and up, offer an integrated biopsychosocial approach for evaluating and treating psychiatric disorders. Both clinical programs involve structured programs implemented by a multidisciplinary team. The team's services include occupational therapy, psychiatric evaluation, medication evaluation and treatment, individual and group therapies, family meetings, educational support, psychological evaluations, expressive therapy, and activities therapy. The staff for these programs include occupational therapists, psychiatrists, psychiatric nurses, psychologists, social workers, special education teachers, counselors, expressive therapists, activity therapists, and trainees in all disciplines.

The average length of stay at this short-term care hospital has been 3–6 weeks. More recently, however, lengths of stay have decreased to less than three weeks. The patient population typically includes a broad range of diagnostic groups: affective disorders, personality disorders, anxiety disorders, schizophrenic disorders, eating disorders, substance-abuse disorders, and psychotic disorders.

For this hospital, occupational therapy is delivered through the rehabilitation services department which provides services to both the adolescent and adult programs through a combination of day, evening, and partial weekend programming. The rehabilitation services department, headed by an occupational therapist, is staffed by three occupational therapists, one certified occupational therapy assistant, one expressive therapist, and two activity therapists. Staff assignments are organized around clinical programs, specific units, and by discipline.

The occupational therapy staff engage fully in implementing the occupational therapy program in coordination with other rehabilitation services staff. The role of the occupational therapist is to screen or evaluate each patient, develop and implement a treatment program, and prepare the patient for their transition back to the community through discharge planning. The occupational therapists contribute to multidisciplinary treatment planning sessions and participate in community meetings and activities of the milieu. They consult with the units on relevant functional and activity-oriented concerns and with other disciplines within their department. Functional concerns may focus on implementing strategies for patients' symptoms management or be aimed toward making environmental interventions at the care-giver level. Occupational therapists also participate in business and staff inservice education meetings with the rehabilitation services staff.

The rehabilitation services department staff represent a collective of occupational, expressive, and activities therapists. Expressive therapy is a therapeutic approach combining modalities such as art, music, movement, and writing into structured, safe, and expressive interactions for facilitating patient communication, awareness, personal growth, and development. Expressive therapy serves to enrich as well as educate and provide therapy. Activities therapy refers to a treatment orientation that uses a variety of activities to enhance psychosocial functioning. This type of treatment employs structured physical, social, and educational interactions to help patients acquire new and/or healthier skills for independent living.

Purpose

The following section will identify and explain what our inpatient model of occupational therapy entails. Specifically, this section will detail our program model by explaining the purpose of occupational therapy in terms of assessment, treatment, health needs for the activity milieu, and discharge planning.

ASSESSMENT

The occupational therapy assessment begins with a systematic process of data collection. Initial data is gathered by chart review, interview, and observation of patient performance in occupational therapy and unstructured and semistructured unit activities.

Chart Review: The first step of data collection is carried out before the initial meeting of patient and therapist. By reading the admission summary and staff notes, the therapist collects information to structure the initial patient-therapist interaction. More specifically, the therapist determines whether the standard evaluation method can be carried out or whether it will need to be adapted. Depending upon such factors as the patient's estimated length of stay and the acute nature of the patient's condition at the time of admission, the occupational therapy assessment may be limited to an initial screening. The occupational therapy screening facilitates the patient's early involvement in treatment, while identifying which performance areas and performance components need to be further assessed. Utilizing further in-depth evaluation tools often depends on availability of occupational therapy staff and other resources such as time, space, and equipment.

Interview: In most cases, the second step is an interview. The interview may take

place within the context of a one-to-one meeting or occur within a structured group specifically designed to orient patients to the occupational therapy program. Patients receive a general written questionnaire when they are first introduced to the occupational therapy program during the initial interview. The general questionnaire is designed to collect historical data about the patient's prehospitalization, adaptive and maladaptive patterns of occupational behavior, and interpersonal and community relationships. The questionnaire also notes the specific daily activities the patients' occupational roles and given environment require and patients' perceptions of their effectiveness and satisfaction in performing these life tasks and leisure interests. Additional questions for specific major life roles (worker, student, etc.) are asked to elicit further data. (See Figure 11.1 for a typical questionnaire.)

A specific section of the questionnaire centers on goals. The patient must identify goals to focus on in the hospital-at-large and during occupational therapy treatment. The goals are directed toward improving performance skills in the areas of socialization, work, leisure, self-maintenance, activities of daily living, and the balance among these. See Figure 11.2 for an example of an occupational therapy goals sheet.

A semistructured interview which includes further history-taking and data clarification follows the completion of the questionnaire and goals section. The interview lays the foundation for the developing patient-therapist relationship and yields rich material related to the individual's occupational performance requirements, skills, and perceptions.

A questionnaire and goals section as components of the interview and assessment provides several advantages. Its' use:

1. Enables data to be collected and organized under a conceptual framework

Figure 11.1. Occupational Therapy General Questionnaire

NAME: _____   DATE: _____

1. Which of the following household chores do you have responsibility for:

    _____ Cooking   _____ Laundry   _____ House Cleaning

    _____ Shopping   _____ Budgeting

    Which one(s) do you have difficulty with?

2. Where do you live? Do you live with others, alone, in a boarding house, etc.?
3. What do you use for transportation?
4. Do you have any fun?
5. What is fun to you?
6. Are there things you would like to do in your spare time that you don't do now? What are they?
7. Do you have any habits which interfere with your daily life?
8. Are there any physical activities you particularly enjoy doing?
9. What kinds of things do you and your family do together?
10. Do you have relatives you get together with fairly often?
11. Do you have any especially good friends you see often? How often? How did you meet them? How do you enjoy spending your time with them?
12. Do you enjoy reading? What?
13. How much time do you spend watching TV?
14. Do you have hobbies or other special interests?
15. Do you belong to any clubs or organizations?
16. How do you spend your weekends?
17. How would you describe yourself to others?
18. What outlets do you use for dealing with feelings?
19. What is your philosophy of life?
20. What do you hope to accomplish by this hospitalization?

---

that will guide its interpretation and translation into a treatment plan.

2. Enables individuals to demonstrate strengths and weaknesses in performance areas and to participate in goal-setting according to the individual's degree of readiness and capability.
3. Enables therapists to assess the patient's task and social skills in structured and semistructured activities.

Because clinical situations exist in which using the questionnaire and goals sheet is not appropriate, data must be elicited by alternate means. Possible reasons for adapting the assessment process include language barriers, illiteracy, blindness, and physical disability. The individual's mental status at the time of assessment is also important. The grossly psychotic or organically impaired patient may not be able to fill out the occupational therapy questionnaire. Because the therapist's ultimate aim is to involve the patient in the assessment process, external and environmental demands and prerequisite psychological, cognitive, sensorimotor, and social skills are factors crucial to the decision of whether or not to use the questionnaire.

Observation of Task Performance: This occurs through observing patients perform a combination of formal, structured occupational therapy activities, such as participating in a cooking group, unstructured use of time, and semistructured unit activities, e.g., tending to self-care and operating the

Figure 11.2.   Occupational Therapy Goals Sheet

In light of your answers on the questionnaire, which of the following goals do you feel the greatest need to work toward in occupational therapy?

_____ To feel more comfortable in groups
_____ To learn to talk more easily with people
_____ To learn to ask for help
_____ To explore the role of social and recreational activities in my life
_____ To do something fun
_____ To learn to structure my time more effectively to include:
_____ Grooming   _____ Social Activities
_____ Household Chores   _____ Recreation
_____ To learn to manage money better
_____ To find an apartment or other living arrangement
_____ To successfully complete a craft project
_____ To learn better skills to organize and complete a task
_____ To clarify career interests
_____ To identify strengths and weaknesses in work skills
_____ To define and assess difficulties in my job
_____ To learn to apply and interview for a job
_____ To look for a job
_____ To learn some ways to relax more
_____ To learn to deal with my feelings more directly and appropriately
_____ To find outlets for angry feelings
_____ To learn to recognize my needs and get them met
_____ To learn more about who I am and what is important to me
_____ To build my self-confidence

---

unit's laundry facilities. The assessment tasks are selected for their ability to elicit data on performance component skills and their effect on functional outcomes. For example, by observing the individual participate in a structured task, therapists can assess the individual's abilities and limitations in performance components such as perceptual-motor, cognitive, and social skills in relation to their impact on functioning. Observing task performance in the areas of work, self-care, and leisure can validate skill in occupational functioning in the functionally intact individual. It can also help identify those areas of occupational dysfunction where more specific assessments and treatment interventions are indicated. Tasks that address the psychological components of roles, values, and interests refer to how the individual experiences, organizes, and responds to the human and nonhuman environment. In this area, tasks enable therapists to evaluate such concerns as the patient's concept of self in society and the obligations that go along with these positions, ideas, or beliefs intrinsically important to the patient and the experience of satisfaction and/or pleasure during leisure or work-related occupations. Habit patterns determine an individual's degree of organization for planning and participating in a balance of meaningful life roles. The social component focuses on interpersonal interactions and environmental and cultural circumstances. The tasks yield data such as the patient's readiness to use available supports and the nature of the patient's value system as it relates to personal time management.

Finally, it is the dynamic interaction between these components—actual performance during work, play, and self-care and the patient's perceptions and wishes about the use of time—that leads to an understanding of the individual's occupational functioning.

The occupational therapy assessment provides a basis for treatment planning and a baseline for reevaluating change during the course of hospitalization. The assessment systematically screens functional skills and limitations. When specific problem areas are identified, a further in-depth assessment may be conducted. In such instances, necessary occupational therapy evaluation tools include standardized tests, activity histories and configurations, interest checklists, activities of daily living performance checklists, and individual or group tasks.

TREATMENT

Occupational therapy treatment is broadly designed to correspond with a short-term hospitalization's overall goals of diagnostic assessment, symptom reduction, and rapid reintegration into the community. The occupational therapy treatment goals are coordinated with and reinforce the treatment team's goals for the patient's hospitalization. The patient collaborates in treatment planning as fully as possible.

Symptom reduction. One of the objectives of occupational therapy treatment with the acutely ill patient is symptom reduction. In our model the problem-oriented intervention for reducing acute symptomatology is applied to restore performance component skills. While in the acute care setting, although symptom reduction is a realistic and attainable short-term goal, we also find it essential to identify longer-term remedial goals that will extend beyond the course of hospitalization.

According to Fidler, in short-term acute settings, activity selection for symptom reduction is "based on those experiences that may be expected, for a given patient, to reduce anxiety, diminish hyperactivity, stimulate response and psychomotor activity, reduce confusion and alert or focus attention" (3). For example, a concrete, success-oriented task may be chosen for the depressed patient because of its tendency to interfere with pathological ruminations and to reduce a sense of worthlessness, both of which are symptoms that can accompany a clinical depression. For the acutely disorganized psychotic patient, an activity may be used to relieve anxiety. Thus the activity serves as an anxiety-relieving agent and is selected because its properties inherently facilitate integrative action which has a positive effect on the overwhelmed person.

Skill development. A second treatment objective is performance skill development. Activities are chosen to facilitate development or learning of skills and attitudes in the areas which will enable the patient to function more effectively in work, leisure, self-care, and socialization. This aspect of treatment involves the patient in a problem-solving process that includes problem identification, goal-setting, planning, and resolution. Depending upon the length of stay, the complexity of patient needs, and the extent of psychopathology manifested, the problem-solving process may reach only the initial phases of implementation in the short-term hospital stay. Carry-over of performance skill development occurs through recommendations for continued outpatient treatment in the community.

While development of major skills can be an unrealistic expectation of a short-term crisis intervention program, increasing the patient's awareness of effective alternatives to a specific and immediate problem may be possible. Treatment may include teaching compensatory techniques or strategies for accomplishing a task. In certain cases, as with patients who have a deteriorating dementia, treatment may be more concerned with both providing education and counseling for the patient's family and environmental manipulation.

Maintenance of intact skills. In addition to restoring and developing skills, occupational therapy is directed at maintaining function and preventing further disability. Intact performance skills are maintained through engagement in activities that provide practice in the skills and reinforce success. Fine notes that "in such instances, the primary concern is for the provision of activities that make it possible for the individual to use existing skills and interests, experience intrinsic gratification and meet basic needs for acceptance, achievement, creativity, autonomy and social interaction" (2).

Lifestyle awareness and development. Another treatment objective is to increase patients' awareness of how they occupied time before hospitalization and increase knowledge of more satisfactory alternatives. An integral aspect of this objective involves teaching, through discussion and experience, the elements and potential value of a balanced routine of work, leisure, self-care, and socialization. Kielhofner states that "balance refers to more than just so much work, play, and rest. Rather, balance recognizes an interdependence of these life spaces and their relationship to both internal values, interests, and goals, and external demands of the environment" (39).

HEALTH NEEDS—THE ACTIVITY MILIEU

By including a variety of activities, the occupational therapy program reinforces the value of a balanced routine or lifestyle (Figures 11.3 and 11.4). For example, the occupational therapy groups and group schedule were designed to fulfill the ordinary human biological need for movement, the psychological need for a product, and the social need for interaction. The patient's daily routine also includes verbal psychotherapy groups balanced with the nonverbal occupational therapy formats such as movement and task-oriented activity groups.

Given our occupational behavior orientation to occupational therapy, the program offered is based on the assumption that problems in doing may arise from a lack of doing. For this reason the activity groups are so designed to first meet healthy needs for movement, action, and productivity. Thus adaptive patterns of behavior are supported and integrated through experiential involvement in the groups.

In several ways the occupational therapy program and its specific groups support an active therapeutic milieu. One way is by building cohesiveness within the patient community in order to facilitate work in the milieu and in the verbal insight-oriented groups. The other is by helping to structure the milieu to meet the patients' health needs. A balanced routine, offering a variety of treatment modalities, fosters active patient participation rather than regression and dependency.

DISCHARGE PLANNING

Discharge planning is recognized as an important objective in a short-term hospitalization. It is essential for maintaining a continuous treatment process from the hospital into the community. Discharge planning involves identifying treatment needs and requires a knowledge of community resources. It is concerned with planning a course of action that recognizes the therapeutic process initiated on the inpatient unit and addresses treatment alternatives to be continued or started postdischarge.

Discharge planning begins when the patient is admitted to the hospital. It may involve evaluating the patient's occupational performance and responsiveness to various occupational therapy formats so that recommendations and referrals can be

Figure 11.3. Rehabilitation Services Adult Program Schedule

Adult Schedule

Monday

12:30–1:30 PM
Stress Management Group

Members are encouraged to identify their individual stressors, their causes and what alleviates them. Problem-solving and effective coping skills are a major focus of the group.

2:00–3:00 PM
Creative Arts Group

An expressive arts group designed to assist patients in finding creative ways to express themselves, work on life issues and get to know other people.

4:00–5:00 PM
Relaxation Group

Specific stress management techniques for relaxation are explored and practiced.

7:30–8:30 PM
Occupational Therapy Clinic

Individual activities are performed in a parallel task group setting for a variety of therapeutic purposes.

Tuesday

2:00–3:00 PM
Occupational Therapy Clinic

3:00–4:00 PM
Orientation Group

This group offers an introduction to Rehabilitation Services. Members are asked to identify goals from which group referrals are negotiated with individuals.

4:00–5:00 PM
Creative Expression Group

This group uses a different art medium each week to explore a variety of techniques as a means of nonverbal self-expression.

6:30–8:30 PM
Vocational Workshop

An individualized format allows patients to address specific goals related to work, school, and time management.

Wednesday

2:00 to 3:00 PM
Occupational Therapy Clinic

3:30–4:30 PM
Challenge Course

Members participate in a variety of cooperative problem-solving and trust-building physical tasks.

6:30–7:30 PM
Occupational Therapy Clinic

Thursday

2:00–3:00 PM
Occupational Therapy Clinic

3:30–4:30 PM
Work Discussion Group

A group for those who are currently employed or are planning to return to the work force, topics address vocational concerns pertinent to its members.

6:30–7:30 PM
Occupational Therapy Clinic

Friday

12:00–2:00 PM
Cooking Group

Preparing and planning a meal offers members an opportunity to engage in a typical daily activity.

2:00–3:00 PM
Occupational Therapy Clinic

2:30–3:30 PM
Orientation Group

Figure 11.4. Rehabilitation Services Adolescent Program Schedule

---

Adolescent Schedule

Monday

12:30–1:45 PM
Challenge Course

3:00–3:45 PM
Occupational Therapy Clinic

3:30–4:30 PM
Sex Education Group

The group is designed to educate adolescents about anatomy, birth control, sexually transmitted diseases, and interpersonal relationships.

6:30–7:30 PM
Rock 'N' Roll

This is a social activity in which members act as disc jockeys in order to help promote organizational skills and an ability to work cooperatively.

7:30–8:30 PM
Occupational Therapy Clinic

Tuesday

11:00–11:45 PM
Occupational Therapy Clinic

1:00–2:00 PM
Occupational Therapy Task Group

Patients engage in a structured task designed to elicit assessment data. Patients are assisted in identifying goals for hospitalization.

3:30–4:30 PM
Drug and Alcohol Group

An educational group designed to help increase awareness of the potential dangers of substance abuse.

6:30–9:30 PM
Roller-skating Field Trip

A structured recreational activity carried out in the community.

Wednesday

12:30–1:45 PM
Challenge Course

2:00–3:00 PM
Life Skills Group

Topics covered help to explore, develop, and practice daily living skills.

3:00–3:45 PM
Occupational Therapy Clinic

3:30–4:30 PM
Sex Education Group

6:00–7:00 PM
Gym Trip

A structured recreational activity that is held weekly.

7:30–8:30 PM
Occupational Therapy Clinic

Thursday

11:00–11:45 PM
Occupational Therapy Clinic

1:00–3:00 PM
Bowling Field Trip

A recreational leisure activity carried out in the community.

3:00–3:45 PM
Occupational Therapy Clinic

3:30–4:30 PM
Drug and Alcohol Group

6:30–9:30 PM
Movie Field Trip

A leisure trip carried out in the community.

311

Figure 11.4.   Rehabilitation Services Adolescent Program Schedule—*continued*

Friday

11:00–11:45 PM
Occupational Therapy Clinic

2:00–4:00 PM
Swim Trip

A weekly physical activity is offered as optional.

3:00–3:45 PM
Occupational Therapy Clinic

7:00–9:00 PM
The Dance

A dance is provided weekly to offer an opportunity to develop positive peer interactions and leisure skills in a drug- and alcohol-free environment.

---

made for appropriate outpatient care. For example, a socially isolated patient who gradually became less withdrawn through active participation in a structured socialization group may derive similar benefits from an outpatient socialization group. Another aspect of discharge planning may revolve around family education to prepare the family for the patient's reentry into the home activity environment.

Community reentry may involve directing the patient to a community resource. In establishing treatment services aimed at furthering rehabilitation goals, the occupational therapist often acts as a liaison between the hospital and the community. Long-term treatment needs concerning issues of vocational performance, basic life skills, or socialization may require referrals to such institutional resources as partial hospitalization programs and vocational adjustment programs or noninstitutional community resources such as adult education programs.

Methods

PURPOSEFUL ACTIVITY

Occupational therapy's emphasis on the meanings and uses of actual engagement in purposeful activity distinguishes it from other psychiatric therapies. Purposeful activity is a goal-directed doing process. The Fidlers note that *"doing* is a process of investigating . . . responding, managing, creating, and controlling. It is through such action with feedback from both nonhuman and human objects that an individual comes to know the potential and limitations of self and the environment and achieves a sense of competence and intrinsic worth" (55). The value of purposeful activity depends upon its social, cultural, and personal meaning—both real and symbolic—and relevance to the individual.

We suggest that a wide range of purposeful activities be offered in the acute care hospital and attempts made to include many activities with which people fill the majority of their time. The general activity categories include: (*a*) work and prevocational tasks, (*b*) activities of daily living, (*c*) arts and crafts, (*d*) self-expressive or creative tasks, and (*e*) avocational pursuits.

THE NONHUMAN ENVIRONMENT

The nonhuman environment, an essential element in the occupational therapy doing process, refers to all aspects of the external environment that are not human. The nonhuman environment connotes the physical space and the objects, both natural and man-made. On the inpatient unit, it refers to the occupational therapy room, its arrangement of tables and chairs, and the equipment and materials used in the room. It also includes the community environment outside the hospital that the patient will be interacting with after discharge.

Searles (56) examines the relationship children have with their nonhuman worlds as they grow and develop. He explains the role of nonhuman object relationships: they increase the child's awareness of the capacity for feeling, help children safely express feelings and absorb conflicts, facilitate awareness of physical-cognitive abilities and limitations, and serve as a place to practice developing interpersonal skills. These potential meanings are also found in the purposeful activities, and are thereby utilized to accomplish therapeutic aims.

The nonhuman environment can serve as both the means and the end in the occupational therapy treatment process. First, it can be viewed as an entity to be manipulated and mastered. In this instance, the treatment emphasis would be on helping the individual use the nonhuman environment to learn specific performance skills or social roles, i.e., filling out a job application or learning to cook as part of an individual's move toward more independence. The nonhuman environment can also be viewed as a vehicle or bridge for helping individuals acquire greater self-understanding and more satisfying interpersonal relationships. Thus, it is used as a means for learning something else. For example, a creative writing exercise may be used to help individuals identify their feelings, or engaging in a group task may help individuals to recognize how they work with others.

THERAPEUTIC RELATIONSHIP—THE HUMAN ENVIRONMENT

The human environment refers to the interactions, both verbal and nonverbal, between the therapist and the patient. The therapeutic relationship is built upon the therapist's use of self. According to Tiffany, "in the occupational therapy process, the therapist's 'use of self' means bringing together knowledge, skills, caring, and basic personality strengths to help the client overcome difficulties and maximize abilities" (57). In this acute-care setting, the psychoanalytic concept of transference is not used. Rather, therapists establish and maintain their own identities as helpers. The occupational therapist assumes a variety of roles, including teacher, facilitator, counselor, coach, advocate, and supervisor. For example, our experience indicates that for the patient with a borderline personality disorder a consistent approach and clear definition of rules and expectations elicits the most adaptive functioning. For the depressed patient, a supportive and accepting approach is used.

ACTIVITY ANALYSIS

Activity analysis, in a biopsychosocial model, is concerned primarily with the biological, psychological, and sociocultural characteristics of the elements of an activity—the materials, process, and product. The analysis has two major purposes: to identify the capabilities required to engage in an activity and to identify components of the activity that may be emphasized or adapted in promoting development or restoration of function.

Nonhuman environment—materials, process, and product. In analyzing the biological dimension of an activity, we look at the kind and level of sensory-integrative, motor, and cognitive behaviors and actions required for successful completion. Materials are described by such aspects as their sensory input. An analysis of activity process may include identifying levels of thinking (abstract versus concrete) required and the motor actions (gross or fine movements, repetitions, coordination) involved. The product may be analyzed in terms of its adaptive or survival value to a human organism.

Psychological processes of an activity are analyzed along such lines as the potential for self-expression, originality, and creativity; the required ego skills; the affective feeling states potentially generated; and the symbolic and unconscious feelings, needs, and drives associated or gratified by the activity. Materials are described by such properties as resistiveness, pliability, controllability, and symbolic potential for sexual identification and reality testing. In our psychological analysis we are also concerned with identifying potential meanings, both real and symbolic, of the self-created product.

The acquired sociocultural properties of an activity reflect the values and beliefs of individuals and groups of people. Thus the various elements of an activity are analyzed for their symbolic meanings or inferences to gender, religion, age, ethnicity, and socioeconomic status.

Human environment—patient and therapist relationships. In addition to the nonhuman environment, in an activity analysis we also examine the inherent social and interpersonal processes or demands of an activity. In the analysis we ask: how much and what type of relatedness and communication are necessary to successfully complete the activity? Activities may require involving other patients or the therapist or be best suited as solitary occupations.

ACTIVITY ADAPTATION

Activity adaptation refers to the strategic process of grading an activity along a planned continuum. This process operates developmentally and sequentially to facilitate restoring and maintaining functioning and promote new learning and more adaptive behaviors and attitudes. Based on the activity analysis, we now ask: are the properties of the activity meaningful and the processes and product relevant to the patient's life situation, occupational roles, and performance needs, or should they be modified in some way to better suit the patient's needs?

Graded structured activities—individual and group. The following are some general principles we observe in grading activities:

1. The steps of an activity and the requirements for action should proceed from *simple to more complex.*
2. The activity should be initially presented at a level at which the patient can *succeed.*
3. The demands of the activity should increase as the performance skills of the patient increase.
4. The patient should be led away from *inactive behavior towards more active and productive behavior.*

In grading structured activities for the individual, we consider the variability of symptomatology. For example, the depressed patient with an impaired attention span would be more assured of success if he or she were engaged in a short-term task or one that could be separated into smaller achievable steps. For the schizophrenic patient who has difficulty with informational processing and abstract concepts, an environment with limited stimuli and a visual sample of an end product would be beneficial for prompting success.

Group activities, including both modality and content, are graded according to the needs of the group members and the hospital setting in which the treatment takes place. On the short-term unit, where rapid patient turnover exists and patients display a wide range of individual pathology and occupational performance dysfunction, the group program is graded in the areas of activity process and program content. While the heterogeneous groups reflect diverse needs for activities and are graded to be meaningful and accommodate both the higher- and lower-level functioning patients, the homogeneous groups are developed to address common areas of need.

Graded structured relationships—individual and group. In the biopsychosocial model, it is believed that the relationship between therapist and patient is dynamically influenced by the needs and behaviors of the patient and the subsequent response of the therapist. Interpersonal issues such as dependency, hostility, passivity, and need for control are emphasized and dealt with to an extent that is determined on an individual basis.

For example, for the patient who experiences poor vocational adjustment and dysfunctional coworker and supervisory relationships, tasks may be structured to place the therapist in the role of authority figure and supervisor and the patient in the role of coworker with another patient. In such a situation the therapist may model appropriate worker behaviors, give the patient feedback and suggest alternative behaviors, and reality test as needed. If the patient's primary treatment goal is to develop specific occupational performance skills, interpersonal issues would be named and identified as they occur but would not be a major focus of interaction. Rather, the therapist would structure the relationship to focus on the role of the therapist as facilitator or educator and the role of the patient as learner.

Finally, depending on the individual's treatment plan, the therapeutic relationship can be structured to emphasize the ego building and supportive value of individual or group activities rather than their uncovering aspects. The therapist may choose to gently instruct a patient on the processes of a particular activity or devise a plan whereby the patient needs little or no instruction and can instead use written instructional aids such as those given in prefabricated embroidery or window-staining kits.

The choice of activity and its adapta-

bility are finally determined by the constraints imposed by a particular setting. On the short-term unit, one must consider whether it is feasible to adapt an activity or whether it is more economical to select an alternative task. In making such a program decision, we find it necessary to consider the time factor for preparing and completing an activity, the cost of materials, the amount of space required, and staffing demands, needs, and resources.

Our purpose in this section was to describe a model for occupational therapy on a psychiatric inpatient unit. As was just mentioned, therapists face some complex decisions in their daily practice. The following concluding remarks outline some of these problems and point us toward occupational therapy in the future.

CONTEMPORARY PROBLEMS IN OCCUPATIONAL THERAPY

As a profession, occupational therapy has always been concerned with the disabled individual's rights to a meaningful and productive existence. Grounded in our humanistic and existential philosophy has been the general belief that purposeful activities help prevent disease, promote health, and facilitate learning or desired change.

Current "bottom-line health care" management (58) and payment systems based on diagnostically related groups demand efficiency and cost control. Internally, occupational therapists have been debating the relative merits of our various conceptual models, and several have called for a unified theoretical base or paradigm for practice, education, and research. Basing her work on recent advances in neurosciences, Allen (25) convincingly questions and challenges the validity of our basic assumption that activities can prevent or change a psychiatric disease caused by a biologic abnormality. She suggests that given the rapid effectiveness of psychotropic medication, the occupational therapist should focus treatment on the cognitive disability by changing the task rather than attempting to change the patient. Allen calls for a radical shift in acute care—from believing we can treat the cause of a disease to providing programs that detect changes in task performance and compensate for learning and memory after-effects or disabilities.

In addition to these problems, hospital administrators and members of other disciplines often lack an understanding of the educational preparation, role, and value of the occupational therapist. Furthermore, psychiatric patients need rehabilitation programs which may be considered too costly, especially since the mentally ill are not viewed as a profitable market.

Reimbursement patterns are influenced by the type of settings in which occupational therapists work. These patterns in turn affect the kind of services provided. As the length of hospital stays shorten, programs focus more and more on containment through successful activity, evaluation of functioning in activities of daily living, and discharge planning. Outpatient and day services are faced with providing services to help patients find and adapt to the demands of work and self-care and achieve some qualitatively satisfying life through employment, leisure activities, and social pursuits. Unfortunately, resources are limited for aftercare services at this economic time.

The shortage of occupational therapists in the United States is particularly acute in mental health practice settings. Compounding this problem is a lack of understanding of the profession and a growing shortage of role models for future practitioners. The direction in general hospitals toward role blurring and merging occupational and physical therapy departments under the administrative umbrella of "rehabilitation" appears to be having a dire effect. Occupational therapists ordinarily at-

tracted to mental health practice are perhaps lured into other role and specialty areas where their unique contribution to patient care is better defined and they receive fiscal, peer, and administrative support. Fortunately, systematic efforts are underway to understand and exert a positive effect on factors influencing (a) referral rates in psychiatric occupational therapy and (b) the decrease in selecting mental health as a specialty choice in occupational therapy (59–61). In addition, attrition and recruitment of occupational therapists is under serious study (62, 63).

CONCLUSION

The various approaches and model for inpatient occupational therapy outlined in this chapter are based on our best knowledge of theory, research, and practice. As evidence about psychiatric disorders changes, one can expect modifications in the theory and practice of occupational therapy.

It is therefore imperative that a coherent model of occupational therapy be communicated, understood, and valued. This emphasizes the need for occupational therapists to make informed clinical and administrative decisions based on empirical data; hence, the need for more research on both the cost-benefit and cost-effectiveness of occupational therapy and its qualitative value to the individual suffering from an acute psychiatric illness or chronic mental disability, the well person, and the individual at risk for a psychiatric condition.

Based on predicted shortened lengths of hospitalization we also suspect structured, standardized functional evaluations will need to be developed. To assist in discharge and treatment planning, these tools must rapidly produce objective data about what the patient will be able or unable to do in community environments. Occupational therapy programs will emphasize symptom reduction and after-care planning. It is likely that occupational therapy program resources will shift, in part, to community programs and outpatient practice. Finally, we will see the role of occupational therapy in general hospital liaison psychiatry flourish as the occupational nature of individuals is better understood.

This chapter has focused primarily on occupational therapy practice on a psychiatric inpatient unit for adults. We did not address other clinical specialty populations and settings. It should be mentioned that occupational therapists work in the following psychiatric areas not focused on in this chapter: children and adolescents, substance abuse, biological-psychological units, geriatric psychiatry, mental retardation psychiatry, head injury, forensic psychiatry, eating disorders, and long-term care.

REFERENCES

1. Occupational therapy: Its definition and functions. Am J Occup Ther, 26:204–205, 1972.

2. Fine SB: Occupational therapy: The role of rehabilitation and purposeful activity in mental health practice. Rockville, Md., American Occupational Therapy Association White Paper, 1983.

3. American Occupational Therapy Task Group of the APA Psychiatric Therapies, Fidler GS (chair): Overview of occupational therapy in mental health, pp 9–10, Rockville, Md., American Occupational Therapy Association White Paper, 1981.

4. Mosey AC: *Occupational Therapy Configuration of a Profession*, New York, Raven Press, 1981.

5. American Occupational Therapy Association: Standards of practice for occupational therapy. Am J Occup Ther, 37:802–804, 1983.

6. Kielhofner G, Burke JP: Occupational therapy after 60 years: An account of changing identity and knowledge. Am J Occup Ther, 31:674–689, 1977.

7. DeCarlo JJ, Mann WC: The effectiveness of verbal versus activity groups in improving self-perceptions of interpersonal communication skills. Am J Occup Ther, 39:20–27, 1985.

8. Barris R, Kielhofner G, Watts JH: *Psychosocial Occupational Therapy Practice in a Pluralistic Arena*, Laurel, Md., RAMSCO, 1983.

9. Lazare A: Hidden conceptual models in clinical psychiatry. N Engl J Med, 288:345–351, 1973.

10. Kaplan HI, Sadock BJ: *Modern Synopsis of Psychiatry/IV*, ed. 4, Baltimore, Williams & Wilkins, 1985.

11. King LJ: Occupational therapy research in psychiatry: A perspective. Am J Occup Ther, 32:15–18, 1978.

12. Menninger KA: Work as a sublimation, in Sze WC (ed): *Human Life Cycle*, pp 413–425, New York, Jason Aronson, 1975.

13. Neff W: Psychoanalytic conceptions of the meaning of work. Psychiatry, 28:324–333, 1965.

14. Reisman D: The themes of work and play in the structure of Freud's thought. Psychiatry, 13:1–7, 1950.

15. Walder R: Psychoanalytic theory of play in Schaefer CE (ed): *Therapeutic Use of Child's Play*, pp. 79–93, New York, Jason Aronson, 1976.

16. Mosey AC: A model for occupational therapy. Occup Ther Ment Health, 1:11–31, 1980.

17. Meyer A: The philosophy of occupational therapy, Arch Occup Ther, 1:1–10, 1922.

18. Mosey AC: An alternative: The biopsychosocial model. Am J Occup Ther, 28:137–140, 1974.

19. Clark PN: Human development through occupation: Theoretical frameworks in contemporary occupational therapy practice, Part 1. Am J Occup Ther, 33:505–514, 1979.

20. Kaplan K: Short-term assessment: The need and a response. Occup Ther Ment Health, 4:29–45, 1984.

21. King LJ: A sensory-integrative approach to schizophrenia. Am J Occup Ther, 28:529–536, 1974.

22. King LJ: 1978 Eleanor Clarke Slagle lecture toward a science of adaptive responses. Am J Occup Ther, 32:429–437, 1978.

23. Vander Roest LL, Clements ST: *Sensory Integration: Rationale and Treatment Activi-*

ties for Groups, Grand Rapids, Mich., South Kent Mental Health Services, Inc., 1983.

24. Ross M, Burdick D: *A Sensory Integration Training Manual for Regressed and Geriatric Patients,* Middletown, Conn., Connecticut Valley Hospital, 1978.

25. Allen CK: *Occupational Therapy for Psychiatric Diseases: Measurement and Management of Cognitive Disabilities,* Boston, Little Brown & Co., 1985.

26. Azima H, Azima FJ: Outline of a dynamic theory of occupational therapy. Am J Occup Ther, *13:*215–221, 1959.

27. Fidler GS, Fidler JW: *Occupational Therapy: A Communication Process in Psychiatry,* New York, Macmillan, 1963.

28. Holmes C, Bauer W: Establishing an occupational therapy department in a community hospital. Am J Occup Ther, *24:*219–221, 1970.

29. Briggs AK, Duncombe LW, Howe MC, Schwartzberg SL: *Case Simulations in Psychosocial Occupational Therapy,* Philadelphia, F. A. Davis, 1979.

30. Hemphill BJ (ed): *The Evaluative Process in Psychiatric Occupational Therapy,* Thorofare, N.J., Charles B. Slack, 1982.

31. Hyman M, Metzker JR: Occupational therapy in an emergency psychiatric setting. Am J Occup Ther, *24:*280–283, 1970.

32. Mosey AC: *Activities Therapy,* New York, Raven Press, 1973.

33. Llorens LA: *Application of a Developmental Theory for Health and Rehabilitation,* Rockville, Md., American Occupational Therapy Association, 1976.

34. Mosey AC: Recapitulation of ontogenesis: A theory for practice of occupational therapy. Am J Occup Ther, *22:*426–432, 1968.

35. Mosey AC: The concept and use of developmental groups. Am J Occup Ther, *24:*272–275, 1970.

36. Florey LL: Intrinsic motivation: The dynamics of occupational therapy theory. Am J Occup Ther, *23:*319–322, 1969.

37. Reilly M: A psychiatric occupational therapy program as a teaching model. Am J Occup Ther, *20:*61–67, 1966.

38. Reilly M: The education process. Am J Occup Ther, *23:*299–307, 1969.

39. Kielhofner G: Temporal adaptation: A conceptual framework for occupational therapy. Am J Occup Ther, *31:*235–242, 1977.

40. Black MM: Adolescent role assessment. Am J Occup Ther, *30:*73–79, 1976.

41. Florey LL, Michelman SM: Occupational role history: A screening tool for psychiatric occupational therapy. Am J Occup Ther, *36:*301–308, 1982.

42. Kielhofner G, Henry A, Walens D: A user's guide to the occupational performance history interview, The American Occupational Therapy Association. Rockville, Md., 1989.

43. Matsutsuyu JS: The interest checklist. Am J Occup Ther, *23:*323–328, 1969.

44. Moorhead L: The occupational history. Am J Occup Ther, *23:*329–334, 1969.

45. Neville A: Temporal adaptation: Application with short-term psychiatric patients. Am J Occup Ther, *34:*328–331, 1980.

46. Shannon PD: The work-play model: A basis for occupational therapy programming in psychiatry. Am J Occup Ther, *24:*215–218, 1970.

47. Howe MC, Briggs AK: Ecological systems model for occupational therapy. Am J Occup Ther, *36:*322–327, 1982.

48. Kielhofner G (ed): *Health through Occupation Theory and Practice in Occupational Therapy,* Philadelphia, F. A. Davis, 1983.

49. Mosey AC: Meeting health needs. Am J Occup Ther, *27:*14–17, 1973.

50. Reed KL, Sanderson SR: *Concepts of Occupational Therapy,* ed 2, Baltimore, Williams & Wilkins, 1983.

51. Reed, KL: *Models of Practice in Occupational Therapy,* Baltimore, Williams & Wilkins, 1984.

52. Fidler GS: The task-oriented group as a context for treatment. Am J Occup Ther, *23:*43–48, 1969.

53. Howe MC, Schwartzberg SL: *A Functional Approach to Group Work in Occupational Therapy,* Philadelphia, J.B. Lippincott, 1986.

54. Charles River Hospital, Wellesley, Mass., 02181.

55. Fidler GS, Fidler JW: Doing and becoming: Purposeful action and self-actualization. Am J Occup Ther, *32:*305–310, 1978.

56. Searles HF: *The Nonhuman Environment in Normal Development and in Schizophrenia,*

New York, International Universities Press, 1960.

57. Tiffany EG: Psychiatry and mental health, in Hopkins HL, Smith HD (eds): *Willard and Spackman's Occupational Therapy,* ed. 6, p. 295, Philadelphia, J.B. Lippincott, 1983.

58. Levey S, Hesse DD: Sounding board: Bottomline health care? N Engl J Med, *312*:644–646, 1985.

59. Strauss H: Factors Influencing Psychiatrist Referral to Occupational Therapy: A Pilot Study. Master's Thesis Research, Tufts University, Boston School of Occupational Therapy, Medford, Mass., 1990.

60. Ezersky S, Havazelet L, Scott AH, Zettler CLB: Specialty choice in occupational therapy. Am J Occup Ther, *43*:227–233, 1989.

61. Wittman PP, Swinehart S, Cahill R, St Michel G: Variables affecting specialty choice in occupational therapy. Am J Occup Ther, *43*:602–606, 1989.

62. Bailey D: Reasons for attrition from occupational therapy. Am J Occup Ther, *44*:23–29, 1990.

63. Bailey D: Ways to retain or reactivate occupational therapists. Am J Occup Ther, *44*:31–37, 1990.

Child and Adolescent Treatment

Gordon P. Harper, MD
Nancy S. Cotton, PhD

Inpatient psychiatric treatment of children and adolescents differs from inpatient treatment of adults in the following ways:

1. The goals of hospitalization;
2. The diagnostic process;
3. The treatment methods used;
4. The role in treatment of nonpatients (family, schools, agencies);
5. The core dilemmas in treatment;
6. Controversy over the use of hospitals for children and adolescents: Are some children and adolescents hospitalized unnecessarily? Are others who need hospital treatment going without it?

Through case example, this chapter will discuss and illustrate each of these differences.

THE GOAL OF HOSPITALIZATION

The *goal* of hospital treatment determines interventions employed and, consequently, the length of stay. Therefore, the goal must be stated explicitly. Practitioners frequently assume there is more agreement about the goal than really exists: asked about the goal, one team member may say "Detox"; another says "Help the patient change schools;" and a third interjects, "So he can get an assessment."

Defining a goal is more complicated in child and adolescent treatment than in adult psychiatry, for several reasons. First, children and adolescents come to the hospital for a wide range of troubles—from acute symptoms to developmental arrest. Second, treatment is directed not just at the hospitalized child, but at the child-and-family together (and often at child-and-family-and-agencies). (The exception to this rule, long-term hospitalization aimed at personality restructuring of the child, is discussed below.) Third, by themselves, categorical diagnoses do not explain admissions in child psychiatry; admission is the result of "disorder-plus-something else." Finally, fantasy goals emerge more frequently: among professionals, the rescue fantasy (1); among families, fantasies that the child will be magically "fixed" or certified as "damaged goods" and taken off their hands.

Short- and Long-Term Hospitalization

The goal of hospitalization is different in *short-term* (length of stay = 20–40 days) and *long-term* (length of stay = months–years) treatment.

Short-Term Hospitalization: Focal Treatment

For several decades in the literature and in practice, "hospital treatment" meant long-term treatment. Today, in both general hospitals and free-standing psychiatric hospitals, hospital treatment is short-term (2, 3). Short-term hospitalization is a form of crisis intervention—the crisis consisting of the events leading to admission and the hospitalization itself (4).

In contrast to long-term treatment, short-term hospital treatment does not attempt to reconstruct the child's personality. It responds to acute crises, intervenes in child-and-family (and agencies), and readies the child for nonhospital treatment. The goal of short-term treatment is to make those minimal changes necessary for the child to return to the community (5). This approach is called Focal Treatment (6).

Short-term hospital treatment aims toward providing one or more of the following:

1. *Respite/protection/cooling-off*
2. *Assessment/relabelling/linkage* (7)
3. *Acute stabilization* (5)
4. *Initiation of change*

The following cases illustrate the goals of short-term hospital teratment.

Hospitalization for Respite/ Protection/Cooling-Off

CASE 1: Emily, a 6-year-old girl beaten and abandoned by her natural parents by age 5, had poor affect modulation with occasional tan- trums thereafter; she became increasingly assaultive with her foster mother in the months after the foster mother gave birth. When additional outpatient therapy appointments did not help, Emily was hospitalized after badly biting her foster mother. Relevant factors included the girl's status in the family (as foster child lacking both biological family and pre-adoptive family), her poor modulation of rage at deprivation (intensified by the birth of the foster sibling) and the foster mother's exhaustion, depression, and ambivalence about caring for the girl. During a ten-day admission, both parties cooled off. The girl practiced an exercise developed on the ward called "Bagging Your Anger and Taking Your Time," in which she filled small garbage bags when annoyed and large garbage bags when enraged, and took time-outs when she broke a rule. Time, a break from day-to-day contact, and the change in the girl helped the foster mother feel less overwhelmed, get treatment for her own depression, and recommit to the child's care. Post-discharge outpatient treatment would focus upon permanency planning, interactions in the family, and the girl's continued emotional growth.

Hospitalization for Relabelling

CASE 2: A 13-year-old girl was hospitalized for defiance and suicidal behavior by her maternal grandparents. They had raised the patient, the child of a delinquent daughter long estranged from the family. Asked where the girl would live after hospitalization, the grandparents indicated they were torn between the wish to redo the unhappy adolescence of their own daughter, the girls' mother, and the wish to get rid of the child as "hopeless, just like her mother." The girl was equally ambivalent about herself, her identification with her mother, and her prospects for living with her grandparents. For both the girl and the grandparents, mother and daughter were hard to tell apart. The problem was redefined to include the family's confusion about the girl and her mother. Treatment was then redefined as helping the girl and the grandparents "find the girl" amid the painful memories of the mother and facilitating their grieving for what had been lost and what could never be. With this redefinition of the work, to be pursued in outpatient treatment, the girl's suicidal behavior and defiance subsided, allowing discharge.

Hospitalization for Assessment and Linkage

CASE 3:   Ed, a 9-year-old possibly psychotic boy, was hospitalized for mute withdrawal and severe tantrums at school. In the hospital, he began to talk, allowing diagnosis of a previously unrecognized language disorder with secondary emotional reaction but no psychosis. With the diagnosis, the parents felt relieved, then guilty; the boy felt better to have a problem, not just to feel "dumb" or "bad." He excelled at charades and was sought out by others for his dramatic nonverbal abilities. The discharge plan included referring the boy for language therapy, introducing different ways of managing the boy at home, modifying the school program, psychoeducation for the family, and psychotherapy for the boy. The family began to play charades at home.

These three cases illustrate the principle of *parsimony* in treatment planning. Clinicians were aware of many problems needing treatment; they could have recommended weeks or months of additional inpatient treatment. By focusing on the specific dysfunction that required admission (the Focal Problem, discussed below) and maintaining a good relationship with the outpatient treaters (the "horizontal alliance," see below), hospital staff prevented the rescue fantasy ("We will make him all better"), mobilized the patient's and families' strengths, and limited the length of stay.

The following cases illustrate acute stabilization and initiation of change.

Hospitalization for Acute Stabilization

CASE 4:   Karen, a 14-year-old with a restrictive eating disorder, was hospitalized after frenzied dieting and family struggles led to a 20% weight loss. In the hospital the girl broke out of her established eating patterns and gained back half the lost weight. Her thinking became clearer. Family treatment offered hope that the old patterns would not recur at home. Family and individual therapy, previously devoted to discussions of calories and weight, now concentrated on everyone's fears of the patient's growing up.

Hospitalization for Initiation of Change

CASE 5:   George, an 11-year-old with a history of severe withdrawal and delusional preoccupations in early childhood, had, with outpatient treatment, made gains in his ability to stay engaged with peers in school and at play. At home, however, frequent tantrums, with screaming and throwing, persisted. Parents' resourceful attempts to prevent the tantrums distorted family life; for example, to support the boy's perceived need to discharge tension through action, the family room was frequently converted to a gym, regardless of what his brother and sister were doing there at the time. Although the parents' distress and tension were evident, they could not acknowledge their disappointment and rage or the fear and anger the other children felt toward George. A trial of stimulant medication made no change in his behavior and may have contributed to decreased appetite and linear growth. Desperate not to give up anything that might help, the parents insisted on continuing the medicine. The system was "stuck."

An inpatient admission initiated change by (a) interrupting ongoing interactions, giving the boy a chance to learn new ways of managing frustration, and giving the parents a chance to see the boy functioning differently from what they had accepted as inevitable; (b) discontinuing the stimulant medication; (c) encouraging the boy to eat more; (d) through playing a game, "Twister," letting George and his siblings practice competition and asserting rules safely, with George acting increasingly normal; and (e) once the pressure of daily coping was lifted, letting the parents acknowledge how difficult life had been, as a prelude to working on new ways of managing everyone's frustration and anger.

Admission Criteria

Many suggested criteria for admission to short-term hospitalization are available; those recommended by the American Academy of Child and Adolescent Psychiatry appear in Table 12.1.

Table 12.1.   Admission Criteria for Children and Adolescents

A disorder impairing daily functioning in at least two areas of a child's life (school, peers, family);
Proposed treatment is relevant to these problems and likely to help;
Outpatient approaches are not available, deemed unlikely to help, or have been tried and not helped.

(Adapted from Policy Statement, American Academy of Child and Adolescent Psychiatry, June 1989)

Long-Term Hospitalization

The goal of long-term hospitalization is *personality restructuring*. This model of treatment is based on psychoanalytic psychotherapy. It differs from outpatient treatment in the types of patients treated and in the therapeutic use of the patient's life outside the therapy office. "Life-space" treatment, encompassing the concepts of "containing," "holding environment," "therapeutic management," and "clinical exploitation of life events," is discussed below. Long-term hospital treatment has been recommended for more disturbed patients whose symptoms cannot safely be managed in the community, who do not change in outpatient treatment, and whose use of destructive action-oriented defenses (running away, substance abuse, promiscuity) precludes their engaging in outpatient treatment (8–10).

The course of long-term treatment is divided into three phases, built around a hoped-for "corrective emotional experience" in which the patient reworks distorted object relations, particularly failed separation-individuation (8–10). In the first phase, self-harming behavior used to avoid personal vulnerability is confronted. In the second, "working through," patients establish relationships through which they can understand and accept their authentic needs and begin to tolerate ambivalence toward those they care about. This is the hoped-for "corrective emotional experience." In the third phase, "separation," the relationships made in the hospital are gradually given up and new attachments made outside the hospital.

In long-term treatment, the disorder under treatment "exists" in the hospitalized patient. Accordingly, treatment is directed at the child. The family is offered less intensive treatment in which psychoeducation is prominent.

Outcome studies of long-term treatment are mixed. Maintenance of and the "undoing" of gains made in long-term hospital treatment once the child has returned to the community are both reported (11, 12). The reader is referred to other sources (8–10) for further description of long-term hospital treatment of children and adolescents. The remainder of this chapter will refer to short-term treatment.

DIAGNOSIS

Categorical Diagnoses: Uses and Limitations

In inpatient child psychiatric treatment a categorical diagnosis is necessary but not sufficient for treatment planning. Categorical diagnoses define disorders in descriptive, non-etiological terms. Necessary for epidemiologic and administrative purposes, they guide treatment, especially biomedical treatments. They do *not* differentiate patients requiring hospitalization from those who do not, and they are not adequate for comprehensive treatment planning. Moreover, overemphasizing the child's categorical diagnosis may lead clinicians to squeeze the child into a poorly fitting slot and neglect context, such as family interactions, parents' constructions of the child's behavior, cultural and socioeconomic factors, and treaters' roles. The following case illustrates these risks.

CASE 6: Four-year-old Mark had three psychiatric hospitalizations in four months for reported unmanageable behavior, including defiance of his parents, urinating on his toys, disrobing, and breaking glass and trying to eat it. His parents, especially his mother, described him as a "monster" and felt that only a categorical diagnosis, preferably one with a biological basis, would validate their experience. Diagnostic efforts in the first two hospitals focused on the child; categorical diagnoses of Attention Deficit Hyperactivity Disorder, Major Depression, and Bipolar Disorder, NOS, led, respectively, to trials of stimulants, antidepressants, and haloperidol. The parents' distress with the child's behavior did not change. They became alienated from treatment and pursued diagnoses such as food allergy. In the third hospitalization, developmental assessment of the child showed fluctuations of ego functioning and difficulty in managing anxiety characteristic of borderline children (13). The interaction between the boy and his mother was notable for the mother's exasperation and ineffectual management of the boy, resulting in increased anxiety and disorganization in both. Working two jobs, the father was at home very few hours to dilute the interaction between Mark and his mother. For the parents, reporting the boy's symptoms was an attempt to get validation of a desperate situation. Definitive intervention followed appreciation of the boy's difficulties in self-regulation *and* the parents' need for help in feeling good about themselves as parents and safe with their son. They then could reclaim a positive view of their son from the "monster" with whom he had become identified.

To avoid such risks in similar cases, a comprehensive assessment, not just a categorical diagnosis, is needed.

The Comprehensive Assessment

The comprehensive assessment includes the present illness, a developmental assessment, family assessment, and educational assessment. Work with families is discussed later in this chapter. The developmental and educational assessment are important because underdiagnosed learning problems and language disorders are common among child psychiatric inpatients. Cognitive and projective psychological testing should be used selectively, depending on the patient's needs and the treatment goals (see Table 12.2).

With data from the comprehensive assessment, the clinician has considerable information about the patient but is at risk of drowning in data and losing task orientation. Length of stay is then likely to be prolonged and patients can regress (6). The task of the clinician is to decide where to focus.

Table 12.2. Psychological and Educational Tests for Children and Adolescents*

Developmental—General
  Gesell and Amatruda Developmental Scales
    4 weeks–6 years
  Compares child's development to age norms for personal-social, language, adaptive, and gross and fine motor development.
Neuropsychological
1. Halstead-Reitan Battery
   5–14 years
   Assesses brain function via Wechsler Intelligence Scale for Children-Revised (WISC-R) and specific tests of motor coordination and visual-motor integration.
2. Luria-Nebraska Neuropsychological Battery
   8–12 years (Children's Version)
   13+ years (Standard Version)
   Assesses brain function, gives 11 summary scales for motor rhythm, tactile, visual, receptive and expressive language, writing, reading, arithmetic, memory, intellectual processes. Screens for brain damage and lateralized brain defects.
Perceptual-Motor
1. Bender Visual-Motor Gestalt Test
   4–12 years
   Nonverbal test assesses perceptual-motor maturity through child's copying geometric designs.
2. Beery-Buktenica Test of Visual-Motor Integration (VMI)
   2–15 years
   Similar to Bender, well-suited to young children
Cognitive
1. Wechsler Preschool and Primary School Intelligence Scale (WPPSI)
   4–6 years
   Modification of WISC-R for younger children.

Table 12.2. Psychological and Educational Tests for Children and Adolescents*
—continued

2. Wechsler Intelligence Scale for Children-Revised Version

   6–16 years

   Full-Scale IQ derived from verbal and performance subscales; assesses various aspects of intelligence; screens for learning disabilities, developmental disorders, and perceptual dysfunctions.

3. Wechsler Adult Intelligence Scale (WAIS)

   16 years and above

   Modification for older adolescents and adults

4. Peabody Picture Vocabulary Test (Revised)

   2.5–18 years

   Screens intelligence in nonverbal or language-impaired children.

Academic Achievement

   Wide-Range Achievement Test (WRAT)

   5 years to adult

   Screens reading, spelling, arithmetic; most widely used.

Personality

These "projective" tests assess reality testing, imagination, handling of affects, personality structure, core conflicts, views of self in family, and interpersonal relatedness.

1. Rorschach Test

   4+ years

   Children describe what they see in 10 inkblots.

2. Thematic Apperception Test (TAT)

   6+ years

   Children tell stories prompted by pictures of children and adults in ambiguous situations.

3. Children's Apperception Test (CAT)

   3–7 years

   Modified for younger children, using pictures of animals.

4. Draw-a-Person, Draw-a-Family Test

   4+ years

   A graphomotor projective test; child draws a picture; assesses body-image, self-concept, attitudes toward sexual development and gender identity.

5. Tasks of Emotional Development (TED)

   5+ years

   Uses pictures with developmentally designed interactions; age norms exist.

6. Sentence Completion Test

   6–18 years

   Child completes partial sentences; assesses current stressors, worries, and coping devices.

Adaptive functioning

1. Vineland Adaptive Behavior Scales (VABS)

   Birth to maturity

   Parent interview, reviewing child's adaptation in 5 areas; produces scores usable on Axis V of DSM-IIIR (*Diagnostic and Statistical Manual of Mental Disorders*, ed. 3, revised).

*See also references 14 and 15

The Focal Problem

The *Focal Problem* is the problem requiring the child to be in the hospital. Because it is the basis for the treatment alliance, the Focal Problem should be noncontroversial, stating the reason for admission in ordinary language (free of psychiatric jargon) that team members, patient, family, and referring clinicians can accept. To distinguish the inpatient from others with the same disorder who do not require hospitalization, the Focal Problem usually includes not just a symptom or disorder, but some aspect of the child's overall functioning and *context*. Although the Focal Problem may include the categorical diagnosis, it does not need to. The criteria for the Focal Problem are listed in Table 12.3. The differences between Referring Problem, Focal Problem, and related terms are listed in Table 12.4.

The following case illustrates the Referring Problem, Focal Problem, Developmental Assessment, Formulation, Empathic Diagnosis, and Categorical Diagnosis.

Case 7: Greg, a 14-year-old whose school avoidance is not responsive to outpatient treatment, threatens his mother with a knife when she insists on yet another emergency ward visit for medical assessment.

Referring Problem: Outpatient therapist: "Threatening behavior to mother." *Chief Complaint*, according to mother: "There's something wrong with him, but he won't let me help him any more"; according to patient: "I just want to be left alone, and she keeps hassling me."

Focal Problem: Panicky threats to his

Table 12.3. Criteria for Focal Problem

Gives real reason child is in hospital;

Distinguishes hospitalized child from child with same disorder not in hospital;

Written in language one can share with patient, family, and referring clinicians;

Written in language that will enhance the alliance;

Refers to actual dysfunction in child;

Defines the work of hospitalization parsimoniously.

Table 12.4. Common Terms and Their Definitions

Referring Problem/Chief Complaint: the reason for referral in the words of the referring party or the parent or child.

Focal Problem: the specific dysfunction that requires the child to be in the hospital.

Developmental Assessment: Summary of the child's development, both descriptively (observable cognitive, linguistic, motor, and social milestones) and in terms of *developmental lines* (16), referring to integration of drives and affects, and to the development of the ego and of the components of the self.

Formulation: a narrative statement of the child's situation, summarizing description and etiological hypotheses (17, 18).

Empathic Diagnosis (Central Theme): a concise statement in everyday language, on a level acceptable to the patient, of the patient's current pain and longstanding conflicts (19).

Categorical Diagnosis: a disorder or syndrome, not specifying etiology, from a diagnostic system such as the DSM-IIIR or the ICD-9.

mother by a 14-year-old boy with long-standing school and peer avoidance, who resents his mother's frightened insistence that what he needs is another medical examination to "check out his innards."

Developmental Assessment: A 14-year-old with above-average cognitive development, but greatly delayed social development, poor differentiation from his mother, fear of passivity, and brittle control of his rage.

Formulation: A 14-year-old boy with long-standing separation anxiety, afraid of his wishes to be cared for, who experiences transient panic, fear of fragmentation, and rage when his mother intrudes and is not emotionally responsive. His knife threats to his mother are seen both as a breakthrough of primitive rage and as a defense against fragmentation in a boy with an overly enmeshed and stimulating mother-son relationship.

Empathic Diagnosis: "You want to live a full life, but for a long time you have not felt well enough to go to school; you and your mother, although you are very devoted to each other, have had a hard time managing disagreements and differences. When things between you get too heated, it feels like you're going to explode or fall apart and you threaten to strike out. Now you're scared that you might hurt someone."

Categorical Diagnosis:
Axis I: 309.21 Separation Anxiety Disorder
         312.39 Impulse Control Disorder, NOS
(The Categorical Diagnoses do *not* explain why this patient is in the hospital.)

Referring Problem, Undisclosed Problems

The Referring Problem may be a clue (the "entry ticket" or a "cry for help") to a more serious problem, as yet undisclosed. For example, "school refusal" may be the Referring Problem of a child with incipient panic state, psychosis, or undisclosed abuse or molestation. The possibility of abuse or molestation requires special attention, as in *Case 8.*

CASE 8: Diana, a 14-year-old living in the North with her parents for two years after being raised in the rural South by her grandparents, was admitted in a highly agitated state after ingesting a small amount of bleach and saying she wanted to die. She had become agitated when an aunt, who had discovered her and a female cousin viewing a sexually explicit video, threatened her with trouble "when I tell your father." The girl's agitation and rapid affective shifts (from tearful pleading for help to angry denial that she needed any help at all) were clarified when the girl disclosed physical abuse and sexual molestation by her father. Redefinition of the problem led to protective and clinical intervention, and the girl's agitation and suicidal behavior subsided.

Given the high prevalence of abuse and molestation in psychiatric patients (30–80% in selected populations, compared to 10–30% in the general population), the team must consider seriously in *every admission* the possibility of undisclosed abuse. The child should be asked explicitly about abuse or unwanted touching. Since many abused and molested children deny abuse when first asked, indirect evidence must be considered as well. Such evidence may appear in behavior toward adults or in play with peers, or in play therapy, expressive therapy, or psychological testing.

Focal Problem, Factors, and Strengths

Once the Focal Problem is defined, one lists the possible *Factors* contributing to its origin or persistence. The Factors can be drawn from any domain of the child's life (biological, individual-developmental, family life, school, treatment systems). They express explicitly the elements of a formulation.

The Factors summarize *not* the history, but those aspects of the history and the current psychosocial state most likely contributing to the Focal Problem. For example, in *Case 8*, the *history* includes such items as the following:

- Born in the South;
- Benign gestation and delivery;
- Left by mother with relatives at 3 months, when mother moved North;
- Development recalled as "fine, like the others";

and so on.

In contrast, the *Factors* contributing to the Focal Problem ("Agitation with suicidal ideation and ingestion of bleach") are such as these:

- Alleged molestation by father, only disclosed in hospital, denied by father;
- Intimidating behavior by father;
- Possible knowledge of molestation by mother—"family secret";
- Patient's acute confusion (guilt, shame, fear, torn loyalties, relief) following disclosure;
- Lack of parental alliance regarding need for individual or family mental health services.

Strengths are listed separately to avoid a pathocentric view of the patient and family. The Strengths are resources of the child and her situation that mitigate the Focal Problem, contribute to the child's resilience, or help the child and family to use treatment.

In *Case 8*, Diana's strengths included:

- Engaging, animated personal style;
- Makes friends easily;
- Wish to find a way to protect self and also be loyal to family.

TREATMENT

Treatment consists of coordinated interventions directed toward an agreed upon and articulated Goal. Consensus, articulation, and coordination are necessary lest each member of the team start "doing therapy" with only a clinician-specific or a discipline-specific goal in mind, which amounts to multiple-therapies-in-parallel. In contrast, when the elements of inpatient treatment are coordinated toward a single articulated Goal, the *synergy* of individual, family, and life-space treatment is unrivaled in its therapeutic power.

According to the rule of parsimony, treatment aims to make those *minimal* changes in the Focal Problem that will allow the patient to enter a less intensive level of care. This rule reflects economic realities and the principle of treating the patient in the "least restrictive" setting; it does, however, violate the wish of inpatient clinicians to "do the whole job" of treatment.

Interventions are chosen by identifying the Factors that contribute to the problem requiring hospitalization then *selecting* those Factors that need to be changed during this admission.

Selecting Factors and Defining Interventions

Factors are selected according to the following criteria:

- A difference in them is likely to ameliorate the Focal Problem;

• They are likely to change during the available treatment.

For example, if the Focal Problem is major depression with suicidal ideation and lack of consensus about the treatment needed, the goal is decreased suicidal risk and increased consensus about the treatment. The relevant Factors are

• Major depression, inadequately treated;
• Child's feeling no one understands the extent of her despair;
• Parents' estrangement from treatment, underappreciated by treaters.

Case 9 illustrates Factors, Strengths, and the selection of Factors in treating a chronically psychotic teenager.

CASE 9:   Kareem, a 17-year-old inner city youth with paranoid schizophrenia, was hospitalized after spending nights on the streets, preoccupied with dangers there and his personal mission to "save other Black youths from gang violence." He lived with his paternal grandmother, who felt intimidated by his threatening behavior and acceded to his noncompliance with neuroleptic medication. The family lived in a neighborhood where drugs were sold freely and five homicides had occurred in the previous four months. Family background was notable for chronic poverty, a father who had recently committed suicide after years of serious mental illness, a mother who had abandoned the family some years before, and hypertension in the grandmother.

In the hospital, the team acknowledged the family's grief at the death of Kareem's father and the grandmother's bravery in maintaining hope and in parenting a disabled grandchild against the background of the death of her son who had despaired of life and an environment in which many despaired.

Factors identified and addressed included:

• Chronic schizophrenia, exacerbated, secondary to inconsistent use of perphenazine;

• A neighborhood stimulating and validating fears of danger;
• Grandmother, important support, but intimidated and not supporting medication use now;
• Kareem and grandmother grieving recent death of father.

Strengths included the grandmother's courage and Kareem's caring, protective nature and interest in the vulnerability of his peers.

Not all Factors identified were selected for *intervention.* Some, such as violence in the neighborhood, were acknowledged to Kareem and his grandmother. Others, such as the grandmother's hypertension, were left to other treaters. And others, such as the learning disabilities that had contributed to Kareem's dropping out of school, were left to outpatient evaluation and vocational rehabilitation.

The admission was used to assess with Kareem and his grandmother the nature of his illness; to reach a new consensus regarding his treatment needs (especially the use of neuroleptics); to reinstitute medication; and to contract (and to practice) with grandmother and Kareem ways that they could feel comfortable with her supporting his treatment needs, including the times when he became threatening or intimidating.

The Background of Treatment: Containment

Admission begins the process of containment. It interrupts interactions which have exhausted child and parents. It protects the child from his own or others' impulses. And it offers hope.

Containment is the hospital equivalent of what Winnicott termed the "holding environment" (20), conveying to patient and parents a sense of purpose and safety, by demonstrating that the inpatient unit and staff are willing and able to absorb anxiety and contain impulses.

With containment begins what Gutheil (21) calls "the therapy in clinical administration," meaning that the treatment of disturbed patients begins with "administrative" interventions directed at the patient's person: confinement, restriction, restraint, medication. Similarly, in Cotton's description of "therapeutic management," the first phase "constructs the framework" in which treatment can take place, a "therapeutic holding environment" (22). Such measures provide from the outside the impulse control, organization, or self-protection patients cannot provide for themselves. Admitting a child or adolescent also provides such control for the family.

Table 12.5 lists the ways that seclusion and physical containing may be helpful to the overwhelmed child. Table 12.6 lists criteria for its use.

For some patients, like Emily in *Case 1* above, "holding" and the passage of time are enough to allow a return to the community. The goal of Respite/Protection/Cooling Off has been met.

Beyond Containment: Therapeutic Management

Therapeutic management has several components: (*a*) the overall structure of the ward and the program designed to contain individuals and the patient group; (*b*) individual interventions meant to contain maladaptive responses and induce readiness for change; and (*c*) individual interventions fostering recovery and growth by providing alternatives to the presenting problems.

Table 12.5.   Potential Benefits of Seclusion for the Overwhelmed Child

1. Protects child and others.
2. Protects physical and therapeutic environment.
3. Demonstrates that adults care and can take control when the child can not control himself or herself.
4. Introduces skills such as leaving the scene, seeking solace in quiet, using privacy to reflect, waiting before reacting, taking consequences gracefully, and using adults before trouble gets worse.
5. Prevents greater violence and destruction (with consequent guilt and shame).
6. Channels blowups away from peers so that child can calm down without loss of face.
7. Decreases outside stimulation so that the child can replenish himself or herself inside.
8. Uses room boundaries to help the child restore inner boundaries.

Table 12.6.   Criteria for Use of Seclusion or Restraint

Seclusion or restraint must be:
1. Part of a process to support the patient's own controls;
2. Defined in written policies and procedures;
3. Conducted in a consistent manner;
4. Exercised for predictable reasons;
5. Clinically indicated;
6. Explained to the child before and after its use;
7. Supervised by trained direct-care staff, humanistically oriented;
8. Supervised and monitored by child psychiatric staff;
9. Maintained in a safe, attractive, and soothing space.

Table 12.7.   Therapeutic Management: A Four-Phase Model

Phase I: Starting Out and Feeling Safe
1. Holding environment for safety and containment (design of physical space, unit culture, value system); staffing pattern, daily schedule and routines; rules and discipline system.
2. The Empathic Formulation: understanding patient and family through individualized dynamic-development assessment.

Phase II: Responding to Trouble: Controls from Without
1. Containing at times when the child is overwhelmed: quiet room or open-door seclusion; physical holding; (locked-door) seclusion; mechanical restraint, reactive contracts.
2. Techniques as the child is able to use them: time-outs, privilege system, life-space interview, preventive contracts, staff support and praise.

Phase III: Introducing New Ways: Controls from Within
1. New strategies for problem-solving, controlling anger, getting along with peers.
2. New meanings: stories children read and tell about themselves, understanding their lives through books, drama.

Phase IV: Leaving: Taking it Home
1. Saying Goodbye: special group meetings, "goodbye books," calendars.
2. Taking it all home: transitional passes, overnights, practicing new routines with parents, transition groups.

Therapeutic management invites clinical imagination. From the child's symptoms, the meanings of the symptoms to the child and others, and the clinician's own understanding of child development, one tries to create safe and facilitating "play spaces" in which the child can learn new ways of coping and regain the capacity to play that is the hallmark of psychological health.

A program was designed for 4-year-old Mark (*Case 6*), seen by parents (and himself) as a monster, called "Getting to Know My Monster." It included bibliotherapy (the story, "There's a Nightmare in my Closet"), proactive contracts (therapeutic holding during tantrums), concrete anticipatory guidance (e.g., going to amusement parks only when Mark was well-fed and rested), and practice home visits, in which Mark tried out new ways to signal distress and his mother tried new ways to listen. The program carried out the principle that the rage expressed in the tantrums needed to be reworked and integrated, not banished. This spirit was expressed in the saying, "When you get to know a monster, you can even like him; and when the monster feels liked, he can show you his other parts."

One technique used in therapeutic management, the reactive contract, is de-

Table 12.8. Reactive Contracts: Post Crisis Components and Rationale

1.	Description of Behavior	Specifies impact, rule broken; avoid jargon and shaming or judgmental language
2.	Reparative Words (drawing, for young children)	Making amends lets the child rebuild ties, rejoin the group
3.	Reparative Deeds	Second step in making amends; turns guilt and fear into constructive action; ties to group, builds self-esteem
4.	Penalty	Atonement diminishes guilt; use natural consequences when possible
5.	Rechanneling	Fosters acceptance of feelings, provides adaptive and safe expression; fosters feeling/action distinction and new solutions for old problems. Use phrases such as "Just think of . . . ;" "Try to;" avoid "I'll never . . . again"
6.	Teaching	Indicates how to avoid future trouble; spells out rules, consequences; emphasizes impact on others

Table 12.9. Sample Reactive Contract

(after a patient assaulted another patient and staff member)

I, Ed, understand that hurting people is against the rules of the Unit and not a safe way to tell people that I am angry. Because I sat on Paul's legs and hurt him and then punched Stacey in the arm and scratched her in the eye, I will need to do the following:

____/ 1. Take 20 minutes of time-out in the Quiet Room.

____/ 2. Do Paul's chore after supper.

____/ 3. Do a chore for Stacey.

____/ 4. Write an apology letter to Paul.

____/ 5. Write an apology letter to Stacey.

____/ 6. Punch the punching bag 50 times.

____/ 7. Miss snack outing tonight.

____/ 8. List 3 ways to safely tell people that I am angry:

       1._____

       2._____

       3._____

If I do not obey this contract:

      I will be unable to rejoin the group and watch TV with them this evening.

                signed: (Ed)_____

                witness: (Stacey)_____

scribed in Table 12.8. The contract used with Ed, in *Case 3* above, is presented in Table 12.9.

Ingredients of Treatment: Pharmacotherapy

As with adults, pharmacotherapeutic treatment of young inpatients depends on the symptoms: neuroleptics for psychotic symptoms, tricyclics for depression, lithium carbonate or neuroleptics for mania, stimulants (or the newer alternatives, desipramine or clonidine) for attention-deficit disorders, and beta blockers or neuroleptics for posttraumatic symptoms (23). Like all inpatient efforts, pharmacotherapy must be coordinated with the Goal and anticipated length of hospitalization. At times, medication may only need to be introduced, not provided on an inpatient basis for an entire trial.

A special problem in the inpatient pharmacotherapy of children and adolescents is managing transient states of ego disorganization characterized by agitation, rage, paranoid thinking, and aggression in children with features of borderline or severe narcissistic disorders who are not psychotic between episodes. Pharmacological management is used in these states because of the observed loss of reality orientation during the episode. In addition, patients themselves, as well as others affected by the episodes, often request pharmacological help in preventing or containing these incidents. Some patients with such episodic breakdowns respond to nonneuroleptic sedatives (an antihistamine such as diphenhydramine or the benzodiazepine lorazepam) which are the drugs of first choice. However, many patients will require neuroleptics: chlorpromazine, haloperidol, thioridazine. Because evidence from controlled clinical trials is lacking, such practice is based on clinical experience.

Providing medication to such patients should not distract the inpatient clinician

Table 12.10. Commonly Used Medications

Name	Dose/Day (mg/kg)	Doses/Day
Neuroleptics:		
Chlorpromazine	3–8	1–2
Thioridazine	3–8	1–2
(lower-potency, more sedating, less neurol SEs)		
Haloperidol	0.1–0.5	1–2
Perphenazine	0.1–0.5	1–2
(higher-potency, less sedating, more neurol SEs)		
Antidepressants:		
Imipramine	2.0–5.0	1–2
Amitriptyline	2.0–5.0	1–2
Desipramine	2.0–5.0	1–2
(also used in attention-deficit disorder)		
Fluoxetine	0.5–1.0	1
Trazodone	4–10	1
Anti-Obsessive-Compulsive Disorder:		
Clomipramine	not established for children	
Stimulants:		
Dextroamphetamine	0.3–1.2	2–3
Methylphenidate	0.5–2.0	2–3
Pemoline	1.0–3.0	1
Anti-Tourette's Syndrome		
Haloperidol	0.1–0.2	1–2
Clonidine	3–10 **mcg**/kg	2–3
Antimanic:		
Lithium Carbonate	10–30	1–2
(treat to serum level of 0.5–1.5 mEq/L)		
Carbamazepine	10–20	2
(treat to serum level of 6–10 mcg/ml)		
Antianxiety:		
Clonazepam	0.01–0.04	1–2
(especially for social anxiety)		
Lorazepam	0.04–0.09	3
(adjunctive to neuroleptic in psychosis)		
Alprazolam	0.02–0.06	3
(short-acting; may synergize with antidepressant)		

from the *nonpharmacological* elements of managing agitation or ego disorganization: pay attention to the possibility of nonconsensus among clinicians, therapeutic management including specific ego-mobilizing activities, and physical restraint or seclusion as needed.

Medications and the appropriate doses for children and adolescents appear in Table 12.10.

ROLE OF NONPATIENTS IN HOSPITAL TREATMENT

In hospital treatment of children and adolescents, one works with families, schools, and agencies as well as with individual children. Clinicians who work only with the child, such as child clinicians who restrict their view of treatment only to what they see in the office, are fundamentally ill-informed.

Families

THE COLLABORATIVE ATTITUDE WITH PARENTS

The team *works for* the parents. The appropriate role for the team is that of partners who consult with parents. Alternative models are presented in Table 12.11. A team that starts to feel a loss of partnership (e.g., competitive, judgmental, or displacing) needs to examine its reaction to the parents. This does not mean the team should ignore actual shortcomings of parents or parental pathology, including domestic violence, that affect the child. It does mean that such observations should be acknowledged, empathically described, and addressed proactively in the treatment plan. Evidence that

Table 12.11.   Models of Parents' Role During Hospitalization

Parents' Role	Participation
1. Parent as Pathogen	No contact at first, then restricted visiting; therapy outside hospital.
2. Parent as Inpatient (24)	Parents admitted along with child, work together on the ward.
3. Parent as Outpatient	Family therapy, parent support groups, multifamily groups, sibling groups
4. Parent as Team Member	Parents meet with treatment team, join in key decisions (admission, goal, treatments to use, discharge plan), including contact with child, and in behavior management; parents take part on ward (routines, chores, groups, and school).
5. Parent as Learner	Psychoeducation, training in child management, practicing on the ward.

parents are injuring children or have abandoned them should be discussed openly and any indicated clinical, protective, or legal action taken. Otherwise such feelings, unexpressed, distort treatment.

Defining (Together) the Problem, Goal, and Treatments

Treatment begins with reaching consensus about the problem to be treated. Because the range of possible goals in inpatient treatment is so great, the potential is great for disagreements about what is to be done. Treatment goals should be stated openly and clearly. The American Academy of Child and Adolescent Psychiatry recommends that families contemplating inpatient treatment ask explicitly about the goals of the proposed treatment (25). Length of the proposed hospitalization and interventions to be used should also be discussed.

Sensitive aspects of treatment need to be specified at the outset. These include the parents' role in treatment (required meetings, visiting on the ward, multifamily groups) and the administrative aspects of the child's care (privileges, restrictions—including use of seclusion and restraint—and use of psychotropic medication).

Empowering the Parents

Parents deciding to hospitalize their child often feel depleted, helpless, and demoralized. These feelings are sometimes masked by anger at the child or the staff. The anger may or may not be expressed openly. Such anger usually abates in a few days; its persistence suggests problems in treatment, such as inadequate orientation to the program or consensus development, or the possibility of undisclosed family problems such as abuse or molestation. Whatever feelings the parents present, one of the goals of the hospital treatment is to empower them positively.

Empowerment begins with the language of the formulation. The problem to be treated should be stated in language one can share with the parents. If you feel like describing the problem in terms you can*not* share with the parents, you have not yet found the right words.

Parents are also empowered through contact with other parents, especially in multifamily groups for all the families on the ward (26). Cutting through shame and alienation, parents give each other support in a way that professionals cannot. Parents see in other families dilemmas and points of view they have not been able to see in their own.

Psychoeducation also empowers. This approach contrasts to the "find-out-the-cause," parent-blaming tradition of family treatment. Psychoeducation starts with the idea that the patient has a serious disorder, regardless of etiology, and views sympathetically the challenge families face in coping with this kind of disorder. It provides information about the child's disorder and facilitates problem-solving regarding managing the child in the hospital and beyond.

Managing Nonalliance

Nonalliance between treatment teams and families is a common occurrence in inpatient treatment. Sometimes the nonalliance is present from the start, such as when parents bring their child to the hospital reluctantly, feeling coerced, for instance, by protective services. At other times the nonalliance develops in the course of treatment. The three principles of managing nonalliance are (*a*) *acknowledgement*, implying that we want to work together ("We are not working together; what can we do to get back on track?"); (*b*) *defining the limits of consensus* (for instance, we may agree on the child's behavior, but not on whether it is a problem; or agree on a problem, but not on the proposed solution); and (*c*) *clarity re-garding expectations*, particularly expectations for parent participation. Such expectations need to be reconciled with parents' schedules; when the hospital is far from home, participating in treatment requires a major sacrifice.

When parents are not allied with or empowered, one typically sees the "adoption process" ensue, with negative consequences for child, family, and hospital (27).

Schools

The hospitalized child or adolescent should receive an educational assessment and educational services. Such children and adolescents have more learning problems, frequently undiagnosed before admission, than the general population.

Assessment should include a school history, a test of educational achievement (see Table 12.2) and observation of the way the child approaches learning. Contact with the child's home school, by phone and in writing, is necessary. While some hospitals provide only tutoring for instruction, it is ideal to have a classroom where the child's interactions with teachers and peers may be observed.

For children with both learning and behavior problems, the classroom may be the crucial setting for accurate diagnosis and intervention.

CASE 10: Burt, a 12-year-old with rage attacks and intermittent suicidal behavior, was regarded differently by clinicians and parents once his low threshold for distraction in noisy classrooms was appreciated. Before hospitalization, he had managed his difficulty at school but would "fall apart" on the playground or at home. Recognition of this problem in the hospital classroom led to preferential seating and modification of the acoustic demands in the classroom. Behavioral improvement followed.

For other children, educational assessment during hospitalization indicates that they have been overachieving in school, without family, child, or school recognizing this. This factor can contribute to serious mood or eating disorders as children identify with their parents' goals and feel ashamed at falling short. Reducing academic demands may be the key to the child's recovery.

Agencies

A third of hospitalized children and adolescents receive services from state departments of social service, child protection, mental health, or youth corrections. Among more disturbed children, this proportion reaches 100%. Treatment and aftercare planning depend on the relationship between the inpatient clinicians and these agencies.

Hospital-agency relationships are not always smooth, for several reasons. First, hospital and agency have different missions regarding the child. For example, when an out-of-home residence is not available, agencies may regard a child's prolonged hospitalization more benignly than does the hospital staff. Second, cutbacks in human services have reduced states' resources below even the level to which inpatient clinicians had become accustomed. In addition, for inpatient teams caring for deprived and needy children, already beleaguered state agencies make an easy target for projecting the feelings of inadequacy inevitable in such cases.

CASE 11: Dena, a four-year-old in foster care for several months after her abusive and drug-using mother lost custody, was hospitalized following a fire in the foster home in which another foster child died. The hospitalized girl was suspected of having set the fire. In the hospital, she had little to say, even indirectly, about the fire, but was grieving the loss of both homes. While the hospital team tried to judge the risk this child would present in the future, agency problems unrelated to the case delayed assignment and home-finding. The hospital team

members spent several meetings focusing on the agency's deficiencies until they recognized their own difficulty in bearing the feelings of inadequacy such a child and history arouses and the tendency to blame a particular person or agency.

Sometimes the tension is overt such as in the case above. Sometimes it is more subtle, as in this case.

CASE 12: Hoang, an orphaned suicidal teenager of Vietnamese background who lived with relatives, was recovering from a depression. No one on the hospital team knew about community resources for immigrants and assumed the resources were inadequate. Without knowing exactly what resources were available, a team member said, "It doesn't look too good for him out there."

Disparagement of outside treatment implies that the patient should "stay here with us." It undermines the patient's belief that he or she can live out of the hospital.

Inpatient teams need a *horizontal alliance*—a consciously felt partnership—with outside providers. To facilitate this alliance, it is useful for inpatient staff to attend meetings at the agency or visit outside facilities.

CORE DILEMMAS IN INPATIENT TREATMENT OF CHILDREN

1.   Home or Hospital?

For decades, child psychiatric hospital units have looked even less like medical hospitals and more like residential units than general psychiatric units have. Schoolrooms, cottage-like dormitories, and gymnasia and outdoor play spaces deliberately convey the message, "You are an active, growing child of diverse talents; we want to provide for you here what all children need (individualized bed spaces, schooling) and scope for activities that help you grow." Not only broken limbs but broken spirits and fractured egos heal better when exercised than when immobile (28). An added message—"Your personal dignity, your individuality, and your capacity to respond to beauty are important to us"—is illustrated in the color pictures of the Sonia Shankman School appearing in Bettelheim's book, *A Home for the Heart* (29). The "residentializing" of inpatient treatment reached its height in the 1950s, an era in which inpatient treatment hardly meant hospital treatment at all (30–31).

In the current era of "remedicalization" of inpatient treatment, the challenge is to maintain within our new hospital programs the many modes of mobilizing children's strengths for recovery that were developed in nonhospital settings.

2. To Take in Children without Adopting Them

The child's experience of the hospital as a second home is a powerful therapeutic tool.

CASE 13: Tina, a chronically dysphoric, irritable 13-year-old, had not responded to outpatient treatment of psychotherapy and adequate trials of two antidepressants. She was alienated from her family and quarrelsome with friends. She frequently expressed discouragement about herself and hopelessness about her future. She and her parents concurred that the most helpful part of her hospitalization was her experience of having a "fresh start" with staff and peers among whom she found recognition and validation of positive interests and personal qualities she had felt she had lost.

The risks attendant to "fresh starts" are those of "adoption": the child not only experiences the hospital as a second home, but the child, staff, and family together start to act as if the patient were really the child of the hospital and the hospital staff (27). Parents withdraw, staff let them withdraw, and staff start speaking as if their job is to replace the parents. The child also complies by providing the clinicians a view of herself as a normal child lacking only a home.

3. Accepting Limits on Care verses Advocating for Care

Inpatient clinicians must realistically match the therapeutic agenda to the time available. For example, starting a course of treatment heedless of the limited number of hospital days available is wasteful and cruel. In this situation the clinician's role is to help child and family do what can be done with the resources available.

Clinicians may also take an advocacy role in cases where benefit managers deny authorization for hospital care the clinician judges to be essential. Collaboration with the family and the hospital administration is essential in such cases. Patient advocacy with benefits managers, state regulators, or professional associations must be balanced with the role described above of helping the family accept what is available.

4. Validating Adversity versus Sentimentalizing and Externalizing

Hospitalized children and adolescents often have known horrible life circumstances. The inpatient staff may support the child's sanity and sense of self by acknowledging and labelling, sometimes for the first time, the abuse, victimization, and abandonment the child has experienced.

The risk inherent in such validation of the external facts of the child's life (especially if done in a one-sided way) is of underdiagnosing the child's intrinsic psychopathology. Children's own contributions to their problems may be neglected, which supports unhealthy externalization and increases guilt (for making these nice people see only the bad side, say, of parents). Success in helping children find ways to affect their own fate can be compromised.

Balancing a validation of external adversity while also supporting the child's mastery, instrumentality, and responsibility is the art of therapeutic practice.

CONTROVERSY OVER TREATMENT NEED AND ACCESS TO TREATMENT

Child and adolescent inpatient treatment has been a matter of controversy in the past decade. Statements in the sociological literature and the media and at congressional hearings have alleged that: (*a*) large numbers of children and adolescents are hospitalized unnecessarily; (*b*) adolescents are committed to hospital treatment without due process; and (*c*) the rapid growth of private hospitals (whose admissions of adolescents rose from 17,000 in 1980 to 38,000 in 1986) has exceeded need (32).

The profession has responded to these allegations in several ways (32).

First, the American Academy of Child and Adolescent Psychiatry has developed and distributed criteria for admission and guidelines for hospital treatment (see Table 12.1). These address the process of commitment and the bases for admission.

Second, the Academy has supported parent empowerment and consumer education by distributing an information sheet called "Facts for Families" that includes "Eleven Questions to Ask" when considering hospital treatment (33).

Third, epidemiological data indicate that approximately 15% of children and adolescents have a diagnosable psychiatric disorder and 1–2% have a disorder serious enough to require intensive treatment (34). In the current U.S. adolescent population of 30 million, 1% is 300,000; the roughly 60,000 admissions of adolescents per year (38,000 admissions to private hospitals and approximately 20,000 to general and public hospitals) do not appear to exceed the need. On the other hand, those admitted to these units are more likely to have private insurance; the uninsured are more likely to find treatment in the state systems at a time when state services are being reduced (2, 32).

More likely than an excess of admissions is the problem of an overall *shortage* of inpatient services. Greater shortages exist among selected populations such as the uninsured and individuals living in states without mandated psychiatric benefits or very limited benefits. Shortages also exist in alternatives to hospitalization such as partial hospitalization and nonhospital treatment settings. State efforts to broaden the service spectrum (by developing pre- and posthospital services) remain forever vulnerable to fiscal retrenchment.

REFERENCES

1. Eckstein R: *Children of Time and Space, Impulse and Action,* New York, Appleton-Century-Crofts, 1966.

2. Jemerin JM, Philips I: Changes in inpatient child psychiatry. J Amer Acad Child Adolesc Psychiatry, 27:397–403, 1988.

3. Harper G, Geraty R: Hospital and residential treatment, in Michels R, Cavenar JO, et al. (eds): *Psychiatry,* Philadelphia; J.B. Lippincott, 1987.

4. Parad HJ (ed): *Crisis Intervention: Selected Papers,* New York, Family Service Association of America, 1965.

5. Nurcombe B: Goal-directed treatment planning and the principles of brief hospitalization. J Amer Acad Child Adolesc Psychiatry, 28:26–30, 1989.

6. Harper G: Focal inpatient treatment planning. J Am Acad Child Adolesc Psychiatry, 28:31–37, 1989.

7. Doherty MB, Manderson M, Carter-Ake L: Time-limited psychiatric hospitalization of children: A model and three-year outcome. Hosp Community Psychiatry, 38:643–47, 1987.

8. Masterson J, Costello JL: *From Borderline Adolescent to Functioning Adult: The Test of Time,* New York, Brunner/Mazel, 1980.

9. Rinsley D: *Treatment of the Severely Disturbed Adolescent,* New York, Jason Aronson, 1980.

10. Bleiberg E: Stages in the treatment of narcissistic children and adolescents. Bull Menninger Clin, 51:296–313, 1987.

11. Blotcky MJ, Dimperio TL, Gossett JT:

Follow-up of children treated in psychiatric hospitals: A review of studies. Amer J Psychiatry, 141:1499, 1984.

12. Lewis M, Lewis DO, Shanok SS, Klatskin E, Osborne JR: The undoing of residential treatment: A follow-up study of 51 adolescents. J Amer Acad Child Psychiatry, 19:160–171, 1980.

13. Robson KS (ed): *The Borderline Child*, New York, McGraw Hill, 1983.

14. Adams PL, Fras I: *Beginning Child Psychiatry*, New York, Brunner/Mazel, 1988.

15. Anastasi A: *Psychological Testing*, ed. 5, New York, Macmillan, 1982.

16. Freud A: *Normality and Pathology in Childhood: Assessments of Development*, New York, International Universities Press, 1965.

17. Perry S, Cooper A, Michels R: The psychodynamic formulation: its purpose, structure, and clinical application. Amer J Psychiatry, 144:543–550, 1987.

18. Shapiro T: The psychodynamic formulation in child and adolescent psychiatry. J Amer Acad Child Adolesc Psychiatry, 28:675–680, 1989.

19. Mann J: *Time-Limited Psychotherapy*, Cambridge, Harvard University Press, 1973.

20. Winnicott DW: *The Maturational Processes and the Facilitating Environment*, New York; International Universities Press, 1965.

21. Gutheil TG: On the therapy in clinical administration: Parts 1–3. Psychiatr Q, 54:3–25, 1982.

22. Cotton NS: *Therapeutic management*, San Francisco, Jossey-Bass, to be published in 1991.

23. Popper CW: Child and adolescent psychopharmacology, in Michels R, Cavenar J, et al. (eds): *Psychiatry*, Philadelphia, J.B. Lippincott, 1985.

24. Nakhla F, Folkart L, Webster J: Treatment of families as inpatients. Fam Process, 8:79–86, 1969.

25. American Academy of Child and Adolescent Psychiatry: *Facts for Families*, Washington D.C., American Academy of Child and Adolescent Psychiatry, 1989.

26. Koman SL: Conducting short-term inpatient multiple family groups, in Mirkin MP, Koman SL (eds): *Handbook of Adolescent and Family Therapy*, New York, Gardner Press, 1985.

27. Palmer AJ, Harper G, Rivinus TM: The "Adoption Process" in the inpatient treatment of children and adolescents. J Amer Acad Child Psychiatry, 22:286–293, 1983.

28. Erikson JM: *Activity, Recovery, Growth: The Communal Role of Planned Activities*, New York, Norton, 1976.

29. Bettelheim B: *A Home for the Heart*, New York, Knopf, 1974.

30. American Psychiatric Association: *Psychiatric Inpatient Treatment of Children*, Baltimore, Lord Baltimore Press, 1957.

31. Barker P: *The Residential Psychiatric Treatment of Children*, New York, Wiley & Sons, 1974.

32. Wiener, JM: The challenge: Need and efficacy, perceived and demonstrated, in Inpatient Child and Adolescent Psychiatry. Paper presented at Annual Meeting, American Academy of Child and Adolescent Psychiatry, New York, October 11, 1989.

33. American Academy of Child and Adolescent Psychiatry: *Facts for Families*, Washington, D.C., American Academy of Child and Adolescent Psychiatry, 1989.

34. Offer D, et al.: Epidemiology of mental health and mental illness among adolescents, in Call J, et al. (ed): *Basic Handbook of Child Psychiatry*, vol. 5, New York, Basic Books, 1987.

The Clinical Laboratory

Peter Herridge, MD
Joel R. L. Ehrenkranz, MD
A. Carter Pottash, MD
Mark S. Gold, MD

INTRODUCTION

This chapter reviews the clinical laboratory, its use in evaluating the patient with psychiatric disease and its role in monitoring psychiatric treatment. The chapter is organized into three sections: using the laboratory in the differential diagnosis of patients with altered mental status; evaluating medical complications in psychiatric disease; and monitoring psychiatric treatment and its complications. The chapter is intended as a practical guide and based on the authors' extensive clincial experience. The laboratory services discussed are in standard practice and routinely available. No esoteric and research tests of unproven utility in clinical practice, such as measuring endorphin levels in biological fluids or hair radioimmunoassay for drugs of abuse (1–4), are included. The chapter is directed toward the psychiatric clinician responsible for evaluating and treating patients with psychiatric disease. It assumes only a basic understanding of internal medicine and its

subspecialties. Recommendations on when to seek specialty consultation, based on abnormal lab tests, are made.

DIFFERENTIAL DIAGNOSIS OF THE PATIENT WITH PSYCHIATRIC DISEASE

Brain mechanisms that subserve mood, cognition, and thought are exquisitely sensitive to dysfunction caused by systemic factors. These include pharmacologic and environmental toxins, endocrine and metabolic imbalances, nutritional deficiencies, infectious and immunologic factors, organ system dysfunction, and neurologic disease. Accordingly, the evaluation of every patient with psychiatric disease begins with a comprehensive physical examination, including detailed medical, psychiatric, and drug history; measurement of height, weight, and vital signs; and thorough examination of all organ systems. The physical exam generates a differential diagnosis. Correct use of the laboratory involves confirming or eliminating elements from this differential. Unfortunately, because psychiatric symptoms and signs are rarely specific, the lab is crucial for identifying whether, for instance, paranoia is secondary to thyrotoxicosis, amphetamine abuse, or schizophrenia.

Toxicology

The ongoing epidemic of substance abuse requires that every psychiatric patient be screened for substance abuse. Not only are abused drugs a common cause of psychiatric symptoms, their use is frequently encountered in patients with a primary psychiatric disease. All psychiatric patients at the time of their initial evaluation, during periods of symptom exacerbation, and with the onset of new psychiatric symptoms must be screened for the following classes of drugs: amphetamines, barbiturates, benzodiazepines, opiates, cocaine, glutethimide, placidyl, phencyclidine (PCP), cannabinoids, and ethanol. It is important that the laboratory provide comprehensive screening within each class of drugs in order that Xanax abuse, for example, is detected in the benzodiazepine screen and oxycodone use is detected in the opiate screen. Additionally, the laboratory should provide quantitative screening results based upon the sensitivity of the lab method used. The laboratory must not establish arbitrary cutoffs and report as positive only those specimens with drugs in excess of an arbitrary cutoff. For instance, no known human physiologic condition is associated with benzoylecgonine, the primary cocaine metabolite, in the urine. Accordingly every urine specimen that contains benzoylecgonine, no matter what the concentration, is clinically significant. Arguments whether low concentrations could result from passive exposure, such as breathing in exhaled air from a crack smoker, are also irrelevant in this regard. Whether or not the individual

willfully ingested drugs, the drug still affects the central nervous system. With the exception of alcohol, urine is the biological fluid of choice for documenting previous illicit drug use (5). Unfortunately, urine is not useful for indicating acute toxicity nor do urine drug concentrations correlate with the degree of impairment. In comparison, blood is a good indicator of acute toxicity and is used primarily to determine whether the person is under the influence of alcohol or abused drugs at the time of examination. Although alcohol can be measured in urine as well, methodologic problems caused by alcohol's prompt excretion and volatility commonly result in false negative results and are not reliable (6). To diagnose chronic alcohol abuse, other lab studies that reflect chronic alcohol exposure and toxicity, such as mean red blood cell volume and liver function tests, are of some value (7).

Drug testing in psychiatry involves initial screening of the urine specimen for categories of drugs described above using immunoassay procedures. All immunoassay methods, including enzyme-linked (EMIT), fluorescent polarization (FPIA), and radioimmune assays (RIAs) have clinically comparable sensitivity and specificity. Because immunoassays cannot reliably distinguish over-the-counter compounds such as appetite suppressants, decongestants, or poppy seeds from drugs of abuse, all immunoassay positives must be confirmed by the extremely sensitive and specific assay method, gas chromatography/mass spectroscopy (GCMS) (8). Assay methods, such as thin layer chromatography, are useful only in the emergency screening of a biological fluid for a potential toxin; because of poor sensitivity and lack of quantification, such crude methods are rarely required.

GCMS confirmation of all immunoassay positives will eliminate virtually all false positive screening results. However, false negative drug tests are a more commonly encountered problem (Table 13.1).

Table 13.1.   Reported Methods for Urine Sample Tampering in Drug Testing

Tampering Agent	Assay Affected	Detection Method
Sample Substitution (e.g., diet Mountain Dew[R], Gatorade[R], bogus urine)	All	Peak detecting urinary thermometer
Sample dilution	All	Peak detecting urinary thermometer, creatinine, specific gravity
Vinegar	EMIT marijuana	pH
Table salt	EMIT amphetamines	Specific gravity
	EMIT barbiturates	
	EMIT cocaine	
	EMIT opiates	
	EMIT benzodiazepines	
	EMIT PCP	
Oxidizing agents (e.g., bleach)	EMIT amphetamines	Peak detecting urinary thermometer
	EMIT barbiturates	
	EMIT cocaine	
	EMIT opiates	
	EMIT marijuana	
	RIA amphetamines	Peak detecting urinary thermometer
	RIA opiates	
	RIA PCP	
	FPIA amphetamines	Peak detecting urinary thermometer
	FPIA opiates	
	FPIA PCP	
	FPIA marijuana	
Liquid drain cleaner (e.g., Drano[R])	EMIT amphetamines	pH ± peak detecting urinary thermometer
	EMIT barbiturates	
	EMIT cocaine	
	EMIT opiates	
	EMIT marijuana	
Golden-Seal Tea	EMIT marijuana	Specimen inspection
3H	All RIAs	Negative control assay
Liquid handsoap	EMIT barbiturates	Specimen inspection
	EMIT benzodiazepines	
	EMIT marijuana	
	EMIT PCP	
Eyedrops (e.g., benzalkonium chloride)	EMIT benzodiazepines	Positive control assay
	EMIT marijuana	
	FPIA marijuana	
Bicarbonate	EMIT opiates	pH
Vitamin C	FPIA cocaine	Positive control assay
Flagy[R]	All EMIT	Negative control assay
Fluorescein dye	All FPIA	Negative control assay

Drug users will go to great lengths to generate false negative urine drug tests and thus avoid detection of their own drug use. They may substitute drug-free urine for their own or adulterate their urine with hypertonic fluids, soaps, or strong acids or bases in an effort to defeat the analytical methods used (9–13). Self-catheterization and instilling drug-free urine into the bladder before testing has even been described as a method for cheating on drug tests. Ac-cordingly, measures must be taken during urine collection for drug testing to ensure that a fresh, unadulterated specimen is in fact obtained from the individual being tested. Observed urination, practiced by the military, criminal justice systems, the Olympics, and some drug treatment programs, can be defeated. Historically, urine sample tampering appears to have originated in screening for diabetes mellitus during the course of life-insurance and pre-employment physical examinations. During World War II, military inductees would add pineapple juice to their urine to mimic glycosuria and thus avoid conscription. Ongoing federal and transporation department employee drug-testing programs are generally regarded of little value because of widespread urine sample tampering (14). Measuring peak urine temperature at the time of voiding and checking specimen pH and specific gravity (10, 13, 15), eliminates urine sample tampering as a cause of false negative drug tests. Urine temperature less than 96.4°F indicates sample substitution, while temperatures above 100.4° suggest fever, hyperthermia, or urine sample adulteration with oxidizing agents. Drug tests performed on urine specimens with pH outside the range 5–8 or specific gravity less than 1.002 or in excess of 1.040 are likely to be invalid and should be repeated. Use of nonpeak detecting temperature sensing devices, such as placing liquid crystal strips on the outside of the specimen bottle or dipping a mercury or electronic thermometer into a urine specimen are unreliable for distinguishing fresh from substituted urine (14). These methods are inappropriate for use in clinical practice.

Steroid hormone abuse represents a special form of substance abuse that may present to the psychiatrist as a primary mood or behavior problem (16). It should be suspected in all male and female athletes, especially if characteristics such as temporal balding, voice deepening, increased acne, muscular hypertrophy, or gonadal atrophy are noted. Because of the variety of self-treatment regimens steroid hormone abusers employ, obtain endocrine consultation for all suspicious steroid-abuse cases.

In addition to screening for abused drugs, perform a standard urinalysis during evaluation of every psychiatric patient. Urinalysis should include measuring specific gravity and pH, as described above, tests for hemoglobin, protein, and leukocytes, and

microscopic inspection of the urine sediment if clinically indicated.

ENVIRONMENTAL TOXINS

Many thousands of environmental toxins potentially cause psychiatric symptoms. Most of these toxins are related to industry or the products of industry. In this chapter we will discuss only some of the more common toxins that may affect psychiatric patients. These are (*a*) heavy metals—lead, mercury, manganese, arsenic, and aluminum; (*b*) pesticides; and (*c*) organic solvents; gasoline, cleaning solvents, and toluene.

HEAVY METALS

Lead is one of the msot common and perhaps most toxic heavy metal in the environment. The metal is easily absorbed, the exposure is cumulative, and the effects can be devastating especially on children (17, 18). There is good reason to believe that lead levels formerly thought to be nontoxic (< 25 ug/dl) may damage children and cause behavioral problems. This may suggest that standards of toxicity developed for use in medicine may be crude and underestimate brain or behavioral levels of toxicity. Acute lead intoxication (e.g., from eating paint chips) may cause apathy, irritability, anorexia, and encephalopathy. Testing for lead entails a blood lead level or a 24-hour urine collection. It is also possible to mobilize lead stores with a chelating agent such as calcium disodium edetate and then to perform a 24-hour urine collection. Some researchers working with children have measured lead levels in deciduous teeth. A good test for chronic lead intoxication is measuring the free erythrocyte protoporphyrin (FEP) levels.

Many other metals can cause neuropsychiatric symptoms. One commonly encountered is mercury. This metal can be absorbed through skin, inhaled, or ingested as inorganic or organic mercury-containing compounds such as fungicides. Exposure to mercury can also occur in many industrial processes and may cause psychosis, emotional lability, impaired memory, fatigue, headache, and apathy. Mercury levels are commonly measured in urine and blood.

Arsenic exposure can occur from contact with certain pesticides, rodenticides, herbicides, and other chemicals from industrial processes. Inhaling sawdust or smoke from wood treated with copper arsenate can cause considerable arsenic exposure. Although arsenic can be measured in blood, serum, urine, hair or nails, urine yields the most accurate sample for acute exposure. Arsenic poisoning can cause hyperkeratosis of the palms and soles, hair loss, fatigue, and anemia.

High serum aluminum levels may produce a dementia-like picture and can occur during renal dialysis if the water has not been cleared of aluminun. This metal may be measured in serum or urine.

Exposure to organic solvents may be deliberate (in order to "get high") or inadvertent (e.g., work-related). Chronic exposure to organic solvents may cause organic personality disorders sometimes called "solvent encephalopathy." Toluene abuse can cause loss of gray-white matter differentiation and frank brain atrophy. Other organ systems can be damaged as well, including kidney, liver, lungs, and bone marrow.

PESTICIDES

Two major types of pesticides are in common use today; chlorinated insecticides and cholinesterase inhibitor pesticides. Typical of the former group is DDT whose mechanisms of poisoning are not known. However, DDT acts chiefly on the cerebellum and motor cortex causing hyperexcitability, tremors, and convulsions. Cholinesterase inhibitors are more toxic and act by inactivation of cholinesterase which allows large amounts of acetylcholine to accumulate; effects are widespread, including po-

tentiation of postganglionic parasympathetic activity, neuromuscular block, and CNS stimulation followed by depression and convulsions.

Chronic exposure to these agents may produce various neuropsychiatric syndromes. However, little is definitely known about the precise neuropsychiatric effects of cholinesterase inhibitors. Some investigators believe that chronic exposure to cholinesterase inhibitor pesticides may in some rare individuals cause episodes of impulsive violence.

Although it may be difficult to find laboratories that can analyze these chemicals, state departments of public health can often help.

Metabolic and Endocrine Factors

ELECTROLYTES, ELEMENTS, AND METABOLITES

Determine serum concentrations of sodium, potassium, chloride, bicarbonate, urea nitrogen, creatinine, calcium, magnesium, phosphate, and glucose on every patient with psychiatric disease. Hyponatremia (i.e., serum sodium less than 135 meq/liter) which invariably produces fatigue and depression, may be a sign of neurologic, endocrine, cardiac, liver, or renal disease; water intoxication; or diuretic abuse. Hypernatremia (sodium greater than 145) produces confusion and encephalopathy and indicates underlying neurologic disease or overmedication. Hypokalemia (serum K+ less than 3.5) is often associated with general weakness and usually indicates diuretic or steroid excess. Bothy hypo- and hyper- (greater than 5.5) kalemia may be signs of endocrine or renal disease. Low concentrations of chloride (less than 95) also are associated with generalized weakness and suggest diuretic use or prolonged vomiting. Low serum bicarbonate frequently results in anxiety and suggests underlying medical illness or significant prescription drug use.

Low urea nitrogen suggests malnutrition, while elevations in urea nitrogen are associated with dehydration. When accompanied by an elevated creatinine, an elevated BUN (blood urea nitrogen) suggests renal disease. Patients with these metabolic abnormalities may present with fatigue and depression. Low serum calcium and magnesium, frequently found in malnourished or alcholic patients, produces anxiety and increased muscle tone and cramping. Low serum magnesium may also produce depression and organic brain syndrome-like (OBS) symptoms. Even mild elevations in serum calcium produce depression. Patients found to have abnormalities in the serum concentration of electrolytes, elements, or metabolites should have prompt medical consultation.

Hyperglycemia, defined as a fasting blood sugar over 140 mg/% or a random blood sugar in excess of 200 mg/%, indicates glucose intolerance. This may signify diabetes mellitus or other conditions associated with glucose intolerance, such as obesity, Cushing's syndrome, pheochromocytoma, acromegaly, or diuretic use. Hyperglycemia produces fatigue and listlessness and may present as depression.

Hypoglycemia, defined as a blood sugar less than 40 mg/%, is a life-threatening condition associated with characteristic neurologic signs and symptoms that are promptly relieved (i.e., within minutes) by ingesting glucose. Hypoglycemia is markedly overdiagnosed in psychiatry and almost never accounts for food intolerances or vague and nonspecific meal-related complaints of depression, irritability, restlessness, or fatigue (19). In fact, a chief complaint of "hypoglycemia" by a patient is almost diagnostic of psychiatric and not metabolic disease. To rule out hypoglycemia, draw a blood sugar at the time of the patient's symptoms. If the blood sugar is less than 40 mg/%, endocrine evaluation is indicated. If the value is greater than 40, re-assurance is all that is required. Never order a glucose tolerance test to evaluate suspected hypoglycemia; an abrupt fall in blood sugar—termed "reactive hypoglycemia"—any time after the second hour, even to levels less than 40, is a normal variant and of no clinical concern.

THYROID DISEASE AND THE TRH STIMULATION TEST

In 1972, Prange et al. first reported a blunted TSH (thyroid-stimulating hormone) response to TRH (thyrotropin-releasing hormone) in euthyroid depressed women. Since then this finding has been repeatedly confirmed and seems to occur in approximately 25% of otherwise healthy depressed patients (20).

The test is generally performed by injecting 500 ug of TRH intravenously at time zero. Serum TSH levels are then measured at baseline and at intervals from 15–90 minutes thereafter. In most individuals TSH peaks at approximately 25 minutes postinjection. The greatest change in TSH from baseline to maximum value is called Δ max TSH. Most investigators have defined a blunted response as a Δ max TSH of less than 5.0 uIU/ml. Subclinical hypothyroidism (a commonly overlooked cause of depression) is identified by an incremental TSH rise of greater than 35 miu/ml in a patient who may also have a goiter and circulating antithyroid antibodies or euthyroid forms of hyperthyroidism (characterized as an incremental rise of 0 miu/ml TSH) can be diagnosed. Preliminary evidence suggests that patients whose Δ max is greater than normal may be less responsive to tricyclic antidepressants.

The TRH stimulation test directly measures the responsiveness of the pituitary thyrotroph cells to stimulation by TRH. In patients with thyroid disorder this is the most sensitive possible index of hypo- or hyperthyroidism, and, of course, the original purpose of the TRH stimulation test is to determine thyroid status. The precise cause of a blunted Δ max TSH in euthyroid depressed patients is unknown. However, this finding has been used as a research and clinical tool in the differential diagnosis of psychiatric illness for many years. When used to confirm a psychiatric diagnosis the test has many serious limitations which must be carefully taken into account in order to obtain a useful result. Its first limitations is its low sensitivity of approximately 25%. This renders the test less useful in populations either likely or very unlikely to have mood disorder. Limted sensitivity also makes the TRH stimulation test absolutely unsuitable as a screening test for affective disorder in any population. Whether or not the results of the TRH test are valid for detecting depression in adolescents is unclear, unlike the DST (dexamethasone suppression test) (21).

Medical illness and recent medication use may seriously affect the TRH stimulation test. The most obvious problem is the presence of any thyroid disorder; even mild hyperthyroidism will cause a blunted response. Other factors that may influence the TRH test are age, gender, chronic renal failure, Klinefelter's syndrome, recent weight loss, dementia, repeated administration of TRH, and recent administration of thyroid hormone, glucocorticoids, somatostatin, and dopamine.

While the test is apparently not affected by tricyclic antidepressants or neuroleptics, chronic lithium administration can increase the TSH response after TRH most likely through its direct antithyroid activity. This test may have utility in early diagnosis of lithium-induced hypothyroidism. Several commonly used drugs can cause blunting of the TSH response, including steroids, aspirin, barbiturates, opiates, cocaine, amphetamines, theophylline, and bromocriptine.

Of course, detailed knowledge of a patient's medical history and recent use of medications or drugs of abuse is essential before even considering using the TRH stimulation test to assess mood disorders.

TRH TEST IN OTHER PSYCHIATRIC DISORDERS

In addition to depression, several other psychiatric disorders are associated with a blunted TSH response to TRH in some patients.

Alcoholism

Approximately 50% of patients in acute alcohol withdrawal show blunting of the TSH response. However, in about one-third of alcoholic patients the blunting may persist long after all withdrawal symptoms have remitted. Thus, blunting may be a trait marker in alcoholism.

Borderline Personality Disorder

Several investigations have found a blunted TSH response in patients with borderline personality disorder. In at least some of these patients there were no depressive symptoms at the time of testing or in the past and no history of substance abuse.

Mania

Several investigators have studied the TSH response in mania. One study found that 18 out of 30 mania patients had a blunted response (Δ max TSH less than 7.0 uIU/ml).

Schizophrenia

Most investigators have found that schizophrenic patients rarely have a blunted TSH response to TRH injection. In one study 31 of 41 unipolar depressed patients (76%) showed a blunted response, but only one of 14 schizophrenic patients did.

CLINICAL USE OF THE TRH STIMULATION TEST

The phenomena of blunting of TSH response to TRH administration is of great theoretical interest and an important investigative tool. For the clinician this test has two uses. As a marker of mood disorder, the blunting phenomena can be useful in diagnosing carefully selected patients if the results are thoughtfully evaluated in the full clinical context. However, after many years of extensive clinical experience with the test and a careful review of the literature, we believe that the greatest use for the TRH stimulation test in the psychiatric population is its ability to detect extremely subtle thyroid disease which may otherwise go undetected; thus the test may play an important role in diagnosing and treating many patients. For example, even a marginally elevated Δ TSH on a TRH stimulation test may indicate subclinical hypothyroidism. We routinely obtain both antithyroid and antimicrosomal antibodies on patients with elevated Δ TSH. The presence of subclinical hypothyroidism may be a major factor in treatment resistant depression.

Because thyroid function disorders are the most common treatable medical cause for psychiatric disease, thorough laboratory testing of thyroid function is indicated in every psychiatric evaluation. Although the symptoms of hypothyroidism include depression, fatigue, lightheadedness, memory loss, dementia, jocularity, changes in personality, confusion, and altered mental status, these symptoms are by no means specific. Additionally, although the manifestations of hyperthyroidism may include restlessness, anxiety, insomnia, irritability, paranoia, weakness, personality intensification or apathy, these manifestations are also variable and not diagnostic. Accordingly, it is our practice to measure indices of both hyper- and hypothyroidism, including total T_4 concentration, T_3 resin uptake (an index of thyroid binding globulin concentration), total T_3 concentration, and TSH levels, routinely in all patients' initial evaluation.

Although interpreting thyroid function tests is usually straightforward, medication effects that interfere with T_4 binding or T_4 to T_3 conversion, malnutrition associated with the euthyroid sick syndrome (low T_3 RIA, low/normal T_4, normal/slightly elevated TSH), and subtle forms of thyroiditis can complicate thyroid function test interpretation. Accordingly, we obtain endocrine evaluation on all patients found to have abnormal thyroid function.

The first laboratory sign of primary (as opposed to pituitary or hypothalamic induced) hypothyroidism is an exaggerated TSH response to TRH. Some call this stage "subclinical" hypothyroidism. Next, is an elevated basal TSH level, followed by a low T_4 and decreased free thyroid index (defined as $T_4 \times T_3$ resin uptake). Finally, a low T_3 RIA is encountered. In hyperthyroidism, first is a flat TSH response to TRH, followed by an elevated T_3 and then an elevated free thyroid index. In hyperthyroidism, a suppressed level of TSH is only seen when ultrasensitive assays of TSH are employed; otherwise TSH concentration in hyperthyroidism falls into the normal range. Approximately 20% of acutely ill psychiatric patients hospitalized on an inpatient psychiatric unit will present with elevations in T_4 and free thyroid index at the time of admission (22). This is usually transient and not associated with increased levels of T_3 by RIA or accompanied by other signs of thyrotoxicosis. It is important that the psychiatric clinician recognize this entity to insure that appropriate endocrine evaluation is obtained.

ADRENAL DISEASE

Both hyper- and hypocortisolism may present as a primary psychiatric disturbance. In fact, Harvey Cushing, who discovered the syndromes of adrenal hypersecretion, found his first series of patients with bilateral adrenal hyperplasia secondary to a basophilic adenoma of the anterior pituitary. He was working with inpatients from the Northampton, Massachusetts, State Mental Hospital (23). Although classic endocrine clinical teaching suggests that endogenous hypercortisolism presents as mania and exogenous (i.e., secondary to medication) hypercortisolism as depression, the symptoms of hypercortisolism are in no way specific. Any patient with a mood disorder, obesity, hypertension, glucose intolerance, or cutaneous stigmata of steroid excess should be screened for hypercortisolism. Screening is conveniently done through an overnight endocrine dexamethasone suppression test. One mg of dexamethasone is given p.o. at midnight and a single serum specimen drawn at 8 AM the next morning. Cushing's Syndrome is ruled out if this value is less than 5 micrograms %. Unfortunately, frequent false positive results are encountered, especially in a psychiatric population, because depression, alcoholism, liver disease, and a variety of medications can all yield 8-AM values in excess of 5 mcg % despite otherwise normal adrenal function. Because the evaluation of the patient with suspect hypercortisolism is intricate, we advise endocrine evaluation of all patients whose 8-AM serum cortisol exceeds 5 mcg % after 1 mg of dexamethasone at midnight.

Adrenal insufficiency may present as chronic fatigue and depression. Acute adrenal insufficiency has on occasion been misdiagnosed as a severe bereavement reaction (24). This diagnosis is based on a low AM serum cortisol level (less than 5 mcg %) and an insufficient cortisol rise in response to exogenously administered ACTH (adrenocorticotropic hormone). Consider the diagnosis of adrenal insufficiency and order appropriate lab tests in patients with otherwise unexplained weight loss and depression, especially when accompanied by hyponatremia or hyperkalemia.

THE DEXAMETHASONE SUPPRESSION TEST

During the past 10 years the dexamethasone suppression test has become the most extensively studied biological test in psychiatry. It is widely used to evaluate overactivity of the hypothalamic pituitary adrenal axis in psychiatric patients with a variety of diagnoses. Numerous reviews of the test exist in the literature (25, 26). Because so much clinical experience with the DST has accumulated it is now possible to be more precise and realistic about the current status of the test.

Method. The procedure most widely used for administering the DST for psychiatric purposes begins with oral administration of 1.0 mg of the potent synthetic steroid dexamethasone at 11:00 PM on day one. Dexamethasone administration should suppress the release of plasma cortisol for at least 24 hours by blocking release of corticotropin-releasing factor (CRF) from the hypothalamus and ACTH from the anterior pituitary. On day two, plasma cortisol levels are sampled at various times. The most common sampling times are 8:00 AM, 4:00 PM, and 11:00 PM. Other sampling times may be used; in fact, an elevated plasma cortisol level in any blood sample drawn between 9 and 24 hours after administering dexamethasone indicates a failure of normal suppression of cortisol levels and is an abnormal or positive result. A cortisol level above 5 ug/dl or 50 ng/ml is generally considered to constitute an elevated level.

A recent study suggests that the diagnostic utility of the DST can be significantly increased by expressing serum cortisol as a function of serum dexamethasone (27). This technique helps control for individual variations in dexamethasone pharmacokinetics and may have considerable promise.

There seems to be consensus that when properly performed in selected patients the DST can be useful in evaluating and assessing treatment response of patients with psychiatric illness. However, the sensitivty of the test is fairly low, its predictive power is limited, and many drugs, medications, and medical conditions may interfere with its results. It seems that Carroll summed it up well when he wrote in 1988 that "the DST is a promising beginning in psychiatry . . . , but one must expect and hope that better tests eventually will replace it."

Perhaps the most comprehensive overview of the current status of the DST comes from the review performed by the APA Task Force on Laboratory Tests in Psychiatry (25). The task force concluded that the rate of a positive outcome or nonsuppression of cortisol in patients with major depression was 40–50%. The rate of nonsuppression may be higher (60–70%) in patients with very severe affective disorder, especially if psychotic symptoms are present, including mania and schizoaffective disorder.

In normal controls the specificity or true negative outcome of the DST is high and may be above 90%. However, it may be considerably worse than this and perhaps below 70% in psychiatric patients with a wide variety of diagnoses including dementia.

Acute treatment with antidepressants, neuroleptics, or lithium may stimulate HPA (hypothalamic-pituitary-adrenal) axis secretion enough to cause a false positive DST result in some patients. On the other hand, chronic use of tricyclic antidepressants, neuroleptics, or alcohol may, in time, produce false negative DST results. Anticonvulsants, carbamazepine, and estrogens often produce false positive DST results; even cold medication, oral contraceptives, large amounts of caffeine, and minor illness may do the same (28).

DST nonsuppression may exist for up to three weeks following abrupt discontinuation of antidepressants, lithium, neuroleptics, benzodiazepines or alcohol. This may also occur following withdrawal of narcotics, sympathomimetics, anticholinergics, antihistamines or MAOIs (monoamine oxidase inhibitors). Although nicotine use may affect the DST, little data supports this. Clearly, in order to assess the validity of a DST result, it is essential to know in detail the patient's recent use of psychotropic medications; all other medications, including over-the-counter drugs; drugs of abuse, including alcohol; caffeine; and nicotine (29).

Does the DST have significant predictive power in mood disorders? Unfortunately the available literature suggests that although the DST may be useful, the test's predictive power is less than originally hoped for. To be specific, a positive initial DST result does not seem to increase significantly the likelihood of antidepressant response. Because of the test's limited sensitivity, a negative test result is a virtually useless indication for deciding whether or not to treat with antidepressants. However, patients who are DST-positive may be significantly less likely to respond to a placebo than DST-negative patients. Perhaps the most intriguing possibility is the likelihood that a DST-positive patient who fails to convert to normal suppression of cortisol after an apparent clinical recovery from depression may be at increased risk for early relapse or suicidal behavior.

The DST appears to be as valid and useful a test for depression in adolescents as it is in adults (30, 31). This can be extremely useful in the differential diagnosis of an adolescent with conduct disorder-like behavior who does not fully meet the criteria for major depression. As most clinicians know, depression may often present in an atypical or masked manner in adolescents. In our experience the ability of the DST to help support a diagnosis of depression in these cases has been its most useful clinical service.

The DST can also be performed using saliva instead of plasma. Comparison studies of plasma and cortisol DST results suggest that this method may be reliable enough to use clinically when use of plasma is not possible (32).

Diseases of the adrenal medulla associated with excess catecholamine production may also present to the psychiatrist. Pheochromocytoma can manifest as paroxysmal episodes of anxiety that may mimic a panic attack or generalized anxiety disorder. The triad of paroxysmal headaches, sweats, and palpitations in association with hypertension or arrhythmias suggests catecholamine excess. The traditional screening test for pheochromocytoma is to measure 24-hour urinary excretion of a battery of catecholamine metabolites, including VMA (vanillylmandelic acid), metanephrine, norepinephrine, and epinephrine. Although assay methodologies currently in use do not require dietary restriction, false positive screens from prescription drugs, such as beta blockers, or acute stress are not infrequent. Patients with elevated urinary catecholamine levels should be referred for additional endocrine investigation.

GONADAL DYSFUNCTION

As the understanding of the biological basis for sexual function increases, the need increases for psychiatrists to evaluate a potential medical cause for decreased libido or impotence in the male or anhedonia, anorgasism, or hypersexuality in the female. At a minimum, obtain serum testosterone, prolactin, thyroid function tests, and glucose measurements to rule out the most common causes of male sexual dysfunction. Although the endocrine basis for decreased libido is less well understood in the female than in the male, as a rule if a woman is having regular ovulatory menstrual cycles, the likelihood of underlying endocrine disease is small. On the other hand, however, increased libido and hypersexuality in a woman is often a sign of androgen excess; measure serum testosterone and DHEA-S* (the major adrenal androgen) and perform an overnight DST.

NUTRITIONAL DEFICIENCY

During the 19th century, pellagra was a frequent cause of chronic psychiatric disease (33). Fortunately, niacin and other nutritional deficiencies are now rare causes of psychiatric disease. However, clinicians should keep in mind the possibility of vitamin deficiencies producing psychiatric symptoms in patients with starvation and malnutrition secondary to anorexia or bulimia nervosa, alcoholism, pica, or social deprivation. B_{12} deficiency represents a difficult diagnostic challenge to this day; patients with B_{12} deficiency may lack objective evidence of the problem (34). Specifically, these patients may lack megaloblastosis, hypersegmented polymorphonuclear leukocytes, or low serum B_{12} levels, measured by RIA. However, such patients tend to demonstrate other clinical factors, such as absent gastric tissue, terminal ileum, or antibodies to intrinsic factor, suggesting the diagnosis. It is our practice to measure B_{12} levels in patients exhibiting any of the above clinical features, which may include depression or atypical psychosis, and treat for B_{12} deficiency even if serum levels measured by RIA are in the low-normal range.

Although serum vitamin profiles can be measured commercially, we have found these assays to be unreliable. Based on clinical suspicion, we treat psychiatric patients with vitamin supplements; we routinely administer B_1 with glucose, folic acid, and vitamin K to most, if not all, chronic alcoholic patients. There is little risk in supplementing vitamins in patients at risk for vitamin deficiencies.

---

*dehydroepiandroepiandrosterone-sulfate

Infectious Disease

Although many infectious illnesses have neuropsychiatric manifestations, these are usually acute in onset, rapidly progressive, associated by systemic signs, accompanied by a clouded sensorium, and rarely present as a primary psychiatric disturbance. However, certain infections—such as HIV, syphilis, viral encephalopathy, Lyme disease, and brain abscess—have a primary psychiatric component as a presenting feature.

Perform HIV tests on every psychiatric patient in the following categories (35):

1. Men who have had active or passive oral or anal sexual intercourse with other men.
2. People who have shared needles or other paraphernalia related to injecting drugs that might have been contaminated with blood.
3. People who have had sexual intercourse (vaginal, oral, or anal) with individuals known or suspected of having AIDS or HIV infection.
4. People who have engaged in sex for drugs or money.
5. People who have had, or may have had, sexual intercourse with individuals in any of the above categories.
6. People who have received blood or blood products (not including immune serum globulin or albumin) between 1978 and mid-1985, particularly those who received multiple units of blood or blood products or products containing pooled blood from multiple donors.
7. Psychiatric patients with a history of:
   a. Tuberculosis
   b. Any sexually transmitted disease between 1975 and the present
   c. Hepatitis B or non-A, non-B hepatitis
   d. Dementia
8. Women of high risk groups who are planning pregnancy or who are pregnant.

In some states informed consent and counselling must precede HIV testing. HIV testing routinely uses serum and is screened with an ELISA (enzyme linked immunosorbent assay) immunoassay. Positives are confirmed with Western blot analysis. All individuals who test positive for HIV antibodies should be referred for counselling and medical evaluation.

Diagnosing viral dementia or brain abscess as a cause for psychopathology relies upon radiographic, neurodiagnostic, and cerebrospinal fluid analysis. All cases in which an infectious etiology on clinical grounds is considered should have medical and neurological evaluation.

Tertiary syphilis, previously one of the major treatable causes of psychiatric illness, will be seen more frequently because of the changing epidemiology of sexually transmitted disease. Every psychiatric patient at the time of initial evaluation should be screened for syphilis with either VDRL (Veneral Disease Research Laboratories) or RPR (rapid plasmin reagin) testing. If positive, perform FTA (fluorescent treponemal antibody) testing to rule out false positives, such as occurs with other treponemal or rheumatological disease. Medically evaluate all FTA-positive patients.

Lyme disease, particularly when chronic, can present with depression or dementia. Suspect Lyme disease in patients with significant antibody titers to the etiologic agent for Lyme disease, Borrelia burgdorferi. If antibodies are present, medically evaluate the patient.

A number of newly specified presumptively infectious clinical entities, including systemic candidiasis and chronic fatigue syndrome from Epstein-Barr virus infection, have been described as causing chronic psychiatric complaints, particularly depression. These syndromes are not accepted as discrete clinical entities at this time and laboratory evaluation does not appear to be indicated.

Rheumatologic Disease

Systemic lupus erythematosus may present as psychiatric disease. It is characteristically associated with an abnormal electroencaphelogram (EEG) and other laboratory manifestations of vasculitis, such as an elevated erythrocyte sedimentation rate (ESR) and decreased complement levels; renal or hematological impairment are usually apparent. In patients with lupus and concurrent psychiatric complaints, a normal EEG and ESR will rule out lupus cerebritis as a cause of psychiatric symptoms.

Gastrointestinal Disease

Hepatic encephalopathy may present to the psychiatrist as depression or dementia; perform liver function testing, including AST[a] (SGOT)[b], ALT[c] (SGPT)[d], LDH[e], gamma glutamyl transaminase, alkaline phosphatase, and bilirubin measurement on all patients who present for psychiatric evaluation, independent of whether a history of alcohol abuse is present.

Wilson's disease, an autosomal recessive deficit in ceruloplasmin synthesis, includes hepatic, psychiatric, and neurologic manifestations. In a patient with abnormal liver function tests and a movement disorder, Wilson's disease is easily excluded by measuring the serum concentration of ceruloplasmin.

Acute intermittent porphyria is a well-known cause of intermittent psychosis (36). It is traditionally associated with acute abdominal pain and peripheral neuropathy. During an attack, 24-hour urine concentration of delta aminolevulinic acid and porphobilinogen is increased. During and in between attacks, erythrocyte uroporphyrin-ogen-1-synthetase, a red blood cell enzyme, is decreased. This is a convenient marker for porphyria in otherwise asymptomatic individuals.

Hematological Disease and Malignancy

Hematological disorders encountered by the psychiatrist include anemia and malignancies. A complete blood count and differential should be obtained on every patient with psychiatric complaints. If low hemoglobin or hematocrit is encountered, measure iron, B_{12}, and folate levels.

Malignancies may produce psychiatric symptoms through a number of mechanisms, including weight loss and malnutrition, electrolyte abnormalities, brain metastases, or as a paraneoplastic phenomenon. CBC, electrolytes and minerals, liver chemistries, ESR, and serum protein concentrations are reasonable laboratory screening tests for underlying malignancy in psychiatric patients, in addition, of course, to the history physical exam and any indicated radiological testing.

Organ Failure

Altered mental status and associated psychiatric complaints frequently accompany renal, cardiac, and pulmonary disease. Dysfunction of these organ systems is diagnosed during the physical examination or with routine laboratory studies.

Genetic Disease

Among children and adolescents, psychiatric symptoms, including antisocial behavior, personality and conduct disorder, and arrested psychosocial development may be the initial manifestations of chromosomal abnormalities or inborn errors of metabolism. To screen for genetic syndromes, obtain a karyotype with Giemsa banding. This need only be done once dur-

---

[a] aspartate aminotransferase
[b] serum glutamic-oxaloacetic transaminase
[c] alanine aminotransferase
[d] serum glutamic-pyruvic transaminase
[e] lactate dehydrogenase

ing a patient's life. Consider inborn errors of metabolism when a dysmorphic appearance, skeletal, cardiac, hepatic, or other congenital anomalies are encountered. Refer such patients for appropriate speciality evaluation.

Neurological Disease

The subject of neurological disease is an extensive one and largely beyond the scope of this chapter. However, several neurological syndromes are of great interest to the psychiatrist because they can present with primarily psychiatric symptoms. These are:

1. Degenerating—demyelinating disease
2. Seizure disorders—especially temporal lobe epilepsy
3. Structural lesions—AVMs (arteriovenous malformations), tumors, strokes, hematomas
4. Infectious agents—brain abscesses, some viral infections

If any element of the history, physical exam, or clinical presentation suggests the possibility of neurological disease the psychiatric clinician has several tools available. The most commonly used are magnetic resonance imaging (MRI), computed tomography (CT), and several types of EEGs.

The indication for ordering an MRI or CT scan in a psychiatric patient are broad and include:

1. Focal neurologic finding or confusion, delirium or impaired cognition on mental status exam
2. Abnormal EEG or history of seizures
3. Onset of mood disorder or personality change after midlife (age 45)
4. First psychotic episodes
5. History of significant head trauma
6. Anorexia nervosa, movement disorder, or catatonia

Although the MRI is relatively new technology and considerable experimental work needs to be done, it seems to be superior to the CT in several important ways. The MRI may be better able to image the changes of demyelinating disorders and dementia and to evaluate seizure focii especially of the temporal lobe. The CT may be superior to the MRI in evaluating pituitary lesions or calcified lesions or subarachnoid or parenchymal hemorrhages (37).

THE ELECTROENCEPHALOGRAM

The EEG has for many years been a useful tool in the differential diagnosis of psychiatric and organic mental disorders. However, the EEG is an insensitive and rather nonspecific test and must be interpreted with caution. For example, even a sleep-deprived EEG may have less than a 20% chance of detecting seizure activity in a patient with known temporal lobe epilepsy. The likelihood of detecting this and other subtle seizure disorders may be increased by repeated EEGs or a 24-hour ambulatory EEG recording which can include video recordings to document seizure activity.

The EEG may be very useful in differentiating between organic delirium and functional psychiatric illness. Although the EEG may also be a helpful test in cases of dementia, strokes, tumors or subdural hematomas, the sensitivity and specificity are low in these conditions.

The use of the sleep-deprived EEG and nasopharyngeal leads may well increase the sensitivity of the test to seizure disorders.

Sleep EEG or polysomnography have value for the psychiatric clinician as aids with nocturnal penile tumescence tests and in diagnosing affective and sleep disorders and some types of sexual dysfunction.

Although the relatively new technology of CT mapping of EEG data is an exciting research tool, generally accepted clinical applications are not clear at this time.

MONITORING MEDICAL COMPLICATIONS OF PSYCHIATRIC ILLNESS

Abnormal patterns of behavior resulting from ongoing psychiatric disease can affect every organ system and produce medical complications. Eventually overt clinical manifestations will develop, however. The clinical laboratory can provide early objective evidence and confirmatory data that systemic pathology secondary to psychiatric disease is ongoing. Clinical laboratory aspects of acute, life-threatening psychiatric complications such as overdose, asphyxiation, or lacerations are outside the scope of this chapter.

Substance Abuse

The clinical pathology of substance abuse is extensive and new complications are described regularly. Intravenous substance abuse, independent of the drugs abused, is associated with acute infections, including hepatitis, endocarditis, sepsis, osteomyelitis, and abscess formation; opportunistic infection, including HIV, TB, fungal, and parasitic etiologies; and venereal disease. Vascular and embolic diseases are also a direct complication of parenteral substance abuse. Screen every substance abuser for infectious complications, with a comprehensive physical examination, RPR/VDRL, HIV, and hepatitis testing. Hepatitis testing requires the screening of serum for hepatitis B, non-A, non-B, and E antibody and antigen.

Substance abuse, especially alcohol and inhalant abuse, is frequently associated with hematologic abnormalities. These can be direct toxic effects, such as ethanol-induced bone marrow suppression; nutritional effects as seen, for example, in folic acid deficiency secondary to malnutrition in heroin addicts; or secondary to organ dysfunction, such as with thrombocytopenia secondary to splenomegaly caused by alcoholic cirrhosis. Accordingly, measure of liver function and CBCs are part of the laboratory evaluation of every patient with a history of substance abuse.

Other organ systems affected via abused substance toxicity include reproductive endocrine effects such as unwanted pregnancy, pseudocyesis, hyperprolactinemia, hypogonadism, oligospermia, and anovulation. If a female psychiatric patient of reproductive age has a history of ongoing menses or potential exposure to any teratogen, perform a urine or serum pregnancy test. However, base additional laboratory investigations on the patient's history and physical examination.

Insufflation of illicit drugs, especially cocaine, is a common route of exposure, making a chest x-ray part of the routine substance-abuse workup. Because cardiac complications such as alcoholic cardiomyopathy or cocaine-induced ischemic heart disease are so frequent in substance abuse, a 12-lead EKG is part of evaluating the substance-abusing psychiatric patient. Additional cardiac testing, such as echocardiogram, Holter monitoring, or stress testing, is based upon clinical or EKG findings.

Affective Illness

Medical complications of affective illness form the basis of the panoply of syndromes encountered in psychosomatic medicine. The workup of each syndrome, whether it is colitis, gastritis, or headache, is based on the clinical presentation these patients often present to nonpsychiatric physicians.

The clinical laboratory is especially helpful in evaluating patients with affective illness associated with severe nutritional deficiencies, such as anorexia nervosa, depression, or bulimia. Measuring serum albumin, carotene, white blood cell count, and thyroid function tests are good indictors of nutritional status. Perform serum amylase, electrolytes, and fecal occult blood testing on all patients with a history of purging. Anxiety disorders, especially panic attacks, can produce not only functional laboratory abnormalities—such as elevated white blood cell count, cortisol, and prolactin levels, and hyperthyroxinemia—but may also exacerbate underlying psychiatric disease, making thyroid testing essential. Additionally, patients with anorexia nervosa or depression may have CNS mediated derangements in water metabolism, detected by measuring serum electrolytes.

Psychosis and Thought Disorders

Bizarre behavior seen in patients with thought disorders can result in a wide array of medical and surgical disease. Infectious, hematologic, endocrine, and metabolic complications, as described above with substance abuse and affective illness, also occur in psychotic patients. Additionally, severe functional abnormalities such as pica, paranoid fear of contaminated food and water, or food fetishes can yield bizarre hematologic profiles, liver chemistries, or metabolic abnormalities.

Dementia

All patients with a dementing illness should have comprehensive medical and neurological evaluations at the time of initial presentation to ensure that no treatable illness is overlooked. As the dementing process progresses, a number of complications requiring laboratory evaluation may occur. These include infections secondary to incontinence, pressure ulceration, aspiration, septicemia, and metabolic abnormalities, especially in patients unable to feed themselves. Perform CBC, chemistry screening (incluidng electrolytes, minerals, renal function, glucose, and liver enzymes), and urinalysis on a regular basis in all patients with progressive dementia.

MONITORING PSYCHIATIRC TREATMENT AND ITS COMPLICATIONS

The final major role of the clinical laboratory in psychiatry is to monitor toxic effects and complications of medications used in psychiatry.

Tricyclic Antidepressants

Electrophysiologic effects of tricyclic antidepressants on the heart represent the major source of toxicity with this group of medications. Abnormalities commonly encountered include PR and QT interval elongation, QRS widening, and rate-related ischemia. All patients started on tricyclic antidepressants after the age of forty (this does not include heterocyclic agents such as fluoxetine) should have a baseline EKG and repeat EKGs performed if cardiac symptoms occur at times of dosage increases. Perform ECG monitoring more frequently in patients with underlying heart disease. Emergency EKG monitoring is indicated in all patients with tricyclic overdose.

Hepatic, endocrine, and metabolic toxicity from tricyclic antidepressants occurs infrequently enough not to require laboratory surveillance.

The laboratory can be extremely helpful to the clinician treating a patient with antidepressants by providing plasma level measurements. According to the American Psychiatric Association Task Force on the use of laboratory tests in psychiatry (38), plasma level measurements of imipramine, desmethyl imipramine (desipramine), and nortriptyline are *unequivocally* useful in certain situations. Some of the most common are:

1. Patients showing questionable compliance

2. Patients with a poor response to normal doses of a given antidepressant
3. The existence of an important clinical reason to establish a therapeutic plasma level as soon as safely possible
4. Patients who need the lowest effective dose of the TCA (tricyclic antidepressant) because of unusual sensitivity to side effects
5. Patients who appear to experience serious side effects at a very low dose

It is also an excellent safety procedure to recheck even stable plasma antidepressant levels whenever changes are made in other medication the patients may be taking. For example, concomitant use of neuroleptics or anticonvulsants can markedly increase or decrease plasma TCA levels. Difference in bioavailability of different preparations even at the same dose may also affect plasma levels. This can be a far more powerful phenomenon than many clinicians realize if a patient changes brands of medication (39).

Many laboratories will establish plasma level ranges for most or all antidepressants, even those that do not have generally accepted therapeutic plasma levels. These ranges cannot be relied upon to dictate dose changes. However, obtaining plasma levels of any antidepressant can always be useful to (a) detect slow metabolizers who may develop extreme high levels on small doses; (b) check for compliance and monitor long-term changes in plasma levels that may result from alteration in metabolism or changes in other medications.

Blood samples for TCA levels and their antidepressants should be drawn 12 hours from the last dose. It generally requires five half-lives to establish steady state levels. This means approximately 10 days must pass on a steady dose before the measured level of a TCA can be compared to the steady state values found in the literature.

The therapeutic levels of three tricyclic antidepressants as suggested by the APA Task Force are:

1. Imipramine (sum of IMI & DMI) < 200 ng/ml
2. Nortriptyline (therapeutic window) 50–150 ng/ml
3. Desipramine < 125 ng/ml

The so-called "therapeutic window" is well-established for nortriptyline and may also occur with desipramine. However, we recommend confirming blood levels of all antidepressants after initiation of therapy for compliance.

Monoamine Oxidase Inhibitors

These agents can rarely be associated with liver function abnormalities. As with tricyclic antidepressants, the frequency of clinical laboratory abnormalities is sufficiently rare not to require regular screening. The laboratory does have a place in obtaining maximal therapeutic benefits from MAOIs. These agents may be most effective when the blood platelet MAO inhibition is greater than 80%. However, this may only be valid for phenelzine.

Major Tranquilizers

Although certain antipsychotics such as chlorpromazine produce liver function abnormalities, they are not necessarily of any clinical significance and do not require laboratory testing unless specific symptoms occur. On the other hand, other agents such as clozapine can produce such severe and life-threatening abnormalites—e.g., agranulocytosis—that mandatory CBCs are required despite the relative infrequency of severe complications. Other laboratory side effects of major tranquilizers, such as elevations in serum prolactin, are part of these drugs' basic pharmacology and should not be measured unless specific clinical indications exist. Obviously for patients with underlying or preexisting liver or cardiac disease, close monitoring of liver and cardiac function during therapy is in order.

A unique complication of major tranquilizers is the neuroleptic malignant syndrome. This acute and life-threatening drug reaction consists of hyperpyrexia, autonomic instability, basal ganglion dysfunction, and encephalopathy. Laboratory abnormalities include myopathy with an increase in serum creatine phosphokinase (CPK) and myoglobin levels. When extreme elevations in these enzymes occur, close laboratory monitoring of renal function (e.g., BUN and creatinine) is required to detect myoglobinuric renal failure. An enormous amount of information exists regarding the blood levels of various antipsychotics and their metabolites. However, at this point no consistent therapeutic levels or clear therapeutic windows for any of the antipsychotics have been established with certainty.

Lithium

Major laboratory abnormalities associated with lithium therapy include hypothyroidism, nephrogenic diabetes insipidus, and leukocytosis. The significance of lithium-induced hypothyroidism must not be underestimated or overlooked. It is our practice to screen all patients on lithium by measuring TSH at least every three months and institute T_4 therapy while maintaining the patient on lithium as soon as any rise in TSH outside the normal range occurs.

Lithium may induce thyroid function changes in 5–15% of patients on long-term lithium therapy. The likelihood of lithium-induced hypothyroidism may be increased by preexisting autoimmune thyroiditis. Therefore, determining the presence of antithyroid antibodies before instituting long-term lithium therapy may be useful, especially in patients where thyroid disease is

suspected. At times, lithium treatment may also affect parathyroid function.

Many clinicians believe that the slowly progressing hypothyroidism that lithium may cause may have profound effects on the severity and pattern of the mood disorder under treatment. Bipolar patients may cycle more rapidly and appear to be less responsive to lithium over time or they may spend more and more time in a chronic dysphoric state.

Lithium may have significant effects on kidney functions; determine BUN serum creatinine, urinalysis, and serum electrolytes before starting lithium. It is reasonable to include a creatinine clearance and a 24-hour urine volume in patients with a history of kidney disorder or when initiating long-term treatment.

Significant polyuria and polydipsia secondary to lithium-induced nephrogenic diabetes insipidus respresents a significant clinical side effect. Diabetes insipidus can be diagnosed by finding a 24-hour urine output in excess of 5 liters per day or a first morning void urine osmolarity less than 150 milliosmols/liter. If either of these are equivocal or inconsistent with clinical findings, formal dehydration testing can be performed. Perform urine and serum osmolarity and serum electrolytes and renal function tests when symptoms of polyuria or polydipsia occur in patients on lithium.

Elevations in the leukocyte count not associated with any infectious or hematologic abnormality are so common in patients on lithium that routine CBCs are not required. It is essential for any woman of child-bearing potential to receive a pregnancy test before starting lithium treatment.

Lithium may cause T-wave flattening or inversion and can cause sinus node dysfunction such as sinus arrest or sinoatrial block. All patients with any history of cardiac disease should have an EKG before lithium treatment.

The monitoring of serum lithium levels is essential for obtaining maximum therapeutic benefit. The generally accepted range of therapeutic lithium levels is 0.8–1.2 meq/liter. Acutely manic patients may improve more rapidly with higher levels such as 1.2–1.4. However, many patients, especially older ones, may begin to experience signs of toxicity at levels of 1.2 or above. Most patients have pronounced toxic symptoms at levels of 2.0 or more and levels of 3.0 or above indicate a medical emergency and require immediate medical consultation. Dialysis may be required for serious poisoning.

Lithium levels are always obtained 12 hours after the last dose. Steady state serum lithium levels are achieved in approximately five half-lives or in 5–8 days. It is our practice to start patients on 300 mg b.i.d. or t.i.d. and obtain lithium levels three times a week for the first two weeks. It is usually possible to guess accurately what dose a given patient will require after the first two levels are back even though steady state is not reached. The vast majority of healthy patients require from 1200–1800 mg total lithium per day. However, even without renal disease a few patients will obtain therapeutic levels on 900 mg or less per day. As an acute manic episode resolves, the dose required to produce a given serum level may decrease. The phenomenon may be powerful enough to produce toxic effects unless serum levels are determined during the resolution of a manic episode.

Although lithium levels of 0.6–0.8 can be effective as a maintenance dose, in most patients it makes sense to maintain levels of 0.8–1.2.

It is important to remember that various medications, especially diuretics and nonsteroidal anti-inflammatory agents, can markedly elevate serum lithium levels even to toxic levels.

Anticonvulsants

In the past decade or so the remarkable effectiveness of several anticonvulsants for treating certain psychiatric disorders has become generally recognized. Tegretol, the most widely used anticonvulsant is well established as effective for treating bipolar mood disorders and several other conditions. In the U.S. during the early 1980s, sodium valproate began to be prescribed for psychiatric patients. This medication can be very effective in treating atypical and rapid cycling bipolar disorder (40). The most recent anticonvulsant to enter common use in psychiatry is clonazepam (Klonopin). This long-acting benzodiazepine can be used to treat acute mania and is a superb medication to detoxify patients from other benzodiazepines, especially Xanax. Although all three of these drugs are fairly safe, tegretol and sodium valproate can cause potentially serious medical complications that must be carefully watched for.

TEGRETOL

Tegretol can produce aplastic anemia but the prevalence is extremely low, approximately 1/30,000. Tegretol also produces transient leukopenia in 10% of patients. Our procedure for starting a patient on tegretol is fairly typical. Pretreatment tests include CBC with platelet and reticulocyte count, liver function test, serum electrolytes, and EKG. The patients WBC count is checked every week for the first two months of treatment and every 2–3 months thereafter. If the WBC count falls below 3000/mm, tegretol is stopped and the patient observed for signs of infection and to see if the WBC count returns to normal. Any patient on tegretol should have an immediate CBC if pallor, petechiae, or any signs of infection occur.

Although tegretol rarely produces the syndrome of inappropriate antidiuretic hormone release, serum electrolytes need to be measured when suggestive clinical symptoms occur.

Tegretol can produce toxic effects on the liver with elevation of liver functions. Tegretol may also cause abnormal thyroid hormone release which may necessitate formal endocrine evaluation.

A powerful effect of tegretol is its ability to alter the metabolism of other medications. It may increase or decrease levels of other drugs to a marked degree. Because it also tends to induce its own metabolism, serum levels tend to fall at a constant dose.

The serum levels used for treating psychiatric disorders are roughly the same as the levels for treating seizure disorders. However, many clinicians believe that for treating psychiatric disorders the serum levels should be toward the high end of the therapeutic range.

SODIUM VALPROATE

The most serious medical problem resulting from using sodium valproate is hepatotoxicity which may range from mild dysfunction to fatal hepatic necrosis. Serious hepatic necrosis occurs most often in children under two years when valproate is combined with other anticonvulsants. Sodium valproate can cause bone marrow suppression and acute hemorrhage pancreatitis and may alter thyroid function tests.

Pretreatment tests should include a CBC, liver function, total protein, serum albumin, prothrombin time, partial thromboplastin time, and thyroid function. Liver functions and CBC should be checked every week for the first month, biweekly for the next three months, and then once every 3–4 months.

Levels used to treat psychiatric illness should run toward the high end of the therapeutic range for seizure control. When using sodium valproate it is important to remember that it contains potent self-induc-

tion properties. A patient's level will fall steadily at a fixed dose for mamy weeks or months, requiring frequent monitoring and adjustment of dose.

ELECTROCONVULSIVE THERAPY

A typical "pre-ECT" workup is outlined:

1. CBC
2. Sequential multichannel autoanalyzer-12 or 23
3. Chest x-ray
4. Spinal x-ray
5. Urinalysis
6. Electrocardiogram
7. CT scan or MRI—only indicated if patient has any suggestion of space-occupying lesions

Vitamin, Hormone, and Nutritional Supplements

Excessive ingestion of a variety of nutritional supplements can produce distinct laboratory abnormalities. Check serum calcium levels every three months in all patients taking calcium supplements, especially if the supplement also contains vitamin D. Measure liver function tests at six-month intervals in patients on estrogen replacement. Although excess consumption of vitamins A, B_1, B_6, C, and D may produce laboratory abnormalities, they are of no pathological significance unless linked with associated clinical symptoms. Rarely, patients will ingest excess amounts of iron or copper. Although discrete pathology is thought to occur only in patients with predisposing abnormalities in carrier proteins (e.g., hemochromatosis or Wilson's disease), abnormally high serum iron or copper levels should indicate that dosage reduction is appropriate.

Excessive thyroid hormone ingestion, so-called thyrotoxicosis factitia if the patient is responsible or thyrotoxicosis medicamentosa if the prescription specifies too high a dose, will present with clinical signs of hyperthyroidism. Because of mood elevating and weight reducing properties of thyroid hormone, psychiatric patients frequently abuse these medications. Most patients on appropriate doses of T_4 will require serum T_4 levels in the slightly hyperthyroid range to be clinically euthyroid.

It is our practice to measure serum-free T_3 concentration (the primary biologically active form of thyroid hormone) in patients on T_4 to assess adequacy of treatment. Patients found to have free T_3 concentrations above normal are ingesting excess thyroid medication and must have their dose reduced.

REFERENCES

1. Rapaka RS: Opioid peptides: An update. NIDA Res Mongr, 87:1–232, 1988.

2. Bailey DN: Drug screening in an unconventional matrix: Hair analysis. JAMA, 262:3331, 1989.

3. Baumgartner WA, Hill VA, Blahd WH: Hair analysis for drugs of abuse. J Forensic Sci, 34:1433–1453, 1989.

4. Graham K, Koren G, Klein J, Schneiderman J, Greenwald M: Determination of gestational cocaine exposure by hair analysis. JAMA, 262:3328–3330, 1989.

5. Hawks RL, Chaing CN: Urine testing for drugs of abuse. NIDA Res Monogr, 73,1986.

6. Chasnoff IJ, Landress HJ, Barrett MZ: The prevalence of illicit drug or alcohol use during pregnancy and discrepancies in mandatory reporting in Pinellas County, Florida. N Engl J Med, 322(17):1202–1206, 1990.

7. Watson RR: Diagnosis of Alcohol Abuse. Boca Raton, Fl., CRC Press, 1989.

8. Hoyt DW, Finnigan RE, Nee T, Shults TF, Bolter JJ: Drug testing in the workplace—Are methods legally defensible? JAMA, 238(4):304–309, 1987.

9. Taylor L, Faulkner D: Living on the Edge, p 158, New York, Times Books, 1987.

10. Mikkelsen SL, Ash KO: Adulterants causing false negatives in illicit drug testing. Clin Chem, 34(11):2333–2336, 1988.

11. VuDuc T: EMIT tests for drugs of abuse: Interference by liquid soap preparations. Clin Chem, 31(4):658–659, 1985.

12. Pearson SD, Ash KO, Viry FM: Mechanism of false negative urine cannabinoid immunoassay by Visine® eyedrops. Clin Chem 35(4):636–638, 1989.

13. Warner A: Interference of household chemicals in immunoassay methods for drugs of abuse. Clin Chem, 35(4):648–651, 1989.

14. Person NB, Ehrenkranz JRL: Evaluation of urine temperature measurement methods to screen urine specimens for drug testing. Clin Chem, 35(6):1181, 1989.

15. Person NB, Ehrenkranz JRL: False urine samples for drug analysis: Hot, but not hot enough. JAMA, 259(6):841, 1988.

16. Wilson JD: Androgen abuse by athletes. Endocr Rev, 9(2):181–199, 1988.

17. Needleman HL, Gunnoe C, Levitan A, et al.: Deficits in psychologic and classroom performance of children with elevated dentine lead levels. N Engl J Med, 300:689–695, 1979.

18. Bellinger D, Levitan A, Waternand C, et al.: Longitudinal analyses of prenatal and postnatal lead exposure and early cognition development. N Engl J Med, 316:1037–1043, 1987.

19. Palardy J, et al.: Blood glucose measurements during symptomatic episodes in patients with suspected postprandial hypoglycemia. N Engl J Med, 321(21):1421–1425, 1989.

20. Herridge P, Gold MS: TRH stimulation test in psychiatry, in Lerer B, Gershon S (eds): New Directions in Affective Disorders, New York, Springer-Verlag, 1988.

21. Khan AU: Sensitivity and specificity of the TRH stimulation test in depressed and nondepressed adolescents. Psychiatry Res, 25:11–17, 1987.

22. Ingbar SH: The thyroid gland, in Wilson JD, Foster DW (eds): William's Textbook of Endocrinology, p. 722, Philadephia, W.B. Saunders, 1985.

23. Rushing H: The Pituitary Body and its Disorders, Birmingham, Ala., Classics of Medicine Library, Gryphon Editions, Ltd., 1979.

24. DeMilio L, Dackis C, Ehrenkranz JRL, Gold MS: A case of Addison's disease initially diagnosed as bereavement and conversion disorder. Am J Psychiatry, 141(12):1647, 1984.

25. The APA Task Force on Laboratory

Tests in Psychiatry: The dexamethasone suppression test: An overview of its current status in psychiatry. Am J Psychiatry, *144*:1253–1262, 1987.

26. Arana GW, Mossman D: The dexamethasone test and depression. Endocrinology of Neuropsychiatric Disorders, *6*:21–39, 1988.

27. Arana GW, Reichlin S, Workman R, et al.: The dexamethasone suppression index: Enhancement of DST diagnostic utility for depression by expressing serum cortisol as a function of serum dexamethasone. Am J Psychiatry, *145*: 707–711, 1988.

28. Kraus RP, Grof P, Brown GM: Drugs and the DST: Need for a reappraisal. Am J Psychiatry, *145*:666–674, 1988.

29. Meador-Woodruf JH, Greden JF: Effects of psychotropic medication on hypothalamic-pituitary-adrenal regulation. Endocrinology of Neuropsychiatric Disorders, *6*:225–234, 1988.

30. Casat CO, Arana GW, Powell K: The DST in children and adolescents with major depressive disorder. Am J Psychiatry, *146*:503–507, 1989.

31. Evans DL, Nemeroff CB, Haggerty JJ, et al.: Use of the dexamethasone suppression test with DSM-III criteria in psychiatrically hospitalized adolescents. Psychoneuroendocrinology, *12*:203–209, 1987.

32. Harris B, Watkins S, Cook N, et al.: Comparison of plasma and salivary cortisol determinations for the diagnostic efficacy of the dexamethasone suppression test. Biol Psychiatry, *27*:897–904, 1990.

33. Snyder SH: *Brainstorming,* p. 188, Cambridge, Harvard University Press, 1989.

34. Lindenbaum J, et al.: Neuropsychiatric disorders caused by cobalamin deficiency in the absence of anemia or macrocytosis. N Engl J Med, *318*(26):1720–1728, 1988.

35. Allen JR: Screening and testing asymptomatic persons for HIV infection, in DeVita VT, Hellman S, Rosenberg SA (eds): *AIDS,* Philadelphia, J. B. Lippincott Co., 1988.

36. Kappas A, Sassa S, Anderson KE: The porphyrias, in Stanbury JB (ed): *The Metabolic Basis of Inherited Disease,* New York, McGraw-Hill, 1983.

37. Rosse RB, Giese AA, Deutsch SI, Morihisa JM: *A Concise Guide to Laboratory Diagnostic Testing in Psychiatry,* Washington, D.C., American Psychiatric Press, 1989.

38. APA Task Force on the use of laboratory tests in psychiatry: Tricyclic antidepressants—blood level measurements and clinical outcome. Am J Psychiatry, *142*:155–162, 1985.

39. Preskorn SH: Tricyclic antidepressants: The whys and hows of therapeutic drug monitoring. J Clin Psychiatry, *50*(7 suppl):34–42, 1989.

40. Herridge PL, Pope HC: Treatment of bulimia and rapid cycling bipolar disorder with sodium valproate: A case report. J Clin Psychopharmacol, *5*(4):229–230, 1985.

14

Psychological Assessment

John F. Clarkin, PhD
Steven Mattis, PhD

Hospitalization for a psychiatric disorder is an especially traumatic time in the life of the patient (and the family). However, the occasion presents an opportunity for thorough assessment, psychoeducation, and effective planning for acute treatment and treatment needed following discharge. Since patients who need hospitalization are often those who failed to follow outpatient treatments and since those inpatients who obtain outpatient treatment upon discharge have the best prognosis, thorough assessment and education about the need and nature of treatment is a major goal during any hospitalization. Psychological testing and feedback to patient and family about the findings can play a major role in this endeavor.

In this chapter we are concerned with standardized tests and other assessment instruments as they are used in formulating treatment plans for adult psychiatric inpatients (either in general or psychiatric hospitals). We will provide an overview of psychological tests, and then consider the major areas of assessment essential for hospital treatment planning and which tests are most useful in each area.

DEFINITION AND DEVELOPMENT OF PSYCHOLOGICAL TESTS

Psychological tests are basically standardized situations that enable the clinician to gather information about the individual patient (1). Test data can be compared with the same information on other patients and nonpatients, thus generating norms and normative comparisons. Technical criteria enable one to assess the usefulness of a test. Unless tests meet certain criteria, they should not be used in the clinical setting. Chief among these technical criteria are the requirements of reliability and validity. Essential for establishing reliability is the standardization of the test administration and scoring. Reliability can be assessed in various ways. For example, a test can be readministered a second time to ascertain if individual scores remain stable. This is referred to as test-retest reliability. Alternatively, one can assess whether or not the test yields a score in one subgroup of items comparable to another subgroup of items; this is referred to as split-half reliability.

After establishing reliability, evidence must prove that the test scores adequately reflect what they are intended to measure. *Content validity* is demonstrated when the content of the test adequately samples the area of interest. Criterion-related validity refers to the test's relationship to independent criteria *(concurrent validity)* or the correlation of the test score to samples of future behavior *(predictive validity)*. *Construct validity* is achieved by demonstrating that the test measures a theoretical construct of interest and that the scores on the test are related to scores on comparable tests of the same construct.

GOALS OF ASSESSMENT DURING HOSPITALIZATION

Our focus in this chapter is not on psychological testing in general, but on those assessments most useful during a psychiatric hospitalization. The hospitalization of an individual will occasion the possibility of three kinds of assessment focus: (*a*) treatment planning for the hospitalization itself, (*b*) progress in goals of treatment during hospitalization, and (*c*) assessment for discharge planning and treatment of the patient upon discharge.

The central goal of testing is to assist in developing an individualized treatment plan for the patient (and family). Treatment planning is complicated in psychiatry; the relationship between diagnosis and treatment is not simple because of the nature of psychiatric difficulties, in which multiple causal pathways lead to the end-stage of symptomatology, and the impreciseness of our current treatments.

Five areas of patient functioning need to be evaluated to adequately inform treatment planning (2). (*a*) Assessing patient symptoms. These symptoms often form complexes or syndromes classified as Axis I disorders. This phenomenological description of symptoms is just that, and often the etiologies and pathogenesis of these symptoms are unknown. (*b*) Assessing personal-

ity traits and disorders. Classified as Axis II syndromes, personality disorders have substantial impact upon the treatment and prognosis of Axis I disorders and may form the focus of treatment in and of themselves. Personality traits, including patient strengths, are also crucial for treatment planning; individual strengths may be more important than the disorder in treatment response. (*c*) Assessing cognitive abilities and functioning. Cognitive malfunctioning may be part of the diagnosed disorder (e.g., thought disorder) or a potent variable in what treatments (e.g., psychoeducation, insight) can be accomplished. In certain subgroups of patients (e.g., drug addicts and the depressed elderly), cognitive malfunction may play an important role and need attention in treatment planning. (*d*) Assessing patient psychodynamics and therapeutic enabling factors, patient variables enabling the patient to engage in various kinds of treatments. (*e*) Assessing environmental demands and social adjustment. The patient is a social being; the demands of the social environment may affect how the patient copes with the psychiatric condition or may aggravate the condition. Under each of these five categories we will describe the patient areas to be assessed and discuss tests commonly used for assessment.

ASSESSMENT OF SYMPTOMS

Usually patients are hospitalized because of intense, frequent, and debilitating symptoms, especially symptom complexes involving thought disorder, depression, and anxiety. Assessing the symptoms in terms of dimensions (intensity and duration) and categories (DSM-IIIR [*Diagnostic and Statistical Manual of Mental Disorders*, ed. 3, revised] symptom categories) is central to treatment planning and measuring the effectiveness of treatment interventions.

In general, two types of instruments assess symptoms: (*a*) omnibus measures of symptoms and (*b*) instruments targeted toward assessing a specific symptom constellation such as substance abuse, depression, anxiety, suicidal behavior, thought disorder, and aggressive behavior (see Table 14.1 on this page). The instruments used for overall measurement of symptom patterns in hospital settings typically include the MMPI-2 (Minnesota Multiphasic Personality Inventory), MCMI-II (Millon Clinical Multiaxial Inventory) the SCL-90 (symptom checklist), the BPRS (Brief Psychiatric Rating Scale), and semistructured interviews for Axis I assessment such as the SCID (Structured Clinical Interview for the DSM-IIIR) and the SADS (Schedule for Affective Disorders and Schizophrenia) (3–8).

The MMPI-2 is a good example of a carefully developed psychological test with attention to the details of reliability, validity, and normative information. This is a recent revision of the MMPI which had become a standard of practice since its first development in the 1940s. The MMPI-2 yields both validity scales and clinical scales. The clinical scales include the traditional ones plus new content scales. New content scales include anxiety, fears, obsessiveness, depression, health concerns, bizarre mentation, anger, cynicism, antisocial practices, type A behavior, low self-esteem, social discomfort, family problems, work interference, and negative treatment indicators.

Another relatively new instrument gaining in usage in hospital settings is the MCMI-II. This is an 175-item, true and false inventory which yields scores on clinical personality pattern scales (e.g., schizoid, avoidant, dependent, histrionic, etc.), severe personality pathology scales (schizotypal, borderline, and paranoid), clinical syndrome scales (anxiety disorder, somatoform disorder, bipolar manic disorder, etc.), and severe clinical syndrome scales (thought disorder, major depression, and delusional disorder). A major advantage of this self-report instrument, which has computerized scoring and computer-generated reports based upon normative data, like the MMPI-2, is that it provides scaled scores for both Axis I symptom patterns and Axis II personality disorders. While some debate ensues about the relative congruence between the

Table 14.1. Instruments for the Assessment of Symptoms

Instrument	General Classification	Description
Omnibus Measures		
Minnesota Multiphasic Personality Inventory-2	Self-report	566-item checklist, true/false format
Symptom Checklist-90	Self-report	90-item checklist, 5-point intensity checks
Brief Psychiatric Rating Scale	Clinical interview	16 items, 7-point severity scales
Schedule for Affective Disorders and Schizophrenia	Semistructured interview	7-point rating scales of symptoms
Structured Clinical Interview for Diagnosis	Semistructured interview	3-point rating scales of symptoms
Assessment of Specific Symptom Areas		
State-Trait Anxiety Inventory	Self-report	Two 20-item scales, 4-point frequency ratings
Fear Questionnaire	Self-report	17 items reflecting specific phobias rated on 9-point avoidance scales
Beck Depression Inventory	Self-report	20 items, 4-point intensity scales
Hamilton Rating Scale for Depression	Clinical interview	17–24 items, 3- to 5-point severity scales
Suicide Intent Scale	Self-report	15 items, 3-point categorical scales
Reasons for Living Inventory	Self-report	6 factors

test scales and their match with DSM-IIIR categories, the fact that the test yields scores along symptom and personality disorder trait dimensions is an asset.

Instruments useful in assessing specific symptom patterns should be mentioned. For substance abuse there are self-report instruments for abuse of alcohol, drugs, and food (e.g. *Eating* Attitudes Test [EAT] and the Alcohol Use Inventory [AUI] (9, 10). Specific scales assessing anxiety and depresssion include the State-Trait Anxiety Inventory and the Beck Depression Inventory (11, 12). Thought disorder can be assessed by either semistructured interviews (e.g., the SADS or SCID) which yield ratings of such behavior as reported or reviewed in the interview situation or from Rorschach productions through such scales as the Thought Disorder Index (13). The latter is more useful when thought disorder is suspected but not clinically prominent or questionable through interview assessment.

ASSESSMENT OF PERSONALITY TRAITS AND DISORDERS

Some patients are admitted to the hospital for severe personality disorders with associated Axis I symptoms (e.g., borderline personality disorder with depression). In other situations, although the patient has a major Axis I symptom disorder, a co-morbid Axis II disorder becomes a focus of intervention or a moderating variable in the treatment of the Axis I disorder. Evidence is

growing, at least in treating depression, that the presence of an Axis II disorder indicates slower response to symptom treatment. It should also be noted that certain personality traits of a positive or adaptive nature may be important variables in treatment planning; the prognosis for treatment is sometimes less dependent upon the severity of the symptoms and more dependent upon coexisting or premorbid strengths and personality characteristics (see Table 14.2 on this page).

ASSESSMENT OF COGNITIVE ABILITIES AND FUNCTIONING

In general, one assesses cognitive abilities in psychiatric patients for one of two reasons: (a) to document a specific disorder in cognition referable to a specific class of psychiatric disorders; e.g., intrusion of task-irrelevant items in thoughts of patients complaining of delusional or obsessive ideation or disturbances in recall in patients with major affective disorders, or (b) to document disorders in cognitive skills referable to alternative or concomitant neurogenic disorder; e.g., discriminating between a thought disorder and a language disorder or the mnemonic deficits of a depression versus a dementia.

While the field of cognitive and experimental psychology may offer an almost limitless number of different cognitive functions capable of being defined and measured in the adult, only a finite number ap-

Table 14.2. Instruments Assessing Personality Traits and Disorders

Instrument	General Classification	Description
Eysenck Personality Inventory	Self-report	57 yes/no items, parallel forms
Personality Research Form	Self-report	352 items
Millon Clinical Multiaxial Inventory-II	Self-report	175 items, true/false format
Structural Inteview for the DSM-IIIR Personality Disorders	Semistructured interview	3-point rating scales
Personality Disorder Examination	Semistructured interview	Semistructured interview for patient and self-report by family members on the patient

Table 14.3. Instruments for Assessing Cognitive Functioning

Instrument*	Description	Time
Wechsler Adult Intelligence Scale-Revised	11 subtests of complex intellectual abilities.	1 hour
Wide Range Achievement Test	Reading, spelling, and arithmetic achievement.	25 minutes
Continuous Performance Test	Vigilance test; hits, false alarms, and reaction time noted.	10–15 minutes
Wechsler Memory Scale-Revised	Attention, verbal, and nonverbal memory subtests.	30 minutes
Benton Test of Visual Retention	Reproduction from memory of 10 items (30 geometric designs).	10–15 minutes
Benton Line Orientation Test	Target lines at given orientations must be detected from among a radial display of lines. Two forms, 30 items each.	10 minutes
Benton Face Recognition Test	Target face detected from among similar faces. Correct choice can be identical or same individual in different profile.	15 minutes
Goldman-Fristoe	Auditory perception measured under three different conditions of ambient noise.	20 minutes
Category Test (Booklet)	Concept formation task. Patient informed about impending change of rules.	30–40 minutes (short forms available)
Wisconsin Card Sorting Test	Concept formation task. Patient not informed about impending change of rules.	30–40 minutes
Conceptual Level Analogies Test	Verbal analogies test.	15–20 minutes
Raven Progressive Matrices	Spatial analogies test using patterned visual stimuli.	30–40 minutes
Trail-Making Test	Set switching. Connect dots in ascending numeric order, then in alternating alpha-numeric order.	5–10 minutes
Purdue Pegboard	Fine motor task. The number of pegs placed in 30″ by either and both hands.	5 minutes

*All instruments are objective measures.

pear, at present, to be clinically useful. In one form or another, most psychological assessments of cognitive processes evaluate the presence of disorders in the following abilities: general intelligence, attention and concentration, memory and learning, perception, language, conceptualization, constructional skills, executive-motor processes, and affect (see Table 14.3 on this page).

General Intellectual Abilities

In general, most psychological assessments include both an estimate of premorbid general intellectual abilities and some measure of present intellectual abilities in order to gauge the severity of disturbance of cognition. The most commonly used measure of general intelligence is the WAIS-R (Wechsler Adult Intelligence Scale-revised) (14). The WAIS-R takes about one hour to administer, contains 11 subtests, and offers a verbal, performance, and full scale intelligence quotient (IQ). Because of the length of administration, abbreviated versions of this measure are often employed either by using only some of the subtests or fewer of the specific items and weighing each response. Alternatively, different briefer measures may be employed, e.g., Ammons quick test or Shipley-Hartford (15, 16). Premorbid intelligence may be estimated by assessing those cognitive abilities that do not rapidly deteriorate with dementing processes such as the general fund of information and vocabulary measured by subtests of the WAIS-R or reading recognition measured by the wide range achievement test reading subtest (17). It is also common to estimate premorbid intelligence on the basis of educational and vocational background. The validity of a number of different estimates of premorbid intelligence based on demographic data have been demonstrated.

Attentional Disorders

Attentional disorders are among the most common findings in psychiatric patients since attention and concentration will be effected by both psychologically determined processes such as anxiety, depression, and personal preoccupations and neurogenic compromise of brainstem and limbic structures caused by toxic-metabolic disorders or direct structural impairment. Attentional processes are most commonly measured by the WAIS-R subtests constituting the "distractibility" triad—digit span, mental arithmetic, and digit symbol. In digit span the patient is asked to repeat a string of digits of increasing length and then, separately, repeat a string of digits in the reverse order in which they were presented. The digit string cannot be repeated by the examiner; lapses in the patient's attention result in repetition of only the shorter strings. In the arithmetic subtest, the patient is asked to solve arithmetic problems of increasing difficulty without pencil and paper. Selecting and monitoring the appropriate arithmetic operation while storing partial solutions are easily disrupted by alterations in arousal and attention. The digit symbol subtest presents the patient with the digits 1–9 and assigns each digit a separate very simple geometric design. The digits are then randomly sequenced in rows across the page and the patient must draw the appropriate design beneath each digit. The number of designs correctly drawn in 90 seconds is noted. This task is not only affected by impairment of the attentional system but is very sensitive to fine motor tremor and extrapyramidal impairment secondary to neurotoxins.

In addition to the above, a number of variants to these procedures and other specialized procedures are in common practice. Through cancellation tasks the patient is required to cross out a given letter or design presented within rows of randomly distributed other letters or designs. An advantage of such tasks is that they can be strung together to form a lengthy continuous performance task of 10–15 minutes, determining variation in accuracy across discrete 20-second epochs. The increasing use of computer-assisted examinations has popularized a continuous performance test Rosvold developed (18, 19). This task presents the patient with a randomly selected letter in midscreen at fixed intervals and directs the patient to push a button (or press the space bar) when a given letter appears. One notes the number of correct responses (hits), misses, false alarms (the number of times the bar is pressed in response to a nontarget item) and correct rejections. The advantage of this computer-assisted approach to measuring attention lies in its flexibility and accuracy in recording responses and presenting stimuli. One can measure reaction time of each response and note fluctuations in reaction time over the duration of the task. One can systematically alter stimulus characteristics such as stimulus duration, speed of presentation, and even target size and duration of task. A good deal of clinical research has been conducted using such a procedure to explore the attentional characteristics of children with ADHD (attention-deficit hyperactivity disorder).

Research in attentional processes has long used a procedure called dichotic stimulation (20) which presents dissimilar auditory stimuli simultaneously to each ear and requires the patient to report both stimuli. Thus the patient might hear the number "one" in the right ear and "four" in the left at the same time. Strings of three such pairs might be presented to adults and the patient asked to report all six digits. The competing stimuli can be matched for such stimulus characteristics as time of onset, offset peak amplitude, etc., making it a very difficult speech sound discrimination task and attentional measure.

Memory and Learning Disorders

Note that none of the subtests of the WAIS-R measures the nature and severity of memory and learning disorders occurring in patients with amnesic and dementia syndromes. Thus in studies of classical alcoholic Korsakoff syndromes, care is taken to select patients with profound amnesic syndromes whose performance on measures such as the WAIS-R are clearly within normal limits. The memory disorder of particular interest to the clinician is the one which affects "recent" memory and is generally referable to impairment of limbic system functioning. Operationally, one seeks to present the patient with a specific set of information or events, divert attention so that the data cannot be rehearsed, and then require the patient to reproduce the material or recognize it among distractor items, demonstrating that the patient has encoded and stored the target information. Thus recall of brief paragraphs or reproduction of geometric designs from memory are often used to assess mnemonic processes.

Among the most commonly used standard tests of memory are the Wechsler memory scale-revised, which presents both verbal and nonverbal material as the to-be-remembered items, and the Benton test of visual retention, which presents only geometric designs (21, 22). Free recall of recent events has been found to be among the most sensitive of memory processes. Unfortunately, in many instances free recall—found to be quite fragile and vulnerable to disruption from affective arousal, depres-

sion, and motivational factors—may present many "false positives" when one is discriminating between neurogenic and psychogenic diagnostic considerations. It has been suggested that mechanisms other than free recall might be employed to assess the integrity of encoding and storage processes. Recognition memory techniques, in which the patient is asked to detect a recently presented word or design from among distractor items, have been successfully used to discriminate patients with major affective disorders from those with organic amnesias such as progressive dementia. In patients presenting with a major depression, for example, free recall might be quite consonant with patients suffering from Alzheimer's disease, although recognition memory remains intact and consonant with normal controls.

It should be noted that neurologic patients with focal lesions might present only a verbal or nonverbal recent memory defect depending on the locus of lesion. Therefore, only in patients with bilateral or diffuse neurogenic impairment does one find amnesic disorders in both realms. Thus both verbal and nonverbal memory must be assessed independently with the finding of asymmetric dysfunction strongly suggesting focal neurologic impairment (23, 24).

Perceptual Disorders

Very little evidence exists for a high prevalence of perceptual deficits in a psychiatric population when care is taken to exclude significant problem-solving components from the task and exclude the presence of concurrent toxic metabolic disorders in the patients. Nonetheless, it is probably a good idea to rule out the presence of perceptual deficits. This is done most frequently by noting the integrity of perceptual processes measured by more complex tasks completed for other screening purposes; e.g., one can presume intact visual and visuospatial perception from above average performance of complex constructional tasks or drawings or excellent "form level" in response to the ambiguously organized Rorschach blots. If one cannot make such a presumption, visual perceptual processes can be assessed with tasks such as the Benton line orientation tests (25) which requires the patient to match a target line at a given orientation to true vertical with alternative lines presented at various orientations. Another such test is the Benton face recognition test (26) in which a photograph of a face is presented as the target and the patient is requested to detect this face from alternatives. In this task the correct face is presented as an identical photograph as well as the same individual in various profiles. Both of these tests validly measure the integrity of posterior cerebral, primarily nondominant hemisphere functioning. Auditory perception tends to be difficult to assess without hardware. However, the fidelity available in small portable "Walkman" type tape recorders with ear phones affords the clinician a wide range of excellent auditory stimuli. Tests such as the Goldman-Fristoe test of speech sound discrimination (27) assesses the effectiveness of speech sound detection with and without background noise. The use of dichotic stimulation tests as measures of speech sound discrimination has been mentioned above.

Subtests of the Seashore battery of tests of musical abilities (28), especially the timbre discrimination and tonal memory subtests, are used as measures of auditory perception of nonverbal material.

The study of disorders of somatosensory perception have a long history in the field of psychophysics and the techniques evolved from this early literature comprise a large part of the standard neurologic examination for peripheral and central nervous system disorder. Measures of pressure threshold (Von Frey hairs and Semmes-

Ghent-Weinstein pressure asthesiometer), two-point discrimination, joint position sense, finger agnosia, finger order and differentiation, graphesthesia, and stereognosis are common assessment procedures for the presence of disorders of parietal lobe functioning.

Disorders of Language

Among the more sensitive indices of neurogenic impairment is the presence of a language disorder. For almost all right-handed individuals and half of left-handed individuals, focal or diffuse impairment of the left hemisphere is likely to result in an aphasia, i.e., a disorder of language comprehension and/or usage. Moreover, the study of the aphasias provides some of the "hardest" evidence in the mental status exam of the presence and locus of brain impairment. Needless to say, many well-constructed tests exist for aphasia. In general, all such tests are multidimensional, comprising measures of verbal labeling or word finding skills, language comprehension, imitative speech, and motor-expressive speech. Many such tests also include specific measures of reading and writing. Among the most commonly used multifactorial instruments are the multilingual aphasia examination, neurosensory center comprehensive examination for aphasia, and the Boston diagnostic aphasia examination (29–31). Among the most widely used screening instruments for assessing aphasia is the Halstead-Wepman aphasia screening test (32).

Conceptualization Disorders

The question whether or not the patient can assume an abstract attitude is often critical to diagnosis and treatment planning. The question arises most often when the differential diagnostic considerations include diffuse brain damage and, to some degree, schizophrenia.

Perhaps the most direct measure of

the concept of abstract or categorical thinking is the similarities subtest of the WAIS-R which presents patients with perceptually dissimilar items and asks them to determine the category to which both items belong; e.g., "How are north and west alike?" Proverb explanation has a long history in the psychiatric mental status exam as a task designed to measure abstract reasoning and is included among the items of the comprehension subtest of the WAIS-R; e.g., "Shallow brooks are noisy." However, some consider explanation of proverbs too dependent on general intellectual abilities and sociocultural factors to be a specific measure of concretization of thought. Analogistic reasoning can also be gauged through such tasks as the conceptual level analogies test for verbal reasoning and the Raven progressive matrices or test of nonverbal abilities for nonverbal or spatial analogistic reasoning (33, 34). Two measures of concept formation arising from the neuropsychologic literature have recently been applied to psychiatric patients. The data to date indicate that schizophrenic patients, like patients with frontal lobe lesions, have particular difficulty with the booklet categories test and Wisconsin card sorting test described below (35–37).

Constructional Disorders

Perhaps the quickest estimate of the integrity of the central nervous system can be obtained by asking the patient to draw a complex figure. Posterior sensory, central spatial, and anterior planning, monitoring, and simple motor skills must all be intact, integrated, and appropriately sequenced for this task to be successfully completed. One can alter the degree to which psychological and dynamic factors and initiative or executive planning play a role by modulating both task structure and design complexity. For example, asking patients to draw a person or draw their family requires a maximum level of planning, initiative, and decision making; does not put any limit on the degree of complexity of the figures; and chooses a subject matter fraught with complex feelings and attitudes. Patients without structural impairment but with conflictive feelings about family or disordered thinking that affects planning and execution will have difficulty with such tasks. However, asking a patient to draw a clock and setting the hands to a specific time, e.g., ten minutes to eleven, also requires complex planning and initiative but without the conflictive overlay. Similarly asking the patient to copy a complex design, e.g., the Rey-Ostereith figure (38), minimizes initiative, limits (but does not eliminate) planning, but maintains assessment of high levels of spatial constructional skills. Contrasting patients' figure drawing to their clock and copy of geometric figures often validly infers the presence and locus of CNS impairment and the degree to which affective and psychiatric factors impair otherwise intact cognitive skills. Quite often construction tasks other than drawing, such as the block design and object assembly subtests of the WAIS-R, are used for the same assessment goals.

Disorders of Executive-Motor Skills

Assessing disorders in executive skills requires one to detect the presence of perseveration in motor activity, thought, and/or affect. Perseveration of motor activity is often elicited by starting the patient on a simple repeated task and then altering one of the motor components. Instructing the patient to perform a simple diadochokinetic task, such as alternating palm-up–palm-down and with palm-up–palm-down–fist, may result in repeated performance of only two components of the task. Similarly, instructing the patient to write in script alternating *m*'s and *n*'s will also elicit simple motor perseveration. Perseveration of thought or set is often quickly elicited by shifting task instructions. For example, in a task developed by Luria (39) for assessing frontal lobe dysfunction, the patient is told, "When I raise one finger you raise one finger, and when I raise two fingers you raise two fingers." After a number of successful completions, the patient is told, "Now when I raise one finger you raise two fingers, and when I raise two fingers you raise one." Patients with dorsal lateral frontal lobe lesions have a great deal of trouble with such tasks. The trail-making test (40) is a connect-the-dots type task; the patient must first connect the dots in ascending numerical order (trails A) and then connect the dots in alternating sequence of numbers and letters (trails B), e.g., 1 to A to 2 to B to 3 to C, etc. Time for completion and number of errors is noted. Disorders in evolving or shifting more complex ideas can also be measured quite accurately. Concept formation tasks such as the category test and Wisconsin card sorting task differ in specific directions and stimuli; however, both present a series of specific examples of a class of events and require the patient to induce the concept or rule exemplified (35–37). The rule changes over time. Thus, one might observe the failure of the patient to induce the first concept or perseverate the same rule well past its utility. The number of perseveration errors is among the scores obtained on both tests.

Disorders in Motor Skills

Disorders in simple motor skills are among the common concomitants to most toxic-metabolic disorders and structural lesions of the extrapyramidal and pyramidal systems. Examination is usually exceptionally brief and the results quite reproducible and valid. One can measure line quality parameters of copied geometric drawings (41). In addition, one can present simple fine motor coordination tasks such as the Pur-

due pegboard or the grooved pegboard (42, 43). The Purdue Pegboard measures the number of slim cylinders (pegs) one can insert in a row of holes in 30 seconds. One notes the number of pegs placed with the right hand alone, left hand alone, and pairs of pegs placed using both hands simultaneously. The number of pegs placed simultaneously has proven to be a sensitive measure of frontal dysfunction. The Grooved Pegboard uses pegs that contain a flange on one side so that the pegs fit into a keyhole-shaped hole. The keyholes are placed in differing orientations on the board. One notes the total time to place all the pegs with each hand alone. Given the greater fine motor component to the grooved pegs, the Grooved pegboard tends to be a more sensitive measure of tremor than the Purdue.

ASSESSMENT OF PSYCHODYNAMICS AND THERAPEUTIC ENABLING FACTORS

The assessment of patient factors relevant to the focus of psychodynamic treatment approaches has a long and rich history in the psychological testing literature (see Table 14.4 p370). The stimulus for developing and using the standard battery in psychological testing originated in the efforts of clinical psychologists to assess unconscious wishes, conflicts, and defenses. This standard battery included an intelligence test and projective tests such as the Rorschach and the thematic apperception test (TAT) (44, 45). Both of these projective tests are still widely used to examine patients for a range of ego functions and dynamic factors. Recent advances include the development of reliable and valid scoring systems for various psychological constructs (46) as assessed by the Rorschach test. Originally developed by Murray, the TAT is a

Table 14.4.   Instruments for Assessing Psychodynamics and Patient Enabling Factors

Instrument	General Classification	Description
Rorschach Inkblot Test	Unstructured or projective test	10 ambiguous inkblots, responses scored on multiple criteria
Thematic Apperception Test	Unstructured or projective test	30 ambiguous scenes

set of 30 pictures used as a projective device to assess the patient's self-concept in relationship with others. Stories generated by patients can be scored for individuals' needs as represented by characters in the stories.

We use the term "patient enabling factors" to refer to those patient dimensions important for treatment planning and engaging in particular forms of psychological intervention. For example, quite possibly the patient's defensive structure, coping style, and interpersonal sensitivity influences the kind of psychological intervention the patient will accept (47). Some patients accept the straightforward directions and input from psychoeducational and cognitive/behavioral treatments, while others experience these approaches as intrusive. The latter may respond better to nondirective and more dynamic approaches. The pattern of elevations on the MMPI-2 scales may be useful indicators of these different coping and defensive styles.

ASSESSMENT OF ENVIRONMENTAL DEMANDS AND SOCIAL ADJUSTMENT

It is commonly assumed that the environment (both positive and negative) exerts an impact on symptom occurrence and maintenance. This relationship between environmental stressors and symptoms is now acknowledged in the standard diagnostic system (DSM-IIIR) by a rating on Axis IV. It is especially with seriously disturbed patients who are the most likely to be admitted to hospitals that environmental stressors

may have the most impact. The empirical data explicating the deleterious impact of toxic family environmental variables such as overinvolvement and a critical atmosphere (high expressed emotion or EE), as assessed on the Camberwell family interview (CFI) (48), is most relevant here. Thus, evaluating the toxic elements in the family of a hospitalized patient, especially patients with schizophrenia and major affective disorder, is most relevant for discharge treatment planning. Under ordinary circumstances, it is probably not clinically feasible to use the CFI because it is time-consuming and reliable scoring is a problem. However, the CFI interview schedule may be a useful guide for clinically evaluating the family.

The term "social adjustment" refers to the capacity and skill of the patient in handling interpersonal situations in typical environments such as home, school, and work. The term, also used more broadly to refer to the community and social adjustment of seriously disturbed psychiatric patients, is quite relevant for hospitalized patients. Instruments to note in this regard are the social adjustment scale (SAS) and the Katz adjustment scale-relatives' form (KAS) (49, 50). The SAS and its companion self-report version covers the patient's instrumental and affective behaviors in role performance, social and leisure activities, relationships with extended family, marital role, parental role, family unit, and economic independence. Norms are available for nonpatient community samples, acute and recovered depressed outpatients, schizophrenics and drug addicted samples.

The KAS, a self-report inventory from

the perspective of the relatives of the patient, evaluates the symptomatic behavior and social adjustment exhibited by the patient in the community. The scale covers symptoms, social behavior, performance of socially expected tasks, relatives' expectation for the performance of these tasks, free-time activities, and relatives satisfaction with the performance of free-time activity.

SPECIFIC DIAGNOSES AND PSYCHOLOGICAL TESTING

A further consideration in reference to psychological testing in an inpatient setting is the type of patients (described by age, sex, specific diagnoses, and severity level of diagnoses) that are hospitalized. In these days of shortening hospital stays, only the most severely disturbed patients are hospitalized for even a relatively brief period of time. Typically, patients with schizophrenia, major affective disorder, severe personality disorders, and dually diagnosed with affective disorder and substance abuse are hospitalized. The psychiatric diagnosis, which is basically a phenomenological description of the cross-sectional and sometimes brief history of the symptom pattern described in DSM-IIIR, can be one but not the only guidepost in planning treatment. The diagnostic pattern helps in treatment planning by indicating the typical *mediating goals* of treatment (51). The treatment mediating goals are intermediary goals that must be achieved in a certain sequence in order to reach the final goal of symptom resolution and social readjustment. These mediating goals are different depending upon the diagnosis of the patient, co-morbid factors, and history of the severity of the disorder. The inpatient chart delineates the mediating goals for each patient; psychological testing can both clarify these goals and measures their accomplishment.

SCHIZOPHRENIA

Once the patient is accurately diagnosed as suffering from schizophrenia, areas of strength and pathology must be assessed in order to tailor the treatment to the specific patient. Diagnosis of schizophrenia covers a heterogeneous group of patients that have different strengths, symptom constellations, and courses of illness. In addition, it is now documented that the particular family environment and nature of this milieu markedly influences the course of the disorder, a factor quite relevant to treatment planning in the hospital and upon discharge. The typical mediating goals of treatment for a patient diagnosed as schizophrenic would include treatment of positive and negative symptoms of the disorder, improving social skills, vocational training, and adjusting to the family environment.

The balance of positive and negative symptoms in a particular patient can be assessed with the scale for the assessment of positive symptoms (SAPS) and the scale for the assessment of negative symptoms (SANS) (52, 53). Many patients with schizophrenia also present with a history of alcohol and substance abuse; this can best be assessed by clinical interview. Although role-playing tests have been used to assess the social skills of schizophrenic patients (54), outside of research settings, observations of the patient's interactions on the unit and by occupational therapy staff can be used to accurately assess the need for assistance in social skills.

During the inpatient schizophrenic's assessment, it is not unusual to find significant decrements in WAIS-R IQs. Decrements in both verbal and performance IQ of as much as 30 points over a 10-year period are not uncommon in patients diagnosed as simple undifferentiated. Such deterioration in any other population would significantly raise the index of suspicion of a progressive dementing neurologic disease with widespread neocortical and subcortical components. However, with the exception of extrapyramidal signs secondary to treatment with neuroleptics, the patients are intact on the vertebrate sensory and motor neurologic exam, ruling out extensive white and gray matter destruction. However, assessing cognitive processes often reveals disorders associated with frontal lobe dysfunction such as inattention, perseveration of thought, intrusion of nonlist items on verbal and nonverbal memory tasks, motor impersistence and perseveration, a word-finding disorder in discursive speech but not on confrontation naming, and concretization of thought. Therefore, disorders are frequently found on concept formation tests such as the category and Wisconsin card sort, complex figure drawings and constructions, free recall of verbal and nonverbal material on the Wechsler memory scale, and tests assessing fine motor coordination and sustained attention such as the various pegboard tests and trail making. Treating the acute psychotic phase is associated with increments in many, but not all, of the cognitive disorders; in part, prognosis for relapse is directly related to the integrity of intellectual abilities.

Semistructured interviews such as SAS can assess social functioning. CFI is the classic semistructured interview for assessing the family environment and the toxic factor of high EE. The time necessary for reliably rating the data from this instrument probably prohibits routine clinical use. However, as a guide the interview can help clinicians who wish to assess in a more or less standardized fashion the family environment and its potential need for intervention, typically with psychoeducation and cognitive behavioral family intervention. Co-morbid depression and related suicidal ideation and behavior is quite common in schizophrenic patients; the standard assessment instruments for depression which

have been noted elsewhere in this chapter can be utilized.

MAJOR AFFECTIVE DISORDER

Major depression. The typical mediating goals in treating patients with major depression include reducing the depressive mood, reinstituting the regular sleep cycle, reducing hostility, assessing and alleviating cognitive dysfunction, alleviating severe interpersonal conflict often existing with spouses and other family members, and coping with stressful life events and traumatic situations. The symptoms of depression can be quite accurately assessed through structured interviews such as the SCID and the SADS, self-report instruments such as the MMPI-2 and the SCL-90, and observer ratings such as the Hamilton rating scale of depression (HRSD) (55).

As noted by many clinicians acquainted with both psychiatric and neurologic patients, patients with a major depression present with many cognitive features similar to those presenting with subcortical impairments. That is, patients in clinical depression do not present the aphasias, apraxias, and agnosia seen with neocortical impairment, but rather with the long latency of response features, general retrieval deficits, and relative inability to mobilize attentional and motivational processes to sustain "effortful" tasks. Indeed, these features of a depression, especially the specific retrieval deficiencies, are capitalized upon in differentiating depression from dementia in the elderly patient. For example, on memory tasks, retrieval of recent information or events is equally poor in depressed patients and demented patients early in the course of their illness. However, one can circumvent the retrieval process and reduce the "effort" required of free recall by providing a recognition paradigm. The depressed patient, unlike the demented patient, has relatively robust recognition memory even after a substantial delay. The analogy between the depressed patient and the subcortical dementia is inexact. For example, during the depth of their episode depressed patients can present as inordinately concrete on such tasks as the similarity subtest of the WAIS-R and perform at apraxic levels and in an apraxic manner on construction tasks such as WAIS-R block design.

Some patients with depression have either a situational or historical malfunction in their cognition described best by Beck (56). This involves a pessimistic view of oneself, the future, and one's environment. A number of self-report instruments have been devised to assess these cognitions; the results can be used to target and track the response to the cognitive treatment of this aspect of depression (57, 58). These tests would include the automatic thoughts questionnaire (ATQ) and the dysfunctional attitude scale (DAS) (59, 60).

When the depressed patient is married, concomitant marital conflict either as a contributing cause or result of the major affective disorder is quite common and can be assessed by a variety of self-report instruments such as the marital satisfaction inventory and the Locke-Wallace (61, 62). In addition, the instrument for assessing comorbid Axis II conditions such as the SCID-II are helpful in treatment planning.

Bipolar disorder. The mediating goals of treatment in bipolar disorder are alleviating manic and depressive symptoms, psychoeducation about the causes and course of the disorder and need for further treatment, assessing social skills and vocational functioning, and assessing the family environment. A family environment characterized by high EE is probably as disruptive for bipolar patients as it is for schizophrenic patients. In addition, the premorbid level of functioning of the bipolar patient is the best predictor of discharge functioning. Vocational assessment and subsequent training will be needed for bipolar patients

with poor premorbid social and vocational history. An assessment of Axis II pathology by semistructured interview is relevant although it may be difficult to accomplish especially in those cases where bipolar symptoms have not subsided substantially by the time of hospital discharge.

The bipolar patient has not been as well-studied during the manic phase as the unipolar patient or the bipolar patient during the depressed phase. In general, the profile of cognitive disabilities of the manic phase patient appears more similar to the schizophrenic than the depressed patient. That is, the most prominent features are intrusion of nontarget items on recall and recognition tasks, difficulties on concept formation tasks, and motor and ideational perseveration.

SEVERE PERSONALITY DISORDERS

The severe personality disorders likely to appear in an inpatient setting are borderline personality disorder, (BPD) for which hospitalization is often occasioned by depression and/or suicidal behavior, and antisocial personality disorder, for which patients are hospitalized for situational depression and/or concomitant substance abuse. Mediating goals of hospital treatment for BPD patients often includes (*a*) controlling acting out and suicide; (*b*) decreasing depression; and (*c*) resolving transference-countertransference stalemates with therapist. Co-morbid Axis II conditions are the rule rather than the exception for patients hospitalized with BPD. These co-morbid conditions can be adequately assessed through a semistructured interview for Axis II.

SUBSTANCE ABUSE

Beyond the typical goals of detoxification and acute management of substance abuse, the patient must be assessed thoroughly for likely personality disorders and co-morbid conditions such as depression. Instruments mentioned earlier for assessing these two areas can be utilized. A number of self-report questionnaires may be useful in providing details about the substance abuse and suggestions for treatment planning. For example, the AUI (10) is a multiple choice questionnaire developed as part of an extensive research program to identify personality types and drinking styles of alcoholics. The resulting test factors seem to be related to condition on follow-up and differential response to treatment intervention.

Assessing cognitive abilities is critical to diagnosing and treating the substance-abuse patient. Three main issues arise with this group of patients:

1. The extent to which a delirium secondary to the abused substance or its withdrawal is present. Measures of sustained attention, working memory, and rapid sequenced fine motor movements are among the most sensitive indices of mild toxic-metabolic disorders. Such assessments are rapid, valid, noninvasive, and can be administered serially to chart the course of detoxification during hospitalization and the presence of a toxic state after discharge.

2. The extent to which premorbid or concomitant cognitive deficits are present. A frequent history of early substance abuse and dropping out of school does not allow the clinician an accurate estimate of premorbid abilities and the presence of possible premorbid contributing factors. Many substance-abuse patients present histories and profiles of cognitive disabilities consonant with developmental learning disabilities and borderline intellectual abilities. Moreover, during the course of this illness, an inordinately high incidence of events will likely result in multifocal cerebral impairment secondary to traumatic brain injury and diffuse cerebral impairment secondary to anoxia. The "yield" for the presence of fixed cognitive deficits is sufficiently high to suggest that cognitive abilities be routinely assessed in the substance-abuse population.

3. The extent to which general intellectual and academic achievement factors will alter treatment planning. Most of the more successful rehabilitation approaches are heavily psychoeducational in nature and the treatment and life planning approaches within this framework require assessment of acquired skills, talents, and knowledge as well as the potential for their acquisition in order to aid in personal and vocational guidance.

CLINICAL DECISION TREE

Use of Screening Tests on Short-Term Units

The rapid tempo of hospitalization and discharge in the current scene has changed the process of psychological testing. One method of adapting testing to this tempo is the use of computer-scored self-report tests. These enable the clinical team to obtain testing information rapidly at minimum staff manpower costs. The results can be combined with clinical interviews to make treatment plans.

A number of the tests in Tables 1–4 are self-report tests that can be computer scored. Some of them have accompanying computer generated verbal reports. Butcher (63) discusses the pros and cons of these computer-generated reports. Logical foci for screening tests on an acute inpatient unit include symptom patterns, suicidal ideation, personality strengths and weaknesses, environmental stressors, and family adjustment.

Typical Indications for Assessment Beyond Screening

The general indication for testing beyond screening is insufficient information on the five areas needed for treatment planning mentioned earlier. A number of typical situations arise on the clinical scene for additional information from tests.

Since children and adolescents have a brief history of psychopathology, more extensive testing is often indicated to delineate the areas of pathology not yet totally manifested and to obtain baseline information. Situations in which the child or adolescent is going back to a school district that wants testing by the Committee on Special Services* also call for further testing. Placement upon discharge in halfway houses, sheltered workshops, and day hospitals may also necessitate testing in order to assist the patient in meeting the admissions criteria for these services.

Patients whose diagnoses are unclear upon clinical interview and screening tests may need further testing. This often includes patients with suspected but unconfirmed thought disorder and patients with both affective and thought disorder symptoms. Further testing is often indicated when clinical interview suggests that the patient is suffering from neuropsychological deficits such as memory dysfunction, thus raising the differential question of depression and/or dementia. The use of tests with normative data for memory and cognitive functioning are most useful here.

Using Test Results Over Time to Chart Change

Third party payers are exerting increasing pressure on mental health profes-

sionals to provide evidence of patient pathology and indicators of clinical change. In addition, good clinical care suggests the need for assessing patient functioning and change along the specific mediating goals of hospital treatment. Thus, the use of multiple testing along specific dimensions of pathology targeted for change during an inpatient stay is indicated. Self-report instruments with normative data and computerized scoring lend themselves to this assessment task. We suspect that this area of testing will begin to increase in use. Although little literature in this area is available, we have utilized three forms of repeat testing. First, we have used repeat neuropsychological evaluations to assess delirium secondary to toxic-metabolic disorder secondary to substance abuse. Second, we have used repeat MMPIs on a substance-abuse unit to ascertain the change in symptomatology and to assess more characterological traits as the patient comes out of detoxification. In general, although the level of severity of symptoms decreases, the personality pattern profile remains relatively stable (64). Third, we have utilized repeat SCL-90s assisted by scanner scoring on a weekly basis on patients in an extended treatment division. Clinically useful profiles of symptom decay emerge. For example, one pattern emerges in which psychoticism decreases while anger rises, at least temporarily. And, finally, we encourage using using nurses' rating scales on a regular basis to chart patient change. These ratings are often more reliable and helpful to the clinical team than extensive nurses' chart notes. With the introduction of computerization, scores can easily be entered and plotted on a regular basis. An example of this type of development is the Cornell nurses' rating scale, a brief rating of patient behavior across areas of salient patient pathology (65).

---

*Designated group of school professionals who decide on special needs for identified children.

REFERENCES

1. Anastasi A: *Psychological Testing,* ed. 5, New York, Macmillan, 1982.

2. Clarkin JF, Hurt SW: Psychological assessment: Tests and rating scales, in Talbott J, Hales RJ, Yudofsky S (eds): *Textbook of Psychiatry,* pp. 225–246, Washington, D.C., American Psychiatric Press, 1988.

3. Butcher JN, Dahlstrom WG, Graham JR, Tellegen A, Kaemmer B: *Manual for the Restandardized Minnesota Multiphasic Personality Inventory: MMPI-2. An Administrative and Interpretive Guide,* Minneapolis, University of Minnesota Press, 1989.

4. *Millon T. Millon Clinical Multiaxial Inventory-II (MCMI-II),* Minneapolis, National Computer Systems, 1987.

5. Derogatis LR: *The SCL-90R,* Baltimore, Clinical Psychometric Research, 1977.

6. Overall JE, Gorham DR: The brief psychiatric rating scale. Psychol Rep, *10*:799–812, 1962.

7. Spitzer R, Williams J, Gibbon M: Structured Clinical Interview for DSM-IIIR (SCID). New York State Psychiatric Institute, Biometrics Research Department, 1987.

8. Spitzer RL, Endicott J: Schedule for Affective Disorders and Schizophrenia (SADS), ed. 3, New York, New York State Psychiatric Institute, Biometric Research Division, 1977.

9. Garner DM, Garfinkel PE. The eating attitudes test: An index of the symptoms of anorexia nervosa. Psychol Med, *9*:273–279, 1979.

10. Horn JL, Wanberg KW, Foster FM: *The Alcohol Use Inventory,* Baltimore, Psych Systems, 1983.

11. Spielberger CD, Gorsuch RL, Luchene RE: Manual for the State-Trait Anxiety Inventory. Palo Alto, Consulting Psychologists Press, 1976.

12. Beck AT, Ward CH, Mendelson M, et al: An inventory for measuring depression. Arch Gen Psychiatry, *4*:561–571, 1961.

13. Johnston MH, Holzman PS: *Assessing Schizophrenic Thinking,* San Francisco, Jossey-Bass, 1979.

14. Wechsler D: *Wechsler Adult Intelligence Scale, Revised,* New York, The Psychological Corporation, 1981.

15. Ammons RB, Ammons CH: The quick test (QT): Provisional manual. Psychol Rep, *11*:111–161, 1961.

16. Shipley WC: *The Institute of Living Scale,* Los Angeles, Western Psychological Services, 1946.

17. Jastak S, Wilkinson GS: *The Wide Range Achievement Test, Revised,* Wilmington, Jastak, 1981.

18. Rosvold HE, Mirsky AF, Sarason I, Bransome EB Jr, Beck LH: A continuous performance test of brain damage. J Consult Psychol, *20*:343–350, 1956.

19. Mirsky AF, Kornetsky C: On the dissimilar effects of drugs on the Digit Symbol Substitution and Continuous Performance Tests: A review and preliminary integration of behavioral and physiological evidence. Psychopharmacologia, *5*:161–177, 1964.

20. Kimura D: Functional asymmetry of the brain in dichotic listening. Cortex, *3*:163–178, 1967.

21. Wechsler D: *The Wechsler Memory Scale, Revised,* New York, Psychological Corporation, 1987.

22. Benton AL: *Visual Retention Test,* New York, Psychological Corporation, 1955.

23. Squire, LR: Shimamura AP: Characterizing amnesic patients for neurobehavioral study. Behav Neurosci, *100*(6):866–877, 1986.

24. Mattis S, Kovner R, Goldmeier E: Different patterns of mnemonic deficits in two organic amnestic syndromes. Brain Lang, *6*:179–191, 1978.

25. Benton AL, Hannay HJ, Varney NR: Visual peception of line direction in patients with unilateral brain disease. Neurology, *25*:907–910, 1975.

26. Benton AL, Van Allen MW: Impairment in facial recognition in patients with cerebral disease. Cortex, *4*:344–358, 1968.

27. Goldman R, Fristoe M, Woodcock RW: *Auditory Skills Test Battery,* Circle Pines, Minn., American Guidance Service, 1976.

28. Seashore CE, Lewis D, Saetveit DL: *Seashore Measures of Musical Talents, Revised Edition,* New York, Psychological Corporation, 1960.

29. Benton AL, Hamsher K: *Multilingual Aphasia Examination,* Iowa City, University of Iowa, 1976.

30. Benton AR, Spreen O: *Neurosensory*

Center Comprehensive Examination for Aphasia, Victoria, B.C., University of Victoria, 1969.

31. Goodglass H, Kaplan E: *Assessment of Aphasia and Related Disorders,* Philadelphia, Lea & Febeger, 1972.

32. Halstead WC, Wepman JM: The Halstead-Wepman aphasia screening test. J Speech Hear Disord, *14:*9–15, 1959.

33. Willner AE: Towards development of more sensitive clinical tests of abstraction: The analogy test. Proceedings of the 78th annual convention of the American Psychological Association, *5:*553–554, 1971.

34. Raven JC: *Guide to the Standard Progressive Matrices,* London, HK Lewis, 1960.

35. De Fillipis NA, McCambell E, Rogers P: Development of a booklet form of the Category Test: Normative and validity data. J Clin Neuropsychol, *1:*339–342, 1979.

36. Berg EA: A simple objective test for measuring flexibility in thinking. J Gen Psychol, *39:*15–32, 1948.

37. Heaton RK: *Wisconsin Card Sorting Test Manual,* Odessa, Fla., Psychological Assessment Resources, 1981.

38. Rey A: L'examen psychologique dans les cas d'encephalopathie traumatique. Archives de Psychologie, *28*(112):286–340, 1941.

39. Luria AR: *Higher Cortical Functions in Man,* New York, Basic Books, 1966.

40. Lezak M: *Neuropsychological Assessment,* New York, Oxford Press, 1969.

41. Mattis S, French JH, Rapin I: Dyslexia in children and young adults: Three independent neuropsychological syndromes. Dev Med Child Neurol, *17:*150–163, 1975.

42. Costa LD, Vaughan HG, Levita E, Farber N: Purdue pegboard as a predicator of the presence and laterality of cerebral lesions. J Consult Psychol, *27:*133–137, 1961.

43. Klove H: Clinical Neuropsychology, in Forster FM (ed): *Medical Clinics of North America,* New York, Saunders, 1963.

44. Rorschach H: *Psychodiagnostics,* New York, Grune & Stratton, 1949.

45. Murray HA: *Thematic Apperception Test,* manual, Cambridge, Harvard University Press, 1943.

46. Exner JE Jr: *The Rorschach: A Comprehensive System (Volumes 1 and 2),* New York, John Wiley & Sons, 1974, 1978.

47. Beutler LE, Clarkin JF: *Systematic Treatment Selection,* New York, Brunner/Mazel, 1990.

48. Brown GW, Rutter M: The measurement of family activities and relationships: A methodological study. Hum Relations, *19:*241–263, 1966.

49. Weissman MM, Bothwell S: Assessment of social adjustment by patient self-report. Arch Gen Psychiatry, *33:*111–115, 1976.

50. Katz MM, Lyerly SB: Methods for measuring adjustment and social behavior in the community: I. Rationale, description, discriminative validity and scale development. Psychol Rep Mono, *13:*503–535, 1963.

51. Clarkin JF, Frances A, Perry S: *Treatment Choices in Psychiatry: Differential Therapeutics and DSM-IIIR,* Washington, D.C., American Psychiatric Press, (in press).

52. Andreason N: *The Scale for the Assessment of Positive Symptoms (SAPS),* Iowa City, The University of Iowa, 1984.

53. Andreason N: *The Scale for the Assessment of Negative Symptoms (SANS),* Iowa City, The University of Iowa, 1983.

54. Bellack AS: Recurrent problems in the behavioral assessment of social skill. Behave Res Ther, *21:*29–42, 1983.

55. Hamilton M: A rating scale for depression. J Neurol Neurosurg Psychiatry, *12:*56–62, 1960.

56. Beck AT: *Cognitive Theory and the Emotional Disorders,* New York, International Universities Press, 1976.

57. Hammen C, Krantz SE: Measures of psychological process in depression, in Beckham EE, Leber WR, (eds): *Handbook of Depression: Treatment, Assessment and Research,* pp 408–444, Homewood, Il., Dorsey Press, 1985.

58. Beck AT, Rush AJ, Shaw BF, Emery G: *Cognitive Therapy of Depression: A Treatment Manual,* New York, Guilford Press, 1979.

59. Hollon S, Kendall P: Cognitive self-statements in depression: Development of an automatic thoughts questionnaire. Cog Ther Res, *4:*383–396, 1980.

60. Weissman AN: The dysfunctional attitude scale: A validation study. Doctoral dissertation, University of Pennsylvania, 1979.

61. Snyder DK, Willis RM, Keiser TW: Empirical validation of the Marital Satisfaction

Inventory: An actuarial approach. J Consult Clin Psychol, *49*:262–268, 1979.

62. Locke HJ, Wallace KM: Short marital-adjustment and prediction tests. Their reliability and validity. Marr Fam Living, *21*:251–255, 1959.

63. Butcher JN (ed): *Computerized Psychological Assessment*, New York, Basic Books, 1987.

64. Hurt SW, Clarkin JF, Morey L: An examination of the stability of the MMPI personality disorder scales. J Pers Assess, *54* (1 & 2): 16–23, 1990.

65. Evans S, Brown R, Glassman M, Larson K: The Cornell Nurses' Rating Scale. Presented at the annual meeting of the American Psychiatric Association, Washington, D.C., May 1986.

15

Legal Issues in Inpatient Psychiatry

Harold Bursztajn, MD
Thomas G. Gutheil, MD
Bonnie Cummins

INTRODUCTION

Any contemporary textbook on inpatient psychiatry would be incomplete without a substantial section devoted to the legal issues that exert an impact on inpatient clinicians. The past 20 years have spawned a changing but increasingly expanding body of legislation and case law regarding the rights, care, and treatment of the mentally ill. One result of this growth has been an expansion of the contact points between psychiatry and the law, especially in the areas of criminal, victim compensation, and family law. Since numerous books have been written on these classical contact points, we will focus on those emerging areas of contact where the inpatient psychiatrist's understanding of medicolegal issues is critical to the care of *any* hospitalized patient. In particular, the exercise of good judgment and careful understanding of today's most pressing legal issues regarding informed consent, liability, and patient rights are a must if these developments are going to enhance rather than compromise the quality of hospitalized patients' care. Therefore,

this chapter will focus on integrating emerging legal requirements into the clinical process. Matters of documentation, an essential aspect of all medicolegal activity, are addressed in the next chapter.

INFORMED CONSENT

Informed Consent: From Pro Forma to Process

When we approach informed consent as a form to be signed by the patient in order to meet legal requirements, both the clinician and patient experience it as little more than a manipulation: clinical utility is absent and its legal value is dubious. On the other hand, when we understand that the criteria for informed consent derives meaning from a two-person process, the criteria can help build the doctor-patient alliance.

Quality care and the informed consent process are the wheel and axle of the vehicle of psychiatric inpatient diagnosis and treatment. The inpatient psychiatrist is legally mandated to obtain and document informed consent before administering all diagnostic and treatment interventions. The doctrine of informed consent stipulates that the patient must consent to the procedure(s) before it is performed and that this consent is predicated on *voluntary* acceptance and *competence* in understanding reasonable *information* about the procedure or treatment. Failure to obtain patient consent may legally constitute battery; failure to meet the criteria for informed consent may constitute negligence. We can satisfy the criteria for informed consent by determining the patient's voluntariness of consent and capacity to take part in the informed consent procedure.

A patient's signed consent form is not considered evidence of voluntariness or competence. As such it is not a substitute for either the exploration we recommend or for documentation that such exploration took place. Its major use is as a reminder that exploration and documentation are necessary. When consent forms are routinely substituted for these, both quality of care and risk management suffer.

VOLUNTARINESS

In relation to informed consent voluntariness means, most simply, that the patient made a choice in the absence of coercion. Some would argue that institutionalized individuals cannot "voluntarily" choose since their present needs and future wishes are tied to their caretakers' recommendations. Acceptance of this premise would deny institutionalized individuals the right to make any important decisions and seriously compromise the promotion of individual autonomy that informed consent seeks to achieve. Therefore, voluntariness of consent should be understood as free patient choice in the absence of coercion or undue influence. This applies equally to voluntarily or involuntarily hospitalized patients.

To some extent many psychiatric pa-

tients are either "unduly influenceable" or "uninfluenceable." An example of undue influenceability is the overly dependent patient who is over 18 yet still symbiotically tied to a parental figure and unable to distinguish his own wishes from those of the parent. The psychiatrist must consider whether she has become such a figure for her patient, via the process of transference. On the other end of the spectrum is the overwhelmingly counterdependent and uninfluenceable patient who remains aloof and excludes dialogue.

At times patients may be *both* overly influenceable and uninfluenceable. This can occur when patients are so tied to a real or imagined parental figure that they are unable to exercise a will of their own sufficient to engage in dialogue. Such patients may present as counterdependent to the examiner ("I won't listen to anything you have to say"), while experiencing themselves as powerless, weak-willed, and dependent for their survival on an all-powerful parental figure. Exploring with patients their experienced vulnerability to domination or abandonment is critical to moving beyond such a clinical stalemate. It is also critical to undertake such an exploration in order to safeguard against the legal proceedings that patients may focus on as a substitute for working through clinical conflict.

CAPACITY (COMPETENCE)

"The ability to understand rationally"—i.e., competence—is a legal concept, determined by the court (1). Competence most often refers to the capacity to understand the nature and consequences of one's actions or decisions. Some individuals are recognized as generally incompetent, others as showing specific incompetence. In the latter group, the individual may be competent to arrive at personal decisions but not treatment decisions. The general rule today is that involuntary commitment does not presume incompetence. In fact, a committed mentally ill person is presumed competent unless legally adjudicated otherwise.

It is neither possible (because of limited resources) nor desirable to legally determine competence for each patient before the delivery of clinical services. The process of deciding to obtain a judicial competence evaluation is therefore integrated into the work of the inpatient unit.

Psychiatrists and the courts use several tests for determining competency to consent to treatment. Certain populations appear at risk for incompetency: acutely psychotic patients who might exhibit delirium; chronic (long-term) institutionalized patients who may have lost critical reasoning capacity; organically impaired patients; elderly senile patients; depressed patients who may be generally hopeless about the future; and retarded patients (2). Psychiatrists should assess these groups if competency to consent to treatment is at all in question. To be judged psychologically competent, individuals should: (*a*) show an awareness of their current situation (living circumstances, relationships, health status, etc.); (*b*) possess a factual understanding of the issues (exhibit a clear and realistic comprehension of the facts which bear upon decision making); and (*c*) show the capacity to manipulate data rationally for decision making. Apply these criteria to both general and specific competency assessments.

Implicit in the above criteria is that the patient demonstrate these capacities in the presence of another person, namely, the psychiatrist. As such, competence can be most properly considered in a two-person context. The willingness of the examiner to provide the experience of safety and to engage in alliance building and the patient's ability to take advantage of help by engaging in a dialogue regarding the decisions in question are critical elements in any competency assessment. We may call this ele-ment of competency "interpersonal competency" or competency to engage in a therapeutic alliance (3). For example, keeping in mind that dialogue is a two-person process will give the benefit of the doubt to the foreign-speaking patient by placing the onus for achieving a dialogue on the clinician, who may have to seek an interpreter or bilingual examiner. On the other hand, the competence of a paranoid, aloof patient, who is able to recite "facts" but refuses to engage in a dialogue regarding risks and benefits even with an empathic examiner, becomes far more questionable under this criterion.

A primary concern to psychiatrists regarding competence of patients in an inpatient setting is *consent or refusal of treatment.* Since precise competency standards for the treatment decision do not exist, psychiatrists should examine questionably incompetent patients and document findings. One approach is to use a consent form which has a written information component and an oral dialogue questions component to assess level of patient understanding of information. The dialogue exemplifies the next component of informed consent—that is, the clinician's provision of reasonable information about the procedure or treatment.

INFORMATION

As we have discussed, adequate consent entails *voluntary* behavior, the *capacity* to participate rationally in the process, and must also include reasonable and appropriate *information* conveyed to the patient. The current standard of what kind and how much information is reasonable is that the physician should disclose all information that a reasonable person might want in deciding to accept or reject treatment: what the treatment consists of, benefits and risks; alternatives, with their benefits and risks; and no treatment, with its benefits and risks. Since an exhaustive list of risks and alternatives is by no means practical or even possible in all cases, the clinician may wish to use a modified decision analytic sliding scale approach in determining how to engage the patient in the informed consent process. Stated more simply, the greater the probability of an outcome or the greater the magnitude of the gain or loss associated with the outcome, the more incumbent it is upon the physician to enter it into the dialogue.

Special Situations

The requirements of informed consent do not apply to all situations. Emergency, therapeutic privilege, waiver, and incompetency involve special legal and clinical consideration.

EMERGENCIES

In medical emergencies, physicians may render medical services in the absence of a formal consent, if taking the time to secure consent (from the patient or substitute consent for patient) would pose a life-threatening delay of needed treatment. In psychiatry, treatment may be given in the absence of consent when patients become violent or self-mutilating and require intervention to prevent immediate harm to themselves or others. Unfortunately, the law to date does not generally recognize a broader sense of emergency, which would include depressed patients in severe distress or even psychotic patients in overwhelming psychological pain (if they are nonviolent or not actively suicidal).

THERAPEUTIC PRIVILEGE

Another exception to informed consent is that of therapeutic privilege. If the information about the nature of the patient's condition and treatment might be *directly* damaging to the patient, it can be withheld. However, such information cannot be withheld if the damage would be

mediated solely by the decision of an adequately informed patient to refuse treatment. For example, the clincian's concern that a psychotic patient may refuse neuroleptics when informed of the risk of tardive dyskinesia is not sufficient grounds for withholding that information. In such a case, where the damage of a continuing untreated psychotic state is at issue, a careful competency assessment needs to be undertaken rather than invoking therapeutic privilege.

WAIVER

The right of informed consent can be waived by the patient. The patient may say "Tell me what to do, I don't want to know." This waiver should be respectfully explored by the clinician in order to assess the meaning of the patient's wish *not* to know, which may involve a degree of denial ranging from the healthy to the psychotic. Only such an exploration will suffice to document the patient's competence to waive informed consent. Blind compliance, as much as blind refusal, should alert the physician to potential pathology that may need to be addressed in the course of inpatient treatment.

INCOMPETENCY

Patients who have already been judged by a court to be incompetent cannot then give informed consent. A court-appointed monitor or substitute decision maker must then be obtained for purposes of informed consent.

The decision to petition the court to judge the patient incompetent is not a step to be taken lightly. As all other clinical decisions, it is best made following a dialogue with the patient regarding the impact such judicial action will have on the patient. It is critical to document the clinician's efforts at achieving such a dialogue, especially where such dialogue is severely constricted by the patient's illness. Following judicial action it is important to assess the impact the clinician's initiative has on the therapeutic alliance. As treatment progresses and dialogue becomes possible, it is important to inquire about the impact of the judicial determination of incompetency. The patient needs to be assured that the determination was for purposes of treatment aimed toward restoring the patient to competency as his or her own decision maker regarding treatment. As competency is regained, the clinician is well advised once again to initiate the patient in the judicial review process and prepare the clinical documentation supporting a judicial finding of competency. A common error is for the clinician to initiate only the first part of the process while leaving the latter for legal advocates.

Such a clinical error not only disrupts the therapeutic alliance, it also contributes to the posttraumatic stress disorder which patients suffer as a common, yet often unrecognized, sequela to serious, competence-impairing illness. Moreover, it represents an invitation from the clinician for the patient to turn away from the therapeutic alliance toward a posture of opposition and litigiousness. From a risk-management standpoint, failure to ask for judicial review when the patient is restored to competency leaves the clinician vulnerable not only to legal problems but also to the fact that any subsequent tragic outcome would be considered from the generally accepted higher intensive standard of care required for incompetent patients (4–10).

Summary

In approaching informed consent as a two-person process we seek to turn legal constraint to clinical advantage through the clinical dialogue. In doing so, the therapeutic alliance can be strengthened to withstand the uncertainty which characterizes inpatient treatment of high-risk populations. In sharing uncertainty throughout the decision-making process, one may preserve

realistic hopes in the patient without fostering magical wishes for omnipotence. The disappointment of magical wishes by tragic outcomes forms the basis of many a malpractice suit.

MALPRACTICE

Defining Malpractice

Malpractice law is a subcategory of tort law, that branch of civil law concerned with providing redress for damages suffered as a consequence of a breach of duty. Malpractice is negligent or substandard practice by a professional or a failure to perform a duty that results in an injury to patient or client. Psychiatrists are liable for malpractice, though the claims against psychiatrists are fewer than those against other medical specialties. The action taken in a tort is a demand for compensation for damages to the injured party. Four conditions must be met to have a malpractice claim.

DUTY TO CARE

In order for patients to allege that a physician's negligence caused them damage they must first prove that the physician assumed a "duty to care" or a treatment relationship with them. Once a duty to care has been established, the physician is responsible for nonnegligent care. Duty to care can be terminated if the patient is medically discharged or transferred to another facility or physician.

NEGLIGENCE

The physician who takes on the duty to care for a specific patient also takes on the duty to care in a nonnegligent manner. The level of care is generally assessed against what other members of the medical specialty (with similar training and therapeutic orientation) would customarily do in a similar situation, that is, community standards (11, 12). In some jurisdictions, however, the care given has been assessed as negligent in comparison with what a hypothetical "reasonable and prudent" practitioner might do or against an even more abstract risk-benefit standard for care.

The prevailing current standard is the nationally recognized standard for psychiatric care. In practice this is translated by courts to mean that the practitioner or institution "deviated from accepted medical practice expected of a psychiatrist (or institution) in these circumstances." The existence of this standard derives in part from the presence of national journals, meetings, and organizations.

HARM

A physician is liable for damages only in the event that the breach of duty to care directly caused harm of a physical and/or emotional nature.

CAUSATION

A physician who has established the duty to care for a patient in a nonnegligent way and has breached this duty is still liable *only* if the alleged harm can be found to have been the direct consequence of this act or the "proximate" result of the act.

In summary, any patient suing a physician for malpractice must prove these four elements to be true by a preponderance of the evidence.

Historically, psychiatrists have been sued less frequently than other physicians. Among psychiatrists in recent years, the most frequent causes for action alleged in malpractice suits have been psychiatric negligence leading to patient suicide.

The most recent data furnished by the insurers of members of the American Psychiatric Association indicates the frequency of malpractice claims listed in Table 15.1. A comparison of these data with data cited in the previous edition of this chapter indicates that negligent treatment, medication, supervision, and confinement have emerged as leading causes of action during

Table 15.1. Frequency of Type of Claims

Negligent Treatment	19.8%
Suicides/Attempted Suicide	17.1%
Misdiagnosis of Illness	9.9%
Improper Medications	9.9%
Negligent Supervision of Patient	7.4%
Negligent Confinement	5.7%
Undue Familiarity	5.7%
Breach of Confidentiality	2.6%
Lack of Informed Consent	2.2%
Other	15.0%

the interim. These risks can be diminished by integrating the model of *informed consent as process* into the clinical repartee, wherein restoring and enhancing patient competence and minimizing the need for involuntary commitment or treatment are well articulated as *treatment goals* (rather than remaining medicolegal abstractions and the exclusive realm of "patient rightists").

Malpractice Risk Management

SUICIDE

As the evidence demonstrates, suicide poses the second greatest number of malpractice claims against psychiatrists. The cases cited point to suicide as accounting for more than 17% of all malpractice suits. The percentage increases when we include injury from a suicide attempt. A relatively high number of suicides occur among individuals who have seen a therapist in the previous year.

When the risk of suicide is present, as in the chronically suicidal borderline patient, benefits of less restrictive care (e.g., unlocked units or outpatient care) need to be weighed against the risks of being unable to prevent acting out of acute exacerbations of suicidal impulses (e.g., overdose). In such cases, it is useful to engage the patients themselves—and, where appropriate, the family—in the informed consent process. Planned transitions to less restrictive environments, e.g., transfer from closed to open units, provide an opportunity to assess and enhance the patient's capacity for engaging in dialogue and sharing responsibility—a capacity which is at the heart of therapeutic alliance building and the maturational process. For example, hypomanic patients need to be asked what they understand the risks and benefits of any planned transition to be. The clinician needs to monitor how character and psychopathology may shape or distort individual understanding and to confront hypomanic denial of difficulties and risks.

The informed consent process in this way supports the most mature side of the patient's self. By helping patients engage in a dialogue where they are supported in remembering, observing, and anticipating, the therapeutic goals of enhancing these capacities and recruiting them to serve the patients' best interests are advanced. With the understanding of these capacities the patient becomes less vulnerable to being overwhelmed by affect and the acting out of suicidal impulses (11, 12, 13).

The inpatient psychiatrist will more frequently be the target of malpractice action because of treating a select population of more disturbed patients who are at greatest risk for tragic outcomes. By the same token, in treating a population where patient competence and ability to take responsibility are more often at issue, the inpatient psychiatrist needs repeatedly to engage hospitalized patients in a process of assessing their ability to assume responsibility for their own actions. In the absence of such review, the psychiatrist is vulnerable to the assumption that inpatients are less able to take responsibility for themselves than outpatients, and thus an inpatient psychiatrist should be held to a necessarily higher standard of care (14, 15). This blanket assumption ignores the fact that during the course of their hospitalization many inpatients regain their ability to assume responsibility and that inpatient treatment can include an unlocked environment and leaves of absence. For example, by carefully engaging the patient in a dialogue-based informed consent process when leaves of absence are considered, the inpatient psychiatrist gains both a valuable and responsible ally in the patient. This also decreases the likelihood that the hospitalized patient's responsibility for any tragic outcome will, in a jury's hindsight, be automatically discounted, consequently holding the psychiatrist to a higher standard of care than warranted.

Inpatients and outpatient psychiatric populations present different legal dilemmas. With outpatients, a malpractice suit is usually based on the allegation that the treating psychiatrist was negligent for not hospitalizing the patient or negligent in prematurely releasing the patient. These cases are less often successful, as courts do recognize the difficulty in predicting suicide.

For inpatients, documentation of the clinical evaluation and decision to *discharge* is one protection against suit for the suicide of a recently discharged inpatient. When the patient is being discharged against medical advice and the risk of suicide is thought to be chronic but the patient is not deemed committable, this reasoning should be shared with the patient and, when possible, the family. Documentation of the decision-making process, the consultation obtained, and the participation of patient and family is critical.

Inpatients thought to be at *high risk* of suicide constitute another medicolegal problem. Hospital procedures—be they close observation, one-to-one supervision, or some other intervention—should be openly reviewed. Although "suicide-proofing" an inpatient unit remains a concept more platonic than realistic, the inpatient environment itself should be as free as possible of obvious opportunities for suicide, including, for example, insecure windows or access to sharp objects. A shared understanding by staff, patient, and family about what is being done and why in the context of an overall treatment plan is the best protection (15).

Beyond the absence of such "attractive nuisances" for the suicidal, competence-impaired patient, the most important aspect of the inpatient environment is the presence of a trained and continually educated and updated milieu staff capable of communicating and creating a treatment alliance with the frightened and demoralized patient. Whatever the treatment philosophy of the institution (whatever mix of the psychodynamic, behavioral, interpersonal, and biologic orientations), the staff must be aware of the hows and whys and countertransference impediments of communicating with the severely ill patient. The presence of continuing staff education is an important component in creating a risk-minimized environment for the care of the severely suicidal patient (16–18).

Suicide litigation involves two main issues: (a) whether the psychiatrist should have predicted that a patient was likely to commit self-harm, and (b) if the risk was apparent, whether the psychiatrist took adequate precautions to protect the patient from self-harm. If a psychiatrist did not conclude that a hospitalized patient was in danger of self-harm and therefore did not take adequate precautions, the court will ask whether a reasonable and prudent psychiatrist would have predicted the risk. Courts do acknowledge the uncertainty of prediction in this area and will usually not hold a physician liable who exercised reasonable care. When the risk was apparent but the psychiatrist did not prevent the suicide, the courts question the adequacy of precautionary measures taken. The determination of adequacy is difficult for courts and juries acting in hindsight; measures regarded as deterrents to suicide (such as close observation, seclusion, etc.) may, in fact, prove antitherapeutic in the long run, even though they impede immediate self-harm.

Determining the risk of suicide in a given patient is an uncertain matter. Psychiatrists can reduce liability by documenting the decision-making process and the provision of reasonable care, following customary procedures in assessing risk, and noting obtained consultation with colleagues (in difficult cases) (11, 12).

Although the probability of an outpatient as opposed to an inpatient malpractice suit resulting in victory for the plaintiff still seems to be less, both the probability and awards for damages for negligent outpatient care seem to be growing. By the same token, outpatient clinicians have increasingly been named in suits involving the suicide of their hospitalized patients when evidence exists of prior negligent outpatient care. The mere hospitalization of a patient does not absolve the outpatient clinician of responsibility either for prior care or subsequent outcome.

BEARING TRAGIC OUTCOMES

"Outreach" by the hospital treatment team to families of a patient who commits suicide or homicide (2) is an important clinical practice. Though clinicians are barraged by their own feelings of failure, anger, and sadness in the face of such clinical tragedies, to whatever extent possible the clinician can and should try to put these feelings temporarily aside and offer support to the family. Attending funeral services for a patient who has committed suicide is appropriate and usually appreciated by the family. Most importantly, this practice is good, humane care. It is also legally sound behavior. This supportive family "postvention" decreases the likelihood that the grieving family will act out its guilt, displace the anger directed at the deceased onto the psychiatrist and treatment team, and then sue for malpractice.

Homicide perpetrators pose different types of problems. The inpatient staff will need to face fears for their own safety in order to provide quality clinical care. Anger aroused by the crime (in the treatment team) must never be translated into less-than-appropriate treatment. Outreach with the family (who may be related to the victim) again is both a humane act and a form of malpractice prevention (2). By the same token, the perpetrator's family may also need support.

In addition to direct risk-management considerations, providing supportive care to the surviving family and facilitating the referral process for longer-term care can be helpful in protecting the survivors from the sequela of bereavement resulting from the suicide of a relative (24). In practice, such sequelae tend to have the characteristics of posttraumatic stress disorder. The emerging national standard is to provide supportive care, education, and referral for families of survivors (25). Failure to inform the family of an anticipated posttraumatic stress disorder and refer for treatment, even where no negligence exists in the treatment of the now deceased patient, leaves the institution and practitioner liable for damages consequent to such a failure, if it can be demonstrated that a treatment relationship also exists with the family. Although circumstances vary, in the cases of some seriously ill patients, a treatment relationship could be inferred to customarily exist with the immediate family.

MEDICATION SIDE EFFECTS

Informed consent as an ongoing process (19) is particularly critical in an area as anxiety provoking to patients as medication side effects. We shall focus on how to apply the process of informed consent to prescribing antipsychotic medication and its possible side effect of tardive dyskinesia. However, the following discussion applies to any medication with potentially serious side effects (e.g., antidepressants and cardiac toxicity, antianxiety agents and addiction, lithium and renal toxicity). The process

of informed consent allows the clinician the opportunity to turn legal constraints into clinical advantage (20).

Tardive dyskinesia (movement disorders of face, tongue, and extremity muscles) is now an established side effect of antipsychotic medication. The development of tardive diskinesia (TD) does not reflect negligence in adminstering antipsychotic drugs, for it can occur under optimal neuroleptic drug regimes. However, failure to warn patients of the risk of TD (as of any major side effect likely to occur) has in the recent past led to huge out-of-court settlements and in-court awards (21, 22). Therefore, clinical care and malpractice liability concerns insist that psychiatrists fully inform patients of this side effect, obviously in an unthreatening and supportive fashion. Some researchers (recognizing the potential for malpractice suits in this area) suggest that written rather than oral informed consent be used with patients at high risk for TD (23). However, progress notes which document an ongoing process of review may be more clinically sound and no less a safeguard against suit.

Consent and liability issues with neuroleptics are of major import (26–28). The timing of consent is critical. If a patient is, by reason of psychosis, acutely incompetent and in need of emergency treatment, treat the patient and attempt to convey the relevant information; if treatment results in a restoration of competency, informed consent should await recompensation and should then be definitively obtained if and when further neuroleptic treatment is indicated (29). In addition to a legal necessity, a doctor-patient dialogue regarding the risks and benefits of acute and chronic neuroleptic treatment can engage the patient in an educational process in itself alliance-building and potentially capable of restoring self-esteem. Ego capacities of remembering, observing, and anticipating are also exercised by the consent process. The patient can learn to report any change which might indicate the reappearance of psychosis or the emergence of the earliest symptoms of tardive dyskinesia and thus provide an "early warning" system for re-evaluating neuroleptic therapy. Moreover, the extent to which patients can improve their ego capacities in the course of treatment is itself a useful indicator of the ongoing process of recovery. In fact, improvement in the capacity to participate in the informed consent process may be an indicator that the neuroleptic dose can, *ceteris paribus* (all other things being equal), begin to be tapered. If the patient remains chronically unable to engage in such a dialogue, the clinician may have to take sole charge of monitoring, which can entail supplementing the clinical examination for tardive dyskinesia with periodic formal tests, e.g., the AIMS test (an abnormal involuntary movement scale).

Our empirical research at the Program in Psychiatry and the Law at the Massachusetts Mental Health Center has demonstrated that psychiatrists' willingness to prescribe neuroleptics varied depending on whether they were asked to "risk" or to "accept" a particular probability of side effects (30). Moreover, court judges in our survey grossly overestimated the probability of tardive dyskinesia occurring as a side effect. Obviously, clinicians must pay careful attention to the language in which they engage in the informed consent dialogue. Furthermore, psychiatrists face the major task of educating the legal profession regarding the actual balance of benefits and side effects of neuroleptics.

Review of the emerging case law with high awards may be instructive. In what is becoming a landmark case, *Clites v. Iowa* (31), the Iowa court of appeals awarded $760,000 to a mentally retarded man who had been treated with neuroleptics for his aggressive behavior. The plaintiff alleged that the physicians had both used the drugs negligently (lack of patient monitoring, ab-

sence of drug holidays, neuroleptics used as tranquilizers to control behavior) and had not secured informed consent.

A second case, *Faigenbaum v. Cohen* (32), involved the failure to warn about and diagnose tardive dyskinesia. In this case, tardive dyskinesia was misdiagnosed as Huntington's chorea. The plaintiff sued the hospitals, drug companies, and physicians. The original verdict awarded $1.5 million to the plaintiff. (The current appeal is based on the state's claim of immunity from suit for its hospitals and physicians.) The drug companies and private practice physicians have already settled.

A third case, *Hedin v. U.S.* (33), awarded $2.1 million to a veteran and an additional amount to his wife (for loss of companionship) on the basis of negligent prescription of neuroleptics by Veterans Adminstration physicians.

Two of these three cases found for the plaintiff partly on the basis of inadequately obtained informed consent or lack of any informed consent. The message to inpatient psychiatrists should be clear: always obtain informed consent before nonemergency treatment with neuroleptics.

Chronic patients needing high doses of neuroleptics constitute a population at high risk for tardive dyskinesia. General counsel for the APA urges reobtaining informed consent every six months for those patients on high doses of antipsychotic drugs. Only in an emergency should these drugs be used without consent. Therapeutic privilege, which holds that informed consent can be withheld if the physician believes that knowledge of risks would be directly detrimental to the patient, is another exception. However, most courts accept only extremely narrow instances of therapeutic privilege. As a rule, substitute consent from a legal guardian should be obtained instead of using therapeutic privilege.

Psychiatrists are also well advised to

follow the APA guidelines on tardive dys-kinesia (28). These guidelines include (a) using the lowest effective dose of neurolep-tics for a given patient, and (b) examining for early signs of tardive dyskinesia every 3–6 months; if signs of tardive dyskinesia appear, a review should be held to consider whether lowering the dosage, changing to a more benign drug, or stopping treatment is contraindicated. Tardive dyskinesia litiga-tion in the future may shift from a com-munity standard of care to a standard of strict liability (22). At the very least such a shift would mean that the burden of proof would be on physicians to prove that they did not act negligently rather than on the plaintiff to prove that the physician did. In a more extreme form, the treating psychia-trist may be held responsible for the patient suffering tardive dyskinesia irrespective of any proof of nonnegligent prescribing.

As newer antipsychotic agents are de-veloped and approved for clinical use and as their side-effect profile may involve a lower risk of TD and a higher risk of other potentially irreversible serious side effects, the clinician is responsible for reviewing the options and weighing their risks and bene-fits for the chronically ill patient. Where ongoing family treatment is part of the thera-peutic approach to the chronically ill pa-tient, the informed consent *process* can be extended to include the family. Psychiatrists in the often ambiguous role of medical back-up to a nonmedical therapist should insist on meeting with the patient on an on-going basis and be actively involved in ed-ucating *both* the patient and the nonmedical therapist about treatment options (34, 35). "Blind prescribing" carries with it not only the risks of negligent clinical care but also leaves open the possibility that the in-formed-consent process will be aborted, leaving the clinician open to liability for negligently administering medication.

The initial use of high dosages of a high-potency neuroleptic and the failure to attempt to gradually wean the patient from such high dosages after a crisis represent a special quality of care and risk-management problem. For example, *Leal v. Simon* (542 N.Y.S. 2d 328, 1989) resulted in a jury award of $2 million for the patient's pain and suffering as a result of the excessive use of haloperidol and $500,000 for care and maintenance services. In this case the ap-pellate courts acted to reduce jury awards; however, it is not unusual for the damages to be assessed in excess of $1 million.

IMPROPER DIAGNOSIS

This category deserves explanation, for we are all aware that clinical diagnostic errors and ambiguities are inevitable. How-ever, malpractice involving improper diag-nosis does not pertain to human error in judgment. Rather, it applies to negligence, as in failing to use the diagnostic procedures and equipment that a prudent, competent psychiatrist would use to reach a diagnosis. An example of diagnostic negligence would be treating as a psychiatric disorder an or-ganic disorder that should have been sus-pected and failing to obtain an internal medicine consultation.

HOMICIDE AND THE PROBLEM OF CONFIDENTIALITY

Although cases in which a psychiatric patient commits a violent act against a third party do not occur frequently, they may re-sult in large financial awards. The parallel to suicide cases is apparent: both involve the uncertainty which surrounds the accurate prediction of violence. Furthermore, cases of violence raise questions about whether and how the psychiatrist took prophylactic measures to prevent a potentially violent patient from causing harm. Courts have been less sympathetic towards psychiatrists' difficulties in predicting dangerousness to-wards others than they have in cases in-volving violence towards the self (suicide).

A number of cases involve identifiable

victims and the *duty to protect (or to warn)*. These cases involve both outpatients and recently released inpatients. The outcome of most of these cases has held the psychiatrist liable for injuries to the victim when (*a*) the psychiatrist knew or should have known that a patient was likely to harm a specific individual and (*b*) the psychiatrist failed to warn or otherwise protect that individual. An often-quoted and, by now, famous case that held a therapist liable for failing to prevent a violent act towards a patient's victim was *Tarasoff v. Regents of the University of California* (36). In this case, a former student contacted a school psychologist for therapy. The psychologist tried to initiate civil commitment of the young man based on the supposition that this patient might harm his exgirlfriend, Tatiana Tarasoff. The university police who subsequently interviewed the young man decided on their own that he should not be committed. He murdered Tatiana Tarasoff several months thereafter. The family sued the university and the involved clinicians on the basis that they should have done more to protect the young woman. The California Supreme Court held that once a therapist does in fact determine, or under applicable professional standards reasonably should have determined, that a patient poses a serious danger of violence to others, the therapist bears a duty to exercise reasonable care to protect the foreseeable victim of that danger. The duty to protect (or warn) exists in many states, when specific threats are made against specific victims. Some states go even further than the Tarasoff decision, holding that psychiatrists may be liable even if their patients harm persons not specified in advance (37).

The court's creation of a therapist's duty to protect third parties was expected by some psychiatrists to harm the therapeutic alliance needed to treat patients by negating the confidentiality of the patient-therapist relationship. The courts were ac-cused of creating a situation whereby either the patient leaves treatment (and may then be more likely to continue to act out violent impulses) or more patients are civilly committed (38). No recent evidence reliably demonstrates that these fears have proved valid. We have elsewhere attempted to show how the effects of the Tarasoff decision on the care of a potentially violent patient can be turned to clinical advantage. In selected cases it has been possible to foster the therapeutic alliance by engaging patients in a process similar to informed consent and thus enabling them to explore their ambivalence about the destructive act (20). The essential point here is to remember that the clinician's ally is that side of the patient that wants to retain control. The clinician is thus not counterposed to the patient, merely to that *side* of the patient prone to violence.

While the courts have often found the clinician liable in cases in which (from hindsight) the violation of confidentiality would have resulted in saving the life of a third party, an opposing trend is also noted. Recently both Massachusetts and New Hampshire courts indicated that in nonemergency cases, the clinician may be found liable for breaking confidentiality (39, 40)! In view of these opposing trends, clinicians can avoid court-created paralysis by carefully documenting their reasoning and, when in doubt, seeking consultation.

A number of states, Massachusetts among them, have attempted to avoid court-induced paralysis with legislation that clearly spells out a therapist's duties and therapeutic options for discharging such duties. While such legislation is often initiated by state psychiatric societies in conjunction with other disciplinary societies and highly touted as a panacea for judicial intrusion into the treatment domain, it remains to be proven whether the substitution of legislative for judicial limitation of clinical autonomy and treatment options in high-risk cases truly decreases the risk of liability following a tragic outcome.

SEXUAL MISCONDUCT AND OTHER BOUNDARY VIOLATIONS

On an inpatient unit the intensity of affect and the states of regression of many patients often favor various boundary violations. These include inappropriate socialization with patients, fraternization by staff, exchange of gifts and money, special favors, and the entire spectrum of sexual misconduct. While most of these are problems of therapy and administration, the last has an additional weight.

While charges of sexual misconduct have been brought against physicians in various specialties, a psychiatrist who engages in sexual contact with a patient is clearly betraying the patient's trust. The rule clearly stated by the American Psychiatric Association code of ethics is that any sexual activity between patient and therapist represents improper behavior on the therapist's part (2). More recently, the breach of ethics has been extended to cover sexual relations with former patients. In addition, both civil and criminal prosecution for battery may be charged when such misconduct, however rationalized, occurs. It should be noted that the current malpractice insurance policy offered to APA members specifically excludes coverage for liability incurred on the basis of sexual misconduct.

Inpatient clinicians should be particularly sensitive to the vulnerability of hospitalized patients and staff to respond to feelings of frustration, hopelessness, and helplessness by a flight toward sexualization. Clinicians should be aware that under the doctrine of *respondeat superior* (the vicarious responsibility of superiors), they may be held liable for sexual acting out with patients by staff members under their direct supervision.

The doctrine of *respondeat superior* continues to enlarge in scope. Where sexual acting out has occurred by treatment team staff, the treating clinician, clinical administrator, and host institution may all be considered negligent. Where the early cases of negligence involved the failure to prevent such sexual contact once it came to light, the most recent trend clearly points to a finding of negligence irrespective of professed ignorance on the part of the supervising clinician or institution. Failure to provide an educational program and ongoing clinical supervision regarding the ethical issues and countertransference feelings raised in the course of treating seriously ill (and often previously abused) patients and failing to probe credentials thoroughly is well below accepted standards for supervision (41).

Inpatient units treating populations at high risk for sexual exploitation (e.g., adolescents or substance abusers) can meet the standard of care only if they provide adequate psychiatric supervision of clinical staff. Staff should be supported in understanding sexually provocative patient behavior and their own fantasies and feelings as transference and countertransference reactions to be clinically addressed.

Malpractice Prevention

While the delivery of quality care, documentation, and consultation are critical avenues of malpractice prevention, they are not the limits of preventive approaches. Physician sharing of the uncertainty of diagnosis, treatment, and outcome with patients is yet another malpractice prevention strategy (19). Malpractice suits in medicine often result from patient and family disappointment and helplessness in the face of tragic outcomes, rather than negligence. Informed consent, when practiced *pro forma*, often carries the suggestion of a guarantee and leads to unrealistic hopes. Instead, we recommend that informed consent be used as a starting point in establishing a true therapeutic alliance. Uncertainty is then mutually acknowledged and clinical decision making becomes a dialogue which is characteristic of the psychiatrist-patient relationship at its best. Such a dialogue is particularly critical in those areas where paradoxical legal trends have dramatized the conflict between societal needs, such as the need for protection of third parties (illustrated above) and of individuals' rights, such as the right to protection of confidentiality (20).

PATIENT RIGHTS

When beginning treatment or when therapeutic impasse has been reached or even when the patient has made genuine progress, the clinician may hear the patient speak the language of "rights": "I signed myself into the hospital so I have a right to sign myself out." Perhaps the most important reason for the inpatient clinician to understand the legal context of patient rights is to diminish the anxiety engendered by such assertions in order to allow for clinical exploration of their meaning. It is useful for the clinician to remember that while the legal model invokes the adversarial posture of "your rights versus my rights," the same position in psychiatric treatment indicates a narcissistic lesion in the doctor-patient alliance which needs to be explored. In the course of such an exploration one may often find the patient harboring the fear that the doctor-patient relationship will reproduce past relationships in which the only protection against domination and exploitation was to act oppositionally. Here again patient rights can best be protected if they are integrated into the informed consent process. By this process patients truly come to understand the risks and benefits of exercising their rights. Informed consent can only proceed if the clinician is guided by the psychodynamic model of man in conflict with himself, rather than the legal model of defendant versus plaintiff rights. A clinical alliance rather than a legal adversary process must always be the goal of treatment.

Admission to the Hospital

VOLUNTARY ADMISSION

Voluntary admission is defined by statute. Statutory law often explicitly prescribes conduct. Examples of statutory law are the setting of speed limits and the rules of civil commitment. In general, statutes are enacted at the state level. Medicine has recently come to be increasingly regulated by statutory law.

The majority of hospitalized psychiatric patients have voluntarily signed themselves into the hospital. Even incompetent patients can be "voluntarily" admitted by their guardians. Some patients voluntarily request hospitalization, knowing that commitment procedures will be started if they refuse voluntary admission. In this context critics have questioned the meaning of "voluntary" in the face of impending commitment proceedings. Most states do not require legal competence for voluntary admission. While voluntary admission is permitted, leaving the hospital at will is not. In some states voluntarily admitted psychiatric patients, upon entering the hospital, must sign a form acknowledging that they may be detained (for a period of time that differs state by state, e.g., New Hampshire, 24 hours) beyond the request for discharge. Involuntary commitment procedures may be initiated during this time, if necessary.

Voluntary admission is favored by many mental health professionals because it usually indicates that patients recognize that they need care and that the institution is capable of delivering treatment. However, voluntary patients should understand that in most jurisdictions they cannot impulsively leave the hospital at any time. Upon admission, staff should inform all voluntary admittees about procedures required if they then wish to leave against medical advice and about what restraints may be placed upon their leaving under those circumstances. Failure to do so would represent breach of informed consent (42). The clinician who is unaware of the statutes governing voluntary admission and the nature of the admission process is at risk of running afoul of the law. However, more important from a clinical perspective, such knowledge is critical in understanding the patient's expectations upon entering the hospital (43).

The inpatient clinician must know what information the patient has been given in order to evaluate the patient for the presence of distortions of reality (such as denial) and to alert the clinician of potential pitfalls in other emotionally charged areas. Referring to the initial understanding can also be an aid in maintaining a doctor-patient alliance on what has been termed a situational basis, e.g., "Here are the rules that you and I have to live by" (44). Such a clinico-legal situational alliance can serve as a safe haven to return to when navigating through the storms of transference and countertransference that buffet psychiatric treatment.

INVOLUNTARY ADMISSION

During the past 15 years the standards by which a noncriminal person can be involuntarily hospitalized have significantly altered. Traditionally, the state's power to commit a mentally ill person was based on two principles—*parens patriae* (the state as having a parent's power for a class of its citizens, e.g., those unable to care for self) or the police power doctrine (e.g., dangerous to others) (45). Civil commitment statutes in most states now require dangerousness either to self or others, coupled with mental illness, as the basis for the restriction of liberty that hospitalization is argued to represent. In states where the courts changed the civil commitment standard to that of dangerousness, many psychiatrists have regarded this change as a devaluation of the traditional medical concept of illness and need for treatment (45). The reemergence of *parens patriae* considerations along with implicit support for patient's "right to treatment," join risk management and self-protection among the values which guide psychiatric decision making in initiating the procedure to involuntarily commit seriously ill patients (46).

Involuntary commitment standards vary from state to state and are constantly changing among the states; states also vary as to who can commit (e.g., physicians, psychologists, judges). Inpatient clinicians should keep abreast of the recent statutes in their states. A general summary follows.

Most states have provisions that allow for short-term emergency hospitalization until a court hearing is held. In most states at least one physician must sign the commitment certificate. Some states allow the police or courts to sign in the absence of a physician. The criteria for emergency commitment are usually the same as those for court-ordered commitment. All states have stringent time limits for the emergency commitment, but sometimes the bureaucratic lag between emergency commitment and mandatory court review practically extends this limit (47).

At the end of the emergency commitment period, commitment can only continue upon a petition to the court. Most states currently require a judicial hearing for nonemergency commitments, and patients considered for civil commitment may be represented by attorneys. The psychiatrist's role is one of initiating a petition for commitment or assisting the court in the commitment process. It is the court that decides the commitment question.

It is important to note that the judicial process by which a patient is committed may have an impact upon the patient as well as upon the therapeutic alliance. Educating the patient about the process, emphasizing the temporary nature of any commitment, and exploring with the patient the meaning of involuntary commitment are the best antidotes to the demoralization, helplessness, and even suicidal ideation that can follow such a judicial determination (16).

ADMISSION AND THE INCOMPETENT PATIENT

Committability and incompetency are no longer legally synonymous. Mental patients are presumed legally competent unless adjudicated otherwise. However, some states are beginning to require psychiatric competency evaluations performed on new admittees and guardianship petitions filed on those suspected of incompetency.

Treatment

MEDICATIONS

Under the doctrine of informed consent both voluntary and involuntary patients must be given a reasonable explanation of the treatment which the psychiatrist proposes. As earlier noted, informed consent must include risks, benefits, and side effects of the treatment; other treatment options; and the probable course of the disorder without treatment. In many jurisdictions, since commitment no longer presupposes incompetence, both voluntary and involuntary patients have the right to accept or refuse the proposed treatment upon receiving this information. The right to refuse treatment is waived only if: (*a*) such a narrowly defined emergency exists that failure to treat the patient would result in a substantial likelihood of physical harm to the patient or others, or (*b*) the patient has been adjudicated incompetent.

If the patient refuses treatment and is thought to be incompetent, the process of finding a legal guardian should be started. Under *Rogers v. Commissioner*, the now fa-

mous Massachusetts right-to-refuse-treatment case, a mental patient may refuse treatment until and unless adjudicated incompetent by a judge (48). If the patient is found incompetent, the judge *(not the psychiatrist, not the guardian)* decides for the patient whether the patient, if competent, would have consented to be treated by antipsychotic drugs (this is termed a substituted judgment standard). This ruling is an example of the increased adjudication of patient care. Fortunately, other jurisdictions have relied more heavily on clinical judgment for patient treatment determinations when incompetence has been established (49). Clinicians should familiarize themselves with locally relevant cases and regulations.

ECT, PSYCHOSURGERY, AND OTHER MODALITIES

Today most psychiatrists are exceptionally careful about informed consent when proposing electroconvulsive therapy (ECT). This caution was prompted by suits for failure to obtain informed consent and liability for injury. Despite the fact that ECT is safer today and much less likely to cause injury (injury is a precondition for negligence and liability), historically documented ECT abuse (overreliance on ECT and inappropriate usage of ECT) has led several states to design regulatory controls on its use (50). However, before a general right to refuse treatment was recognized, the statutory right to refuse certain kinds of treatment such as ECT, psychosurgery, and aversive conditioning was protected by law. In effect, even if patients do consent to one of these treatments, statutes closely guard their usage.

SECLUSION AND RESTRAINT

Seclusion and restraint represent the maximum restriction on space and movement for inpatients. Seclusion as a treatment technique provides protection to seriously ill patients who are acting out and may harm themselves or others. By minimizing sensory stimuli, seclusion can allow the patient an opportunity to regain self-control in the absence of other people. Seclusion and restraint (like ECT and psychosurgery) have court-ordered restrictions on their use (51). Familiarity with the restrictions in your state is essential.

Before using seclusion or restraint, the clinician must consider and document trials of less restrictive alternatives such as medications and voluntary space restrictions (e.g., an open "quiet room" to decrease stimulation). It is essential to carefully monitor any patient in seclusion or restraint. Monitoring should be both medical (e.g., "periodic checks of vital signs") as well as behavioral (e.g., "observation checks"). When a patient is being removed from a restricted environment (e.g., by increasing periods of time out of seclusion), monitoring should also include examination for any evidence of a recurrence of the behavior that necessitated the original seclusion. All restrictions must be time-limited and subject to periodic review at times often specified by statute. Periodic review is not only legally necessary but also clinically essential. The milieu staff involved in restricting the patient and helping to wean the patient from such restrictions must have clear written guidelines for these procedures. Documentation of the reasoning involved in both initiating and weaning the patient from such restricted environments is an essential legal and clinical communication tool. Postseclusion "debriefing" of patient and staff fosters high clinical standards.

DISCHARGE FROM HOSPITAL

A critical treatment period for inpatient hospitalization is the time around discharge, be it planned or unplanned. "Pure" voluntary admittees (check your state definition) can leave the hospital when they wish, limited only by reasonable hours.

"Conditional" voluntary patients (again, check local statutes for precise terms) usually must give anywhere from 24 hours to several days notice of their desire to leave; time is allotted for staff to conduct an evaluation of commitability and to initiate commitment procedures if indicated (52). If a patient desires discharge and is *not* commitable but staff feel it is inadvisable for the patient to leave, some slight medicolegal protection derives from having the patient sign a form acknowledging awareness of the physician's opposition to discharge. A leave against medical advice form (AMA) offers some modest protection to physicians in the event that a discharged patient unpredictably proceeds to commit self-harm or harms a third party. In cases where a high degree of uncertainty surrounds whether the physician should petition for commitment or release the patient AMA, a second opinion from a colleague or, if available, a forensically trained psychiatrist is warranted.

Involuntary patients (civilly committed, emergency committed, or criminally committed) may attempt to obtain a writ of habeas corpus for discharge. The patient appears in court (immediately), and the state must find that the criteria for commitment continue to be met.

An *involuntary discharge* occurs when a patient wishes to remain in the hospital and the physician recommends discharge. Such discharge also may result from a legitimate response to a serious rule infraction by the patient (e.g., smuggling in drugs, assaults, etc.). It is important to document the *clinical indications* for discharge in this situation, because discharge may mobilize narcissistic rage and threats to sue on the part of the patient and family.

An example of an indication for involuntary discharge is a borderline patient for whom uncontrollable regression on an inpatient basis may be of higher risk than the benefit of continuing hospitalization and who is not judged to be acutely harmful to self or others (53). Occasionally the narcissistic rage mobilized in such patients by the discharge may be of sufficient intensity that plans may need to be changed and the patient transferred on an involuntary commitment to a state facility. If the patient has an involved family, they should be contacted with the patient's permission, educated about the reasons for discharge, and informed of alternative sources of emergency care and any conditions that might need to be met for readmission. The sobering alternative of hospitalization in a state facility may be a regression-limiting and, at times, even a lifesaving alternative for the patient who has previously exploited the private or general hospital as a "hotel."

SPECIAL PATIENT POPULATIONS

Several special patient populations add unusual circumstances and concerns to established medicolegal constraints. In defining these groups and elucidating certain general considerations, we seek to aid the clinician in turning these constraints to clinical advantage.

Alcohol Abusers

The alcohol abuser or alcohol-dependent patient presents special medicolegal concerns. These individuals suffer social, familial, occupational, and/or behavioral/legal (driving while intoxicated (DWI), violence while intoxicated) complications of alcoholism. Of special note to inpatient clinicians is a recent Florida case which found a cause of action against the hospital and physician for damages incurred by an inpatient receiving treatment for alcoholism; when on leave of absence from the hospital, the patient was involved in an automobile accident while driving intoxicated (54).

Clearly, any patient with a recent history of driving while intoxicated should be carefully evaluated for risk when granted a hospital leave. One possible safeguard for

patients with a history of DWI is to make leaves contingent on not driving while on leave. Another is to have the patient's initial leave be followed by a drug and alcohol screen. When sufficient progress has occurred during the course of the patient's treatment that driving while on leave is indicated as part of the patient's rehabilitation, permission to drive must be preceded by careful clinical evaluation. It should also be noted that alcohol and other substance abusers represent a population particularly vulnerable to affective and other psychiatric disorders. Failure to accompany detoxification with proper psychiatric evaluation is clearly substandard care. In the case of a tragic outcome, it may lead to a cause for malpractice action.

Substance Abusers

Substance abusers comprise another special inpatient population. While *substance abuse* is an umbrella term for dependence on opiates, nonnarcotic agents, and alcohol, we will discuss primarily the opioid abuser. Of import to inpatient clinicians is the need to carefully monitor patients (using physiological criteria) for whom methadone is prescribed for heroin withdrawal, because methadone can also be abused. One safeguard is to give each patient the prescribed dose at regular intervals supervised by staff.

Another problem arises with confidentiality. The substance abuser may report a variety of illegal drug use before hospitalization. Here, as with all patients, the clinician is under obligation to maintain the standards of confidentiality, unless the patient poses an ongoing direct threat to a third party (36, 39).

As treatment proceeds a significant number of patients who present with problems of alcohol and other substance abuse and dependence will be recognized as suffering from other significant underlying psychiatric disorders, ranging from manic-depressive illness to personality disorder. As such, failure to obtain an extended psychiatric evaluation for such patients is outside the scope of accepted standards of medical care and therefore negligent. By the same token, upon admission, assessment for drug and substance abuse, including blood and urine testing, is indicated for any patient in a psychotic state presenting for first-time psychiatric hospitalization.

Substance-abuse patients may also enter the hospital with criminal charges against them. Because of the frequency of this problem, it is important to ascertain current legal status and the patient's motivation for seeking treatment. These patients may have transiently impaired judgment during the detoxification period which may affect informed consent. The clinician must evaluate each patient to determine whether the patient has sufficient judgment to grant informed consent or whether the situation can be equated with an emergency. In the latter case, once the acute crisis has passed, patient competency must be reassessed and consent reinstated. For some of these patients competency may not exist because they have permanently impaired judgment caused by chronic organic brain syndromes.

The Antisocial Personality

The hallmarks of the individual with a personality disorder include: apparent inability to experience depression, lack of motivation for change, and absence of anxiety (55). The psychiatric examination of the antisocial personality must include a medicolegal history. Though patients with this disorder may present themselves as victims of family, parents, the law, and previous physicians (56), the clinician should still ask what charges are pending against the patient and who the patient has sued or is currently suing.

More sophisticated individuals with antisocial personalities may view admission to a hospital as an invitation to reach into the physician's or hospital's malpractice insurance "deep pocket." When such an attitude exists it must be confronted. Staff may need to be supported by the unit leadership when they become the subject of repeated malpractice threats.

Individuals with the classical antisocial personality are most often found in public hospitals, have long criminal records, and may wish to use the hospital to avoid jail or even to continue their criminal activities (e.g., drug dealing). Private hospitals may discover what Dr. Leston Havens has described as "white collar" sociopaths (57). These individuals wish to take advantage of what they perceive as vulnerability of inpatient settings to "legal blackmail": "If you discharge me, I'll speak to my lawyer." Whenever a patient is hospitalized under legal coercion, it is critical to clarify the patient's motivation for admission and treatment. In working with patients with antisocial personalities, inform them, from the start, whether you will contact their probation officer, lawyer, etc., depending on the context of the admission. Inform them of your responsibility both to them and the referring agency (e.g., the court). In cases in which you believe that your responsibility to the referring agency would preclude sufficient confidentiality to proceed with treatment, you can refer the patient to a colleague who can serve as the treating psychiatrist.

Borderline Personalities

Patients with borderline personality disorder demonstrate extreme impulsivity, intense anger, unstable relationships and moods, and the inclination towards suicidal behavior. Clinico-legal problems go hand in hand with these symptoms (53). Intense countertransference reactions such as abandonment are common and can lead to frank professional negligence. Furthermore, the impulsivity and suicidal behavior characteristic of this patient group increases the liability risk for their caretakers. Medical decisions with this patient population should involve the patient in sharing the uncertainty. Borderline patients must be encouraged wherever possible to assume responsibility for their behavior and treatment.

Organically Impaired Patients

Organically impaired patients are those whose brain dysfunction results in impaired judgment, intellectual ability, orientation, and memory. Two steps should be taken whenever an organically impaired patient is admitted to an inpatient unit. First, establish the competency status of the patient. Second, if the patient has been legally adjudicated incompetent, ascertain whether prior guardianship has been obtained. If guardianship should be obtained, make that recommendation to the family. It is important to differentiate for the family those conditions that are reversible and require only temporary guardians versus conditions that are irreversible and require permanent guardianship.

Elderly Patients

Not every elderly patient who appears incompetent is incompetent. In cases where incompetence does exist it may result from a treatable organic problem or a depressive pseudodementia. Organic problems are not necessarily irreversible. In order to guard against a premature declaration of incompetency in clinical cases such as these and against the hopelessness that accompanies such a ruling, the clinician should initially petition for temporary guardianship and then reevaluate at a later point in the hospitalization.

Elderly patients represent a population particularly vulnerable to victimization. In some cases they may have suffered abuse or neglect by their family or other caretakers. The regularity of this problem in elderly paranoid patients calls for inquiry into victimization as a part of the full psychiatric assessment. One must differentiate such cases from cases in which victimization is alleged but turns out on closer examination to represent an appeal for help for the loneliness and grief that can accompany illness and aging.

The HIV-Infected Patient

The special problems and needs of the patient infected with human immunodeficiency virus (HIV) on an inpatient psychiatric unit have already been discussed. The clinician who expects clear-cut legal guidelines for risk management will be disappointed. The patient's right to care and privacy, a clinician's duty to protect others from harm caused by the patient, and state-mandated public health reporting statutes must all be considered on a case-by-case basis. When HIV testing of a mentally ill person is clinically indicated, questions regarding voluntariness and capacity arise. An institutionally dependent person facing the "choice" between consenting to testing and discharge may be said to be in a "captive situation" (58). Issues of coercion aside, the patient's capacity to give informed consent must be assessed. The first step in such an assessment is the attempt to engage the patient via an empathic dialogue regarding the risks and benefits of the testing. The patient who demonstrates clear capacity to decide and chooses the testing option should be informed of the results in a context allowing supportive exploration of their meaning. Educational efforts regarding "safe sex" and the risks of i.v. drug use are also part of the accepted standard of medical care. Undertake such efforts on individual, group, and milieu bases. Pay special attention to the meaning of conveying such information to patients already either phobic or reckless about their own sexuality. Distinguish education from puritanical or permissive attitudes.

It is absolutely essential to avoid discrimination against the HIV-positive patient (59). Many such patients come from groups actively discriminated against and carry the stigma (including internalized self-oppression) that are the sequela of such discrimination (60). In an age of universal precautions, it represents good risk management to understand and treat discrimination on an inpatient unit as a clinical phenomenon.

Patients in Overcrowded Facilities

Discharge or transfer of inpatients because of overcrowding deserve special attention. Under these circumstances inpatients may need to be discharged or transferred. Though it may not be the optimal time for discharge for some patients, more seriously ill patients need the space and staff resources. The inpatient clinician may thus be forced into a process of decision making closely resembling the triage practiced among the wounded on the battlefield. An important component of decision making here is the fact that admission to a hospital represents a promise of care. Dangerously overcrowded facilities may need to refuse admission in the interests of care.

A discharge under circumstances of overcrowding may precipitate a charge of abandonment. One must be mindful of countertransference issues and make sure that when patients are chosen for discharge they indeed have a good chance of functioning in an outpatient setting. Inpatient staff must be explicit with patients about reasons for discharge and must monitor their reactions, which can include hopelessness and rage about experienced abandonment. Thoroughly document the rationale for discharge on the chart. Whenever possible, address discharge resulting from over-crowding in the milieu and with the patient's family. Carefully explore alternatives (e.g., transfer) before discharge. When adequate clinical exploration accompanies such discharges, the patient may experience the accompanying difficulties as surmountable and even growth promoting.

The Poorly Insured Patient

The poorly insured patient may not be able to afford an optimal stay in a private inpatient setting (this includes private psychiatric as well as general hospitals). In order to avoid abandonment, explain all decisions regarding transfer to a public facility, and, when possible, include the patient and family in the decision-making process. Provision of adequate follow-up is, as with all patients, critical.

The EAP-referred Patient

Patients often are referred by an employee assistance program (EAP) when their work performance becomes impaired by intercurrent psychiatric illness (61). EAPs which specialize in helping employees with drug and alcohol problems may also refer for admission. In either case, on an inpatient setting, the psychiatrist's first responsibility must be to diagnose and treat the patient, without regard to whether the patient's illness falls within the purview of the referring EAP. For example, a patient referred for admission as a drug abuser must also be evaluated for an underlying depression or some other treatable psychiatric disorder. This must be made clear to both the patient and the EAP. By the same token the patient who says "I was sent here by my boss" needs to be evaluated for motivation for treatment.

Confidentiality can be a problem with EAP patients. The patient's consent must be obtained for all communications, and the patient should be informed from the outset of the extent to which the EAP requires information (e.g., diagnosis, expected length of stay, or prognosis). In order to address the patient's concerns and at the same time insure adequate communication with the EAP, the inpatient staff can clear all communications to the EAP with the patient. The patient can help complete all forms and letters that need to be sent out; telephone communications with the EAP can be held during the patient's therapy sessions; and, when appropriate, meetings with the EAP representative can be held in the patient's presence. If the hospital wishes to supplement these measures by having a nontreating member of the staff be in direct communication with the EAP representative, it should be done only with the patient's consent. Any refusal on the patient's part to furnish such consent should be adequately explored. In certain cases, refusal of consent may compromise the clinician's ability to treat the patient.

Review Liability

An emerging area of liability is liability for review activities. Whether conducting quality review, peer review, or third party utilization review, the reviewing clinician on rare occasions may be liable to charges ranging from conflict of interest and restraint of trade to contributing to the negligent care of patients. As far as utilization review is concerned, the defense of cost containment, although proposed by some legal advocates, cannot be said to justify significant deviations from accepted standards of care for patients with psychiatric or other medical disorders. Patients with serious psychiatric illness are particularly vulnerable to cost-containment-driven cutbacks in care in view of their often inhibited advocacy skills. In general, careful documentation and practicing in good faith are the best touchstones for guarding against liability.

WORKING WITH THE LEGAL SYSTEM

Clinicians who are tempted toward legalistic approaches to psychiatric care are at risk to deliver poor care (62). Clinicians must carefully examine their reactions to their patients whenever the legal, rather than the clinical, aspects of the case have taken center stage. Transference and countertransference resistances are the rule at these moments. On the other hand, the clinician who resists being mindful of the legal constraints within which inpatient therapy proceeds risks vulnerability to malpractice charges. Moreover, denial of legal realities may also indicate a narcissistic alliance with the patient aimed toward satisfying the patient's wish for a caring, omnipotent figure. In either case, whether the clinician overidentifies with the aggressor (by trying to be a good lawyer) or over-identifies with the patient (as victim denying the medicolegal context of inpatient treatment), patient care is sure to suffer.

The Delphic injunction to "Know thyself" must join *primum non nocere* ("first, do no harm") and "do the best for the patient" if clinicians are to turn the legal constraints reviewed here to clinical advantage (63). With psychiatry and the law coming into progressively closer contact, especially in the high-risk populations the inpatient psychiatrist treats, today's climate is one of both crisis and opportunity.

The *crisis* is that of feeling trapped by legal trends which expand clinician responsibility for tragic outcomes while diminishing the physician's authority to provide quality care. Expansion of physician responsibility is well-illustrated by the ever-expanding duties to third parties created by *Tarasoff* and other such cases. A more ominous trend in the expansion of clinical responsibility is the movement toward strict liability. The following passage from a leading work on medical malpractice law exemplifies this problem: "The fact that a patient has begun treatment as the result of a suicide attempt renders liability under the concept of reasonable forseeability virtually automatic in all cases (64).

The diminution of clinical authority in a number of areas has disturbed many clinicians. The most striking example is the trend of allowing treatment refusal by clearly psychotic patients. The inpatient clinician is then left to watch patients "rot with their rights on," as they descend into psychotic regression (65). Similarly, the curtailment of the *parens patriae* justification for commitment has left clinicians with less authority to treat chronically suicidal and homicidal patients.

We have used the term *critogenic* injury to designate any *legally* caused harm the patient may endure (66). Since the legal profession does not have any term for such harm (though medicine has "iatrogenic" for "doctor-caused") we have borrowed from the Greek *crites,* meaning an Athenian presiding judge, to designate legally caused harm. Courts today seem to share a paradoxical pair of assumptions that (a) all inpatients are competent to refuse medications and (b) all inpatients are incompetent to assume responsibility for their own actions (e.g., self-harm or harm to others). Together these views seem to reflect the extremes of either counterdependent grandiosity or infantile dependence which can characterize the extreme positions that disturbed patients can take. If strictly adhered to, this courtroom paradox can make clinical treatment of seriously ill patients legally impossible.

The *opportunity* provided to inpatient clinicians is to begin to engage in an ethical and empirical dialogue with the legal system. Research is growing on biases (such as hindsight) when psychiatric prediction is evaluated by judges and juries (67). It is

hoped research findings will improve the quality of inpatient clinical decision making and give the legal system a more realistic view of the uncertainties inherent in clinical decision making. Perhaps the enforced contact between psychiatry and law, through today's torrent of litigation, will allow each profession to come away with a greater insight into its own presuppositions (68–75).

Enforced contact between psychiatry and law will ultimately be beneficial to patients only if inpatient clinicians who appear in the courtroom appear as *clinicians.* They must avoid either being seduced into the role of playing "lawyer" (thereby identifying with the legal system as aggressor) or playing "hostile witness" (thereby identifying with the oppositional, adversary stance of the injured victim). Only as clinicians in the courtroom can we help the legal system to aid patients and to recognize the potential of patients for injury from legal proceedings we have termed critogenic. Encouraging responses to the "malpractice crisis," such as proposals for arbitration or for creating victim compensation funds, are early signs of success (76). Despite this note of encouragement, inpatient clinicians will only be able to treat their patients by remaining abreast of changing legal constraints and responding clinically with the best that empirical research, professional experience, and ethical theory have to offer (68, 77–79).

Ethical Consultation as Risk Management

Patients at high risk for tragic outcome exemplify the use of ethical consultation for the complex institutional policy and individual treatment issues. Issues which are not simply resolved on the clinical or legal level of discourse may be usefully aired and reflected upon with the aid of a consultant in ethics. Consulting an ethicist and using ethics cases and policy discussions with staff participation is emerging as a valuable tool in staff education. Ethics consultation also helps to maintain an acceptable level of staff understanding *and* of the values necessary for patient care (80).

The value of consulting an ethicist was made apparent when the authors consulted Professor Patricia M.L. Illingworth, currently visiting faculty for the Program in Psychiatry and the Law at Harvard Medical School. Dr. Illingworth emphasizes that an adversarial dimension to the patient-therapist relationship can spur patient growth and development, provided that sufficient attention is paid to the therapeutic alliance. The ability to advocate for oneself, the capacity to distinguish between regressive and mature entitlement, and overcoming narcisstic guilt are all steps in the movement of the self toward healthy narcissism. For the chronically ill patient who has lost the will to advocate, teaching about both moral and legal rights *by* the ethically informed clinician can be a first step in the rebuilding of a healthy self.

Clinical Consultation as Risk Management

The informed consent *process* is the primary risk-management tool in clinical decision making whatever the actual structure of the judgments in question, e.g., heuristic, risk-benefit, or lexical. Although potentially useful, protocols, algorithms, forms, and clinical "efficacy" studies nonetheless require a measure of clinical judgment, interpretation, application, and communication, and are no substitute for any of these (81, 82).

The informed consent *process* needs to be extended at times beyond the confines of the clinician-patient dyad. Whenever possible this extension itself needs to be the subject of the informed consent *process.* The decision to involve third parties, be they family members or clinical consultants, has meanings, risks, and benefits which need to be explored with the patient. Some of the new protection of third parties legislation has specified alternatives to the warning of third parties, such as involuntary commitment (83). However useful knowledge of such legislation is, it is no substitute for clinical judgment informed by a dialogue with the patient and third parties, where indicated, including clinical consultants. The use of clinical consultants is best sought beyond narrow institutional and treatment orientations. This is valuable for adding a new perspective to the clinical process and documenting that the clinician has sought consultation for purposes other than simple confirmation of an already decided-upon course of treatment. Paradoxically, an intra-institutional consultation which disagrees with treatment recommendations and documents the disagreement is a more valid risk-management tool than simple "rubber stamping" consultation. If a patient remains refractory to treatment and intra-institutional consultation has failed to generate viable options, extra-institutional and additional treatment orientation consultation is advised (whether the initial treatment was primarily psychopharmacological, psychoanalytic, or eclectic). In this regard, Alan A. Stone's seminal essay is essential reading for all clinicians (84).

ACKNOWLEDGMENTS

The members of the Program in Psychiatry and the Law continue to provide valuable perspectives on the issues here discussed. We are grateful to Paul S. Appelbaum for his role as a cofounder of the Program. The authors wish to thank Professor Patricia M.L. Illingworth, a medical ethicist and founding member of the Center for Ethics, Medicine, and the Law, McGill University, for her thoughtful articulation of autonomy as a treatment value in Program seminars. In addition to his fundamental contributions to psychoanalysis, psychiatry, and the law, which inform the authors' perspectives, Alan A. Stone continues to inspire the Program and its direction.

REFERENCES

1. *Kaimowitz v Michigan Department of Mental Health,* Div. No. 73-19434 AW, Circuit Court of Wayne Cty, Mich., 1973, 13 Criminal L Rep 2452.

2. Gutheil TG, Appelbaum PS: *Clinical Handbook of Psychiatry and the Law,* New York, McGraw-Hill, 1982.

3. Bursztajn HJ, Hamm RM: The clinical utility of utility assessment. Med Decis Making, 2:161–165, 1982.

4. Bursztajn HJ, Gutheil TG, Mills M, Hamm RM, Brodsky A: Process analysis of judges' commitment decisions: A preliminary empirical study. Am J Psychiatry, 143:170–174, 1986.

5. Gutheil TG, Bursztajn HJ, Brodsky A: The multidimensional assessment of dangerousness: Competence assessment in patient care and liability prevention. Bull Am Acad Psychiatry Law, 14:123–129, 1986.

6. Bursztajn HJ, Gutheil TG, Warren MJ, Brodsky A: Depression, self-love, time, and the "right" to suicide. Gen Hosp Psychiatry, 8:91–95, 1986.

7. Gutheil TG, Bursztajn HJ: Clinicians' guidelines for assessing and presenting subtle forms of patient incompetence in legal settings. Am J Psychiatry, 143:1020–1023, 1986.

8. Pavlo AM, Bursztajn HJ, Gutheil TG, Levi LM: Weighing religious beliefs in determining competence. Hosp Community Psychiatry, 38:350–352, 1987.

9. Pavlo AM, Bursztajn HJ, Gutheil TG: Christian Science and competence to make treatment choices: Clinical challenges in assessing values. Int J Law Psychiatry, 10:395–401, 1987.

10. Gutheil TG, Bursztajn HJ, Kaplan AN, Brodsky A: Participation in competency assessment and treatment decisions: The role of a psychiatrist-attorney team. Mental Physical Disabilities Law Reporter, 11:446–449, 1987.

11. Gutheil TG, Bursztajn HJ, Hamm RM,

Brodsky A: Subjective data and suicide assessment in the light of recent legal developments. Part I: Malpractice prevention and the use of subjective data. Int J Law Psychiatry, 6:317–329, 1983.

12. Bursztajn H, Gutheil TG, Hamm RM, Brodsky A: Subjective data and suicide assessment in the light of recent legal developments. Part II: Clinical uses of legal standards in the interpretation of subjective data. Int J Law Psychiatry, 6:331–350, 1983.

13. Shein HM, Stone AA: Psychotherapy designed to detect and treat suicidal potential. Am J Psychiatry, 125:1247–1251, 1969.

14. Klein JI, Glover SI: Psychiatric malpractice. Int J Law Psychiatry, 6:131–157, 1983.

15. Perr IN: Psychiatric malpractice issues, in Rachlin S (ed): Legal Encroachment on Psychiatric Practice, pp. 47–59, San Francisco, Jossey-Bass, 1985.

16. Bursztajn HJ, Gutheil TG, Brodsky A, Swagerty E: Magical thinking, suicide, and malpractice litigation. Bull Am Acad Psychiatry Law, 16:369–377, 1988.

17. Apter A, Plutchik R, Sevy S: Defense mechanisms in risk of suicide and risk of violence. Am J Psychiatry, 146:1027–1031, 1989.

18. Maltsburger JT: *Suicide Risk: The Formulation of Clinical Judgment,* New York, New York University Press, 1986.

19. Gutheil TG, Bursztajn HJ, Brodsky A: Malpractice prevention through the sharing of uncertainty: Informed consent and the therapeutic alliance. N Engl J Med, 311:49–51, 1984.

20. Wulsin LR, Bursztajn HJ, Gutheil TG: Unexpected clinical features of the *Tarasoff* decision: The therapeutic alliance and the "duty to warn." Am J Psychiatry, 140:601–603, 1983.

21. Gelenberg A: 375,000 for tardive dyskinesia. Biol Ther Psychiatry, 3:41–42, 1980.

22. Appelbaum PS, Schaffner K, Meisel A: Responsibility and compensation for tardive dyskinesia. Am J Psychiatry, 142:806–810, 1985.

23. Davis JM, Schyre PM, Parkovic I: Clinical and legal issues in neuroleptic use. Clin Neuropharmacol, 6:117–128, 1983.

24. Ness DE, Pfeffer CR: Sequela of bereavement resulting from suicide. Am J Psychiatry, 147:279–284, 1990.

25. Dunne EJ: A response to suicide in the mental health setting, in Dunne EJ, McIntosh JL,

Dunne-Maxim K (eds): *Suicide and its Aftermath: Understanding and Counselling the Survivors,* pp. 182–190, New York, W.W. Norton, 1987.

26. Baker B: Expect a flood of tardive dyskinesia malpractice suits. Clin Psychiatry News, *Jan:* 3, 1984.

27. Slovenko R: On the legal aspects of tardive dyskinesia. J Psychiatry Law, 7:295–331, 1979.

28. Tardive Dyskinesia: Report of the American Psychiatric Association Task Force on Late Neurological Effects of Antipsychotic Drugs, APA Task Force Report No. 18, Washington, D.C., American Psychiatric Association, 1979.

29. Muentz MR: Overcoming resistance to talking to patients about tardive dyskinesia. Hosp Community Psychiatry, 36:283–287, 1985.

30. Bursztajn HJ, Chanowitz B, Gutheil TG, Hamm RM: Context specific language effects in the decision to prescribe neuroleptics. Presented at the Fifth Annual Meeting of the Society for Medical Decision Making, Toronto, Ont., Canada, October 2–5, 1983.

31. *Clites v. Iowa,* Court of Appeals of Iowa, June 29, 1982.

32. *Faigenbaum v. Cohen,* reported in Clin Psychiatry News, 5:31, 1985.

33. *Hedin v. U.S.,* reported in Clin Psychiatry News, 5:31, 1985.

34. Vasile RG, Gutheil TG: The psychiatrist as "medical backup": Ambiguity in the delegation of clinical responsibility. Am J Psychiatry, 136:1292–1296, 1979.

35. Bursztajn HJ, Feinbloom RI, Hamm RM, Brodsky A: *Medical Choices, Medical Chances: How Patients, Families, and Physicians Can Cope With Uncertainty,* New York, Routledge, Chapman & Hall, 1990.

36. *Tarasoff v. Regents of the University of California,* 131 Cal Reptr 14 (Calif 76).

37. Appelbaum PS: The expansion of liability for patients' violent acts. Hosp Community Psychiatry, 35:13–14, 1984.

38. Stone AA: The Tarasoff case and some of its progeny: Suing psychotherapists to safeguard society, in *Law, Psychiatry and Morality: Essays and Analysis,* Washington, D.C., American Psychiatric Press, 1984.

39. *Commonwealth of Massachusetts v. Cobrin,* SJC-3671, 1985.

40. In re *Kathleen M.* 493 A2D 472 (April 18, 1985, S.Ct. N.H.).

41. Bursztajn HJ: Supervisory Responsibility for Prevention of Supervisee-Patient Sexual Contact. Presented at the Massachusetts Psychiatric Society, Newton, Mass., March 10, 1990.

42. Halleck SH: *Law in the Practice of Psychiatry,* New York, Plenum, 1980.

43. Appelbaum PS, Mirkin SA, Bateman AL: Empirical assessment of competency to consent to psychiatric hospitalization. Am J Psychiatry, 138:1170–1176, 1985.

44. Gutheil TG, Havens LL: The therapeutic alliance: Contemporary meanings and confusions. Int Rev Psychoanal, 6:467–481, 1979.

45. Stone AA: Mental Health and Law: A System in Transition, U.S. Department of Health, Education, and Welfare Publication 75-176, Rockville, Md., National Institute of Mental Health, 1975.

46. Bursztajn HJ, Gutheil TG, Hamm RM, Brodsky A, Mills M: *Parens patriae* considerations in the commitment process. Psychiatr Q, 39:165–181, 1988.

47. Barton WE, Barton GM: *Ethics and Law in Mental Health Administration,* New York, International Universities Press, 1984.

48. *Rogers v. Commissioner of Department of Mental Health,* 390 Mass. 489 (Nov. 29, 1983).

49. *Rennie v. Klein,* 462 F Supp 1131 (D.N.J. 1979).

50. APA Task Force Report No. 14: Electroconvulsive Therapy, Washington, D.C., American Psychiatric Association, 1978.

51. Soloff PH, Gutheil TG, Wexler DB: Seclusion and restraint in 1985: A review and update. Hosp Community Psychiatry, 36:652–657, 1985.

52. Appelbaum PS, Hamm RM: Decision to seek commitment. Arch Gen Psychiatry, 39:447–452, 1982.

53. Gutheil TG: Medicolegal pitfalls in the treatment of borderline patients. Am J Psychiatry, 142(1):9–14, 1985.

54. *Burroughs v. Board of Trustees of Alachva General Hospital,* 328 So 2d 538, Fla 1976.

55. Vaillant GE: Sociopathy as a human process. Arch Gen Psychiatry, 32:178–183, 1975.

56. Freud S: Some character types met with in psychoanalytic work: "The exceptions," in Strachey J (ed): *Standard Edition*, vol. 14, London, Hogarth Press, 1957.

57. Havens L: Personal communication, 1983.

58. Somerville MA: Refusal of medical treatment in "captive" circumstances. Canadian Bar Review, 63:59–90, 1985.

59. Haimowitz S: HIV and the mentally ill: An approach to the legal issues. Hosp Community Psychiatry, 40:732–736, 1989.

60. Illingworth PML: *AIDS and the Good Society*. New York and London, Routledge, Chapman & Hall, 1989.

61. Brill P, Herzberg J, Speller JL: Employee assistance programs: An overview and suggested roles for psychiatrists. Hosp Community Psychiatry, 36:727–731, 1985.

62. Gutheil TG: Legal defense as ego defense: A special form of resistance in the therapeutic process. Psychiatr. Q, 51(4):251–256, 1979.

63. Stone AA: The new paradox of psychiatric malpractice. N Engl J Med, 31:1384–1387, 1984.

64. Holder RH: *Medical Malpractice Law*, New York, John Wiley & Sons, 1978.

65. Appelbaum PS, Gutheil TG: "Rotting with their rights on": Constitutional theory and clinical reality in drug refusal by psychiatric patients. Bull Am Acad Psychiatry Law, 7:308–317, 1979.

66. Bursztajn HJ: More law and less protection: "Critogenesis", "legal iatrogenesis", and medical decision making. J Geriatr Psychiatry, 18:143–153, 1985.

67. Fischhoff B: Hindsight/foresight: The effect of outcome knowledge on judgment under uncertainty. J Exp Psychol (Hum Percept), 1:288–299, 1975.

68. Bursztajn HJ, Feinbloom RI, Hamm RM, Brodsky A: *Medical Choices, Medical Chances: How Patients, Families, and Physicians Can Cope with Uncertainty*, New York, Routledge Chapman Hall, 1990.

69. Gutheil TG, Rachlin S, Mills MJ: Differing conceptual models in psychiatry and the law, in Rachlin S (ed): *Legal Encroachment on Psychiatric Practice*, San Francisco, Jossey-Base, 1985.

70. Schaffner KF: Causation and responsibility: Medicine, science and the law, in Spicker SF, Healey JM, Englehardt HT (eds): *The Law-Medicine Relation: A Philosophical Exploration*, Washington, D.C., D. Reidel, 1981.

71. Bursztajn HJ, Gutheil TG, Brodsky A: Narcissism revisited: the fantasy of omnipotence in medical practice. Theor Psychiatry, In press.

72. Bursztajn HJ, Gutheil TG, Hamm RM, Brodsky A, Mills MJ, Levi L: Transitions in clinicians' self-reports of the assessment of commitability. Int J Psychiatry Law, In press.

73. Bursztajn HJ, Gutheil TG, Barnard D, Brodsky A: The triage model in hospital psychiatry. Psychiatr Q, In press.

74. Harding HP, Gutheil TG, Bursztajn HJ, Brodsky A: The role of affect in impairing competence. Bull Am Acad Psychiatry Law, In press.

75. Reiser SJ, Bursztajn HJ, Gutheil TG, Appelbaum PS: *Divided Staffs, Divided Selves: A Case Approach to Mental Health Ethics*, Cambridge, Cambridge University Press, 1987.

76. Brodsky A: Doctoring defensively, in The New Republic, p. 6. Aug 19, 1985.

77. Kahneman D, Slovic P, Tversky A (eds): *Judgment under Uncertainty: Heuristics and Biases*, New York, Cambridge University Press, 1982.

78. Modell AH: *Psychoanalysis in a New Context*, New York, International University Press, 1984.

79. Katz J: *The Silent World of Doctor and Patient*, New York, The Free Press, 1984.

80. Bursztajn HJ, Gutheil TG, Cummins B: "Conflict and synthesis: The comparative anatomy of ethical and clinical decision making," in Reiser SJ, Bursztajn HJ, Appelbaum PS, Gutheil TG (eds): *Divided Staffs, Divided Selves, A Case Approach to Mental Health Ethics*, pp. 17–40, New York, Cambridge University Press, 1987.

81. Bursztajn HJ, Hamm RM, Gutheil TG, Brodsky, A: The decision analytic approach to medical malpractice law: Formal proposals and informal syntheses. Med Decis Making, 4:401–414, 1984.

82. Hamm RM, Clark JA, Bursztajn HJ:

Psychiatrists' thorny judgments: Describing and improving decision making processes. Med Decis Making, 4:425–447, 1984.

83. Appelbaum PS, Zonana H, Bonnie R, et al.: Statutory approaches to limiting psychiatrists' liability for their patient's violent acts. Am J Psychiatry, 146:821–828, 1989.

84. Stone AA: Law, science, and psychiatric malpractice: A response to Klerman's indictment of psychanalytic psychiatry. Am J Psychiatry, 147:419–427, 1990.

16

The Psychiatric Medical Record and Issues of Confidentiality

Thomas G. Gutheil, MD

SPECIAL CONSIDERATIONS FOR CASE RECORDS OF INPATIENTS

Many clinicians believe that inpatient psychiatry is a veritable subspecialty in its own right. In effect, this book is an expression of this viewpoint. In an analogous manner, evolving the inpatient case record requires a grasp of certain principles unique to inpatient practice and its documentation.

The inpatient ward may be compared to an intensive care unit in general medicine. Though not always obvious or manifest, issues of life and death usually engross most patients sick enough to require admission, given the high admission threshold most contemporary facilities maintain. These ultimate issues coupled with the manifestations of florid mental illness give to the inpatient's experience a drama, intensity, and urgency rarely seen in outpatient circumstances. In these troubled times such indices invariably connote an increase in potential liability for clinicians and their institutions as well—an issue highly relevant to record-keeping.

A second important consideration, frequently scanted in legal assessments of a given case, is that inpatient clinicians must weigh the effects of interventions on other ward patients as well as on their "own" patient or patients. The hospitalized patient is inevitably a member of a social milieu, an arrangement which contrasts with the unitary model of outpatient practice. The implications for records of a milieu orientation are reviewed in this chapter.

Finally, inpatient psychiatric treatment customarily involves multi-disciplinary care delivered by different personnel whose separate contributions must be orchestrated in constructive collaboration. This poses problems for the record-keeping process different from those encountered in the one patient–one therapist model characteristic of certain outpatient treatments.

Despite inevitable overlap, this discussion is divided into clinical and legal aspects of the record-keeping process. Since confidentiality is a topic intimately related to record-keeping, the third section addresses that subject. Finally the specific organization of the material in the record is outlined in the appendix to this chapter.

CLINICAL ASPECTS

Though fraught with medicolegal implications, the case record is an instrument whose primary purpose is the care of the patient. Reviewed here, the specific functions of the record are in serving the clinical aims of the psychiatric record.

The Archival Function

A major function of the record is the durable storage of information about patients and the care delivered to them by the institution. This storage may be short-term (chart entries may be consulted minutes after they are made, e.g., in a medical emergency) or long-term (decades after a first admission a patient's readmission might require review of the first chart).

The importance of writing the record in language whose meaning will endure is essential for archival reasons. Topical allusions, excessively idiosyncratic abbreviations, or crypticisms, and simple illegibility are all ephemera too transient to serve archival purposes.

CASE 1:   A resident wrote: "LOL in betzopenia with possible 'Big S' admitted from BNH for a Charlie's special." This might be "translated" as: "Little old lady with dementia (facetiously characterized as deficiency of Betz cells) who may have schizophrenia admitted from Bad Nursing Home (i.e., a nursing home whose administration is characterized by a tendency to refuse readmission of the patient after psychiatric intervention, in contrast to a GNH) for that extensive workup of reversible causes of dementia especially favored by the Chief Resident that year, one Dr. Charles."

The "original" is shorter, terser, more richly evocative and, no doubt, almost telepathic in its semantics for those staff on the ward during that particular year. However, we can readily predict that the coherency of this entry will fade rapidly into obscurity with the passage of time. One must write for the ages. Moreover, the breeziness of tone of the case example poses other difficulties discussed later.

The Planning Function

The chart as archive, as a repository of clinical data, observations, reports, results of examinations, etc., is useful only insofar as it generates plans of operation for treatment. We generate the data base in order to identify problems in biological, psychiatric, and social areas and to suggest directions for further exploration or intervention. A statement of the presenting problems, required explorations, and planned interventions constitute the treatment plan—the operational heart of the record.

Like a musical score, the treatment plan orchestrates the contributions from the members of the treatment team into an harmonious, collaborative effort. In addition, the plan points to goals (preferably measurable ones) that the interventions aim to achieve. A goal orientation avoids the twin treatment pitfalls of amorphousness, wherein treatment grinds along directionless or, like Leacock's (1) protagonist, "rides madly off in all directions," and manic grandiosity wherein treatment is aimed at "blue-skies" goals impossible to fulfill in this life.

CASE 2:   A treatment plan read: "All members of the team should get this guy by the lapels, shake some sense into him and turn his life around."

A preferable plan for the case in question might have been: "Psychotherapy for hysterical seizures and medical control of diabetes by psychiatrist; vocational assessment and training in marketable skills by occupational therapist; family therapy by social worker aimed at family's acceptance of severity of his illness; increased socialization by nursing staff."

The improved version, while still brief, specifies who will do what in precise terms that allow for measurable goals. Though the goals are not explicitly spelled out in the example, they may readily be inferred because of the precision of the task definitions. For example, a measure of goal attainment in vocational training of marketable skills would be the patient's suitable employment.

The Documentary Function

The documentary function of the record is linked to its archival and planning functions. Documentation serves to validate the delivery of care, an issue of great clinical and forensic power, further elaborated on in Legal Aspects. The power of this function can best be captured in the axiom: "If it isn't written down, it didn't happen" (2). In countless treatment settings the skilled delivery of care is gainsaid through failures in attention to documentation. Good work deserves credit by careful recording. Complex and difficult decisions made on the firing line deserve the protection from liability that scrupulous documentation provides.

CASE 3:   A malpractice case was lost because of the failure to *note* a patient's condition while in restraints. Though good clinical practice was followed, there was no validation of the indications for, and observations during, the procedure.

It must be stressed that, as often as not, the data to be documented are significant by their absence. Significant negatives such as "*denies* suicidal intent," the *absence* of change, the *absence* of concurrent medical conditions, signs of tardive dyskinesia, or an FTA response can only be conveyed through documentation.

The Justificatory Function

In these times of heightened accountability, data must serve not only to record, guide, and document but also to justify. The need for certain interventions and their clinical, legal, or fiscal (reimbursement) validity will rest firmly only on a foundation of documented information. Among the items requiring justification are examinations, interventions, and, most importantly, the admission itself.

Many patients who are ranting, raving, and out of control in the emergency setting rapidly calm down on the ward. To the inexperienced viewer, they may thus appear ready for discharge the instant they hit the unit. This familiar clinical phenomenon might cast retrospective doubt on the need for the admission unless attention is paid to recording why *no less* a step than admission would provide appropriate clinical care. Many apparently tranquil inpatients simply cannot be responsibly returned to the very outside situation that fostered their decompensation without achieving durable changes in their clinical condition or their extrahospital environment. Furthermore, third-party payers may not allow reimbursement for inadequately justified admissions, resulting in crushing economic effects befalling patient and family.

The Utilization Function

Closely related to the justificatory function, the utilization function addresses aspects of quality control and utilization review (an amalgam of documentation and justification with planning) affecting litigation, reimbursement and other important variables. Utilization review (UR) is an intrahospital "checks-and-balances" mechanism by which patients are evaluated *after* admission about the appropriateness of the decisions to admit and/or treat. The question might be phrased: "Is this patient receiving a level of care appropriate to his or her condition or might lower level (less intense) care serve equally well?" This determination frequently affects third-party reimbursement. At times UR requires a particular form to be filled out addressing the question above.

The principle here is that certain services or procedures must be accounted for in terms of indications, needs, and justification, as earlier noted. Admissions, use of special investigations such as CT scans, or special interventions such as electroconvulsive therapy must be justified in terms of both clinical appropriateness and expense. Professional standards review organizations (PSRO) require similar recording. PSROs are groups of physicians (and sometimes other professionals) who engage in peer review as a form of UR. This function was formerly termed "quality assurance." Again, the issues are checks and balances concerning medical decision-making.

The Educational Function

A good case record should instruct the trainee about etiology, precipitants, interventions, and response. It should be able to serve as a profitable focus in supervisory and training meetings.

More importantly, the act of thinking through one's conceptualization of the case in order to record it is, *in itself,* a vital method of instruction in systematic clinical evaluation and treatment planning. When asked to reread the muddy prose of a chart entry, many a clinically confused trainee has correctly diagnosed, through introspection, the muddy clinical thinking at the core of the problem.

CASE 4: A trainee noted that her chart order that markedly increased a psychotic patient's privileges followed close upon an entry that stressed the patient's profound suicidal ideation. The trainee realized that her countertransference anger at this abusive patient had led her to minimize the patient's lethality. The order could then be corrected.

The Research Function

For obvious reasons, recorded data are the essential raw material for research. The data for research may be gathered from project-specific research instruments or from the actual record, as often occurs in longitudinal studies. For research purposes a premium is therefore placed even on recording observations that seem incidental or uninterpretable at present. Explanatory hypotheses may emerge long after the data are gathered, if available for retrospective review.

LEGAL ASPECTS

As in almost every sphere of modern life, the mental health system has become increasingly involved with the legal and judicial systems. The implications of this involvement are especially relevant to record-keeping. The overlap of this section with its clinical predecessor is profound, largely because of the importance assigned by the legal system to *formal* aspects of care, particularly records. The art of therapy, the role of the unconscious in human functioning, the therapeutic alliance, ambivalence, and the various empathic, experiential, and intuitive elements of psychiatric work are poorly grasped by lawyers. Their ideological heritage stresses concrete matters such as contracts, documents, and explicit testimony, all of which may relate to the psychiatric case record. This difference in conceptual models may lead to misunderstanding. (3).

CASE 5: An attorney agreed to refrain from serving a writ of habeas corpus (for the immediate release of a patient) because the doctor predicted that the patient's condition would probably improve enough over the weekend to permit a Monday discharge. However, the patient's condition worsened unexpectedly over the weekend, and discharge required postponement on *clinical* grounds. At a later commitment hearing, the attorney presented these events as though the physician had promised (i.e., contracted) to discharge the patient that Monday. In conceptualizing the matter as a breach of contract, the attorney failed to grasp the significance of the change in the patient's clinical state as determining the psychiatric decision.

From this general view, we will now turn to particular legal issues relevant to inpatient record-keeping.

Malpractice Prevention versus Fostering Good Practice

The clinician's central concern with good patient care is certainly fostered by good record-keeping. In these litigious times we should not overlook the additional important role of records in preventing suits for negligence and other wrongs as well as in protecting patients' rights. Because the "fostering" and "preventing" aspects of the record are so intertwined they are presented together under the legal rubric.

Inclusions and Exclusions

THE "PROCESS-PROGRESS" DISTINCTION (2–5)

The court subpoena, insurance companies, and other sociopolitical forces conspire to make the record less private than is desirable. Therefore, the record should be written in *all parts* in an objective, descriptive manner. Record the patient's verbal expression and behavior in diplomatic language. Scrupulously eschew unconscious fantasy content, psychodynamic formulations, dream material, and technical descriptive terms or jargon likely to be misunderstood. To put it another way, the record should consist of *progress notes* only. Maintain *process notes*, verbatim accounts, and the dynamic issues just listed, separately in the clinician's private file. A question is sometimes raised about this point when the SOAP (*s*ubjective, *o*bjective, *a*ssessment, *p*lan) record schema is endorsed; "subjective" is often interpreted as verbatim, i.e., a quotation in the patient's own words. Even in this model, compromising words and quotes should be avoided.

CASE 6: Digressing from the main course of examination in a malpractice trial, an attorney seized upon a note mentioning the patient's "homosexually erotized relationship" to the therapist. The attorney then attempted to discredit the therapist by introducing testimony to the effect that the patient had *never* been "gay." Although the attorney had misconstrued the meaning of the phrase, this apparent "contradiction" was damaging to the therapist's credibility.

In keeping with the guideline of careful choice of terminology, one might replace "homosexuality" with "positive feeling" or "identity confusion." Another example would be substituting "developmental" for "infantile" or "primitive" when the recording of these terms is unavoidable in communicating about the patient to subsequent caretakers. In all other cases such material should simply not appear in the "public" record at all.

THE PROFESSIONAL TONE

The professionalism rightly expected of inpatient caretakers should extend to the tone of the written record. In practice this means that the following should be excluded: judgmental or moralistic terms ("the patient is really being evil to the nurses"); inappropriate preciousness ("patient is back to being her sweet widdle self"); facetiousness or sarcasm ("if this patient gets any more grandiose, we'll have to crown him Messiah and be done with it"); casual and pejorative slang ("the patient is being a real brat and a royal pain in the ass"); gratuitous interpolations ("patient plans to work in therapy at being less entitled [hah!] in the future"); and any other lapses of professional demeanor conveyed in written form. No matter how satisfying such entries may be to write or how cute and funny to read to one's colleagues, one must recall (2), first, that the entries are rarely quite so comic when they are read aloud in open court and, second, such material invariably conveys disrespect for the patient; this attitude is destructive to one's actual attitude toward and work with the patient and to the caring posture one would wish conveyed toward that same patient, for instance, at a trial for negligence (3). All the clinical descriptions from the mock examples above can be expressed quite adequately and appropriately in neutral and objective terms. One should recall that the "eyes of the future are upon you" (2).

REFERRING TO OTHER PATIENTS AND STAFF

A patient's interaction with specific other patients may be highly significant and relevant to care; thus it may be important to refer to patient B on patient A's chart. For example, two patients who provoke each other and fight or sexualize will have to be kept apart on clinical grounds. This information should be recorded to guide and inform staff on subsequent shifts in order to prevent harm.

However, if patient A later releases his record to an appropriate reader, that reader is not entitled to gratuitous information about patient B. Therefore, for patient B's protection only the first name and last initial of the "other" patient(s) should be used in order to conceal her identity from future readers. However, current staff will still be able to identify her.

When staff members must be referred to, they should be noted by name and discipline. For example, "patient threatened Ms. Smith, R.N.," instead of "patient threatened Betty."

JUDGMENT CALLS AND THINKING OUT LOUD FOR THE RECORD

Clinical work repeatedly requires exercising clinical intuition, making judgment calls, and taking calculated risks. For inpatients these critical decisions often, but not always, focus around the question of when the patient is clinically ready to leave the hospital or to experience some liberalization of constraints.

The secret of sound documentation and avoiding spending too much time writing is in the notion "don't write more, write *smarter*." Thus one writes less, but more efficiently. Efficiency is achieved by focusing on three pivotal issues:

1. The risk benefit analysis for each alternative. That is, *both* hospitalizing and not hospitalizing, treating and not treating with medications, etc., have both *risks* and *benefits*.
2. "Exercising" clinical judgment at decision points. What did you assess or determine? What was your response?
   The above two areas strongly support the fact that your decision—even if proved wrong by hindsight—was not *negligent*.
3. Finally, recording patients' observed capacity to participate in their own treatment helps clarify patient responsibility for following up on a regimen.

The resulting conciseness is highly desirable for the busy clinician. One exception to this rule of brevity is the high-risk, complex or highly ambiguous clinical situation, requiring a "judgment call."

In such "judgment calls" the usual austerity and restraint that should characterize writing for the record must be compromised. Instead, the clinician should "think out loud for the record" (2, 3). This phrase means that the clinician should go to greater than usual lengths to detail the factual underpinnings and incremental steps of reasoning that lead to the decision in question. Equal care should invest the *explicit* weighing of benefits and risks and advantages and costs that enter into the clinical reasoning.

The essence of judgment calls and thinking out loud relates to the critical distinction between a legitimate error in judgment, on the one hand, and negligence, on the other. Careful decision making based on careful assessment that leads to a regrettable result is not negligence. *Failure* to make such assessment and decision or failure to *record* same is negligent and, given a bad result, thus grounds for malpractice.

CASE 7:   A resident was considering releasing a patient in an AMA (against medical advice) discharge rather than filing for commitment. The patient was a chronically suicidal borderline male intermittently self-lethal and highly resistant to taking responsibility for himself.

In writing up the discharge note, the resident included observations of the patient's state; notations about the goals of treatment in fostering responsibility in this patient; the justifications for this approach; reports of the views of supervisors and consultants; candid acknowledgment of the risk of suicide; review of the disadvantages of hospitalization (regression, absence of an end point, failure of even the hospital to *ensure* safety); iteration of the various extra-hospital supports and safeguards (e.g., "patient was given hospital phone number and instructed to call if situation worsens"); and an outline of contingency plans (2).

While the amount of detail may seem excessive or unnecessary, remember that one is preparing for a calculated risk that may turn out well or for ill, no matter how necessary the plan may be for managing the patient. If well, a slight amount of time is lost. If ill, the presence of details documenting careful assessment and exercise of judgment becomes enormously important.

Recording comments by professional colleagues is also an important step. As an informal "peer review," this documentation demonstrates that the decision on the "judgment call" has the support of at least one or more colleagues in the field, a situation similar to the "second opinion" obtained in general medicine. Professional support for an opinion powerfully refutes the accusation of negligence since the clinician demonstrated care by obtaining consultation and assessed the "community standard" of another "average reasonable practitioner."

AN APPROACH TO FORENSICALLY SIGNIFICANT EVENTS

In the practice of inpatient psychiatry some events are more likely than others to be the focus of medicolegal attention. These include (nonexhaustively): admissions and discharges; assaults, falls, accidents, and injuries; ill effects from treatments, especially sensitive treatment (e.g., electroconvulsive therapy); special procedures (seclusion, restraint); escapes or failures to return from pass; threats or other evidence of dangerousness; concurrent medical conditions (illnesses, allergies); and the like.

These clinical events and their attendant decisions require record-keeping commensurate with their potential forensic significance. At times the documentation requires "significant negatives."

CASE 8:   A patient was inappropriately and without clinical basis sent by a court to a hospital because of alleged dangerousness. Realizing that this issue would adumbrate the eventual discharge, the clinician, in anticipation of discharge, regularly recorded in the progress notes the *absence* of dangerous behavior, threats, etc.

The documentation of forensically significant events should also address any potential future questions. Examples include: Was normal neurological function present after a fall with head injury? Are x-rays indicated? Vital signs? Pupil checks?, and so on.

In a complementary manner, noting evidence *for* dangerousness is useful when a possible future commitment petition is envisioned.

SPECIAL MEDICOLEGAL ISSUES

Certain documents with specific medicolegal significance must clearly be included in the record. These include the legal status paper (voluntary or involuntary admission by court or civil commitment); consent forms for special procedures (the consent form should always be matched by a progress note in the body of the chart outlining the conversation with the patient in which the information about the procedure in question is conveyed. The note should also comment on answers given to the patient's questions, if any. The purpose of these data is to document that consent is truly "informed" [3]); certificates of guardianship and similar papers bearing on matters of competence (3); and the like. For court-committed patients, the relevant court documents should also be included.

Specificity about the sources of data often has medicolegal significance. Direct observation of behavior and speech must be distinguished from secondary sources.

CASE 9:   A record entry read, in part: "4/19/80 5 p.m. I saw Mr. Jones in the day room become agitated and strike Rhonda W. across the face (note that the alleged crime for which Mr. Jones is being evaluated, as reported by the arresting officer on admission, is assault and battery on an older woman)."

Note the distinctions between *primary observations* ("I saw"), *secondary observations* ("as reported"), and the careful use of "alleged" to refer to any actual or potential criminal charges. Note also the use of *time* (as well as date) for recording specific incidents in which time course may be essential (e.g., does Rhonda W. develop neurological symptoms 2, 10, or 18 hours after the injury?).

A more extensive discussion of recordkeeping may be found elsewhere (3, 4).

Confidentiality (3)

DEFINITION

Confidentiality is the term for a person's right not to have revealed to third parties information shared "in confidence" with a second party.

PRACTICAL ASPECTS OF CONFIDENTIALITY

Originally an ethical principle, confidentiality now rests on a number of explicit and implicit legal bases at the core of which lies this principle: *identifiable information about a patient cannot be shared with third parties without that patient's explicit (usually written) consent.*

Implied in this act of consenting are several considerations.

1. Consent should be given for particular data or particular kinds of data, with the amount or degree of detail specified.
2. A single consent is good for a single release of information. A second request, even from the same source, requires a second consent.
3. Even with consent, the clinician is expected to use discretion in how much or what kind of information to release, the standard set by the "needs of the situation," narrowly construed.
4. While acceptable during emergencies and other conditions, oral consent is generally far less desirable than written consent for obvious documentary reasons.

PITFALLS IN CONFIDENTIALITY

The most common breach of confidentiality on inpatient units occurs when staff carelessly discuss patients by name in hospital elevators, corridors, or cafeterias. This harmful practice must be eschewed not only because it is a genuine compromise of confidentiality but also because it is a blow to the morale of other patients in addition to those under discussion. The casual insensitivity thus demonstrated conveys a lack of respect or seriousness of purpose regarding patients in general.

To the surprise of some clinicians, confidentiality extends even to families of the patient, the patient's attorney, the patient's former therapist, and the clinician's professional colleagues who are not directly involved in care of that patient.

On the other hand, supervisors are usually considered part of the treatment team and are thus viewed as within the "circle" of direct information; the same is true for ward personnel directly involved with the patient's care. Thus, ward staff who keep patient-related secrets from each other are not "observing confidentiality" but acting in a manner destructive to good patient care (6).

Clinicians often wonder about the amount of information to share with a consultant when the latter gives advice on a case. It is customary to obtain the patient's permission for the consultation and, hence, for the implicit sharing of information. If some difficulty with this arises—the patient is paranoid, hesitant, reluctant, and ambivalent—I usually recommend that the clinician present the patient anonymously ("The patient is a 50-year-old man") to obtain at least some consultative benefit from a second opinion without compromising confidentiality. This approach also "spares" litigation-shy consultants: because their duty here is to the clinician-consultee, not the patient, the latter cannot sue the consultant for malpractice.

It may be very useful to recall that patients themselves bear no burden of confidentiality: a patient may freely tell anyone anything. This point may serve valuable purposes when the clinician's communications are complicated by conflicts of interests, uncertainty about whose interests one is actually serving, etc.; in sticky situations the patient may pass on information to family, to other caretakers—even to potential victims of his or her own aggression (7).

AIDS

Conceptualizations of both record-keeping and confidentiality in relation to acquired immunodeficiency syndrome (AIDS) are to say the least in flux. Individual jurisdictions vary widely in their regulations and laws on this matter, and clinicians must familiarize themselves with local rules.

In particularly murky situations where laws and regulations provide no illumination, two rules of thumb may be of some help. First, an ethical analysis of competing goods and harms may provide some guidance and justification. Second, one can provisionally treat AIDS as though it were syphilis and invoke public health reporting measures and sanctions via appropriate public health agencies.

EXCEPTIONS TO THE PRINCIPLE OF CONFIDENTIALITY

This topic is extensively covered elsewhere (3). However, a brief outline will serve here to stimulate thought about this important area. Under certain circumstances information from a patient's record may be released without the patient's consent. These include:

1. Emergency needs of the patient (the "best interests" doctrine narrowly construed: patient's lawyer needing to meet with her before an imminent trial and asking if the patient is on your ward, while the patient, through paranoia, refuses release of any information to anyone; the family of a floridly psychotic teenager needing to be queried regarding his possible PCP (phencyclidine) use). In all such incidents, the record should reflect the basis for this (justified) breach of confidentiality. In all such cases an attempt should be made to obtain consent and the effort documented.
2. For incompetent patients, consent of guardian (or next of kin in emergencies) is required.
3. In some jurisdictions but, inconsistently, not in others, the clinician is obligated to breach confidentiality if necessary to

protect third parties from harm from a patient, e.g., in warning the putative victim of death threats without the patient's consent (3). However, the clinician's knowledge of past crimes generally does not mandate reporting.

4. In some jurisdictions reporting requirements govern venereal disease, child abuse, and other issues. Local statutes should be checked.

5. In the interests of the alliance all breaches of confidentiality for one of these emergency reasons should be reviewed with the patient, addressing the necessity of the breach, the impact and consequences, etc. The patients' feelings and the clinical state which necessitated the breach should be reviewed, explored, and worked through as best as possible.

It is hoped that this review of the structure and function of the psychiatric record not only clarifies the complex medicolegal nimbus surrounding "charting" but also offers an insight into the manner in which good clinical care may be fostered by attention to careful recording of clinical data. The appendix which follows addresses some particulars of the chart itself.

REFERENCES

1. Leacock S: *Laugh with Leacock*, New York, Pocket Books, Inc., 1980.

2. Gutheil TG: Paranoia and progress notes: A guide to forensically informed psychiatric record-keeping. Hosp Community Psychiatry, *31*:479–482, 1980.

3. Gutheil TG, Appelbaum, PS: *Clinical Handbook of Psychiatry and the Law,* New York, McGraw-Hill, 1982.

4. Slovenko R: On the need for record-keeping in the practice of psychiatry. J Psychiatry Law, *7*:399–440, 1979.

5. Rappaport RG: The psychiatrist on trial. J Psychiatry Law, *7*:463–469, 1979.

6. Gutheil TG: Legal defense as ego defense: A special form of resistance to the therapeutic process. Psychiatr Q, *51*:251–256, 1979.

7. Wulsin, LR, Bursztajn H, Gutheil TG: Unexpected clinical features of the *Tarasoff* decision: The therapeutic alliance and the "duty to warn." Am J Psychiatry, *140*:601–603, 1983.

Appendix

The Contents of the Psychiatric Inpatient Record

Since the majority of inpatient facilities tend to evolve their own systems of record-keeping in idiosyncratic fashion, we must limit our discussion in this appendix to those general principles defining the purpose—and, hence, the content—of the sections of the record.

THE ADMISSION NOTE

This section heralds the transformation of an individual into an "inpatient." This is a shift of enormous sociolegal impact, rife with implications of changed status, altered rights, liabilities, duty of care, potential stigma, and the like.

In keeping with the seriousness of the patient's passage over this "administrative cliff," this section should emphasize the justificatory aspect of the record. Why was admission the best (or the only, or the only feasible, or the most appropriate) approach? Why would no less a step suffice? What was the "last straw" for this patient that "broke the back" of extrahospital functioning? The answer to these questions must be clear in the note.

Ideally, hospital admission is a carefully planned and weighed prescription. In reality, it is often a precipitous event, partaking of the urgency of a life-or-death emergency room intervention. Like the emergency room workup, the admission note should focus on critical, decisive elements. Deeper, more discursive elaboration must await the definitive write-up. Thus, after identifying data, chief complaints, and a cogent "present illness" have been recorded, obtain a brief history relating social circumstances and family history. Pay particular attention to past *medical* history, noting past and current medical conditions and their pharmocotherapy, if any; current medications, drugs, and alcohol, including O T C preparations; allergies or previous adverse drug reactions; and dietary considerations. The tentative formulation and working diagnosis should guide the early interventions, expressed in goal-directed fashion ("Thorazine 50-mg p.o. test dose, then 50 t.i.d. for hallucinations). Record the working diagnosis and acute interventions together with planned investigations and laboratory tests.

Often the informants or others who accompany the patient are extremely important to the patient, though this may not always be obvious. The admission note should record their names and *phone numbers* as well as similar data for previous mental health or medical and social contacts, if available. If this information is not obtained upon admission it is often far more difficult to track down later.

Of course, a physical examination, including careful neurological assessment, is a central part of each admission workup.

THE STATUS PAPER

This vitally important document is, quite literally, the only indication that what is happening is medical hospitalization and not kidnapping or false imprisonment. Clinical experience reveals the surprising finding that the most dangerously vague status indicators accompany patients sent by the courts. For this reason, carefully scrutinize "the papers" sent with court-ordered patients. Clarify ambiguities as rapidly as possible with the clerk of the court.

THE DEFINITIVE WRITE-UP

Whether termed "case study," "anamnesis," "staffing report," "conference plan," or some similar title, this section of the record should reflect a current detailed portrait of the patient. Rather than merely expanding the admission note, the write-up should describe the result of medical, neurological, and laboratory examinations; reports of detailed family, social, sexual, cultural, religious, educational, and vocational history-taking; data gathered by the various disciplines; and a more confident statement of diagnosis, clinical formulation, and the various planned modalities of treatment, with attention to the utilization perspective noted earlier in chapter 16.

In some institutions this section is maintained separately from the chart as a teaching device. When it is part and parcel of the record, of course, keep in mind the cautions about diplomatic use of terminology.

TEAM TREATMENT PLAN

As the operational core of the chart and the veritable compass of the course of hospitalization, this section should focus on data gathering, task assignment, and goal definition. Often a problem-oriented format helps to organize this section. Regular updating should keep the plan contemporary and up to date with the evolution of the illness, the treatment, the hospital course, newly emerging data, and the pooled wisdom of supervisors, consultants, and others.

PROGRESS NOTES

These regular recordings of the developments of the hospital course should follow the principles outlined in the chapter above. Most of the considerations described apply particularly to progress notes.

Always date progress notes (and for significant events, indicate a time as well) and always sign by name and discipline. Add additional titles when pertinent (e.g., S. Wilson, R.N., night supervisor). Although frequency of entry should be governed by the evolution of hospitalization and treatment, a workable rule of thumb might be: semi-weekly notes for two weeks, weekly thereafter, and—for slow reconstitution/rehabilitation courses—monthly. Make *ad hoc* entries, of course, whenever significant events occur.

THE DISCHARGE SUMMARY

In addition to marking the termination of one phase of total treatment (hospitalization) and the onset of another (aftercare), this section also heralds passage over another "administrative cliff" to outpatienthood. The outpatient state often lacks many of the implicit supports and opportunities for monitoring care that would be present in the hospital. This fact places a burden on the treatment planners to address this deficit, which they must do in the discharge summary.

Many institutions, moreover, send *only* the discharge summary to other caretakers when information is requested (with patient's release, of course). Thus, of the whole record, the discharge summary is "the part that flies." This fact places two potentially contradictory burdens on its author: completeness, since all the critical data must be included, and austerity, since this document is the most "public" piece of the chart by virtue of its transmissibility.

The discharge summary should contain identifying data; chief complaint; brief statement of the admission picture enriched by subsequent information and understanding; a summary of the hospital course specifically including forensically important events (allergic reactions, injuries, etc., as earlier noted) and their outcomes or remedies; a comparison of admission and discharge diagnoses; statements of condition (e.g., "improved") and prognosis (e.g., "guarded"); and a very detailed outline of planned aftercare, preferably including specifics of the first planned outpatient or aftercare appointment.

Example of aftercare plan. Perphenazine, (32 mg h.s. daily) 10 pills were given to pt.; a prescription for 2 weeks' supply given, to be filled by patient's mother. Needs to be monitored by Dr. Smith; pt. has 1st appt. with him on 5/17/85 at 2:30 PM; given appt. slip. Therapy per Jonesville CMHC clinic; case reviewed with Ms. Adams, M S W, who will follow pt. 1st appt. 5/14/85 at 10 AM Pt. given map to clinic.

If some aspect of dangerousness characterized the admission (suicide attempt, homicide threats), assess *present* dangerousness at discharge. If discharge is occurring (as not uncommonly happens) in the context of a calculated risk, meticulously spell out this decision with determinants, risks, and benefits of discharge and benefits of alternative courses of action made explicit. The care with which this is done here may prove decisive (in the event of even an adventitious postdischarge bad outcome) in differentiating a justified judgment call from negligence.

MISCELLANEOUS

Other important parts of the record include: consent forms (witnessed) for special procedures; laboratory and consultation reports; and special forms (e.g., seclusion reports and other statutorily required documents). Have most of these initialled or countersigned by the responsible clinician to indicate they have been reviewed.

Some jurisdictions have mandated special considerations for AIDS and human immunodeficiency virus-related data, such as keeping such information in a separate part of the chart or in an entirely separate chart, and/or requiring separate, specific consent for release of this information. Because of regional inconsistencies in this area consult local regulations.

Quality, Cost, and Contracts: Administrative Aspects of Inpatient Care

Lloyd I. Sederer, MD

Rumor has it a time existed when inpatient clinicians simply had to care for their patients. Rounds, conferences, and clinical conversations attended to the patient's diagnosis and treatment. No urgency existed and contemplation was not only valued, it was possible. Only clinicians questioned the judgments of other clinicians. Vendors, providers, products, and marketing were what obsessed businessmen not doctors and nurses. The "bottom line," I am told, was life and death.

There was a time (library archives can prove it) that a textbook on inpatient psychiatry would not conclude with (or incorporate anywhere) a chapter on administration and economics. What would a chapter like that have to do with clinical practice? However, this chapter is no supplement, nor is it an academic exercise in administrative theory. The administration and finance of health care has become a fundamental aspect of hospital practice. Like a speeding train, our health care industry now hurdles ahead on two tracks—one, the science and humanism of medicine and the other, that of economics and business enterprise.

History has seen stranger bedfellows. This union, in fact, is overdue. Scarce resources such as health care and technology must consequently consider and be informed by a set of economic principles. However, these principles should not govern the practice of medicine. Were this to happen, the ethics of health care would be eclipsed by technocrats preoccupied with cost and efficiency; the social and moral aims and values of health care would be lost. As our medical technologies advance, so must our administrative skills. This chapter is written toward that end. If we are substantially to influence our clinical destinies we will need such skills. To avoid or devalue them is increasingly to hand our fate over to nonclinicians. With both our wheels on the tracks we can best assert the realities of clinical care and vigorously represent the needs of our patients.

UTILIZATION REVIEW AND QUALITY ASSURANCE

Introduction and Definitions

Utilization review (UR) and quality assurance (QA) have become essential aspects of practicing medicine and delivering hospital services. Psychiatry is no exception. Anyone involved in delivering hospital psychiatric services must become highly cognizant of both UR and QA in order to obtain and maintain accreditation and be paid for services provided.

Quality assurance is the determination of whether the treatments that a facility provides to its patients meet specific standards of appropriate and acceptable medical care. These standards are generally defined as minimally accepted standards. *Utilization review* is a review of diagnostic and treatment services for determining if the resources employed were appropriately utilized. Generally, established criteria for resource use are applied. In essence, QA asks "was the service provided any good?"; UR asks "were the services necessary?" or "could a lesser level of care (i.e. less expensive) do?" These definitions of QA and UR will be further developed in the sections that follow.

History of UR and QA

The origins of quality assurance date back to the creation of selective admission requirements to medical school. In effect, medical schools became quality control sites by carefully screening whom they would train and what training they would provide. In doing so, the schools thereby ensured the caliber of their graduates. Subsequently, careful monitoring of the actual education programs of the medical school and standard licensing examinations complemented the admission screening and helped to ensure a properly trained physician. When medical technology began to outpace the careers of physicians, continued medical ed-

ucation (CME) became an essential ingredient of ongoing training and a requirement for licensing renewal.

UR and QA as we know it today is best dated back to the early 1960s (1–3). At that time the federal government entered the business of health care in a major way through congressional establishment of Medicare and the funding of the community mental health center movement. Not long thereafter because of a rapid expansion in costs, the government discovered that cost containment through provider (e.g., hospital) utilization mechanisms was not adequate for achieving fiscal constraint. The financial hazards envisioned were answered by legislation in 1972 that prompted the development of professional standard review organizations (PSROs). The PSROs were defined as local professional organizations for overseeing hospital (and occasionally ambulatory) utilization review and establishing medical care evaluation studies or audits. (This is a true anlage of QA). Some initial debate ensued about whether PSROs stood principally for cost containment or improving quality. This debate waged for some years, concluding in 1977 when administrative control over PSROs was shifted from the Public Health Service to the Health Care Financing Administration (HCFA), a component and fiscal agency of the Social Security Administration. In so doing, PSRO evaluations clearly began to stress dollars saved rather than quality of care.

By 1982 what fiscal hope the PSROs embodied had been overwhelmed by alarming increases in the cost of medical care (4, 5). In fact, the Medicare trust (which funds Medicare) threatened to bankrupt the Social Security Administration. The runaway costs, coupled with organized medicine's steady opposition to the PSROs, led the Reagan administration to eliminate these agencies. Under Reagan, the Congress then passed the Tax Equity and Fiscal Responsibility Act (TEFRA) which established a plan for the creation of peer review organizations (PROs). Simultaneously, TEFRA also created a system of prospective payment for hospital care. Unlike the PSROs which were local, PROs were to be organized at the state level and linked to a system of prospective payment. In 1983, the Deficit Reduction Act mandated an actual prospective payment system in which fixed, prepayment arrangements would replace the cost-reimbursement system that had previously characterized the hospital payment system in this country. We generally know the prospective payment system by its construction of diagnostic related groups (DRGs). DRGs revolutionized the reimbursement system of health care and now pervade general medical and surgical care. Psychiatry has not generally come under DRGs, at least not yet. In 1984, HCFA issued requests for proposals for developing physician-sponsored organizations that could not be affiliated with health care facilities. These organizations are the PROs of today and perform both UR and QA. Many of the current PROs are converted and enlarged PSROs. Many are supported by state medical societies and some are actually run by those societies. The principal task of a PRO is to contain the costs of Medicare payments, though the PROs were also encouraged to enter into similar UR contracts for Medicaid and other third party payers. Physicians have been involved in PROs as members of the board or paid consultants.

The documented objectives of PROs include: (*a*) shifting care from inpatient to ambulatory settings (which tend to be less costly); (*b*) reducing the frequency of invasive procedures and their adverse consequences; and (*c*) reducing the rate of hospital readmission, recognized as a major contributor to the cost of Medicare. Furthermore, PROs were to monitor and validate DRG designations patients received in order to counter what has been called "DRG creep" (hospitals recording higher paying DRG categories in order to receive larger prospective payment). As PROs have matured over the years, their objectives combine utilization review and cost containment with quality of care objectives.

Quality Assurance

Poor quality of care is all too obvious and readily defined. Definitions of genuinely good quality are more elusive. The American Medical Association has characterized high quality as that "which consistently contributes to the maintenance or improvement of health and well being" (6). While recognizing that other variables can affect outcome (e.g., living environments, severity and natural history of the illness, and attitudes towards illness), clinical outcome reflects in good measure the degree to which effective care was rendered by health professionals. For physicians and hospitals, technical competence has been a traditional indicator of quality. In more recent years, patient satisfaction and accessibility to care have also become recognized dimensions of quality care.

Quality assurance is a process that was defined and made an operational reality when the then Joint Commission on the Accreditation of Hospitals (now the Joint Commission on Accreditation of Health Care Organizations) established standards by which hospitals had to identify and resolve problems delivering clinical care (7). The Joint Commission held hospitals responsible for (*a*) identifying target areas that might represent potential problems (e.g., high risk or high volume activity) and (*b*) establishing criteria by which care in those identified areas could be examined to determine if quality was adequate. Any problems discovered through this examination were the responsibility of the health care organization to remedy.

Traditional concepts of quality assurance have been based on three criteria: structure, process, and outcome (3, 6, 8, 9). *Structure* refers to the setting in which the care was rendered. Specifically, structure addresses the nature of the organization's design, the resources and equipment of the facility, and the numbers and qualifications of its staff. *Process* refers to the clinical functions provided by clinicians. Process can include diagnosis, treatment plans, technical aspects of performing treatment, managing complications, and discharge planning. *Outcome* is just that: the results of specific treatments and procedures, adverse effects and complications, and long-term health and functioning.

Until recently, quality assurance was principally reviewed on the bases of structure and process (10). Structure and process measures were especially popular because outcome is difficult to measure; outcomes are difficult to obtain, are generally more costly, and tend to be distant in time from the actual delivery of the care. The problem of face validity also makes outcome assessment difficult. For example, variables such as loss of spouse or residence which are unrelated to hospital care can affect patient outcome; consequently, a poor outcome does not necessarily demonstrate that poor care was rendered. Despite the difficulties with outcome measures, they are now increasingly sought. Expected outcome before care is rendered and the actual result of the intervention can be compared. "Intermediate" rather than "final" outcome allows for realizable measurement and tends to diminish other factors that can effect outcome (7, 11).

A new definition and direction in quality assurance is also emerging. This is a model of "continuous improvement in care" (12–14). Traditional quality control, which aims toward identifying problem areas and poor functioning, can create an ambience of fear and self-protection. Furthermore, inspection and information processing are expensive and easily "gamed." A model of continuous improvement moves away from quality "control" to a vision of seeking defects as "treasures." Instead of relying on surveillance, staff are engaged in a process of always trying to improve on what is being done. Under this method, respect and commitment replace critique and adversity. Initiated in Japan, these concepts are now being adopted by major corporations in the United States. Remarkably, this definition of QA, like its preceding definitions, does not include matters of cost or profit (15).

Quality assurance *criteria* may be either *explicit* or *implicit*. *Explicit* quality criteria are survey- or consensus-established standards the community considers clear, fair, and capable of consistent application. Frequently, explicit criteria are developed by PROs, hospital peer review committees, or government regulatory agencies. *Implicit* quality criteria are the informed clinical judgments of an experienced physician reviewer. Implicit criteria are subjective standards that are case-specific. Their value lies in precluding large-scale "cookbook" medicine.

Quality assurance considerations also must consider the problem of *maximal versus optimal and logical quality*. *Maximal* criteria promote the use of the most advanced knowledge and techniques available. *Optimal* and *logical* criteria aim toward avoiding unnecessary treatment while optimizing efficiency and judiciously allocating limited medical resources.

Because quality measurement can occur along a variety of parameters each with its own distinct alternatives, we must pay particular attention to the critical question of *who* decides whether quality of care should be explicitly or implicitly judged by process or outcome and by maximal or optimal standards? Should doctors decide? Or regulators? Or patients? For the most part, the quality objectives of PROs are judged according to explicit criteria. Who will decide how quality is measured is an open question that physicians must participate in answering, lest this question be answered for them.

Utilization Review

Inpatient utilization review represents the principal site for UR because of the magnitude of the costs of inpatient care compared to ambulatory treatment and specific outpatient procedures. We can expect UR to move increasingly into the outpatient arena as inpatient costs are maximally contained and expenses displaced onto ambulatory care (16). A PRO or UR departments of major insurance companies may carry out the review. Four levels of review may take place, as follows: (4, 5)

First-level review is a clerical review. Administrative clerks check payment requests for completeness, accuracy, and eligibility for benefits.

Second-level review is performed by a medically knowledgeable reviewer—often a nurse, sometimes a social worker. Because this is not considered peer review, the second-level reviewer generally has authority to approve but not deny benefits. This level of review examines for (*a*) medical necessity and reasonableness for hospitalization, especially whether care could have been provided on an outpatient basis; (*b*) appropriateness of the treatment plan; that is, whether effective treatment was provided in a timely manner; and (*c*) timeliness of discharge planning and discharge. Because this is chart review, all judgments are made according to what is written in the chart. As Gutheil has emphasized, "If it isn't written, it didn't happen" (17). (See also Chapter 16).

Third-level review is peer review. Physicians on a consultant status to a PRO, insurance carrier, or proprietary review organization review the work of physician providers. Cases reach third-level review when providers of care appeal second-level review. It is at this level of review that clinical judgment is added to the established criteria for review.

Fourth-level review is a review of a collection of peer review decisions. This level of review may be invoked when a provider (hospital or physician) exceeds expected norms of disallowance or as a check upon the UR committee of a hospital.

An important distinction in the review process arises between *screening criteria* and *criteria for care*. *Screening criteria* are the criteria by which a small number of cases are selected out for review from the total volume of cases. Screening criteria are the tools by which review organizations choose what they will review. Examples include all patients hospitalized in a general hospital psychiatric unit whose length of stay (LOS) exceeds the 75th percentile, all patients receiving more than 20 electroconvulsive (ECT) treatments in a calendar year, and every patient billed for daily psychotherapy on an inpatient unit. *Criteria for care* are the standards by which a given treatment provided is considered an appropriate treatment to administer and whether the treatment was administered properly. Examples include: diagnostic criteria for the use of ECT, guidelines for administering ECT, and guidelines for monitoring lithium treatment.

Finally, review performed before the patient's admission, such as preadmission approval, is termed *prospective review*. Review conducted while the patient is in the hospital is called *concurrent review*. Review performed after the patient has been discharged is *retrospective review*.

MANAGED HEALTH CARE

Managed health care, through prepaid health delivery organizations and by UR, was perhaps the greatest trend in health care in the 1980s (18). It is possible that by the end of the 90s, all health care will be "managed," in one form or another.

Managed health care is a phenomenon that had a modest beginning a generation ago. However, by the 1980s managed care began to expand exponentially. The remarkable growth of managed care is attributed to a variety of economic and social trends (19, 20). The absolute cost of health care in the United States is a primary reason for the development of managed care as a method of cost containment. Currently, more than 11% of the gross national product is spent on health care. This is more than 550 billion dollars, one-third of which the federal government pays (21). The phenomenal costs of health care threaten U.S. business and government with the burden of payment and a consequent diminished capacity to compete in the world market. Remarkably, these vast sums of money—the greatest in the world—are not adequate: 37 million people in the U.S. are not insured and many more are underinsured (22).

A second principal reason for the emergence of alternate delivery systems is the reported oversupply of physicians and hospital beds (21, 23, 24). Too many providers and more than enough beds place those who are seeking and managing services at an advantage because of excess supply. What has been called a "product orientation" to health care is still another factor in the growth of managed care (25, 26). Instead of professional time denoting psychiatry's "product," many services are now called health care products and managed care organizations are their distributional channels.

Another critical factor in the growth of managed care is the failure of the regulation efforts of the 1970s to cut costs. Since health care costs have escalated dramatically and previous efforts at cost containment have failed, a marketplace orientation has emerged as a potential solution. Business, labor, and government are assuming greater control over health care financing and delivery in order to contain what they regard as a runaway system. Managed care has become the enterprise by which medicine, industry, and government are attempting to solve the profoundly complex financial, organizational, and social questions of health care today.

Finally, a chronic, national crisis of malpractice and litigation has added to the cost of health care. Physicians, hospitals, and health care organizations must pay for indemnity policies and litigated judgments. The costs of "defensive medicine" are probably incalculable, but no doubt extensive.

In view of these trends and the fear of continued escalation of costs, policy makers in this country had to respond. The successes of managed health delivery systems and the manifest cost-cutting potential of utilization review organizations (UROs) have given credence to their capacity to contribute to solving some of the problems of health care financing. The real confines of a managed accountability system can yield data and demand clinical problem solving that have heretofore been neglected. Simultaneously, genuine concern exists that unless carefully monitored the financial pressures of managed care will eventually translate into inadequate patient benefits, poor quality of care, and the transfer of liability for these shortcomings onto physicians and health care administrators.

Managed Care

We generally refer to managed care in two ways. *First, as a system of delivering medical services,* such as those offered by health maintenance organizations (HMOs), and second, as a *system of utilization review (and utilization management)* of medical services provided by the HMO or independent companies that control the way benefits are utilized.

The critical need for cost containment

noted above has been central to the development of these organizations. Alternative systems have departed from paying hospitals and professionals on the basis of their costs or on a fee-for-service arrangement. Paying providers on a fee for service basis (for what they did) perennially has been perceived as providing, and in some cases actually has provided, incentives to do more. By doing more, physicians and hospitals could receive greater income. The big buyers of health care, namely the federal government and corporate America, are no longer able to afford to pay the price of traditional health care. Medicare threatened to bankrupt the Social Security Administration and Chrysler Corporation discovered it was paying 10% of the cost of an automobile on health benefits. Estimates indicate that 10–30% of health care benefits can be spent on mental health care (including substance abuse), thereby calling particular attention to psychiatric benefits and treatment. Incentives to be parsimonious and save time and, possibly, to do less, were needed for the recovery of fiscal viability. Such incentives were available in prepaid health care arrangements in which a preestablished fee was set for the care of a particular illness (exemplified by diagnosis related groups) or a fixed dollar amount established to care for a specified number of patients (exemplified by capitation arrangements). Paying providers a set amount in advance for patients (or illness episodes) could achieve a remarkable shift in provider behavior. Instead of doing more to be paid more, the health industry could actually earn more by doing less. The buyers of health care finally had a way of prospectively limiting their budget and influencing providers in a manner previously unavailable through fee-for-service contracts. The marketplace mentality of the 1980s roundly endorsed this strategy. Managed care would be the vehicle for altering provider (and consumer) behavior.

Health Maintenance Organizations (HMO)

An *HMO* is a health care organization that contracts to provide a predetermined set of medical services to a group of voluntary subscribers for a fixed premium. If the HMO meets its budget, it breaks even; if it spends less than projected, it has a profit; if it exceeds its budget it has lost money and is at risk to go out of business. HMOs differ radically from traditional *indemnity* plans. Indemnity literally means protection against hurt, loss, or damage. Indemnity insurance reimburses for whatever costs are incurred. The subscriber is covered, the provider paid, and the insurance carrier guaranteed of its expenses. Should costs exceed budget, premiums will be adjusted to correct for losses.

An emerging area of managed service delivery are provider organizations that deliver only mental health (and substance-abuse) services (so called "carve-outs"). Many are located in California, some in the South. Examples in the East include Psychological Networks (New York) and PsycCare, a subsidiary of Preferred Health Care (Connecticut).

Models of HMO Care

Staff model. In the staff model, the HMO employs physicians and other professional providers on a salaried basis. Typically, mental health services of staff model HMOs are provided primarily by nonpsychiatrist mental health professionals. Primary care physicians (PCPs) generally serve as gatekeepers of this model, responsible for controlling the use of specialist services. Examples include the Harvard Community HealthPlan (HCHP or Harvard Health), Kaiser, and Group Health (Seattle).

Group model. In this model the HMO contracts with a group practice on a negotiated capitation basis. In turn, the physician group provides identified services (in their offices) to the patient population for which it has assumed care. Multi-Group in Massachusetts, recently acquired by Harvard Health, is an example of the group model.

IPA model. The Independent Practice Association is an incorporated group of physicians (practicing in their offices) who have contracted with an HMO to provide medical care to a defined population of HMO subscribers. IPAs show the greatest growth of all the new HMOs. An example of an IPA in Massachusetts is the Tuft's Associated Health Plan (TAHP) which has contract arrangements with more than 19 IPA groups located at as many Massachusetts hospitals. TAHP outpatient mental health services are offered by psychiatrists in the individual IPAs and by nonmedical professionals through a contracted network of local professionals and agencies. Inpatient and partial hospital care is by authorization and must be rendered at designated facilities (when possible) with concurrent, centralized utilization review.

PPO model. The preferred provider organization (PPO) comprises selected providers who the managed entity believes will render effective and efficient care, often at discounted fees. Patients enjoy the option of choice—not available in staff, group, and IPA models—resulting in the popularity of this model. PPOs are generally attractive to psychiatrists because their fees tend to be higher and an enrollment fee may not be required. Many commercial insurance carriers are moving to adopt this model; among them are Hancock, Prudential, Travelers' and Blue/Cross Blue Shield of Massachusetts.

Managed Care through Utilization Review

A growing number of organizations are devoted in part or in full to reducing the costs of mental health incurred by insurance carriers or significant purchasers of insurance benefits (e.g., industry and government). These organizations which work by rigorous utilization review and case management have been effective in reducing health care use and expenditures. Whether the decreases occur in appropriate (i.e. needed) as well as inappropriate services is unclear. In general, the goal of UR is budgetary. Examples of such management companies include American PsychManagement; IntraCorp (which was in partnership with the American Psychiatric Association); Preferred Health Care (through Psychiatric Case Management which may be the largest of its type with more than four million patients under their program); National Psych Reviews; and TAO, Inc., a Blue Cross affiliate in Philadelphia, run by a psychiatrist.

Reimbursement Mechanisms of Managed Care

Reimbursement for medical care under cost-containment management can be understood with a continuum model. At one end of the continuum is payment for full charges. At the other end is capitation. Charge-based payment is exemplified by fee-for-service care and carries with it little, if any, financial risk on the part of the provider. Along the continuum from charges to capitation are methods involving discounting of fees and withholding of partial payment (to be paid at a later time only if budget is not exceeded), flat rates per discharge, per diem rates, and DRGs. Fixed prepayment arrangements entail risk but also allow for profit when the dollars allocated are not spent. Furthermore, risk sharing arrangements can permit flexibility in how service is delivered (e.g., day treatment or crisis intervention instead of hospitalization). Of course, the actual dollar amount negotiated in a contract is crucial, for no measure of clinical creativity can overcome an inadequate budget.

TRENDS IN HEALTH CARE FINANCING AND DELIVERY

We are embarking upon what Relman has called the "third revolution" in health care (27, 28). The 1940s to the 1960s saw a remarkable expansion of medical services. Hospitals proliferated in bed capacity and medical schools enlarged to deliver the doctors needed to staff the hospitals. The technology of medicine grew with startling discoveries and innovations. Private and government insurance, encompassing many more beneficiaries, was better able to finance what was occurring in the hospitals. The first revolution was one of expansion and innovation.

By the 1970s the costs of this expansion had begun to outstrip the buyers' (especially government's) capacity to pay. So began the second revolution, that of cost-containment. The momentum for this revolution only increased as expenditures grew, seemingly immune to the efforts to contain them. Utilization review, PSROs, PROs, prospective payment, and managed care are among the most familiar elements of this second revolution which remains with us today.

The third revolution actually expands upon the second. Relman (and Roper who was instrumental in advancing these ideas in government) characterizes this revolution as one of assessment, effectiveness, and fiscal accountability. In other words, providers of health care will need to demonstrate the effectiveness of particular treatments and interventions before they will be recognized as reimburseable. Outcome-oriented assessment will be instrumental in establishing effectiveness. More than ever (and certainly more than process-orientated quality assurance [see page 422]) we can expect to be subject to "performance based payment" (29).

As this revolution unfolds in the 1990s, a variety of trends are evident among the activities and strategies of the principal players in this complex drama. We can examine these more microscopic trends as they occur in the insurance industry, the world of business, and at the federal government level.

Third-Party Insurers

The function of a third-party insurer is to control expenditures in order to keep premiums affordable, without substantively compromising the quality and access to care beneficiaries seek. This demanding task occurs at a time when expenditures are skyrocketing. Insurers have therefore resorted to a variety of business tactics to achieve these aims (16).

1. Managing the risk pool: If an insurer has a large population of people who are likely to be ill (e.g., the elderly, the poor) or tend to be high users of service, the costs incurred are going to be higher. Managing the risk pool refers to efforts to recruit beneficiaries who are less likely to use services, thereby controlling expenditures. During the 1980s the proliferation of HMOs capitalized on this strategy (as well as selectively providing services that pay well) resulting in what is called *niching* (30). The effect is the creation of many smaller insurers who "cream the crop," leaving high-risk, poorer paying patients to be covered by the federal government, public facilities, and large insurers like Blue Cross/Blue Shield who cannot control their constituency.

2. Designing the benefit plan: Insurers can better control their risk and expenses by limiting which services will be reimbursed and with what shared expense by the subscriber. Mental health benefits provide the best examples. Psychiatric benefits typically restrict the number of

hospital days allowed in a calendar year or in a lifetime and set limits on outpatient benefits, either in dollars or number of visits. Furthermore, benefit design that requires an initial deductible payment and copayments of 20–50% per visit or per hospital day are highly effective in reducing utilization. Should health care become rationed (as is occurring in Oregon), consumers may be asked to rank (and thereby design) which services they value (31, 32). This will eliminate benefits for services that are ranked low.

3. Control of provider payment: Paying the provider (clinician, clinic, or hospital) less and capping payment are already radically changing practice. Provider's fees are often discounted at the start and a percentage of their fee is withheld to make the provider a partner in containing costs. Prospective payment now applies only to hospitals (e.g., DRGs) but could, in time, extend to clinicians who would receive a fixed prepayment for an episode of illness. Still another control is capitation in which the service provider is paid on the basis of number of potential patients. Capitation allows insurers to preset and cap their costs, leaving the provider to shoulder any cost overrun.

4. Relocation of the site of service: Shifting the site where service is rendered can reduce costs, at least initially (33). The remarkable shift from inpatient care to ambulatory treatment best exemplifies this effort. In psychiatry we can anticipate that benefits for inpatient care will become more scarce and incentives created to deliver care in partial hospitals and outpatient centers.

5. Constraining supply: Constraint of supply typically is managed by government regulation agencies, though insurers are increasingly vocal and lobby in this arena. Examples include the numbers of hospital beds and high cost technologies like computerized tomography and magnetic resonance imaging. (As a rule, increased supply of health care results in increased demand and utilization). Offices of technology assessment can also constrain supply by tightening approval of new procedures and treatments, thereby limiting their introduction (34).

6. Managed care: Last on the list, managed care is not at all the least (18). As reviewed earlier in this chapter, this was perhaps the greatest trend in health care financing and delivery during the 1980s. It is possible all health care will be "managed" in some form by the end of the 1990s.

Business: Management and Labor

The uncontrolled increases in health care have added to the erosion of the competitive capacity of corporate America in the world market (35). Compared to Japan, Germany, Britain, and many other nations, the cost of our health care contributes significantly greater costs to our manufactured products. Attempts to transfer some of these costs onto labor (by increasing the employee share of health care) have been the principal issue in recent labor negotiations and actual (and threatened) strikes across this country.

The business community has undertaken a number of initiatives in its efforts to control costs. A coalition of business, labor, and the insurance industry is growing which will have a large voice in making policy decisions at the federal level during the years ahead.

1. Self-insurance: This is a major trend; estimates of 25–50% of medium to large businesses are undertaking control of their health care coverage (36). Although a third party insurer (such as BC/BS, Hancock, Prudential, Aetna) is hired to administer the policy, the business entity defines policy expenditures, benefits,

and utilization arrangements. Because self-insured companies fall under federal regulation, they are exempt from any state-mandated health insurance requirements. The strategies of business, in collaboration with the insurance industry, include many of the elements of cost control detailed above in the insurance section.

2. "Carve-outs," utilization review, and managed care: By tracking costs corporations can identify high costs and services that are rapidly increasing in volume. Mental health and substance-abuse costs have grown in number and cost during the past five to 10 years as we have become better at identifying these disorders, reducing their stigma, and making services accessible and attractive. A "carve-out" is the separating out of a high cost item and transferring its management to a set of services (such as a PPO, an EAP [Employee Assistance Program], or the creation of an inhouse network of services) or to a proprietary utilization management company that will guarantee a reduction in costs (if only temporary).

3. Direct purchasing: As corporations become more familiar with and effective at managing their health care benefits, they will be inclined to eliminate the middle man. This is already happening as some corporations are directly purchasing services for their employees.

Federal Government

The federal government pays one-third of the health care costs in this country, principally through Medicare, Medicaid, federal employee health benefits, Champus, and the Veteran's Administration system. This does not include the substantial revenues it could collect if payment for employee health insurance were to come from taxable, rather than pretax dollars. The Bush administration has targeted health care as a priority, which is to say that more scrutiny and cuts will occur. As noted earlier, this is the era of effectiveness and cost-accountability (28).

1. PROs: Carrying forth on the work of the PSROs, these new organizations answer to the Health Care Financing Administration (HFCA). They have responsibility for controlling costs while demanding quality for Medicare.

2. The Resource Based Relative Value Scale (RBRVS): The RBRVS derives from the Harvard School of Public Health and is funded by HCFA. Based on this scale, physicians' salaries will be revised for Medicare in the early 1990s (37). Other payers will probably follow suit. Payment will be based on measures that assess "resource-inputs" for services and procedures. Though psychiatry may realize a modest gain for some services, other specialties will see marked reductions in their incomes. However, the RBRVS will not solve the larger problem of the growing volume of Medicare services.

3. Performance-based payment, expenditure caps, and the elimination of tax subsidies: Though not yet established, these trendy terms depict what might lie ahead. Outcome and its assessment will be increasingly essential. Outcome will encompass clinical efficacy as well as capacity for cost-effectiveness (i.e. the capacity to deliver services in an economical matter). The most powerful governor of health care costs would be a cap on expenditures. A cap could be absolute or tied to the consumer price index or some agreed upon proportion of the gross national product. The Heritage Foundation has proposed that the tax subsidies the federal government provides for employer-provided insurance be reduced or even eliminated, thereby squarely placing the costs of health care on many of

its buyers (35). This is a type of free-market solution which may not best apply to health care (22). Although radical solutions such as these three may be some time away, change in health care has already outpaced many forecasters.

4. Rationing: Rationing refers to the equitable distribution or division of scarce products essential for living (31, 32). This is quite different from price allocation in which capacity to afford a particular good or service determines distribution. An experiment in rationing of health care services is ongoing in Oregon, though it applies only to the poor. Rationing is another radical solution generally unacceptable to the health care consumer.

5. National health insurance: In order to meet goals of quality care accessible to all at affordable costs, nothing short of a national form of insurance may suffice. Business has subsidized (through insurance) the have-nots for decades by reimbursing hospitals for their costs, which include free care and problems with collections. Business as well as labor and the insurance industry are now looking in an unprecedented manner toward the federal government to relieve them of the financial burden of health care. With a restructuring of Europe and the Communist world and a projected dimunition in defense spending, we may finally be poised to introduce universal health care coverage in the United States.

REFERENCES

1. Nelson JA: The history and spirit of the HMO movement. HMO Practice 1 (2):75–85, 1987.

2. English JT, Kritzler ZA, Schell DJ: Historical trends in the financing of psychiatric services. Psych Annals, 14:321–331, 1984.

3. Sederer LI: Utilization review and quality assurance. Gen Hosp Psychiatry, 9:210–219, 1987.

4. Committee on Peer Review, American Psychiatric Association: Manual of Psychiatric Peer Review, ed. 3, Washington, D.C., American Psychiatric Association Press, 1985.

5. Mintz RS: A peer review primer, in Hamilton JM (ed): Psychiatric Peer Review, pp 142–150, Washington, D.C., American Psychiatric Association Press, 1985.

6. American Medical Association: Council on Medical Service, Chicago, Ill., 1989.

7. Joint Commission on Accreditation of Healthcorp Organizations: The Joint Commission Guide to Quality Assurance, Chicago, Ill., 1988.

8. Mattso MR: Quality assurance: A literature review of a changing field. Hosp Community Psychiatry, 35:605–616, 1984.

9. Donabedian A: Explorations in Quality Assurance and Monitoring, vol. 3, Ann Arbor, Mich., Health Administration Press, 1985.

10. Fauman MA: Monitorintg the quality of psychiatric care. Psychiatr Clin North Am, 13(1):73–88, 1990.

11. Rodriguez AR: Evolutions in utilization and quality management. Gen Hosp Psychiatry, 11:256–263, 1989.

12. Berwick DM: Continuous improvement as an idea in health care. N Engl J Med, 320:53–56, 1989.

13. Deming WE: Out of Crisis, Massachusetts Institute for Technology, Center for Advanced Engineering Study (Monograph), Cambridge, 1982.

14. Deming, WE: Quality, Productivity, and Competitive Position (Monograph), Massachusetts Institute for Technology, Center for Advanced Engineering Study, Cambridge, Mass., 1982.

15. Hillman A, Pauly MV, Kerstein JJ: How do financial incentives affect physicians' clinical decisions and financial performance of HMOs? N Engl J Med, 321:86–92, 1989.

16. Institute of Medicine: Controlling Costs and Changing Patient Care: The Role of Utilization Management, Washington, D.C., National Academy Press, 1989.

17. Gutheil TG: Paranoia and Progress Notes. Hosp Community Psychiatry, 31:479–482, 1980.

18. Sederer LI, St. Clair RL: Managed mental health care and the Massachusetts experience. Am J Psychiatry, 146:1142–1148, 1989.

19. Sharfstein SS, Beigel A (eds): *The New Economic and Psychiatric Care,* Washington, D.C., American Psychiatric Press, 1985.

20. American Psychiatric Association Office of Economic Affairs: *An Economic Survival Manual for Private Practice Psychiatrists,* Washington, D.C., American Psychiatric Press, 1985.

21. Califano JA: The health care chaos. New York Times Magazine, p 44, March 20, 1988.

22. Fein R: *Medical Care, Medical Costs: The Search for a Health Insurance Policy,* Cambridge, Harvard University Press, 1986.

23. U.S. Department of Health and Human Services: Summary Report of the Graduate Medical Education Advisory Committee to the Secretary, vol I, Washington, D.C., Sept 30, 1980.

24. Schwartz WD, Sloan FA, Mendelson DN: Why there will be little or no physician surplus between now and the year 2000. N Engl J Med, 318:892–897, 1988.

25. Sharfstein SS, Krizay J, Muszynski IL: Defining and pricing psychiatric care "products." Hosp Community Psychiatry, 39:372–375, 1988.

26. Stoline A, Weiner JP: *The New Medical Marketplace,* Baltimore, Johns Hopkins University Press, 1988.

27. Relman AS: Assessment and accountability: The third revolution in medical care, N Engl J Med, 319:1220–1222, 1988.

28. Roper WL, Winkelwarder W, Hackbaeth GM, et al.: Effectiveness in health care. N Engl J Med, 319:1197–1202, 1988.

29. Shurtell SM, McNerney WJ: Criteria and guidelines for reforming the U.S. health care system. N Engl J Med 322:463–467, 1990.

30. Kinzer DM: Universal entitlement to health care. N Engl J Med 322:467–470, 1970.

31. Reagan MD: Health care rationing. N Engl J Med 319:1149–1151, 1988.

32. Schwartz WG, Aaron HJ: Rationing hospital care. N Engl J Med 310:52–56, 1984.

33. Goldsmith J: A radical prescription for hospitals. Harvard Business Review, pp 104–111, May–June 1989.

34. Rose M, Leiberleift RF: Antitrust implications of medical technology assessment. N Engl J Med 314:1490–1493, 1986.

35. The Economist, Nov 25, 1989, pp 17–20.

36. Econocast, Psychiatric News, p 20, November 17, 1989.

37. Roper WL: Perspectives on physician payment reform. N Engl J Med 319:865–867, 1988.

Index